TEXTBOOK OF RADIOPHARMACY

NUCLEAR MEDICINE—A SERIES OF MONOGRAPHS AND TEXTS

Edited by Peter H. Cox, Dr Daniel den Hoed Clinic

Volume 1
IMMUNOSCINTIGRAPHY
Edited by L. Donato and K. Britton

Volume 2
NEW PERSPECTIVES IN NUCLEAR MEDICINE
(in two parts)
Edited by Peter H. Cox and E. Touya

Volume 3
TEXTBOOK OF RADIOPHARMACY
Theory and Practice, First Edition
Edited by Charles B. Sampson

TEXTBOOK OF RADIOPHARMACY
Theory and Practice, Second Edition
Edited by Charles B. Sampson

Cover Design by Sarah Sampson and Alfred Sampson

This book is part of a series. The publishers will accept continuation orders which may be cancelled at any time and which provide for automatic billing and shipping of each title in the series upon publication. Please write for details.

TEXTBOOK OF RADIOPHARMACY

Theory and Practice

SECOND EDITION

Edited by

CHARLES B. SAMPSON
Addenbrooke's Hospital
Cambridge, UK

Gordon and Breach Publishers
Australia • Austria • China • France • Germany • India • Japan • Luxembourg •
Malaysia • Netherlands • Russia • Singapore • Switzerland • Thailand •
United Kingdom • United States

First published 1994
Second printing 1995

3 Boulevard Royal
L-2449 Luxembourg

Library of Congress Cataloging-in-Publication Data

Data may be obtained on application to the Library of Congress.

ISBN 2-88124-951-2 (HARDCOVER)
ISBN 2-88124-973-6 (SOFTCOVER) ISSN 0896-0607

CONTENTS

Contents

SECTION II Practical radiopharmaceutics

FOREWORD TO THE SECOND EDITION

The first edition of Sampson's **Textbook of Radiopharmacy** was so well received that the publisher was considering a reprint. Bearing in mind that there had been considerable developments in the field of radiopharmacy in the interim three years it was decided to update the text at the same time. Therefore, whilst retaining the original skeleton, every chapter has been revised and a great deal of new information incorporated. With respect to the professional aspects of radiopharmacy the emphasis is on UK and mainland European practice. Nevertheless the science is international and this book will prove to be a valuable reference source to radiopharmaceutical scientists and nuclear medical practitioners everywhere. I can firmly recommend it.

Peter H. Cox
Rotterdam
September 1933

PREFACE TO THE FIRST EDITION

The **Textbook of Radiopharmacy** has been compiled in response to many requests for a basic guide to the art and science of radiopharmacy. The book is aimed at all those who work with radiopharmaceuticals. It will also be suitable as an adjunct to lectures in schools of pharmacy and technical colleges or, indeed, any institution where radiopharmacy is taught at a basic level. The early chapters deal with basic concepts such as radiation physics, generator systems and the general theory behind the preparation of radiopharmaceuticals. Included in this section is a general discussion on the chemistry of technetium, as well as the principles underlying the formulation of "kit" radiopharmaceuticals. Chapter 4 deals with methods of localisation, and explanations are provided for lung deposition, ion exchange, membrane transportation, phagocytosis and pinocytosis.

Chapter 5 deals with dispensing techniques and incorporates the latest information on standards of cleanliness and the proper storage of radiopharmaceuticals. The various types of dispensing procedures are explained. Operator safety in the handling of radiopharmaceuticals is described in Chapter 6, and this important section explains the various regulations pertaining to dispensing and supply. The recommendations given in *Guidance Notes for the Protection of Persons against Ionising Radiations arising from Medical and Dental Use (1988)*, London, HMSO, are explained. Currently applicable dose limits for employees are described in detail, as well as methods of reducing the radiation dose to the operator. Chapter 7 discusses the importance of quality testing of radiopharmaceuticals, and detailed guidance is given on the parameters necessary as well as the methodology of testing. The principles of paper chromatography, thin layer chromatography, gel filtration and high performance liquid chromatography (HPLC) are explaind. The text incorporates a useful summary of solvent systems and HPLC columns for commonly used radiopharmaceuticals.

Documentation, labelling, packaging and transportation are dealt with in Chapter 8, and the author traces the paperwork needed from receipt of the Isotope Request Form to release of the finished product. Guidance is given on the information required for the labelling of radiopharmaceuticals as well as that needed on the outer packages in order to comply with transportation regulations. Chapter 9 looks at the various factors to be taken into account in the design of a laboratory suitable for the dispensing of radioactive materials. The significance of "supervised" and "controlled" areas is explained, as are the special requirements for the radiolabelling of blood components.

Monitoring of the radiopharmacy for both microorganisms and radiation is an important routinely performed procedure for all who work with radioactive pharmaceuticals and Chapter 10 describes the pieces of equipment needed to carry out these procedures. Chapter 11 outlines the use of Product Licences and Clinical Trial Certificates, and deals with the manufacturing, importing and wholesaling of radiopharmaceuticals. Other topics include the *Health and Safety at Work etc. Act, (1974)*, London, HMSO, and the legal considerations necessary for the supply of radiopharmaceuticals within the National Health Service Scheme.

The chapters on the regulatory requirements in the field of radiopharmacy deal mainly with the legal aspects of dispensing and supplying radiopharmaceuticals. For countries outside the United Kingdom, detailed regulatory information should be sought from local regulatory authorities.

The radiolabelling of blood components is becoming an important function of many radiopharmaceutical laboratories, and Chapter 12 fully describes the techniques required to label erythrocytes, leucocytes and platelets. The text is enhanced by schematic diagrams of the most commonly used procedures. The clinical side of radiopharmacy is next touched upon and Chapter 13 provides a broad overview of the diagnostic information that can be obtained by means of radiopharmaceuticals. Although not part of practical radiopharmacy, this topic has been included so that the reader may obtain a reasonably complete picture of the total field of radiopharmacy.

The final chapters include the latest information on the effects of drugs on the biodistribution of radiopharmaceuticals, adverse and unusual reactions, new radiopharmaceuticals, factors that affect the integrity of radiopharmaceuticals, and dosimetry. The final chapter on paediatric radiopharmacy deals with the preparation of children's doses, documentation, and the different methods for calculating the dose for a child.

In a multi-author volume of this type it is inevitable that there will be some textual overlap. Deletion of duplicated material has deliberately been minimised, as each chapter represents a state-of-the-art review by an acknowledged expert in the field and deletion might affect the total understanding of the particular topic.

Preface

Techniques to radiolabel monoclonal antibodies have not been included in this volume as these procedures have not yet become standard routine practice in the majority of radiopharmaceutical laboratories. Also, radiolabelling techniques are constantly being improved and any review would almost certainly become out-dated within a short space of time. The reader is, therefore, referred to the many excellent review papers for details of radiolabelling methods.

In conclusion, this volume represents a broad outline of the theoretical and practical sides of radiopharmacy and will, it is hoped, be useful for those entering the field of radiopharmacy for the first time as well as those already practising the speciality.

Charles B. Sampson
Addenbrooke's Hospital
Cambridge, UK

PREFACE TO THE SECOND EDITION

Those familiar with the **Textbook of Radiopharmacy** will realise that this edition is considerably enlarged, an increase largely due to the expanded scope of the book. A shortcoming of the first edition was that it did not contain sufficient basic information on practical radiopharmacy. I have tried to correct this imbalance by the addition of new chapters on such important topics as official and non-official radiopharmaceuticals, the use of drugs in the enhancement of nuclear medicine studies, the radiolabelling of antibodies, the use of radiopharmaceuticals as therapeutic agents, and metabolism and pharmacokinetics of radiopharmaceuticals. For those involved in research I have added a review on the use of radiopharmaceuticals in research.

Another valid criticism of the first edition was that the index was not sufficiently comprehensive for the book to be used as a work of reference. Again, I have tried to correct this by the insertion of a greatly expanded index.

Because of the increased number of chapters it seemed logical to divide the text into five separate sections. Section I deals with the theoretical aspects of radiopharmacy and includes updated chapters on basic physics, generator systems and physicochemical mechanisms in the formulation of radiopharmaceuticals.

Section II deals with practical radiopharmaceutics. This section includes the latest information on the design of radiopharmacy laboratories, care being taken to incorporate recent European legislation on standards of air quality. The section on the radiolabelling of blood cells is now divided into two chapters, the first on the theory behind radiolabelling, and the second on the practicalities. The radiolabelling of antibodies is now becoming an important field in many European laboratories and a general review is given on the theory and practice of radiolabelled antibodies. The chapter on quality control has been greatly expanded to include extra information on basic techniques. The latest Transport Regulations are discussed in Chapter 11, and a new and important chapter on waste management has been added. As regards the legal side of radiopharmacy the latest information from the Medicines Control Agency has been inserted into Chapter 15. A general summary of the physical properties of official and non-official radiopharmaceuticals is given in Chapter 16.

Section III deals with the localisation and disposition of radiopharmaceuticals. The first chapter on localisation mechanisms has been expanded and a completely new chapter describing metabolism and excretion has been added. The effect of patient medication on the disposition of tracers has become very important in ensuring accurate diagnosis and a large number of clinical examples of drug interference have been given. As opposed to drug interference, the use of drugs to actually enhance the nuclear medicine test is now becoming an established practice, and Chapter 20 gives a general account of the most widely used interventional drugs and their effects.

Section IV deals with clinical radiopharmacy and the first chapter provides an extended discussion on the diagnostic applications of radiopharmaceuticals. Of particular importance in this section is the new part on the use of radiolabelled leucocytes in the detection of inflammation. Also new is an extensive review on the use of radiopharmaceuticals as therapeutic agents.

The final section, Section V, gives a general up-date of the techniques used in paediatric radiopharmacy.

The compilation of the second edition comes at a time during which major new legislation has come about. This includes the new European standards for air quality, the new Transport Regulations for the carriage and transport of radiopharmaceuticals and the loss of Crown Immunity as regards the hospital preparation of radiopharmaceuticals (in the UK).
I am greatly indebted to all the chapter authors who have taken great pains to ensure that the latest information has been included in their texts. In particular, I should like to thank Mr John Turner of the Medicines Control Agency, United Kingdom, who has been careful to furnish me with the very latest regulatory information as we go to press. I would also like to thank my friends and colleagues in the world of nuclear medicine for their help and encouragement in the compilation of this volume.

And finally, I am indebted to Mrs J. Mackintosh of the Department of Nuclear Medicine, Addenbrooke's Hospital for her help in the preparation of the additional chapters.

Charles B. Sampson
Addenbrooke's Hospital
Cambridge, UK

LIST OF CONTRIBUTORS

Prof Dr P.H. Cox
Director, Department of Nuclear Medicine, Dr Daniel den Hoed Clinic, PO Box 5201, 3008 AE Rotterdam, The Netherlands.

Dr H.J. Danpure
Formerly Research Scientist, MRC Cycotron Unit, Du Cane Road, Hammersmith, London W6, and formerly Lecturer in Radiopharmaceutical Sciences, University of London, UK.

Prof A.T. Elliott
Chief Physicist, Department of Clinical Physics and Bio-engineering, Western Infirmary, Glasgow G11 6NT, UK.

Mr K. Evans
Principal Physicist, Department of Physics, Hospital for Sick Children, Great Ormond St, London WC1N 3JH, UK.

Dr M. Frier
Principal Radiopharmacist, Department of Medical Physics, University Hospital, Queen's Medical Centre, Nottingham NG7 2VH, and Lecturer and Examiner in Radiopharmaceutical Sciences, University of London, UK.

Dr J.R. Gill
Principal Specialist Inspector, Technology Division, Health and Safety Executive, Magdalen House, Trinity Road, Bootle, Merseyside L20 3QZ, UK.

Mrs K. Goldstone
Principal Physicist and Regional Radiation Protection Adviser, Addenbrooke's Hospital, Cambridge CB2 2QQ, UK.

Dr J.G. Hardy
Consultant in Radiopharmaceutical Technology, Pharmaceutical Sciences Department, Nottingham University, Nottingham NG7 2RD, UK.

Dr S.R. Hesslewood
Regional Radiopharmacist, Department of Physics and Nuclear Medicine, Dudley Road Hospital, Birmingham B18 7QH, and Lecturer and Examiner in Radiopharmaceutical Sciences, University of London, UK.

T.E. Hilditch
Principal Nuclear Medicine Physicist, Department of Clinical Physics and Bio-Engineering, Western Infirmary, Glasgow, UK.

Mrs M. Hojelse
Senior Pharmacist, The Isotope Pharmacy, National Board of Health, Frederissundveg 378, DK-2700, Bronshøj, Denmark.

Dr D.H. Keeling
Consultant in Nuclear Medicine, Department of Nuclear Medicine, Derriford Hospital, Plymouth PL6 8DH, UK.

Dr K. Kristensen
Director, Medicines Division, National Board of Health, Frederikssundveg 378, DK-2700, Bronshøj, Denmark.

Dr C.R. Lazarus
Principal Radiopharmacist, Department of Nuclear Medicine, Guy's Hospital, St Thomas' Street, London SE1 9RT, and Lecturer and Examiner in Radiopharmaceutical Sciences, University of London, UK.

Ms S.C.E. Leung
Senior Pharmacist (Radiopharmaceuticals), Pharmacy Department, Queen Elizabeth Hospital, Birmingham, B18 7QH, UK.

Mr P.J. Maltby
Principal Radiopharmacist, Royal Liverpool Hospital, Liverpool L7 8XF, and Lecturer and Examiner in Radiopharmaceutical Sciences, University of London, UK.

Dr S.J. Mather
Principal Radiopharmacist and Head, Nuclear Medicine Research Laboratory, St Bartholomew's Hospital, London EC1A 7BE, and Lecturer and Examiner in Radiopharmaceutical Sciences, University of London, UK.

Dr A.M. Millar
Principal Radiopharmacist, Department of Medical Physics, Royal Edinburgh Infirmary, Edinburgh EH3 9YW, UK.

List of Contributors

D.T. Murray
Principal Radiopharmacist, West of Scotland Radionuclide Dispensary, Western Infirmary, Glasgow, UK.

Dr D.P. Nowotnik
Research Scientist, The Squibb Institute for Medical Research, College Farm Road, PO Box 191, New Brunswick, New Jersey, NJ 08903-0191, USA.

Ms S. Osman
Research Scientist, MRC Cyclotron Unit, Du Cane Road, Hammersmith, London W6, UK.

Dr M. Pillay
Principal Physicist, Dr Daniel den Hoed Clinic, PO Box 5201, 3008 AE Rotterdam, The Netherlands.

Mr C.B. Sampson
Principal Radiopharmacist, Department of Nuclear Medicine, Addenbrooke's Hospital, Cambridge, and Lecturer and Examiner in Radiopharmaceutical Sciences, University of London, and Churchill Fellow 1979 (Pharmacy), UK.

Dr M.D. Short
Principal Physicist, Department of Physics and Bioengineering, University College School of Medicine, Shropshire House, 11–20 Capper Street, London WC1E 6JA, UK.

Dr L. Smith
Consultant in Nuclear Medicine, Department of Nuclear Medicine, Royal Liverpool Hospital, Prescot Street, Liverpool, L7 8XP, UK.

Dr A.E. Theobald
Senior Lecturer and Sub-Dean, Examiner in Radiopharmaceutical Sciences, Chelsea School of Pharmacy, King's College, University of London, and Fellow of the Royal Pharmaceutical Society of Great Britain.

Mr J.L. Turner
Superintendent Medicines Inspector, Department of Health and Social Security, 1 Nine Elms Lane, London SW8 5NQ, UK.

Dedicated to the memory of Dr Derek Sampson
formerly Director of Research, Department of Surgery
Addenbrooke's Hospital, Cambridge

Chapter 1

Basic Principles of Radionuclide Physics

M.D. Short

1.1 INTRODUCTION

During recent years, the availability of new radiolabelled biological and chemical agents has permitted many sophisticated studies of specific physiological and disease processes in the human subject. The use of, for example, various monoclonal antibodies and different types of blood cell labelled with suitable gamma-ray emitting radionuclides has enhanced the study of such processes by external scintillation detection and imaging. Advances such as these have further established the important role of the radiopharmacist in the innovation and development of new techniques for the clinical nuclear medicine environment. This role will undoubtedly continue to be a leading one and will so ensure that the discipline of radiopharmacy remains a major area of endeavour in general pharmacy. The multidisciplinary nature of nuclear medicine however dictates that new entrants to the field of radiopharmacy, such as pharmacy technicians and students, require adequate knowedge of the basic principles of radiation and radionuclide physics. In this first chapter of the textbook, these basic principles are described in sufficient detail to ensure that the reader gains an understanding of the radionuclide principles embodied in the subsequent chapters. Specific subjects dealt with in this chapter include the basic concepts of ionizing radiation, the structure of the atom and nucleus, radionuclides and modes of decay, decay schemes and the radioactive decay law, units of radioactivity, interaction of radiation with matter, radionuclide production processes and a table of the relevant physical data for a number of commonly used radionclides. The chapter concludes with a recommended further reading list.

1.2 BASIC CONCEPTS OF IONIZING RADIATION

Ionizing radiation is radiation which, when incident upon matter, can cause changes in the atomic or nuclear structure of the matter. Its origins may be atomic, by virtue of electron (e) movement between the orbits or shells surrounding the nucleus, or nuclear due to changes in the component particles forming the nucleus.

1.2.1 Electromagnetic Radiation

One form of ionizing radiation is electromagnetic which can be regarded as a wave form composed of transverse electric and magnetic fields propagated at the speed of light. This is shown schematically in Figure 1. This type of radiation includes X-rays (atomic in origin) and gamma (γ)-rays (nuclear in origin) and is highly penetrating in matter.

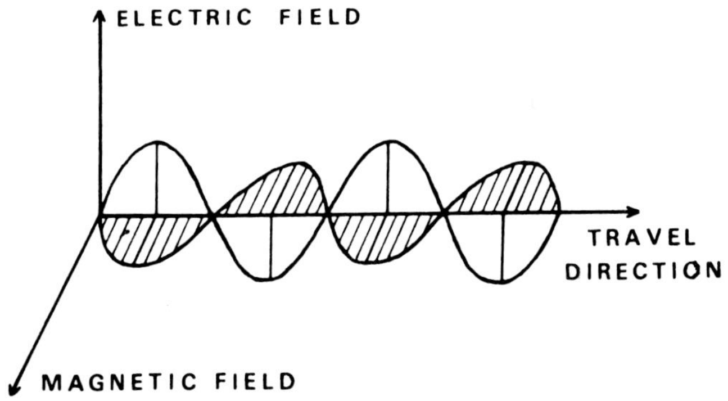

Figure 1. Electromagnetic wave form showing transverse electric and magnetic field components.

The frequency (v) ranges of X and γ-radiation are above 10^{16}Hz (cycles per second and v is related to the wavelength (λ) of the radiation by the inverse relationship

$$v = \frac{c}{\lambda}$$

where c is the velocity of light and equal to $3 \times 10^8 \text{ms}^{-1}$ Under certain situations, electromagnetic radiation may be regarded as being made up of 'packets of energy' which effectively behave as discrete particles. These individual 'packets' are termed X or γ-ray quanta or photons which have an associated energy given by the relationship

$$E = h\,v$$

Where E is measured in joules (J) and h is Planck's Constant equal to 6.63×10^{-34}Js.

Since it it usual to express the energy of radiation in electron volts (eV), it should be noted that

$$1\ \text{eV} = 1.6 \times 10^{-19}\text{J}$$
$$1\ \text{keV (thousand eV)} = 1.6 \times 10^{-16}\text{J}$$
and
$$1\ \text{MeV (million eV)} = 1.6 \times 10^{-13}\text{J}$$

1.2.2 Particulate Radiation

The second type of ionizing radiation is particulate and includes electrons and nuclear particles such as the proton (p), the neutron (n), the alpha (α) particle and the beta (β) particle which can be positively or negatively charged and has the same charge and mass as the electron. These particulate radiations are relatively far less penetrating in matter than electromagnetic radiation. The mass of any of these particles is expressed in atomic mass units (amu) where

$$1\ \text{amu} = 1.66 \times 10^{-27}\text{kg}$$

1.2.3 Equivalence of Mass and Energy

Einstein's principle, developed to explain anomalies in the mass of the nucleus, states that the rest mass of a particle (M_0) is equivalent to an amount of energy E such that

$$E = m_0c^2$$

where c is the velocity of light. In this case, E is referred to as the rest energy. The rest energy of an electron, equal to 511 keV, is commonly used as a natural basic unit of atomic and nuclear energy. Similarly, the total energy of an particle with an inertial mass of m moving at a given velocity may be considered to be a combination of its rest energy and its kinetic energy. This total energy may be written as

$$E = mc^2$$

and the kinetic energy E_k is given by the expression

$$E_k = (m - m_0)c^2$$

1.3 STRUCTURE OF THE ATOM AND NUCLEUS

The atom, the basic unit of all matter, comprises three funadmental particles, the proton, the neutron and the electron. The protons and neutrons, termed nucleons, make up the central nucleus of the atom and the electrons, placed in discrete energy levels or shells, orbit this nucleus. The masses of the proton and neutron are nearly identical and slightly in excess of 1 amu which is about 1840 times the mass of the electron. However, the nucleus is extremely small when compared to the overall dimension of the atom. The nucleus has a diameter of the order of 10^{-14}m and the atom a diameter of 10^{-10}m. In a neutral atom, the number of protons in the nucleus equals the number of orbiting electrons. The proton has a positive electrostatic charge which is balanced by an equal negative charge on the electron. The neutron has zero charge.

1.3.1 Electron Shells

The number of electron shells and the maximum number of electrons in each are limited according to the quantum theory. This theory, first postulated by Bohr in 1913, states that only those orbits for which the angular momentum of the electron has certain discrete values are permitted. The radius of a particular orbit is the mean distance of an electron from the nucleus. The electron is most probably located at this distance but there is also a possibility that it may be found nearer to or further from the nucleus. This "probability distribution" for the permitted orbits helps to explain the processes of electron capture and internal conversion (Sections 1.4.3 and 1.4.7). The quantum theory also states that whenever radiant energy is emitted or absorbed by an atom, this energy is emitted or absorbed in whole quanta of energy of amount hv. Atomic electrons are individually characterised by a set of quantum numbers, including one for spin, such that no two electrons in an atom can exist in the same state, i.e. possess the same set of quantum number values. This concept is known as the Pauli exclusion principle (1925). The electron shells are designated by the letters K to Q and, in line with the exclusion principle, each shell may contain a certain maximum number of electrons. For example, the K and L and M shells may contain maxima of 2, 8 and 18 electrons respectively. Figure 2 shows a schematic representation of a neutral atom with a total of 8 orbiting electrons and hence 8 protons in the nucleus.

1.3.2 Electron Binding Energy

An electron orbiting a positively charged nucleus will have both a potential energy, relating to its distance from the nucleus, and a kinetic energy associated with it (Section 1.2.3). Since the potential energy of the electron in the shell is negative and numerically greater than the kinetic energy, the total energy will be negative. This total energy is usually described in terms of the electron binding energy which is that energy required to remove the electron from the atom. The binding energy is numerically equal to the total energy but of opposite sign such that

$$\begin{aligned}\text{Total Energy }(-) &= \text{Potential Energy}(-)\\ &\quad + \text{Kinetic Energy}(+)\\ &= \text{Binding Energy}(+)\end{aligned}$$

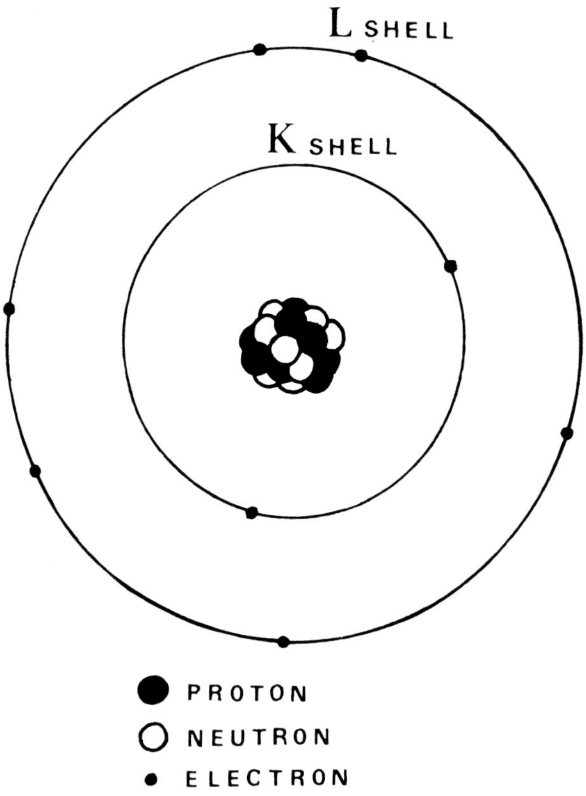

Figure 2. Schematic of neutral atom with 8 orbiting electrons and 8 protons in the nucleus.

Binding energy is greater for those shells closer to the nucleus and also for higher atomic mass. It should also be noted that the shell radii are smaller with increasing atomic mass. Electrons in the inner shells have energies typically in the keV range while those in the outer shells have energies in the eV range. These outer electrons are those involved in the chemical bonding of atoms.

1.3.3 Ionization and Characteristic X-radiation

When a neutral atom loses an electron from one of its shells, the resultant atom, which now has a net positive electrostatic charge, is said to be ionized. Ionization occurs as a result of the bombardment of the atom by external electromagnetic or particulate radiation. Other processes which can cause a vacancy in the shell are electron capture and internal conversion (Section 1.4). In such situations, the vacancy is immediately filled by an electron from an outer shell since partially filled shells are not permitted atomic states when distal shells are full. This electron movement to fill an initial vacancy results in the emission of X-rays (electromagnetic radiation) which are characteristic of the atomic shells between which the movements occur (e.g. L to K, M to K, M to L).

1.3.4 Structure of the Nucleus

Although there is a repulsive force between the protons in an atomic nucleus due to the positive electrostatic charge, there exists a much stronger attractive force within the nucleus which holds it together. This nuclear force, acting over a very short range and therefore confined to the nucleus, acts between all component nucleons. Although the lighter atoms have similar numbers of protons and neutrons, which have no charge, there is a gradual increase in the excess of neutrons over protons in a stable atom as the mass number increases. This is due to the fact that the nuclear force has a limited range which is much smaller than the dimensions of a large nucleus and hence additional neutrons are required to maintain the stability of the nucleus. The nuclear particles also have discrete energy levels associated with them in a similar way to the electron shell energy levels described earlier. The protons and neutrons have separate shells and again the exclusion principle limits the number possible in each one. For example, for both types of nucleon, the maximum number in the respective shells corresponding to the K, L and M electron shells are 2, 6 and 12. Nuclei containing only filled shells have an added stability; one such example is the helium nucleus have two protons and two neutrons which is the α particle (Section 1.4). Nuclei are normally in the ground state but can also exist for a very short period of time in an excited energy state. A return to the ground state occurs with the emission of γ-radiation (Section 1.4).

1.3.5 Characterization of Nuclei

Atomic nuclei are characterized by two numbers, the atomic number (Z), which is the number of protons in the nucleus, and the mass number (A) which is the total number of nucleons (ie. protons + neutrons) in the nucleus. A third number sometimes quoted is the neutron number (N) so resulting in the expression

$$A = N + Z$$

A commonly used notation to describe a nucleus is the form

$$^{A}_{Z}X$$

This denotes a species of atom with a particular atomic number Z, neutron number N(= A − Z) and in a defined nuclear state, usually assumed to be the ground one. This species is termed a nuclide. Nuclides can be stable or unstable, the latter under-going radioactive decay to become stable. One of a group of nuclides having the same proton number is termed an isotope. Such a group comprises different nucleii of the same element since it is the atomic number which defines this. Since isotopes differ only in neutron number, they have the same chemical properties.

1.4 RADIONUCLIDES AND MODES OF DECAY

Most elements have a mixture of stable and unstable isotopes. Nuclides (isotopes) containing an unstable arrangement of protons and neutrons will, at some stage, transform to either a completely stable or a more stable combination of nucleons. Such nuclides (isotopes) are said to be radioactive and are termed radionuclides (radioisotopes). Transformation, or radioactive decay, occurs with either the emission of a charged particle from the nucleus or the capture of an electron from one of the shells surrounding the nucleus. Radioactive decay thus results in a change in the balance between the protons and neutrons and a change in the element. If the product nucleus is left in an excited state, it will de-excite to the ground state with the emission of one or more γ-rays. The initial unstable nucleus is referred to as the parent nuclide and the product nucleus as the daughter nuclide. Throughout the elemental table, there are also many cases of radioactive decay schemes involving a sequence of two or more daughter nuclides prior to achievement of the stable ground state. A schematic representation of a radioactive decay series is shown in Figure 3.

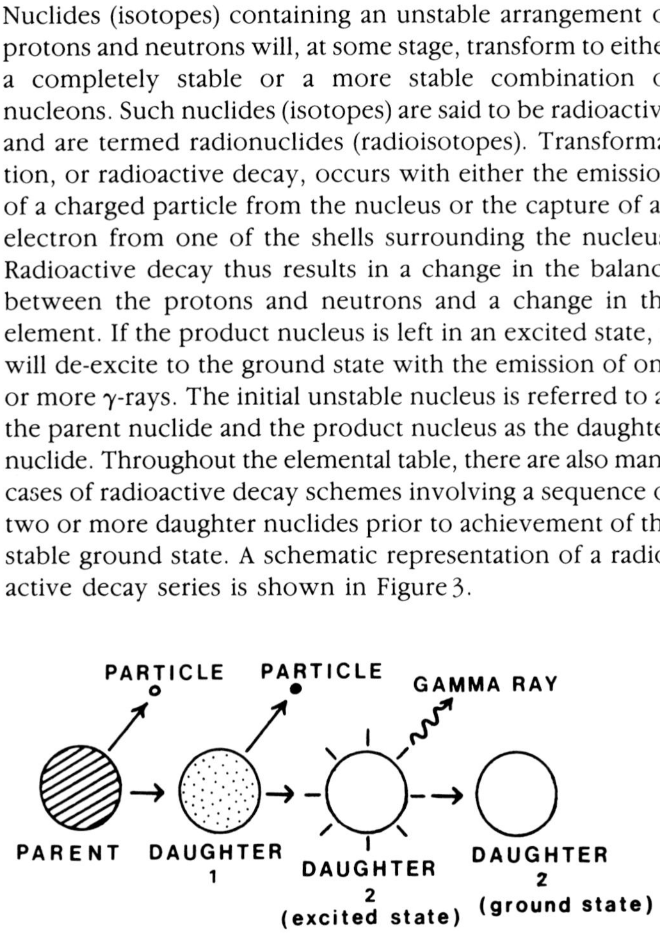

Figure 3. Representation of a radioactive decay series.

Radioactive decay may involve the emission of an electron from a nucleus which has an excess of neutrons or the emission of a positron, a positively charged particle with the same mass as an electron, if the nucleus is deficient in neutrons. This emission of an electron or positron is termed β – decay and these particles are denoted by β^- and β^+ respectively. Electron capture by a neutron deficient nucleus can also occur. Radioactive decay may also involve the emission of a helium nucleus, termed an α particle, from a nucleus with an excess of nucleons. It should be noted that γ-radiation often accompanies these charged particle emissions by a nucleus. Other familiar forms of radioactive decay are annihilation radiation which occurs when an emitted positron combines with a shell electron to produce γ-radiation, internal conversion, where an emitted γ-ray imparts all its energy to a shell electron which is subsequently ejected and isomeric transition where a daughter nuclide remains in an excited state for a significant period of time prior to γ-ray emission. The radioactive decay process of nuclear fission, in which certain high mass radionuclides spontaneously divide into two daughter nuclides of similar mass with the emission of neutrons, is also utilised in the production of certain radionuclides for nuclear medicine.

1.4.1 Conservation Laws

At this stage it is important to note that, in any radioactive decay scheme or radionuclide production process (Section 1.9), there are a number of physical quantities which are always conserved. These include the total charge involved in the transformation, the mass number and the mass-energy relationship (Section 1.2.3). With regard to this relationship, although neither rest mass nor kinetic energy is conserved by itself, their total is always conserved. Momentum (mass × velocity) and spin are two of the other quantities which are conserved.

1.4.2 Beta Decay

Beta decay is a common type of decay which is found throughout the entire range of mass numbers. It produces a change in the atomic number from Z to (Z + 1) for β^- emission and from Z to (Z − 1) for β^+ emission but no change in the atomic mass. These particles do not exist as free particles in the nucleus but are created at the instant of nuclear transformation. For β^- emission, a neutron decays into a proton such that

$$n \rightarrow p + \beta^- + v$$

The particle v, a neutrino, was postulated by Pauli in 1931 as a means of satisfying certain requirements of the conservation laws. This particle is much smaller than an electron and in fact has a zero rest mass and zero charge. For positron (β^+) emission, a proton decays into a neutron such that

$$p \rightarrow n + \beta^+ + v$$

A beta particle can have a kinetic energy of any value up to a definite maximum value which is characteristic of the decay process in question. The general shape of a beta particle energy spectrum is shown in Figure 4. The average energy of decay is approximately one third of the maximum value.

Beta particles encountered in radiopharmacy and associated areas of nuclear medicine cover a wide range of

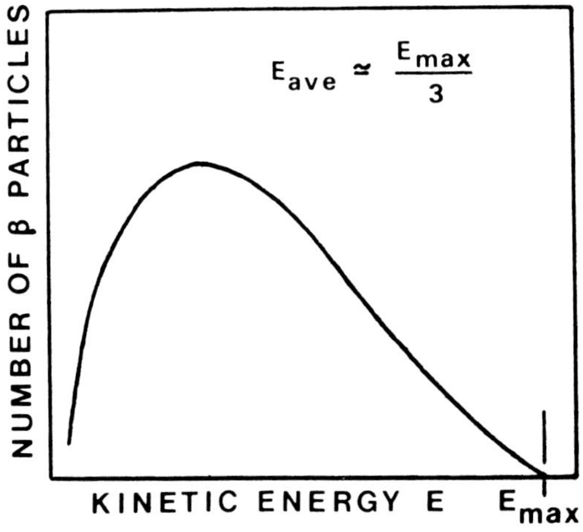

Figure 4. Characteristic β particle energy spectrum.

maximum energies from tritium (H-3) with a maximum of 18 keV to yttrium-90 with a maximum of 2.27 MeV. Although the range of the higher energy beta particle can be several metres in air, the range in tissue is a few millimetres. This means that, for diagnostic in-vivo procedures, beta particle emissions only add to the patient dose and do not provide useful data. However, for therapeutic procedures, this short range type of radiation is a necessary requirement for selective treatment. Two examples of a beta particle decay scheme used in therapy are the transformations of phosphorous-32 into sulphur-32 and yttrium-90 into zirconium-90, both occurring with the emission of a β^- particle. These decay schemes may be written as:

$$^{32}_{15}P \rightarrow ^{32}_{16}S + \beta^- \ (1.71 \text{ MeV}) + v$$

and

$$^{90}_{39}Y \rightarrow ^{90}_{40}Zr + \beta^- \ (2.27 \text{ MeV}) + v$$

1.4.3 Electron Capture

Nuclei which are unstable due to a deficiency in the number of neutrons may, as an alternative to positron emission, capture an electron from a surrounding shell. This process of electron capture may be written as

$$p + e \rightarrow n + v$$

Characteristic X-ray emission then occurs due to the rearrangement of the orbital electrons to fill the vacancy left by the captured electron. There is also the possibility that the X-rays emitted will interact with and eject outer electrons provided that the X-ray energy is greater than the electron binding energy. The ejected electrons have low kinetic energy and are called Auger electrons after the French physicist who first studied this effect.

A radionuclide used in nuclear medicine which decays by electron capture is chromium-51 which decays to vanadium-51 according to the relationship

$$^{51}_{24}Cr + e \rightarrow ^{51}_{23}V + \gamma + v$$

Nine percent of the transformations of Cr-51 result in a gamma-ray with an energy of 320 keV.

1.4.4 Alpha Decay

The emission of a helium nucleus, or alpha particle, leaves the daughter nuclide with an atomic number of (Z−2) and an atomic mass of (A−4) since it comprises two protons and two neutrons. This type of decay is common in very heavy nuclei. One example of alpha decay is the transformation of radium-226 into radon-222 according to the scheme

$$^{226}_{88}Ra \rightarrow ^{222}_{86}Rn + \alpha \ (4.8 \text{ MeV})$$

These particles, usually emitted with energies of several MeV, have a short range even in air (~5 mm) due to their mass and charge and travel only micrometer distances in tissue. For this reason, they have no role in nuclear medicine and, indeed, give rise to exremely high localised radiation dose in tissue. Encapsulated alpha-emitting radionuclides have been used as sealed sources emitting X or gamma-rays for therapy.

1.4.5 Gamma Radiation

Beta and alpha radiation are often accompanied by gamma radiation since the decaying nucleus produces a daughter nuclide which is left in an excited state. Transition to the ground state is virtually instantaneous (less than 10^{-6}s) although there are cases where the excited state is prolonged for a measurable period of time (see Isomeric Transition). The gamma radiation from an excited daughter nuclide has a discrete energy which is characteristic of the daughter. This energy corresponds to the difference between the two energy states of the daughter nucleus following the primary particulate decay process.

1.4.6 Annihilation Radiation

A positron emitted from a nucleus gradually loses kinetic energy during interactions with surrounding atoms. It finally combines with an electron in an interaction in which the rest masses of both particles are given up as electromagnetic radiation in the form of two gamma rays. This process may be written as

$$\beta^+ + e \rightarrow \gamma + \gamma$$

The positron is said to be annihilated and the gamma rays produced, termed annihilation radiation, each have an energy

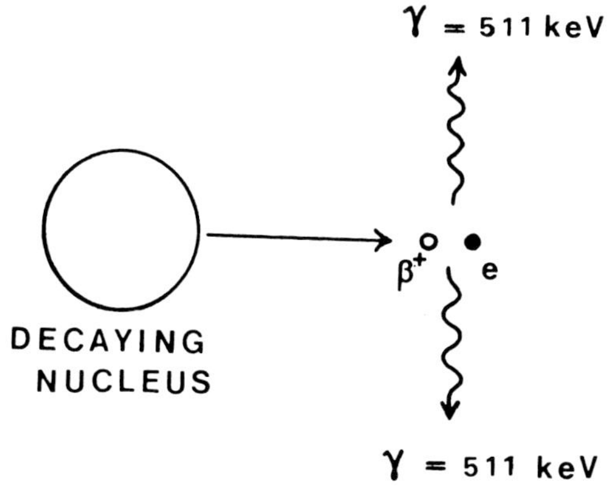

Figure 5. Annihilation radiation decay scheme.

of 511 keV and are emitted at 180° to each other so that the net momentum is zero. This particular property of annihilation radiation, shown in figure 5, has been utilised in the specialized imaging technique of positron emission tomography (PET). Positron emitting radionuclides used in nuclear medicine include

$^{18}_{9}F$ (fluorine-18), $^{52}_{26}Fe$ (iron-52) and $^{68}_{13}Ga$ (gallium-68)

1.4.7 Internal Conversion

When a daughter nucleus is left in an excited state, it de-excites to the ground state by emitting a gamma ray. However, instead of the gamma ray being emitted, it may transfer all its energy to an orbiting electron which is then ejected from the atom. This electron is referred to as an internal conversion electron and has a kinetic energy equal to the gamma ray energy less the electron binding energy. This process is analogous to the photoelectric effect which involves a gamma ray external to the atom with which it interacts. The probability for internal conversion to occur increases with higher atomic number, since the K shell is closer to the nucleus, lower gamma ray energy and longer lifetime of the excited state. There is also characteristic X-ray emission associated with internal conversion due to electron movement to fill inner shell vacancies. These X-rays may then eject outer shell electrons which are the Auger electrons described in the section on electron capture.

1.4.8 Isomeric Transition

A daughter radionuclide which exists in an excited state for a measurable period of time prior to emission of gamma radiation to reach ground state is called an isomer. This prolonged state is referred to as an isomeric state or metastable state and is denoted by the letter m written as a superscript together with the mass number (A) in the notation

$$^{Am}_{Z}X$$

Metastable radionuclides play a major role in nuclear medicine since they form the basis of radionuclide generators in which the metastable daughter may be separated from its longer-lived parent by a simple ion exchange process. These daughter radionuclides, which emit only gamma radiation and no beta radiation, offer the advantage of low radiation dose for patient investigations.

Metastable radionuclides commonly employed in nuclear medicine are $^{99m}_{43}Tc$ (technetium-99 m) and $^{81m}_{36}Kr$ (krypton-81 m) which are produced from the parent radionuclides $^{99}_{37}Mo$ (molybdenum-99) and $^{81}_{37}Rb$ (rubidium-81) respectively. Detailed decay schemes for these two transformations are shown in Section 1.5. Another partent/metastable daughter transformation which has been widely used in nuclear medicine is $^{113}_{50}Sn/^{113m}_{49}In$ (tin-113/indium-113 m).

1.4.9 Fission

Certain heavy nuclei undergo the process of spontaneous fission whereby the nucleus splits into two lighter nuclei of approximately equal mass with the emission of neutrons. Conversely, fission of heavy nuclei may be induced by bombardment with neutrons (Section 1.9). Fission products are rich in neutrons and usually decay by beta particle emission. This characteristic, coupled with a long half-life (Section 1.6), makes many of these products unsuitable for diagnostic nuclear medicine but of use in certain forms of therapy. Radionuclides produced by nuclear fission include

$^{99}_{42}Mo$, $^{131}_{53}I$ (iodine-131), $^{133}_{54}Xe$ (xenon-133) and

$^{137}_{55}Cs$ (caesium-137)

1.5 RADIONUCLIDE DECAY SCHEMES

In this section, decay schemes for a number of radionuclides commonly employed in current nuclear medicine procedures are presented in detail. Data quoted include the modes of decay, the half lives (Section 1.6) of decay schemes and the principal energy levels involved in the schemes. Neutrinos associated with proton/neutron conversions are not shown.

1.5.1 Technetium-99m

This radionuclide is the one most commonly used in diagnostic nuclear medicine and is readily available from commercial molybdenum-99/technetium-99m generators. Technetium-99m, a metastable state, is the immediate daughter product of the parent molybdenum-99. The full nuclear transformation may be written in the form

$$^{99}_{42}\text{Mo} \rightarrow {}^{99\text{m}}_{43}\text{Tc} + \beta^- + \gamma \rightarrow {}^{99}_{43}\text{Tc} + \gamma \rightarrow {}^{99}_{44}\text{Ru} + \beta^-$$

and the detailed decay scheme is shown in Figure 6. Molybeenum-99 has a half-life of 67 hours and decays by beta particle and gamma ray emissions to technetium-99m which has a half-life of 6 hours and decays by isomeric transition to technetium-99 with the emission of a gamma ray with an energy of 140 keV. This gamma emission is that used in nuclear medicine procedures. The very long half-life technetium-99 (2.1×10^5 years) finally decays to stable ruthenium-99 with the emission of a beta particle.

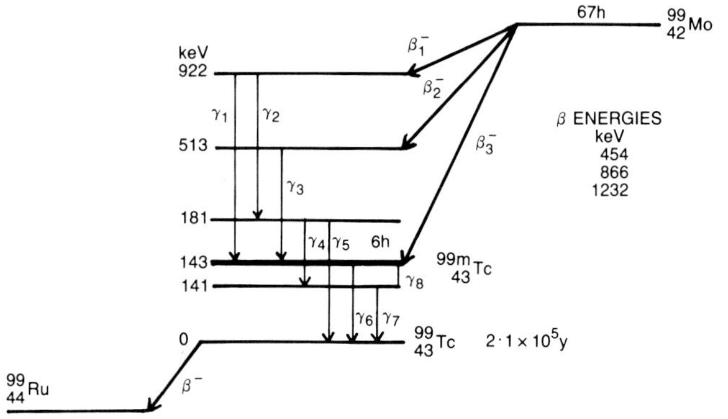

Figure 6. Decay scheme for molybdenum–99/technetium–99 m.

1.5.2 Indium-111

This radionuclide is also readily available commercially and has been widely used to label, for example, various types of white blood cell and monoclonal antibody for imaging studies. Indium-111 has a half-life of 67 hours and decays by electron capture to stable cadmium-111 with associated gamma ray emissions at 173 keV and 247 keV. The transformation process may be written as

$$^{111}_{49}\text{In} + \text{e} \rightarrow {}^{111}_{48}\text{Cd} + \gamma$$

and the detailed decay scheme is shown in Figure 7.

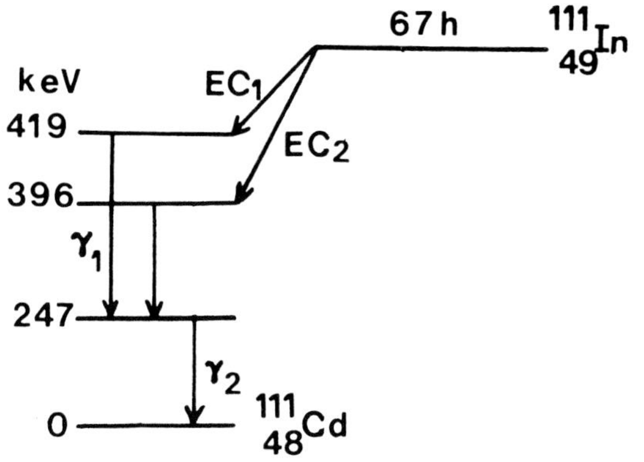

Figure 7. Decay scheme for indium-111.

1.5.3 Iodine-123

This radioisotope of iodine has effectively superseded iodine-131 in diagnostic nuclear medicine and has been labelled to proteins and to a variety of pharmaceuticals that can be iodinated. It has a half-life and gamma emission which make it ideal both in terms of detection efficiency for imaging and reduced radiation dose to the patient. It is, however, relatively expensive to produce with radionuclidic purity and has a limited availability. Iodine-123, like indium-111, decays by electron capture and emits a usable gamma ray at 159 keV. It has a half-life of 13 hours and decays to tellurium-123 which has an extremely long half-life of approximately 1.2×10^{13} years and can thus be regarded as stable. The iodine-123 transformation process may be written as

$$^{123}_{53}\text{I} + \text{e} \rightarrow {}^{123}_{52}\text{Te} + \gamma$$

and the decay scheme is shown in Figure 8.

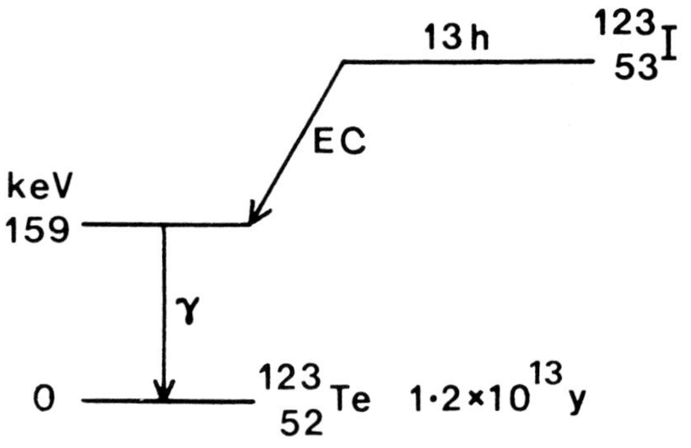

Figure 8. Decay scheme for iodine-123.

1.5.4 Thallium-201

Thallium-201 has been regularly used as a myocardial imaging agent for many years in all nuclear medicine departments undertaking cardiological studies. This potassium analog however is not an ideal agent due to its decay characteristics and, for this reason, there is a continuing search for an appropriate technetium-99m labelled myocardial agent. Thallium-201 also decays by electron capture and emits various X and gamma rays, the maximum energy emitted

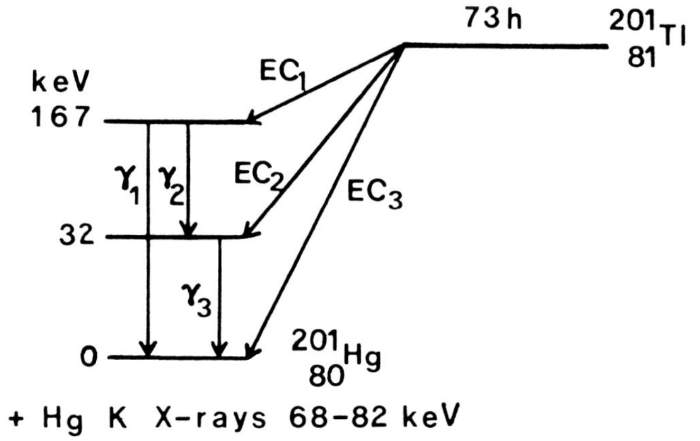

Figure 9. Decay scheme for thallium-201.

being 167 keV. It has a half-life of 73 hours and decays to the stable nuclide mercury-201. The transformation process may be written as

$$^{201}_{81}\text{Tl} + \text{e} \rightarrow ^{201}_{80}\text{Hg} + \gamma$$

and the decay scheme is shown in Figure 9.

1.6 RADIOACTIVE DECAY LAW

The process of radioactive decay, in which a nuclear transformation occurs, is governed by the laws of probability. This means that for a particular radioactive nucleus there is a fixed probability that it will undergo decay within a stated period of time. For a given number of radioactive nuclei with the same atomic mass and number there is no way of ascertaining precisely when one of them will decay and each nucleus is independent of the others with regard to the instant of decay. Hence, there is a statistical fluctuation associated with the number of nuclei decaying within the defined period of time. For a number of identical radioactive nuclei, it may be stated that, on average, a known fraction of them will decay per unit time. The radioactive decay rate is unaffected by the physical or chemical environment of the radionuclide in question, whether it be in a simple or complex molecular structure, at extreme differences in temperature or in different phases.

1.6.1 Radioactive Decay Constant

For a large number of identical radioactive nuclei, suppose that the probability of any particular nucleus decaying in unit time is λ, the radioactive decay constant. The activity of these nuclei, the number decaying per unit time (in a time which is short compared with $1/\lambda$), will be given by $N\lambda$. The rate of depletion of the nuclei, dN/dt, is equal to the activity. Since N decreases with time, a negative sign is inserted in the fundamental relationship

$$\frac{dN}{dt} = -N\lambda$$

which may also be written in the form

$$\frac{dN}{dt} = -\lambda dt$$

If it is assumed that the probability of decay of a nucleus is independent of its age to that λ is independent of t and is constant, then the above expression may be integrated. If there were N_o nuclei present at t = o and N remaining at t = t, then

$$\int_{N_o}^{N} \frac{dN}{N} = -\lambda \int_{o}^{t} dt$$

$$\text{or } \ln\left(\frac{N}{N_o}\right) = -\lambda t$$

where ln signifies natural logarithms.

This equation may be written in the exponential form

$$N = N_o \exp(-\lambda t)$$

where exp signifies e, the base of natural logarithms, which equals 2.718. It should be noted that the exponential decay law signifies that the number of nuclei decaying within a specified period of time is proportional to the number present at the beginning of that period.

1.6.2 Radioactive Half-life

The half-life ($T_{1/2}$) of a particular radionuclide is the period during which half the nuclei initially present will decay. In this case,

$$N = \frac{N_o}{2} \quad \text{and} \quad t = T_{1/2}$$

Substituting these values in the above equation gives

$$\frac{N_o}{2} = N_o \exp(-\lambda T_{1/2})$$

This may be written in the inverse form

$$2 = \exp(\lambda T_{1/2})$$

and in logarithmic form as

$$\ln 2 = \lambda T_{1/2}$$

$$\text{or } T_{1/2} = \frac{\ln 2}{\lambda} = \frac{0.693}{\lambda}$$

Thus, half-life is a constant which is characteristic of a particular radionuclide. Throughout the periodic table of elements, there are some radionuclides with half-lives measured in

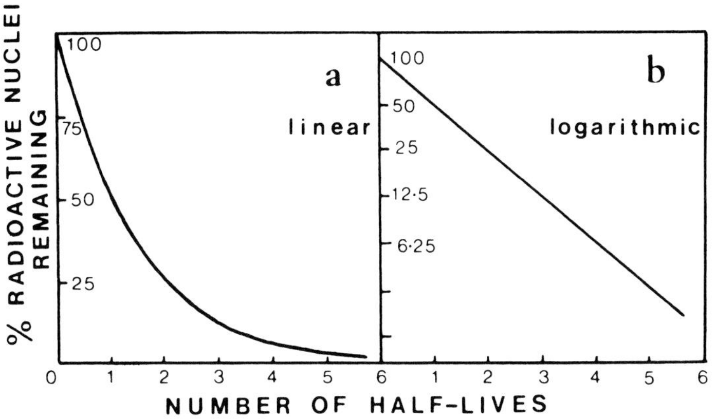

Figure 10. Exponential law of radioactive decay.

fractions of a second and others with half-lives of millions of years. Most radionuclides usefully employed in the practice of nuclear medicine have half-lives measured in hours or days.

Figure 10 illustrates the concepts of the exponential decay law by plotting the percentage of radioactive nuclei remaining against the number of half-lives elapsed on a linear scale (a) and on a logarithmic scale (b) where the slope of the straight line plot is $-\lambda$.

1.6.3 Mean Life

The mean life (T_M) is defined as the average lifetime of a large number of radioactive nuclei and is a quantity which is used in dosimetry calculations. It may be shown that

$$T_M = 1.44 \times T_{1/2}$$

1.6.4 Radioactive Decay Series

A radioactive decay series may be generally represented as

$$P \xrightarrow{\lambda_P} D \xrightarrow{\lambda_D} E \xrightarrow{\lambda_E} F$$

where λ_P, λ_D and λ_E are the decay constants for P parent nuclei and D and E daughter nuclei respectively. There are a number of examples of a radioactive decay series employed routinely in nuclear medicine. Radionuclide generators involve a parent radionuclide decaying into a daughter radionuclide which can be chemically extracted from a generator and used as a suitable radiotracer in clinical studies.

For P parent nuclei and D daughter nuclei present at any time t, the activities are $P\lambda_P$ and $D\lambda_D$ respectively. The rate of change, dD/dt, in the number of daughter nuclei is equal to the supply of a new daughter nuclei due to the decay of the parent less the rate of loss of the daughter due to its own decay. This situation may be expressed as

$$\frac{dD}{dt} = P\lambda_P - D\lambda_D$$

which is the basic equation unerlying the general theory of radioactive decay series. If P_o is the number of parent nuclei present at t = o, then

$$P = P_o \exp(-\lambda_P t)$$

and hence

$$\frac{dD}{dt} = P_o\lambda_P \exp(-\lambda_P t) - D\lambda_D$$

From this differential equation, an explicit solution for the daughter activity $D\lambda_D$ as a function of t may be derived which is of the form

$$D\lambda_D = (P\lambda_P)\frac{\lambda_D}{\lambda_D - \lambda_P}[1 - \exp(\lambda_D - \lambda_P)t)]$$

This expression may be used to calculate activity levels in certain situations, some of which are outlined below.

1.6.5 Ratios of Activity of Parent and Daughter

(a) Daughter longer-lived than parent

If $T_{1/2P} < T_{1/2D}$, then the activity ratio $D\lambda_D/P\lambda_P$ increases continuously with t. Thus, when $\lambda_P > \lambda_D$,

$$\frac{D\lambda_D}{P\lambda_P} = \frac{\lambda_D}{\lambda_P - \lambda_D}[\exp(\lambda_P - \lambda_D)t - 1]$$

An example of this situation is the decay series involving iodine-131 where

$$^{131}_{52}Te \rightarrow {}^{131}_{53}I \rightarrow {}^{131}_{54}Xe$$

$$T_{1/2P} = 1.25d \quad T_{1/2D} = 8d$$

In the extreme case when $T_{1/2P} \ll T_{1/2D}$, the activity of the daughter finally becomes effectively independent of the residual activity of the parent. Thus, for $t \gg T_{1/2P}$ it may be shown that

$$D\lambda_D \approx P_o\lambda_D \exp(-\lambda_D t)$$

(b) Daughter shorter-lived than parent

If $T_{1/2P} > T_{1/2D}$, the activity ratio $D\lambda_D/P\lambda_P$ increases with t at first and then approaches a constant value. For large value of t, the general expression becomes simply

$$\frac{D\lambda_D}{P\lambda_P} = \frac{\lambda_D}{\lambda_D - \lambda_P}$$

When the ratio becomes constant, a particular type of radioactive equilibrium exists known as transient equilibrium. Such a situation is common.

(c) Daughter much shorter-lived than parent

This is the situation relevant to certain radionuclide generators used in nuclear medicine. In this case $T_{1/2P} \gg T_{1/2D}$ and, since $\lambda_P \ll \lambda_D$, the activity ratio is given by

$$\frac{D\lambda_D}{P\lambda_P} = 1 - \exp(-\lambda_D t)$$

The daughter activity increases according to the simple exponential growth curve governed by its own decay constant λ_D. It should be noted that, for $t \gg T_{1/2D}$,

$$D\lambda_D = P\lambda_P$$

This condition, known as secular equilibrium, only occurs if $T_{1/2P} \gg T_{1/2D}$.

1.7 UNITS OF RADIOACTIVITY

Radioactivity is measured in terms of the rate at which nuclear transformations occur or the number of radionuclides decaying in unit time. The SI unit of radioactivity currently in use is the becquerel which is equal to one transformation of distintegration per second. This fundamental unit has the symbol Bq. In practice, larger multiple units of the becquerel are routinely used in nuclear medicine and radiopharmacy. These are as follows:-

1 kilobecquerel (kBq) = 10^3 disintegrations per second
1 megabecquerel (MBq) = 10^6 disintegrations per second
1 gigabecquerel (GBq) = 10^9 disintegrations per second
1 tetrabecquerel (TBq) = 10^{12} disintegrations per second

The multiple units petabecquerel (PBq) and exabecquerel (EBq), equal to 10^{15} and 10^{18} disintegrations per second respectively, have no relevance to the clinical use of ionizing radiation.

Historically, the original unit of radioactivity was the curie (Ci). Although formally replaced by the SI unit, the curie is still widely used and, for this reason, a sound knowledge of the various conversion factors is necessary. The curie, defined as the number of disintegrations per second from 1 g of radium, is a large unit numerically equal to 3.7×10^{10}. More commonly used in nuclear medicine were the millicurie (mCi) and microcurie (μCi) equal to 3.7×10^7 and 3.7×10^4 disintegrations per second respectively. Relevant conversion factors are as follows.

1Ci = 37 GBq
1mCi = 37 MBq
1μCi = 37 kBq

Also, of relevance to low-level counting techniques, the nanocurie (nCi) is equal to 37 Bq.

Alternatively,

1 kBq = 27 nCi
1 MBq = 27 μCi
1 GBq = 27 mCi
1 TBq = 27 Ci

1.7.1 Specific Activity

Specific activity is defined as the radioactivity per unit mass of an element containing a radioisotope. It is important to distinguish between unit mass of the element and unit mass of a compound containing the element since specific activity may refer to either case. Obviously, the quoted value for specific activity per unit mass of element will be much higher. It is also important not to confuse specific activity with radioactive concentration which is simply radioactivity per unit volume.

1.8 INTERACTION OF RADIATION WITH MATTER

1.8.1 Charged Particles

The electrostatic interactions between an incident charged particle and the atoms in an absorbing material give rise to a number of possible mechanisms by which the particle may lose kinetic energy along its track or is deflected from its original path. These mechanisms involve four types of particle interaction. In two of these, the particle may undergo inelastic or elastic collision with atomic electrons. In the former type of collision, usually the predominant mechanism for loss of kinetic energy in an absorbing medium, the major processes involved are ionization and excitation. Ionization occurs when sufficient energy is transferred to an orbital electron to cause its ejection from the atom. Alternatively, if the energy for ionization is not available, the orbital electron will not be ejected but will experience a momentary transition to an excited state (excitation). The density of these inelastic interactions depends upon the mass and charge of the incident particle. During elastic collisions with atomic electrons, the incident charged particle is deflected in the field of the electrons in such a way that energy and momentum are conserved. This type of interaction is only relevant for the case of very low energy incident electrons.

A charged particle may also experience inelastic and elastic collisions with nuclei. During an inelastic non-capturing collision with a nucleus, the charged particle is deflected. In some, but not all, such deflections a quantum of electromagnetic radiation is emitted and a corresponding amount of kinetic energy is lost by the colliding particles. There is also a finite probability of nuclear excitation but this is very small compared to the probability of the emission of radiation. During elastic scattering by a nucleus, although the incident particle is deflected, there is no emission of radiation or excitation of the nucleus. The particle loses only that kinetic energy required for the conservation of momentum between the two particles. Incident electrons have a high probability of undergoing a nuclear elastic collision. The energy deposited per unit length by a charged particle in an absorbing medium is referred to as the Linear Energy Transfer (LET). In tissue, this relates to the biological damage caused. The unit of LET for charged particles is eV (or a higher multiple) μm^{-1}.

1.8.2 Electrons

The major processes involved in the interaction of electrons with an absorbing material are ionization and excitation of atomic electrons (inelastic collisions) and elastic collisions with nuclei. There is also some inelastic scattering by nuclei resulting in the emission of an X-radiation called bremsstrahlung which is described in more detail below. In tissue, the energy lost by an incident electron in inelastic collisions is roughly equally divided between ionization and excitation events. After an ionization, a liberated orbital electron may have sufficient energy to cause further ionizations and excitations and even to produce a separate track. As a result of the multiplicity of interactions of an electron with an absorber, the electron follows a tortuous path such that, although total path lengths in the absorber are similar for monoenergetic electrons, the path length in any given direction varies considerably.

At this stage it is important to distinguish between the path length and range of an electron in an absorber. The range is proportional to the density of the absorber and relates to that thickness which the electron can just penetrate. Conversely, due to the multiple interactions, the path length will be longer and, in practice, has been found to be between 1.2 and 4 times the thickness of absorber traversed. This difference between path length and range of an electron is shown schematically in Figure 11. In part B of the figure, the maximum path length and range are generally obtained by extrapolating the steepest part of each curve to the distance axis.

As stated earlier in this chapter, the range of electrons in tissue is millimetre order of magnitude although the range in air can be several metres in the case of high energy (i.e. > 1 MeV) electroms. The LET values for electrons in a tissue equivalent material are 0.4 and 0.25 keV μm^{-1} for initial electron energies of 100 keV and 1 MeV respectively.

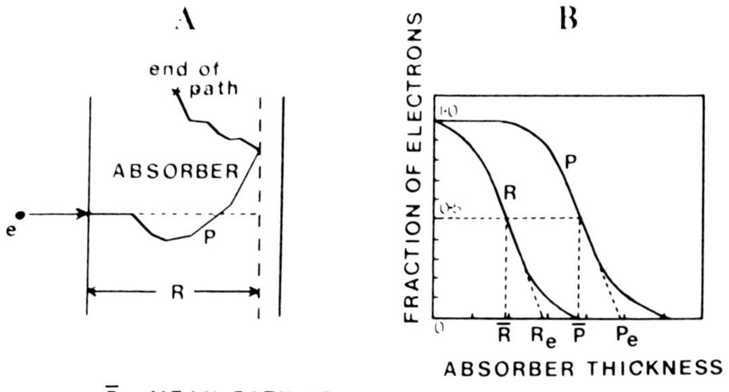

P̄ - MEAN PATH LENGTH
R̄ - MEAN RANGE
P_e - EXTRAPOLATED PATH LENGTH
R_e - EXTRAPOLATED RANGE

Figure 11. Path length and range of an electron in an absorber.

1.8.3 Bremsstrahlung

Whenever an incident electron is slowed down to an inelastic interaction with an absorber nucleus, some of its energy is converted into a type of X-radiation. This X-radiation is in the form of a continuous energy spectrum which is called bremsstrahlung (braking radiation). In this spectrum, the maximum X-ray energy produced is equal to the initial electron energy and occurs when the electron loses all its kinetic energy in a single interaction. Although bremsstrahlung production usually accounts for only a few percent of energy loss, this production varies as the square of the atomic number (Z) of the absorbing material and varies inversely with the square of the mass of the incident particle. This means that protons and alpha particles will produce only about one millionth the bremsstrahlung of an electron of the same velocity. The dependence of bremsstrahlung production on absorber atomic number signifies that a light shielding material such as plastic is more suitable for work with pure beta emitters than high atomic number materials.

1.8.4 Positrons

Positrons interact with matter in a manner similar to that for electrons and their range in an absorber is equivalent to that of an electron with the same energy. At the end of their path, they annihilate by combining with an electron to form two 511 keV gamma rays (section 1.4).

1.8.5 Alpha particles

These particles have a maximum range of less than one tenth of a millimetre and a very high LET in tissue due to their large mass and double charge. For these reasons, they have no application in nuclear medicine.

1.8.6 Electromagnetic Radiation

Unlike charged particles, X and gamma ray photons incident upon matter do not cause ionization directly but can transfer all or part of their energy to atomic electrons by scattering or absorption and it is these electrons which produce ionization. Although charge particles have a definite range in an absorbing material, the range for an individual photon cannot be predicted. However, a well-collimated beam of photons exhibits a truly exponential absorption in matter. This is because photons are scattered or absorbed in a single event. Hence, those collimated photons which penetrate an absorber have undergone no interaction while those absorbed have been eliminated from the beam in a single event. There are a number of interactions with atomic electrons or nuclei which can cause an X or gamma ray photon to be scattered or absorbed and the main ones are outlined below.

1.8.7 Elastic (Rayleigh) Scattering

In this process, the photon is deflected from its path by an atomic electron but suffers no energy loss. For high photon energy and a low atomic number absorber, elastic scattering is negligible in comparison to inelastic scattering. For low photon energy and high atomic number however, elastic scattering is more significant.

1.8.8 Inelastic (Compton) Scattering

During this type of scattering, the incident photon transfers some of its energy to an atomic electron which then recoils. The reduced energy photon is scattered at an angle to its original path which is dependent on its initial energy. This process is shown schematically in Figure 12.

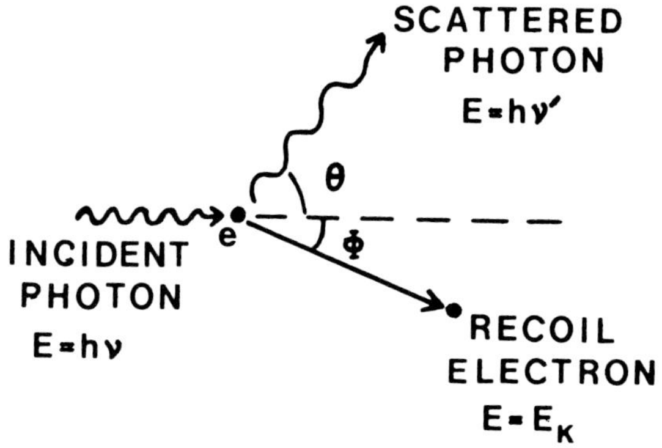

Figure 12. Schematic of Compoton scattering of a photon in an absorber.

Compton scattering is the major type of interaction in low atomic number absorbers such as tissue over a wide range of photon energy. The effect predominates in those cases where the energy of the incident photon is large compared to the atomic binding energy of the electron. In this situation, the electron is effectively free or unbound. For photons with energies of about 50 keV, only the outer electrons in an atom are free whereas, for photon energies of several hundred keV or more, all atomic electrons may be considered thus. The energy and momentum involved in this type of scattering process must be conserved (Section 1.4). If the energies of the incident and scattered photons are hv and hv′ respectively and the kinetic energy of the recoil electron is E_K then

$$hv = hv' + E_K$$

Since momentum is mass × velocity, the incident and scattered photons may be considered to have momenta of hv/c and hv′/c respectively since $E = mc^2$. If the momentum of the recoil electron is mv, then

$$\frac{hv}{c} = \frac{hv'}{c} \cos \Theta + mv \cos \Phi$$

and
$$\frac{hv'}{c} \sin \Theta = mv \sin \Phi$$

1.8.9 Photoelectric Effect

The photoelectric effect, shown schematically in Figure 13, is the predominant mode of interaction in medium and high atomic number absorbers for photon energies up to several hundred keV. In this interaction, the total energy of the photon is used up in ejecting an electron from an atom. This electron is termed a photoelectron. Although an incident photon cannot be totally absorbed by a free electron, total absorption can take place if the electron is initially bound in an atom.

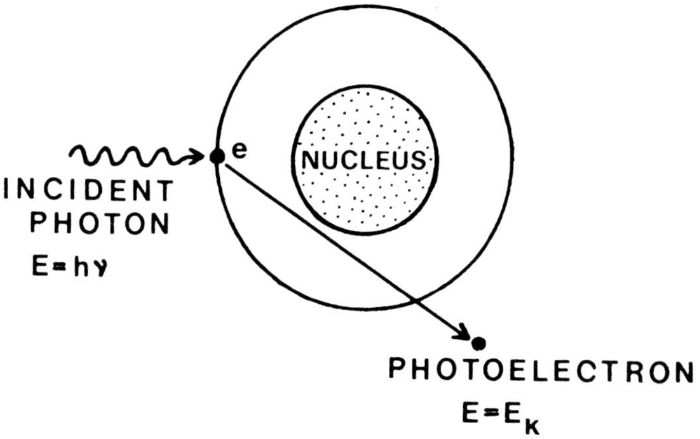

Figure 13. Schematic of the photoelectric effect.

Momentum is conserved by the recoil of the entire residual atom. The photoelectric effect predominates over Compton scattering in those cases where the incident photon energy is comparable to the binding energy of the electron. As expected, the most tightly bound electrons, that is those in inner shells, have the greatest probability of absorbing an incident photon. It has been found that about 80% of the photoelectric absorption processes occur in the K shell provided that the photon energy hv is greater than the K shell binding energy. If E_B is the binding energy of the electron and E_K its kinetic energy following ejection from the atom, then

$$hv = E_B + E_K$$

The remainder of the energy appears as characteristic X-rays and Auger electrons due to electron movements to fill the inner shell vacancy.

1.8.10 Pair Production

When passing through the electrostatic field of a nucleus, an incident photon with an energy greater than 1.02 MeV can create an electron-positron pair whose total energy is just equal to hv, the energy of the photon which ceases to exist. This process is a prime example of the creation of mass from energy and is shown schematically in Figure 14.

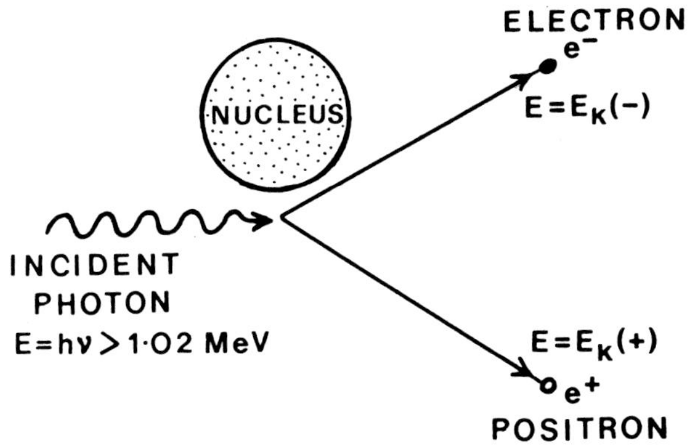

Figure 14. Schematic of the pair production process.

If E_K (−) and E_K (+) are the kinetic energies of the electron and positron respectively and m_oc^2 = 511 keV is the electron rest energy then

$$hv = E_K(-) + E_K(+) + 2m_oc^2$$

The electron and positron lose their kinetic energy by ionization and excitation and the positron finally combines with an electron to create the annihilation radiation of two 511 keV photons travelling at 180° to each other (Section 1.4).

1.8.11 Attenuation of Electromagnetic Radiation

The attenuation of a narrow, well defined beam of X or gamma-ray photons in an absorbing material has two components. These are absorption, when the photon is completely eliminated and scattering, when the photon is deflected out of the beam. This is shown schematically in Figure 15. If the intensity of a monoenergetic beam incident

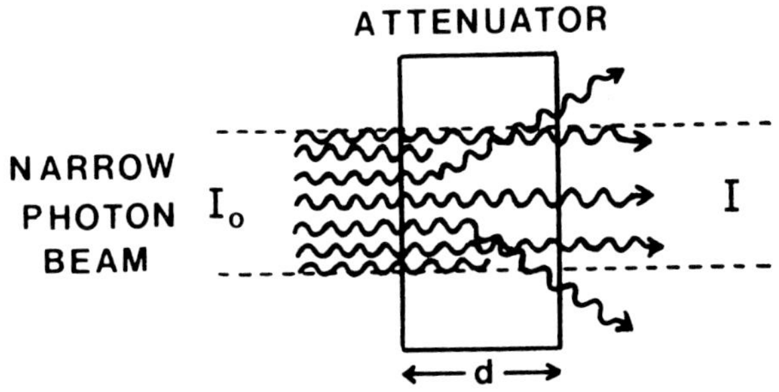

Figure 15. Attentuation of electromagnetic radiation in an absorber.

upon an absorber of thickness d is I_o and the residual intensity after traversing through d is I, then

$$I = I_o \exp(-\mu d)$$

where μ is termed the linear attenuation coefficient and has the unit cm^{-1}. It should be noted that the above exponential expression has an identical mathematical form to that defining the law of radioactive decay (Section 1.6).

The linear attenuation coefficient μ is a measure of the number of incident photons which undergo interactions in the absorber and is characteristic of the photon energy and the absorber density. The coefficient is in reality a total one since there is linear attenuation and an associated coefficient relating to each type of photon interaction described earlier, namely Compton scattering (CS), the photoelectric effect (PE) and pair production (PP). Hence

$$\mu = \mu_{CS} + \mu_{PE} + \mu_{PP}$$

1.8.12 Half-value Thickness

The half value thickness ($D_{1/2}$) is defined as that thickness of an absorber which reduces the intensity of a beam to half its initial value. The relationship between ($D_{1/2}$ and linear attentuation coefficient is the same as that between half-life and decay constant (Section 1.6) and may be written as

$$D_{1/2} = \frac{0.693}{\mu}$$

Half-value thicknesses of water and lead for certain radionuclides commonly used in nuclear medicine are shown in the Table in Section 1.10.

1.8.13 Mass Attenuation Coefficient

This coefficient is of more fundamental value than the linear attenuation coefficient since it is independent of the density and physical state (solid, liquid or gas) of the absorber. The mass attentuation coefficient μ_m is given by the relationship

$$\mu_m = \frac{\mu}{\rho}$$

where ρ is absorber density in gm cm^{-3}. The cm^2g^{-1} unit for μ_m is the one commonly used at the present time. As for the case of linear attenuation coefficient, this total mass attenuation coefficient is given by

$$\mu_m = (\mu_m)_{CS} + (\mu_m)_{PE} + (\mu_m)_{PP}$$

1.9 RADIONUCLIDE PRODUCTION

In addition to those nuclear transformations from those long-lived radionuclides that exist naturally, for example, uranium-235 and 238, radium-226 and potassium-40, other transformations or reactions can be induced by bombarding target nuclei with various particles or other nuclei. The practical ways in which radionuclides for use in nuclear medicine may be produced are by neutron or charged particle bombardment, by nuclear fission and from a radionuclide generator. All radionuclides commonly in use in nuclear medicine are produced via one of these processes.

1.9.1 Neutron or Charged Particle Bombardment

There are a number of factors which dictate whether or not a reaction will occur when a target material is bombarded by particles. The number of reactions which can occur in the material in unit time is proportional to the number of both target nuclei and incident particles. A beam of incident particles is defined in terms of the number passing through unit area perpendicular to the beam in unit time. This is known as the particle flux (ϕ) and has the unit $m^{-2}s^{-1}$. However, before any reaction can take place, the incident particle must have an energy greater than the so-called threshold energy for the reaction. If the particle energy is less than this, the reaction cannot occur. Furthermore, the number of reactions which occur will depend upon the cross section for the particular reaction, which is effectively a measure of the probability that a bombarding particle will interact with a target nucleus. This probability for reaction depends not only on the type of target nucleus but also on the type and energy of the incident particle. Cross-section may be regarded as an area of influence or interaction presented to the bombarding particle. The cross-section (σ) for reaction is zero for all energies less than the threshold energy and is measured in barns where

$$1 \text{ barn} = 10^{-28} m^2$$

Radionuclide production by particle bombardment is the most common method of production and the nuclear transformation may be written in the form

target nucleus (bombarding particle, emitted particle) product nuclus.

An example of this nomenclature is the reaction

$$^{16}_{8}O \text{ (n, p) } ^{16}_{7}N$$

which denotes the bombardment of oxygen-16 by neutrons to produce nitrogen-17 with the emission of a proton.

1.9.2 Neutrons

The most efficient method of producing radionuclides by neutron bombardment and capture is through the use of a nuclear reactor. The nuclear reactor produces neutrons with a range of energy from eV (thermal neutrons) to MeV (fast neutrons) and the energy employed depends upon the requirements of the proposed reaction. If the radionuclide is produced by an (n, γ) reaction and is therefore a radioisotope of the target material, this product is not carrier-free. The ratio of radioactive nuclei to stable nuclei and specific activity are relatively low. Radionuclides produced by neutron reactions which are used routinely in nuclear medicine include chromium-51, iron-59, molybdenum-99 and iodine-131.

1.9.3 Charged Particles

Particle accelerators, such as the cyclotron, employ protons (p), deuterons (^2_1H nuclei), helium-3 nuclei (^3_2He) and alpha particles (^4_2He nuclei) in the production of radionuclides for clinical use. These particles must have sufficient kinetic energy, typically in the range of 1–100 MeV, to overcome the electrostatic repulsion of the stable target nuclei. A significant advantage of producing radionuclides by charged particle bombardment is that the product nucleus is almost certain to be of different atomic number to the target material. This usually ensures that high specific activity and radionuclide purity are obtained provided that the target has

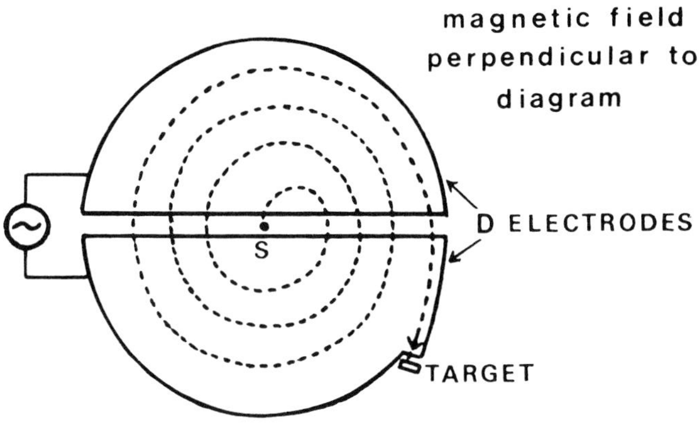

Figure 16. Schematic of cyclotron.

a high nuclidic purity. Radionuclides produced by charged particle interactions are usually neutron deficient and decay by β^+ emission or electron capture. Examples of such radionuclides in current use are the positron emitters carbon-11, nitrogen-13, oxygen-15 and fluorine-18 and the electron capture radionuclides indium-111, iodine-123 and thallium-201. The production reactions for certain of these radionuclides are shown in the Table in Section 1.10.

A schematic of a cyclotron is shown in Figure 16. The device consists of two hollow evacuated metal electrodes, known as D's because of their shape, between which an alternating voltage of several MHz is applied. These electrodes are placed between the poles of a large electromagnet so that the magnetic field is orthogonal to the spiralling path between the surfaces of the electrodes that the particles are constrained to follow. This is achieved by switching the potential to each electrode in turn so that the particle beam is accelerated twice for each orbit. Since the particle velocity increases with each orbit, the beam follows a spiralling orbit rather than a circular one. The particles finally bombard the target which is located at the appropriate position in the beam orbit. The central source of charged particles is usually ions from a simple discharge tube system.

1.9.4 Rate of Production of Radionuclides

An expression may be obtained for the level of radioactivity produced for a given target irradiation time. The production rate will depend on the particle flux ϕ and the cross section σ for the desired reaction. However, the product nuclei are decaying during the irradiation time and this must be taken into account. It may be shown that the radioactivity produced after a time t, R_t, is given by

$$R_t = N\phi\sigma[1 - \exp(-\lambda t)]$$

where N is the number of target nuclei producing the reaction and λ is the decay constant for the product radionuclide. The factor N takes account of the weight of the element in the target, its atomic weight and the fractional abundance of the isotope requried for the reaction. It may be seen that, for very large values of t, R_t approaches a maximum value R_S which is known as the saturation activity. Hence, the above expression may be written in the form

$$R_t = R_S[1 - \exp(-\lambda t)]$$

Figure 17 shows R_t, plotted as a percentage of R_S, as a function of irradiation time t expressed in units of the half-life of the product radionuclide. This plot demonstrates that there is little to be gained by irradiating the target for a time greater than three or four half-lives. Beyond this point, the small increase in radioactivity produced does not justify the continuance of expensive irradiation time.

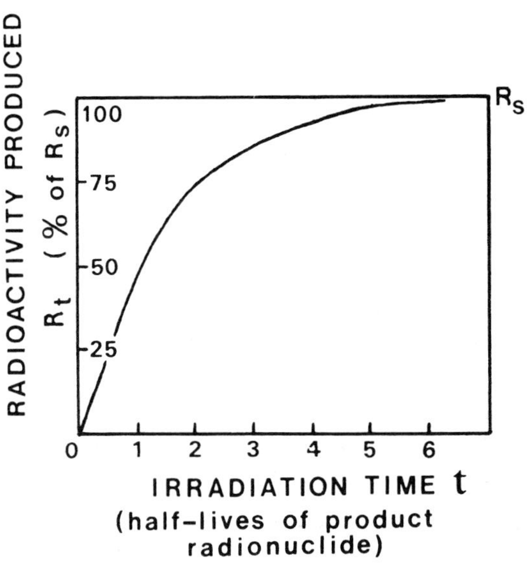

Figure 17. Radionuclide production as a function of target irradiation time.

1.9.5 Target Enrichment

It is important to ensure the presence of as many of the required target nuclei as possible for a specific reaction. This not only permits the production of high specific activities but also reduces the probability of unwanted radiocontaminants being created. Radiocontaminants may be produced from other target isotopes which have similar cross-sections to the nuclide required for the specified reaction. Many elements have a mixture of isotopes and it is often the case that the isotope required has a low natural abundance in the element. This situation could result in the production of far more radiocontaminant than the desired radioisotope. To overcome this problem, it is customary to employ enriched targets in which the abundance of the required target isotope has been artificially increased. However, it should be noted that target enrichment is an expensive process which results in many diagnostic radionuclides having a high cost.

After irradiation, the product radionuclide has to be separated from the target material. The extracted product must be chemically pure, have high radionuclidic purity and be preferably carrier-free. If the product is to be used for administration to patients, a high standard of cleanliness must be maintained throughout the production process to ensure that the final product is sterile and apyrogenic.

1.9.6 Nuclear Fission

The basic features of nuclear fission, which is the division of heavy nuclei into two approximately equal masses, and examples of radionuclides produced by this process have been dealt with earlier (Section 1.4). Only a small number of nuclides are fissionable and the most frequently used reaction is the fission of uranium-235 by neutrons in a nuclear reactor. Since two or three neturons are produced for each fission, it is essential to accurately control the energy release in the reactor in order to avoid a chain reaction. Uranium-235 has less than a 1% abundance in natural uranium compared with uranium-238 and the enrichment of target uranium with the mass number 235 isotope is extremely expensive. However, the incorporation of graphite moderators in reactors to slow down the high energy neutrons emitted by the fission of uranium-235 enhances the probability of fission of this radioisotope whilst reducing the interaction with uranium-238.

1.9.7 Radionuclide Generators

A number of commercially available types of radionuclide generator are in routine use in nuclear medicine. The availability of a generator ensures the ready supply of a suitable short-lived radionuclide which can be chemically separated from a longer-lived parent radionuclide. Metastable radionuclides, which form the basis of a radionuclide generator, have been described in Section 1.4. A more detailed description of the principles of operation and use of radionuclide generator is given in Chapter 2.

1.10 SUMMARY OF PHYSICAL DATA FOR SELECTED RADIONUCLIDES

Table 1 shows physical data for a number of radionuclides which are widely used in nuclear medicine and is not intended to be a comprehensive list. The physical parameters shown are those relevant to the topics covered in this chapter.

Table 1
Relevant Physical Date for Radionuclides Commonly Used in Nuclear Medicine

Radionuclide	*Type of decay*[a]	*Principle emissions (keV)*	*Half-life*	*Half-value thickness (cm)*		*Production process*
				Water	*Lead*	
Gallium-67	EC	γ 93, 185, 300	78.3h	4.7	0.07	Zinc-68 (p, 2n) Gallium-67
Krypton-81 m	IT	γ 190	13s	5.0	0.06	Generator, daughter of Rubidium-81
Technetium-99 m	IT	γ 141	6.02h	4.5	0.03	Generator, daughter of Molybdenum-99
Indium-111	EC	γ 173, 247	67.3h	5.1	0.07	Cadmium-112 (p, 2n) Indium-111
Iodine-123	EC	γ 159	13h	4.6	0.04	Tellurium-124 (p, 2n) Iodine-123
Iodine-131	Beta	β 606 γ 364	8.05d	6.3	0.25	Nuclear Fission
Xenon-133	Beta	β 346 X 30-36 γ 81	5.25d	3.9	0.01	Nuclear Fission
Thallium-201	EC	X 68-82 135, 167	73h	4.3	0.03	Thallium-203 (p, 3n) Lead-201 → Thallium-201

[a]EC – Electron Capture IT – Isomeric Transition

1.11 FURTHER READING

Evans R.D. (1970) *The Atomic Nucleus* 13th edn. New York, Toronto, London: McGraw-Hill Book Company.

Lederer C.M. and Shirley V.S. (Editors) (1978) *Table of Isotopes* 7th edn. New York, Chichester, Brisbane, Toronto: Wiley-Interscience, John Wiley and Sons Inc.

Parker R.P., Smith P.H.S. and Taylor D.M. (1984) *Basic Science of Nuclear Medicine* 2nd edn. Edinburgh, London, Melbourne, New York: Churchill Livingstone.

Amersham (1987) *Nuclear Medicine* England: Amersham International plc.

Chapter 2

Radionuclide Generators

A.T. Elliott

2.1 INTRODUCTION

The first radionuclides used in nuclear medicine had physical half-lives sufficient for transport from the production site to the user hospitals, an example being iodine-131 with a half-life of 8 days. Particularly for those tests where the biological half-life of the radiopharmaceutical is prolonged, these radionuclides gave rise to very high radiation doses to the patient. Materials with short half-lives could only be used close to the production site. The solution to this problem was the development of the radionuclide generator system. Radionuclide generator systems employ a relatively long-lived 'parent' radionuclide which decays to a 'daughter' nuclide, itself radioactive but with a short half-life. For the system to be viable, there must be a method for the easy separation of the daughter from the parent; to facilitate this, the parent should decay by particulate emission so that the daughter is a different element. The usual technique, elution, is to employ a liquid in which the daughter is soluble but the parent is not. Considering the patient radiation dose for diagnostic use, the daughter should decay by isomeric transition (i.e. be a pure gamma emitter) to a stable, non-toxic grand-daughter. The first generator system to have clinical application was the Rn-222/Th-224 system developed by Failla in 1926. This, and several successors, was open to air with associated problems for parenteral administration. The chemical separation techniques developed in Brookhaven National Laboratory led to several generators in the 1950's and 1960's, the most important being the Mo-99/Tc-99m generator (Richards, 1960) which revolutionised the practice of nuclear medicine.

2.2 THEORY OF A GENERATOR SYSTEM

As stated in Chapter 1, the decay of a radionuclide follows the equation

$$A_t = A_O.e^{-\lambda t} \qquad 2.1$$

where A_t is the activity at time t, A_O is the initial activity and λ is the decay constant of the radionuclide. Similarly, the growth of a radionuclide is governed by the equation

$$A_t = A_\infty.(1 - e^{-\lambda t}) \qquad 2.2$$

where A_∞ is the activity which would be present after an infinite time. In the case of a generator system, the decay of the parent is clearly governed by equation 2.1, but the activity of the daughter is subject to a more complex expression than 2.2 since it is decaying as well as being produced. Considering the number of atoms of the parent ($N1_t$) and daughter ($N2_t$) present at time t, the rate of change of N2 with time is given by

$$dN2_t/dt = \lambda_1 N1_t - \lambda_2 N2_t \qquad 2.3$$

where λ_1 and λ_2 are the decay constants of the parent and daughter respectively. The first term on the right-hand side gives the rate of decay of the parent (i.e. the rate of production of daughter atoms), while the second gives the rate of decay of the daughter. By substitution from equation 2.1 into 2.3, it can be shown that

$$N2_t = N2_O.e^{-\lambda_2 t} + (\lambda_1/(\lambda_2 - \lambda_1)).N1_O.(e^{-\lambda_1 t} - e^{-\lambda_2 t}) \qquad 2.4$$

Now, in most circumstances, the start material is a pure sample of the parent radionuclide and so $N2_O = 0$. Thus the first term of 2.4 vanishes to give

$$N2_t = (\lambda_1/(\lambda_2 - \lambda_1)).N1_O.(e^{-\lambda_1 t} - e^{-\lambda_2 t}) \qquad 2.5$$

Now $A = \lambda.N$ and so 2.5 may be rewritten as

$$A2_t = (\lambda_2/(\lambda_2 - \lambda_1)).A1_O.(e^{-\lambda_1 t} - e^{-\lambda_2 t}) \qquad 2.6$$

There are three general cases of parent/daughter pairs to consider, depending on the relative half-lives of the two radionuclides. The first, of no further interest to the present discussion, is when the parent has a shorter half-life than the daughter. In this case, the daughter atoms will eventually decay with their own natural half life as shown in Figure 1.

The second case is when the parent half-life is very much longer than that of the daughter – for example the mercury-195m/gold-195m generator, where the parent Hg-195m has a 67 hour half-life, while the daughter Au-195m has a 30.5 second half life. The constant λ_1 is very small

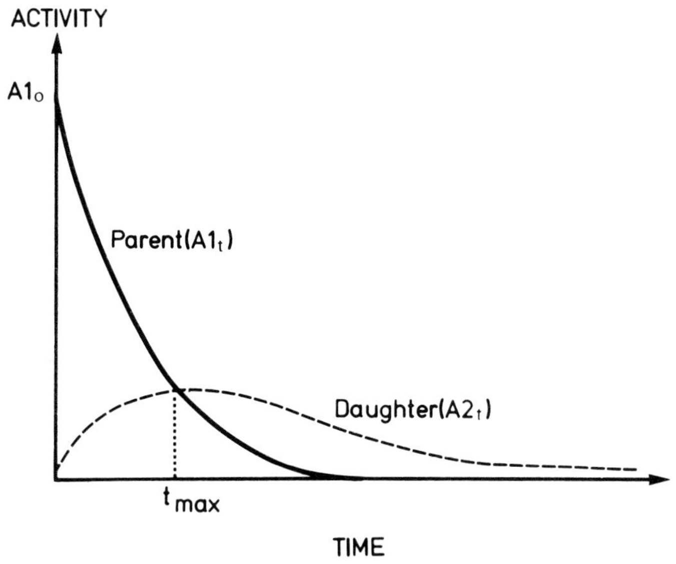

Figure 1. Activity/time curve – type 1 system.

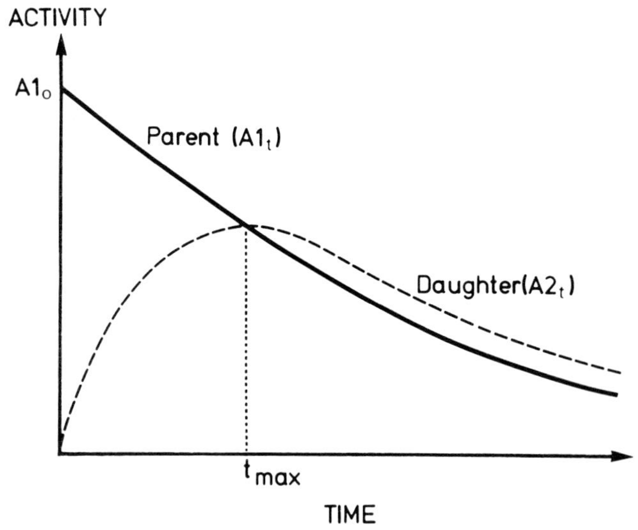

Figure 3. Activity/time curve – type 3 system.

which means that we may assume

$$e^{-\lambda_1 t} \simeq 1 \Rightarrow Al_t \simeq Al_o$$

also $$(\lambda_2/(\lambda_2 - \lambda_1) \simeq 1$$

and so equation 2.6 simplifies to

$$A2_t = A1_o.(1 - e^{-\lambda_2 t})$$

as shown in Figure 2. The limiting decay rate is exactly that of the parent. This situation is termed secular equilibrium.

The third case, in which the parent half life is again longer than that of the daughter, but not sufficiently so to make the simplifications above, is termed transient equilibrium. This is the case with which most readers will be familiar, the best known example being the Mo-99/Tc-99m generator. The corresponding activity-time curves are shown in Figure 3. For the later part of the curve, the second term of equation 2.6 may be neglected, giving

$$A2_t = (\lambda_2/(\lambda_2 - \lambda_1)).A1_o.e^{-\lambda_1 t} \qquad 2.7$$

Now, the decay of the parent follows

$$A1_t = A1_o.e^{-\lambda_1 t} \qquad 2.8$$

and so, by comparison, it can be seen that the decay rate of the daughter is greater than that of the parent by a factor of $(\lambda_2/(\lambda_2 - \lambda_1))$. It can be shown, by setting the derivative of equation 2.6 to zero, that the time at which the daughter decay rate is a maximum is

$$t_{max} = (1/(\lambda_2 - \lambda_1)).\ln(\lambda_2/\lambda_1) \qquad 2.9$$

For the case of the technetium generator, assuming no Tc activity at time zero (i.e. all Tc was cleared from the column at the previous elution), t_{max} is 23 hours.

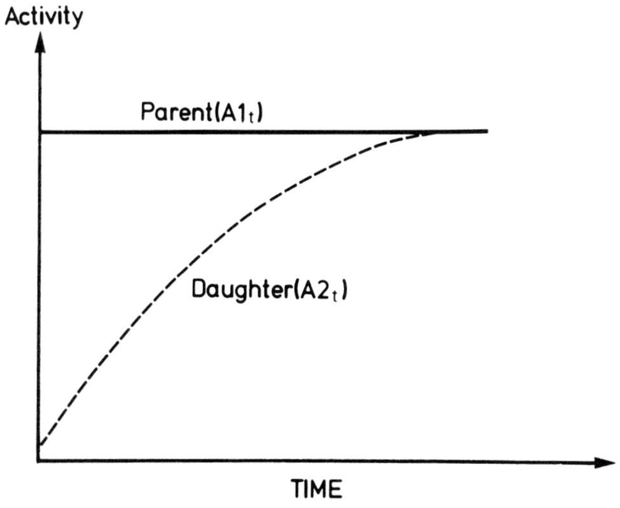

Figure 2. Activity/time curve – type 2 system.

2.3 RADIONUCLIDE SEPARATION TECHNIQUES

Although the ion exchange technique has come to be the most common, there are several methods of separating one isotope from another.

2.3.1 Precipitation

This is the simplest technique, where the parent can be prepared in an aqueous solution and the daughter subsequently precipitated out by addition of a chemical forming an insoluble compound of the daughter. The latter may be separated by filtration or centrifugation. An example is the Cs-137/Ba-137 system, caesium chloride or nitrate being highly soluble. Although the number of barium atoms formed in solution is too small to form a precipitate, the addition of inactive 'carrier' barium in the form of soluble barium sulphate by the subsequent addition of a soluble sulphate.

2.3.2 Distillation

This method is used to separate a volatile daughter from a solution of the parent and is the method used to prepare I-131 commercially from its Te-131 parent. The telluric acid produced by dissolving tellurium in nitric acid is heated gently so that the iodine boils off. The vapour is condensed into water containing a mild reducing agent, becoming entrapped in the form of the non-volatile iodide ion.

2.3.3 Gas evolution

If the parent can be prepared in solution form, with the daughter being a gas, the latter can be separated by bubbling an insoluble carrier gas through the solution. An example in clinical use, the Rb-81/Kr-81m generator, is described in detail below.

2.3.4 Solvent extraction

In this case, the separation utilises two immiscible solvents, the parent being soluble in one while the daughter is soluble in the other. The daughter atoms produced in the parent solution will gradually migrate into the other solvent, but only very slowly. If the mixture is shaken, however, almost all the daughter atoms will be exposed to the second solvent; if the two solvents are then permitted to separate (either naturally or by centrifugation), the daughter activity may be drawn off. An example with which many schoolchildren will become familiar is the protactinium generator used to demonstrate radioactive decay. Protactinium-234 is a member of the decay chain

U-238/Th-234/Pa-234/U-234/Th-230.

Uranyl nitrate can be dissolved in concentrated hydrochloric acid, to which is added pentyl ethanoate (less dense and water-immiscible). Protactinium forms into a complex acid which is soluble in the pentyl ethanoate (thorium is not), so that when the liquids are shaken and allowed to separate, the Pa-234 is extracted into the organic layer.

2.3.5 Sublimation

This was the method used by Perrier and Segre to separate Tc from Mo in 1937 and has been used (Boyd and Robson, 1968) in a large-scale generator system. The parent material is prepared in solid form (usually powder), placed in a temperature-controlled furnace and heated to the appropriate temperature; a carrier gas (oxygen) is blown through the bed and separation achieved because the daughter oxide is volatile at the selected temperature while the parent oxide is not. A terminal filter permits gas containing the daughter activity to pass through but traps any entrained particles of the parent material. In the sublimation Tc generator, oxygen is passed over heated molybdenum trioxide and the resulting technetium heptoxide gas is collected by bubbling through sterile saline. Separation efficiences of 50% can be achieved.

2.3.6 Ion exchange

This technique has come to dominate generator technology because of its convenience (for the user, although not necessarily the manufacturer) and capability of incorporation into closed systems. Although the early materials used were the natural zeolites, most modern exchangers are synthetic. There are both organic and mineral exchange materials, the latter having a superior resistance to radiation damage. The most common mineral exchanger is alumina (Al_2O_3). Most organic exchangers are formed by polymerising styrene; the amount of crosslinking present in the resulting lattice structure is adjusted by the addition of a proportion of divinylbenzene. Exchangeable atoms are then introduced into the lattice at random. To produce a cationic exchanger, free acidic acid groups (such as sulphonic acid) are used to provide replaceable hydrogen atoms while, for an anionic exchanger, quaternary amine groups have replaceable hydroxyl ions. There are approximately 10^{24} exchangeable atoms per kg of exchanger, so that even 1g will exchange up to 10^{21} atoms. The exchanger particles have sizes commonly in the range of 80–160 μm, sometimes referred to as 100–200 mesh. Generators using the ion exchange technique are often termed chromatographic systems, the exchanger material being packed into a glass chromatographic column and held in place by glass frits which permit the passage of liquid.

2.4 GENERATOR SYSTEMS

There are two types of chromatographic radionuclide generator system, positive and negative pressure. In each case, the parent radionuclide is contained within a generator column placed in a lead or (see 2.4.1) depleted uranium shield. The column is usually made of glass and packed with the ion exchange material onto which the parent is adsorbed. Both types of generator are fitted with a terminal 0.22 μm filter to ensure sterility of the eluate; this also traps any particulate material which may escape from the column. The

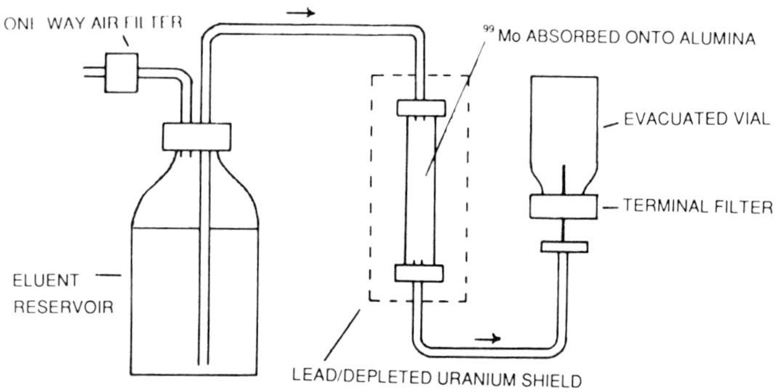

Figure 4. Schematic of negative pressure system.

schematic outline of a standard negative pressure generator system is shown in Figure 4. It is operated by the vacuum initially present in the output (elution) vial, which draws the solvent liquid (eluent) from the reservoir through the generator column. Note that these systems are 'fail safe' in that, if there is any leak in the connecting tubing, air will be drawn in to the elution vial; there is no risk of spillage of radioactive material. Most generators are of the negative pressure design. A positive pressure system is shown in Figure 5. Here, the elution vial is at atmospheric pressure and, instead of an eluent reservoir, a pressurised vial containing the desired volume of eluent is connected to the input side of the generator column; for continuous infusion, the eluent may be pumped through. In this case, if there is any leak in the circuit downstream of the column, radioactive liquid will escape. A plot of the concentration of activity vs volume of eluate is known as an elution profile. This curve has an approximately Gaussian shape, whose peak height decreases and width increases as the volume of exchanger increases. The volume to elute the peak activity and the concentration at the peak are both proportional to the square root of the height of the exchanger bed in the column. For high specific activities, a small volume, low diameter column is to be preferred.

In negative pressure systems, the eluent reservoir can be a glass bottle or collapsible vinyl bag. The latter may introduce trace levels of organic impurities into the eluent, causing a reduction in elution efficiency (Molinski, 1982). Traces of residual glue (cyclohexanone) and disinfectant (propan-1-ol) have been shown to affect elution efficiency (Boyd *et al.*, 1985). It is known that many types of connecting tubing permit the diffusion of air into the lines. The length of tubing in a generator should thus be kept to a minimum. Also in order to reduce the risk of air leaks, the number of joints should be minimised.

Table 1 shows a number of available generator systems. In the following sub-sections, specific examples of generator systems are considered which demonstrate the various factors which have to be considered in generator production and operation.

2.4.1 Mo-99/Tc-99m (molybdenum-technetium system)

This is the most common generator system and many variants are available commercially; schematics of two types

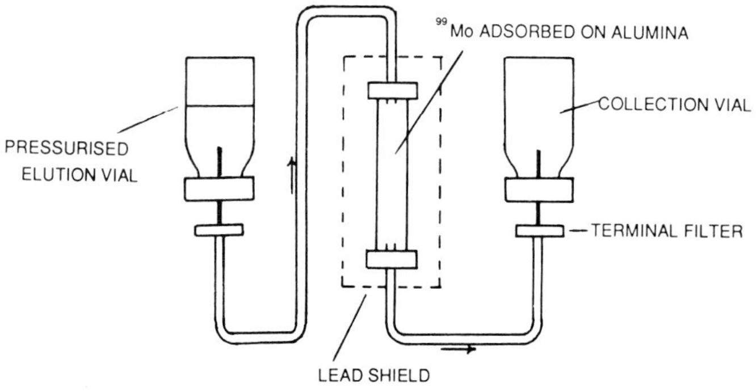

Figure 5. Schematic of positive pressure system.

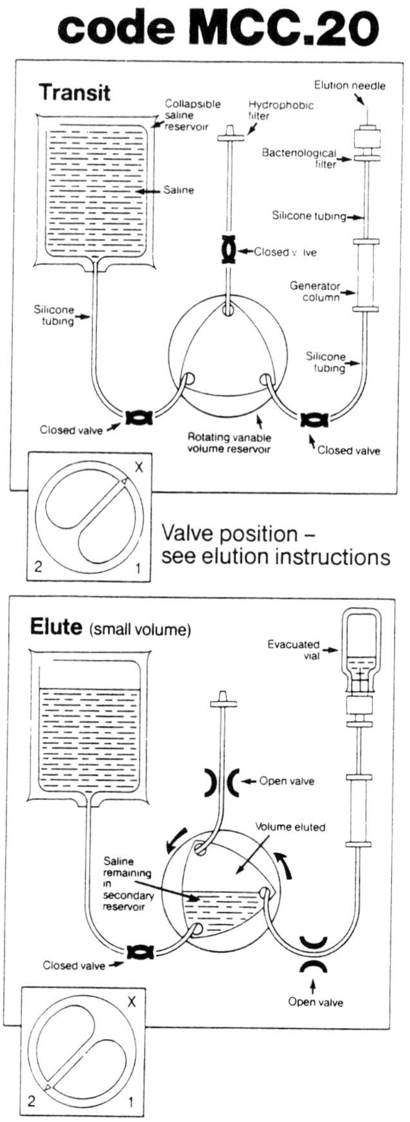

Figure 6. Diagrams of Amersham Tc generator.

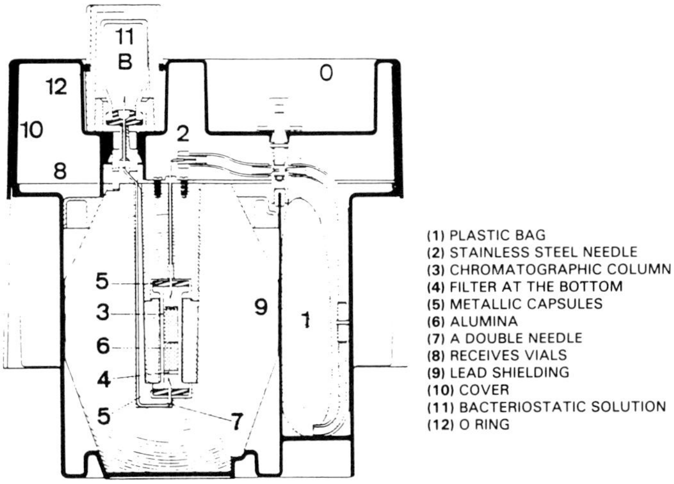

Figure 7. Diagram of CIS (UK) Tc generator.

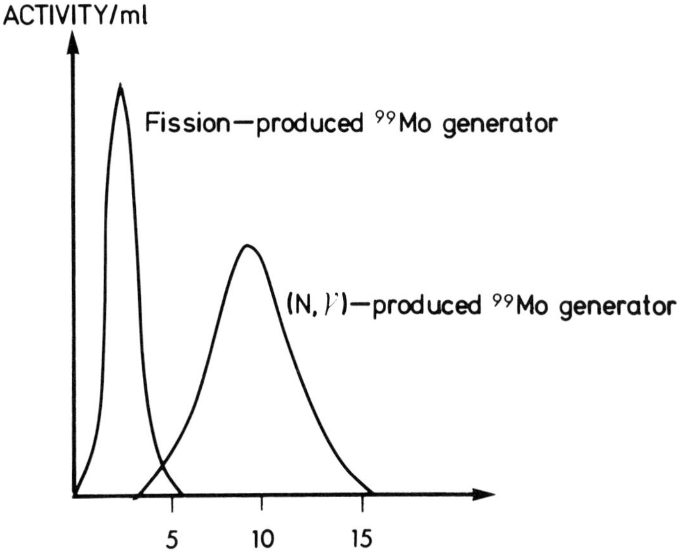

Figure 9. Elution profiles – non-fission and fission columns.

are shown in Figures 6 and 7, with the nuclear data shown in Figure 8. Technetium was first separated from molybdenum by sublimation (Perrier and Segre, 1937) and this process has been used for clinical production of Tc-99m (2.3.5 above). Solvent extraction generators have been used also (Anwar *et al.*, 1968). The molybdenum for early generators was produced by the thermal neutron activation reaction

Mo-98(n, γ)Mo-99

in a reactor or, in a cyclotron, by the charged particle reaction

Mo-100(p, 2p)Nb-99 $\rightarrow$ Mo-99 Mo-100(p, pn)Mo-99

Both methods were expensive due to the requirement for isotopically enriched target materials. The neutron reaction also yielded a product which was not carrier-free; the generator had to be eluted in a relatively large volume (Figure 9). Almost all current generators make use of fission-produced Mo-99. This method requires elaborate processing facilities, together with high-level waste disposal capabilities. The resulting Mo-99 is carrier free and of very high specific activity, allowing the production of high-activity, small-volume columns and permitting elution in a small volume (Figure 9). Even after processing, the column may be contaminated with trace amounts of other fission impurities. Hammermaier *et al.* (1985) found that the most common contaminants present in eluates (other than Mo-99) were I-131 and Ru-103; respective maximum values found were 8 and 7 × 10^{-6}% of the Tc-99m activity. Other contaminants noted were Ba-140 and La-140.

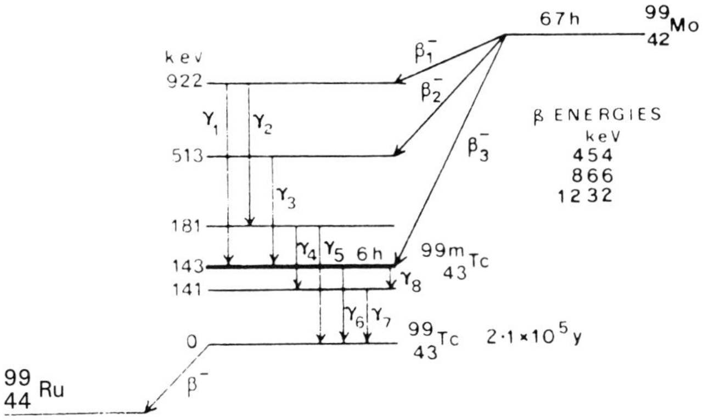

Figure 8. Decay scheme for molybdenum – 99/technetium – 99m.

Table 1
Generator systems

Parent/Daughter	*Half-life* Parent	*Half-life* Daughter	*Gamma emission (keV)*
Mo-99/Tc-99m	67h	6.03h	141
Cd-115/In-115m	53.4h	4.5h	336
Sn-113/In-113m	115.1d	1.66h	392
W-178/Ta-178	21.5d	9.3m	93
Hg-195m/Au-195m	40h	30.6s	262
Rb-81/Kr-81m	4.58h	13.3s	191
Os-191/Ir-191m	15.4d	4.9s	129
Ge-68/Ga-68	287d	68.3m	511, 1080
Fe-52/Mn-52m	8.28h	21m	511, 1434
Zn-62/Cu-62	9.13h	9.7m	511, 1173
Xe-122/I-122	20.1h	3.6m	511, 564
Te-118/Sb-118	6d	3.5m	511, 1230
Sr-82/Rb-82	25d	76s	511, 780
Sr-90/Y-90	28y	64.2h	(beta)
W-188/Re-188	69.4d	16.98h	155 (+beta)
Ra-224/Bi-212	3.6d	60.5m	(alpha)

For generators carrying high Mo-99 loading, over 30GBq, the amount of lead shielding required to reduce the external dose rate to an acceptable level becomes rather cumbersome. Depleted uranium offers a higher atomic number and higher density than lead but, even so, additional external lead shielding may be necessary to further reduce the dose rate. The largest commercially available generators contain 100 GBq of Mo-99 at reference.

Early columns remained full of saline eluent between elutions and the reduction in elution efficiency with time was ascribed to the conversion of Tc VII to a lower oxidation state by the products of radiolysis of water. On this basis, so-called 'dry' column generators (such as that shown in Figure 6) have been developed. In these designs, elution is arranged so that all liquid is removed from the column and so no radiolysis can occur. Boyd *et al.* (1985) have reported that the reduction in elution efficiency can be negated also by the addition of 50 ppm N_2O to the saline or the replacement of the saline by 0.05 M sodium sulphate or 0.15 M sodium perchlorate; these authors postulate that the reduction in elution efficiency is due to the presence of chloride ions. Dry column designs require that the inlet and outlet needles do not penetrate too far into the column, leading to a more stringent specification on components and assembly tolerances.

2.4.2 Sn-113/In-113m (tin-indium system)

The indium-113m system was among the first generators to be developed; it has largely been superseded by the technetium generator but is still in use in areas where routine delivery poses problems. The nuclear scheme is shown in Figure 10. The parent Sn-113 is adsorbed onto a zirconium oxide column and the In-113m eluted with 0.05 N hydrochloric acid. The elution efficiency of this negative pressure generator is 80%, with a parent breakthrough of less than 10^{-4}. Following elution, the column is dried by placing a second evacuated vial on the output needle and drawing air through the system.

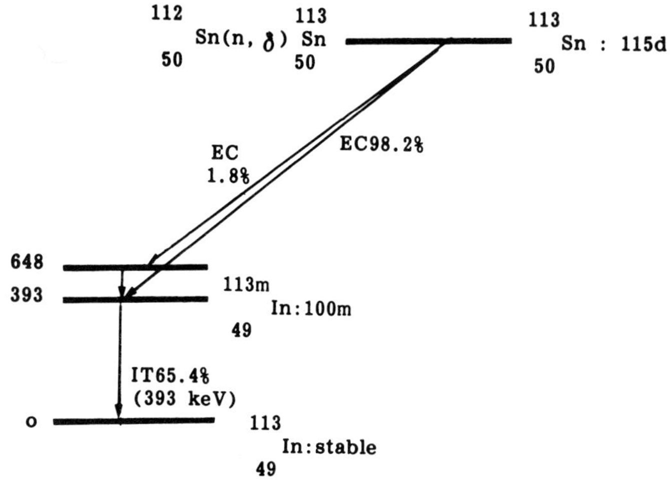

Figure 10. Nuclear data Sn-113/In-113m.

2.4.3 Rb-81/Kr-81m (rubidium-krypton system)

There are two versions of this generator (Clark, Horlock and Watson, 1978), one producing Kr-81m gas for ventilation imaging and the other producing Kr-81m in solution for perfusion studies; both are positive pressure systems. The nuclear scheme is shown in Figure 11. For this and other

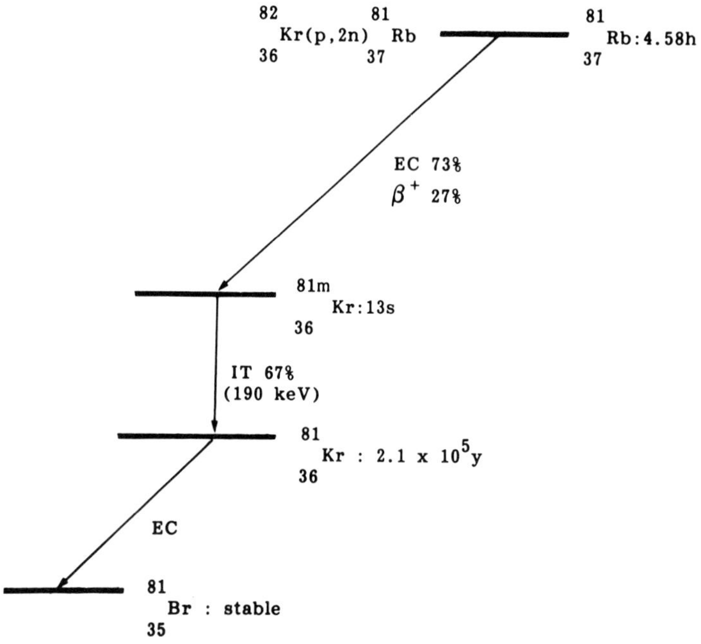

Figure 11. Nuclear data 81/Kr-81m.

ultrashort-lived systems, the half-life does not allow any chemical manipulation of the eluate prior to patient administration. Thus the eluent must be physiologically acceptable (isotonic, neutral pH, non-toxic). Particular care must be taken also in testing parent and exchanger breakthrough (see 2.5) prior to use. The column material for these generators is zirconium phosphate which has a high affinity for rubidium; this permits rapid column loading at high efficiency. For perfusion studies, elution may be carried out with sterile water, but the eluate has to be mixed subsequently with an equal flow of 1.8% saline to render it isotonic. Alternatively, isotonic dextrose may be used as the eluent, but this gives rise to an increased level of Rb-81 breakthrough, necessitating the introduction of a small resin trap column downstream of the generator. If the generator is to be used for ventilation studies, it is eluted using air. Prior to passage through the column, it is essential to ensure saturation of the eluting gas flow or the column will dry out and no Kr-81m will be eluted. Care must be taken to adjust the amount of water in the saturator and the eluting gas flow rate to avoid the deposition of droplets in the delivery tubing. The elution efficiency is in the range 70–80%.

2.4.4 Hg-195m/Au-195m (mercury-gold system)

This generator, whose nuclear data are shown in Figure 12, is one of several which have been developed in recent years to produce ultra-short-lived radionuclides, particularly for use in nuclear cardiology. Others are Os-191/Ir-191 (Treves *et al.*, 1976; Packard *et al.*, 1987), W-178/Ta-178 (Neirinckx *et al.*, 1978; Lacy *et al.*, 1991) described below and the Rb-81/Kr-81m generator described above. The parent material is prepared on a cyclotron using 34 MeV protons, the reaction being

Au-197(p, 3n)Hg-195m

The best column materials have been found to be thiopropyl sepharose-6B and controlled pore glass lipoamide; both are pre-washed with EDTA/sodium acetate solution to chelate any heavy ions. A typical column loading is 4–5 GBq of Hg-195m. The eluent is 2.5 mM sodium cyanide in one design (Elliott *et al.*, 1983), which yields the activity in a volume of approximately 0.5 ml; the chemical form in the eluate is though to be $(Au(CN)_4)^{n-}$. The concentration of cyanide is such that the blood levels do not rise above the normal ranges for non-smokers. This design can be operated in positive pressure mode also for infusion studies. A second design uses 29.8 mg sodium thiosulphate pentahydrate per ml (Panek *et al.*, 1984), with an elution volume of 2 ml and a higher level of parent breakthrough; this latter factor is of crucial importance since the major portion of the radiation dose to the patient is due to the parent radionuclide. Elution efficiencies achieved in practice are in the range 30–45% for both designs. With these generators, the elution protocol is of critical importance since the quantities of Hg-195m and Au-195 in solution increase with time between elutions. In operation, therefore, several elutions at 2-minute intervals must be discarded prior to the elution to be administered to a patient in order to minimise the radiation dose to the patient.

2.4.5 W-178/Ta-178 (tungsten-tantalum system)

The nuclear data for this generator are shown in Figure 13. In its most recent form (Lacy *et al.*, 1991), it is an automated system, the eluate being delivered into a syringe ready for patient administration. The eluent contains 0.03N HCl with 0.1% H_2O_2, the buffer solution being 0.13N Na_2HPO_4. The eluent is passed through the column, and the buffer added automatically to the eluate by a dual-channel peristaltic pump. The activity in a patient dose ranges from 550–3700 MBq, with a breakthrough level of some 0.005%.

2.4.6 Ge-68/Ga-68 (germanium-gallium system)

This is the most widely-used positron generator system and is available commercially; the nuclear data are shown in Figure 14. Others include Zn-62/Cu-62 (Zweit *et al.*, 1992)

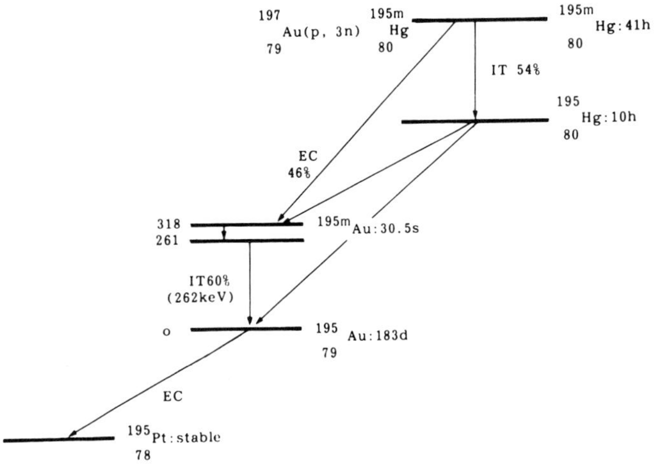

Figure 12. Nuclear data Hg-195m/Au-195m.

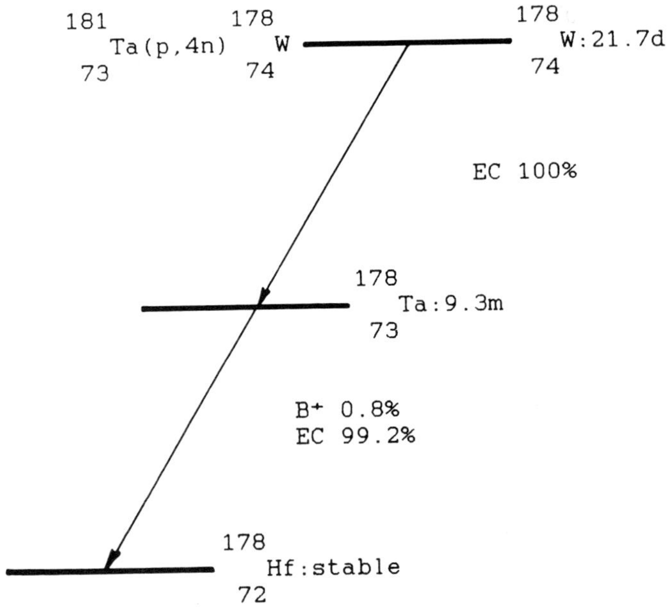

Figure 13. Nuclear data W-178/Ta-178.

and the Sr-82/Rb-82 generator described below. Early systems produced the gallium-68 in a complexed form, requiring an extra step prior to incorporation into radiopharmaceuticals. Loc'h *et al.*, (1980) described a generator which produces ionic gallium. The column material is tin dioxide, the eluent being 1N HCl; the latter concentration was found to give optimum gallium yield (75–80%) with only 0.0002% germanium breakthrough. The level of tin contamination of the eluate is 0.5 μg/ml, which is negligible in comparison to the amount in many radiopharmaceutical preparations. Interestingly, the simplest method of assaying the tin content is by neutron activation analysis of the eluate. The authors found that the generator could be used for up to a year with no reduction in yield.

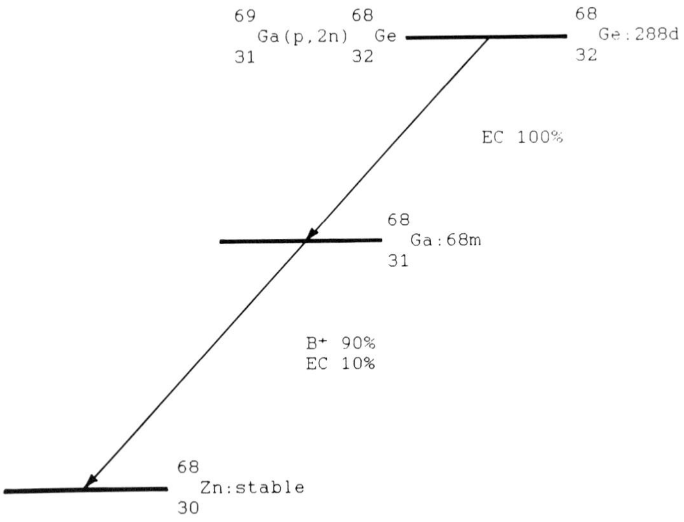

Figure 14. Nuclear data Ge-68/Ga-68.

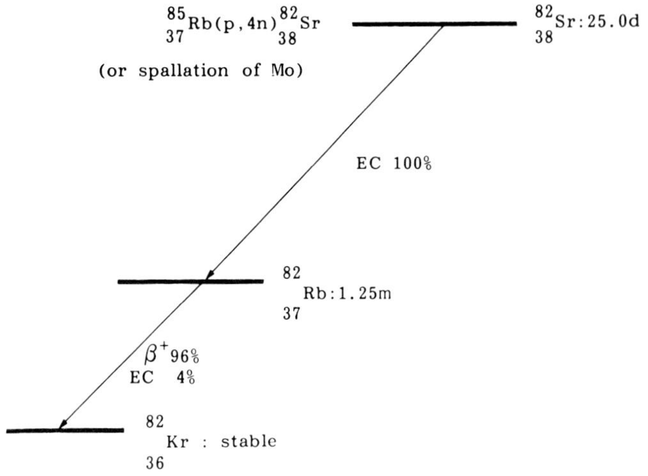

Figure 15. Nuclear data Sr-82/Rb-82.

2.4.7 Sr-82/Rb-82 (strontium-rubidium system)

This is another positron generator, used primarily for cardiac studies. Its scheme is shown in Figure 15. The first generator (Yano and Anger, 1968) used ammonium acetate as the eluent; a more recent microprocessor-controlled design (Yano *et al.*, 1981) employs an alumina column and 2% saline as eluent. The column is loaded with up to 7.5 GBq of Sr-82, which may be contaminated with up to 22 GBq of Sr-85, and eluted until the Sr-82/Sr-85 breakthrough level falls below 1 ppm. The generator has a 3–4 month lifespan and so requires periodic checking of sterility, apyrogenicity and breakthrough levels; should the latter rise above 4 kBq per elution, a small alumina trapping column is placed in series with the active column. The elution efficiency is 85–95%. The generator can be operated in either bolus (27 ml) or constant-infusion modes; in the latter case, the yield is dependent on flow rate, rising to a plateau value within 6 minutes. It is a positive-pressure system, the computer driving the saline through the column via a stepper-motor driving an autoclavable 150 ml pumping system; the operating pressure is 50–100 psi.

2.4.8 Ra-224/Pb-212/Bi-212 (radium-lead-bismuth system)

This is an example of a more complex system, showing that a generator need not be limited to a single stage. Bismuth-212 is an alpha emitter which has been proposed for radiolabelling monoclonal antibodies for therapeutic use. The first generator to produce Bi-212 was developed by Zucchini and Friedman (1982), based on Th-228; a more recent design is described (Gansow *et al.*, 1984), the nuclear data being shown in Figure 16. The Ra-224 parent is dissolved in dilute HCl and loaded onto the primary cation exchange column; this is eluted with distilled water into a 2 ml reservoir to introduce a time-delay to permit the Rn-220 and Po-216 to decay to Pb-212, which is then absorbed onto the secondary column. The secondary column is then eluted with 2M HCl to yield a solution of Bi-212. The breakthrough level of Ra-224 is below the detection limit, while the elution efficiency is approximately 30%.

2.5 ROUTINE QUALITY CONTROL

For reasons of sterility, the Guide to Good Pharmaceutical Manufacturing Practice (GGPMP) suggests that a generator should be stored within a Class I environment. This may be

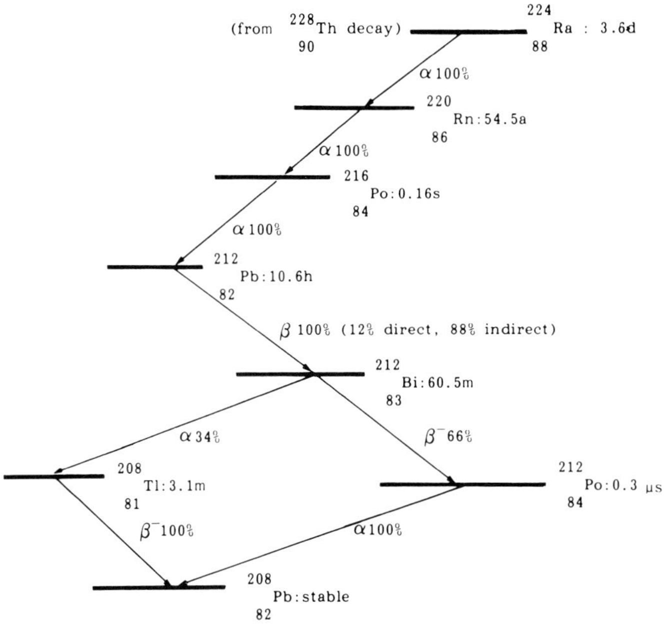

Figure 16. Nuclear data Ra-224/Pb-212/Bi-212.

achieved by a laminar flow cabinet or the new containment cabinets. The manufacturer's instructions as to the frequency of changing the elution needle, needle shield etc must be strictly adhered to. A generator should be eluted on delivery. The daughter activity should be assayed and checked against the expected value and, if possible, a check made that the elution vial contains the expected volume. If these tests are satisfactory, the eluate should be checked for breakthrough of parent radionuclide or column material. For an ultra-short lived generator, the amount of parent breakthrough may be assayed directly by measuring the activity of the eluate immediately after elution and again after some 10 half-lives. By comparing the latter reading against that calculated by decaying the first reading to the time of the second, the amount of parent activity present may be determined. For generators in the transient equilibrium category, it is necessary to utilise some form of spectral analysis to separate the parent and daughter activities. This will usually require the use of a semiconductor detector to obtain the necessary energy resolution. For the technetium generator, where the energy of the gamma emission from Mo-99 is much greater than that from Tc-99m (739 keV vs 141 keV), use can be made of a lead shield whose thickness is chosen to attenuate the Tc-99m emission. The activity contained in the unshielded elution vial is measured in a re-entrant ionisation chamber; the vial is then placed in the special lead shield and re-assayed. The Mo-99 level must be less than 0.1% of the Tc-99m activity at the time of administration. Chemical tests are required to test for breakthrough of column materials; for convenience, an indicator strip method is available for the Tc generator (and others using an alumina exchanger). A standard aluminium solution (10 μg/ml Al^{-3} ion) is supplied, a drop of which is spotted on to the strip, where it reacts to form a red spot. A similar-sized drop of eluate is then tested adjacent to the standard; if the size and intensity of the red spot (if any) caused by the eluate are less than that of the standard, the eluate contains less than 10 μg/ml of aluminium, the permitted level. The detection limit of the test is approximately 10^{-9}g of aluminium ion.

The sterility and apyrogenicity of a generator will be guaranteed initially by the manufacturer. The column and all components will have been autoclaved or gamma sterilised prior to assembly. It is good practice, nevertheless, to submit at least one elution vial to sterility and pyrogen testing (for fuller account see Chapter 9).

2.6 PROBLEMS

This section applies particularly to the negative-pressure Mo-99/Tc-99m system, but the principles apply to other generators. There are several problems which may affect a generator in operation, some of which are amenable to user attempts at correction. The extent of such attempts will be determined by the number and type of patient investigations which would be affected by the generator failure, by the radiation dose levels associated with each corrective procedure and by the level of experience of the staff concerned. Under no circumstances should the column itself be accessed or exposed.

If, on completion of the elution period of a negative-pressure generator, the vial is found to be empty, the first action should be to re-elute with a fresh vial (from a different batch if available). Loss of vacuum from (or non-evacuation of) the vial is the most probable cause of this fault. Should the second elution yield the same result, the seating of the elution needle should be checked. Particularly if the fault occurs on first elution, the integrity of the terminal filter (which may crack if mishandled in transit) and of accessible connections should be checked; this will be possible only if the outer casing can be removed easily and safely.

For a dry column generator, the presence of liquid in the column will reduce the elution efficiency due to radiolysis; this may happen if, for example, an elution vial is removed before the elution is complete. At the next elution, an increased volume will be eluted but the amount of activity present will be less than expected. A possible solution, in a system with a secondary reservoir, is to draw as large a quantity of air through the column as possible to dry it out. The elution efficiency may then recover, albeit not completely.

If the correct colume of eluate is present but the activity is much lower than expected, the reason is almost certainly a phenomenon known as 'channelling'. In this case, the column material bed has been disturbed and a channel has been created allowing liquid to pass through without permeating the column material. There are two possible courses of action, the first being to drop the generator from a height of 150–300 mm on to a hard surface in an effort to compact the column material. The second method is to carry out several maximum-volume elutions in rapid succession, when the flow of liquid may carry particles of column material into the channel to block it.

A generator yielding both low volume and activity may have developed a number of problems. The first action is to re-elute, leaving the elution vial in place for, say, 10–15 minutes. Should this vial contain the correct volume and (roughly) the correct activity, it may be possible to continue to use the generator, although Mo-99 and aluminium breakthrough should be checked carefully on each elution. If not, and the outer casing can be removed easily and safely, a check should be made that there are no airlocks in the connecting tubing. If still no fault can be identified, the most likely cause is the partial blockage of one of the column connections; no further user action should be attempted.

2.7 CONCLUSION

Although the Mo-99/Tc-99m generator continues to dominate nuclear medicine, the impetus for change brought about by the introduction of PET, computerised axial tomography (CT) and nuclear magnetic resonance imaging (NMR or MRI) systems will ensure continued development of new radiopharmaceuticals. New generator systems will play a major role in this development.

REFERENCES

Anwar M., Lathrop K., Ross-Kelly D. and Harper P.V. (1969). J. Nucl. Med., **9**, 298.

Boyd G.E. and Robson J. (1968). *The production of technetium-99m. In* Radioisotope Production, **117**, IAEA, Vienna.

Boyd R.E., Hetherington E.L.R. and Moore P.W. (1985) *Radionuclide generator technology. In* Radiopharmaceuticals and labelled compounds 1984. pp. 79–94, IAEA, Vienna.

Clark J.C., Horlock P.L. and Watson I.A. (1978). *Krypton-81m generators for ventilation and perfusion. In* Clinical and experimental applications of krypton-81m, Special Report No. 15, British Institute of Radiology, London, 1978.

Elliott A.T., Dymond D.S., Stone D.L., Flatman W., Bett R., Cuninghame J.G., Sims H.E. and Willis H.H. (1983). *A Hg-195m/Au-195m generator for first-pass nuclear angiocardiography*, Phys. Med. Biol., **28**, 139–150.

Failla G. (1926). *The development of filtered radon implants*, Am. J. Roentgenol., **16**, 507.

Gansow O.A., Atcher R.W., Link D.C., Friedman A.M., Seevers R.H., Anderson W., Scheinberg D.A. and Strans M. (1984). *Generator-produced Bi-212 chelated to chemically modified monoclonal antibody for use in radiotherapy. In* Radionuclide generators, pp. 215–227, American Chemical Society, Washington.

Hammermaier A., Reich E., Endrulat H.J. and Bogl W. (1985). *Investigations on the quality of eluates from seven fission Mo-99/Tc-99cm generators*, ISH Report 64, Institute for Radiation Hygiene of the Federal Health Office, Neuherberg.

HMSO (1983) *Guide to Good Pharmaceutical Manufacturing Practice 1983*, HMSO, London.

Lacy J.L., Layne W.W., Guidry G.W., Verani M.S. and Roberts R. (1991). *Development and clinical performance of an automated portable tungsten-178/tantalum-178 generator*, J. Nucl. Med., **32**, 2158–2161.

Loc'h C., Maziere B. and Comar D. (1980). *A new generator for ionic gallium-68*, J. Nucl. Med., **21**, 171–173.

Molinski V.J. (1982). Int. J. Appl. Radiat. Isotopes, **33**, 811.

Neirinckx R.D., Jones A.G., Davis M.A., Harris G.I., Holman B.L. (1978). *Tantalum-178 – a short lived nuclide for nuclear medicine: development of a potential generator system*, J. Nucl. Med., **19**, 514–519.

Packard A.B., Treves S.T., O'Brien G.M. and Lim K.S. (1987). *An osmium-191/iridium-191m radionculide generator using an oxalo osmate parent complex*, J. Nucl. Med., **28**, 1571–1576.

Panek K.J., Lindeyer J. and van der Vlugt H.C. (1984). *A new generator for production of short-lived Au-195m radioisotope. In* Radionuclide generators, 3–21, American Chemical Society, Washington.

Perrier C. and Segre E. (1937). *Chemical properties of element 43*, J. Chem. Phys., **5**, 712.

Richards P. (1960). V Congresso Nucleare, **2**, 225–244.

Treves S., Kulprathipanja S. and Hnatowich D.J. (1976). *Angiocardiography with iridium-191m. An ultrashort-lived radionculide (t – 4.9 sec)*, Circulation, **54**, 275–279.

Yano Y. and Anger H.O. (1968). *Visualisation of the heart and kidneys in animals with ultrashort-lived Rb-82 and the positron scintillation camera*, J. Nucl. Med., **9**, 412–415.

Yano Y., Cahoon J.L. and Budinger T.F. (1981). *A precision flow-controlled Rb-82 generator for bolus or constant-infusion studies of the heart and brain*, J. Nucl. Med., **22**, 1006–1010, 1981.

Zucchini G.L. and Friedman A.M. (1982). *Isotopic generator for Pb-212 and Bi-212*, Int. J. Nucl. Med. Biol., **9**, 83.

Zweit J., Goodall R., Cox M., Babich J.W., Potter G.A., Sharma H.L. and Ott R.J. (1992). *Development of a high performance zinc-62/copper-62 radionuclide generator for positron emission tomography*, Eur. J. Nucl. Med., **19**, 418–425.

Chapter 3

Physico-Chemical Concepts in the Preparation of Technetium Radiopharmaceuticals

D. P. Nowotnik

3.1 INTRODUCTION

Commercially-available non-radioactive ('cold') kits are used to transform pertechnetate from the $^{99}Mo/^{99m}Tc$ generator (as described in the last chapter) to a desired radiopharmaceutical. These kits are aseptic, lyophilised formulations held in sealed glass vials. By virtue of extensive development and testing by the manufacturer, they permit radiopharmacists to conduct a series of chemical modifications of technetium within the hospital environment, reliably and in high yield. Complex chemical reactions can often be achieved simply by the addition of generator eluate to the vial, shaking to dissolve vial contents, followed by a short room temperature incubation period.

The simplicity in use of these kits disguises the complexity of the chemistry of technetium. It is the purpose of this chapter to describe some of the processes which occur during the formation of technetium radiopharmaceuticals, and provide an insight into the wide range of technical considerations which are necessary in the development and use of 'cold' kits.

3.2 CHEMISTRY OF TECHNETIUM

3.2.1 Introduction

As element 43 in the periodic table, technetium is placed in group VIIIA, in the second row of the transition metals. As is the case with all transition elements, the chemistry of technetium is dominated by the formation of metal-donor complexes; compounds formed by bonding between the electron-deficient metal and atoms or functional groups which are capable of donating electron pairs. Examples of typical donor groups for technetium complex formation are amine, amide, thiol, phosphine, oxime, and isonitrile. With only minor exceptions, all technetium radiopharmaceuticals are metal-donor complexes.

Compounds which form complexes with metals (termed ligands) may have only one donor group (a monodentate ligand), or two (bidentate) or more (polydentate) donor groups. When two or more donor groups from a single compound bind to one metal center, the term 'chelating agent' is applied to the ligand, and 'chelate' to the metal complex. Examples of technetium complexes from mono-, bi-, and tetradentate ligands are shown in Figure 1; the monodentate t-butyl-isonitrile (TBI) ligand (Abrams *et al.*, 1983) and cyclam (Zuckman *et al.*, 1981) each form a single technetium complex. The bidentate ligand, DMPE can form several complexes (Deutsch *et al.*, 1983). Three DMPE complexes are shown in Figure 1; the primary difference between these complexes is the oxidation state of the metal, which is the topic for the next section.

3.2.2 Oxidation States

The oxidation state (number) of an atom within a molecule is usually considered to be the formal charge on the atom if, hypothetically, all of the molecule is composed of ions. A feature of the transition metals is that each may have multiple oxidation states. For technetium, as a member of this group, all oxidation numbers from 0 to +7 have been reported (Deutsch *et al.*, 1983), and a possible oxidation state of −1 was also suggested (Huggins & Kaesz, 1964). The $^{99}Mo/^{99m}Tc$ generator provides technetium in its highest oxidation state, +7. While complexes of technetium in this oxidation state are known, the oxidation states which dominate the chemistry of technetium are +1, +3, and +5 (Deutsch *et al.*, 1983). Lowering of oxidation state is a prerequisite of complex formation and in 'cold' kits, the

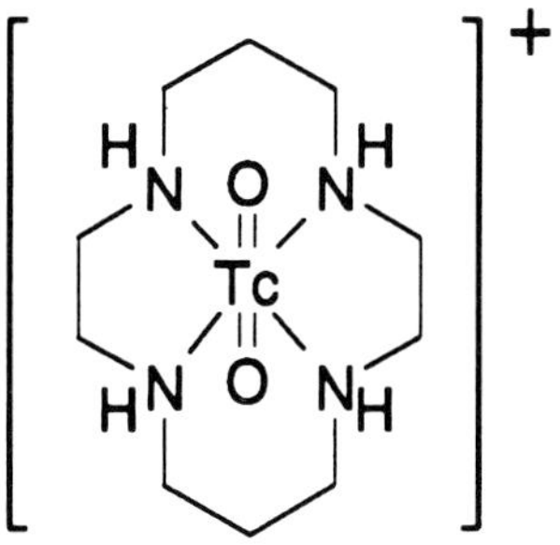

$Tc(V)O_2$(cyclam)

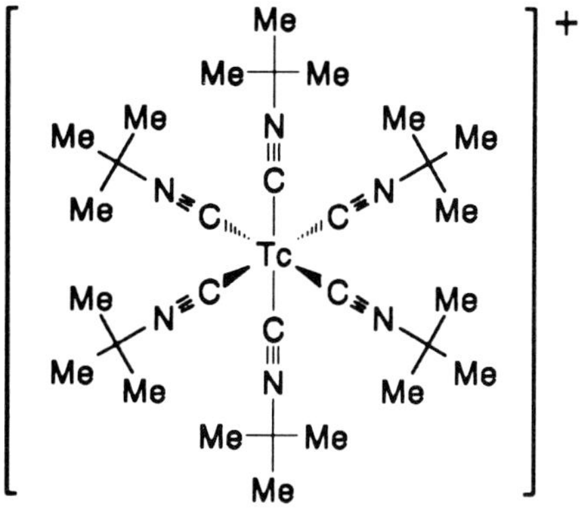

Tc(I)TBI

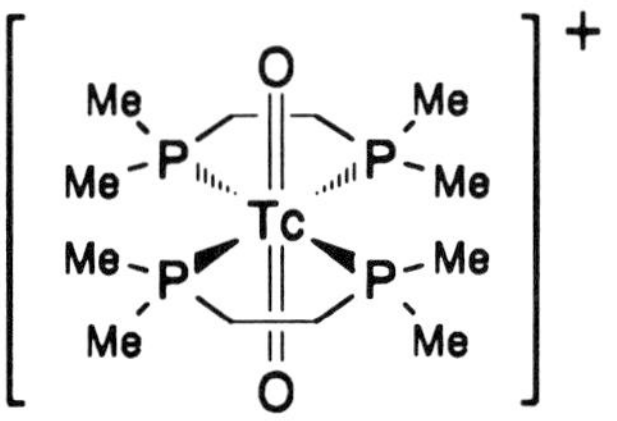

$Tc(V)O_2(DMPE)_2$

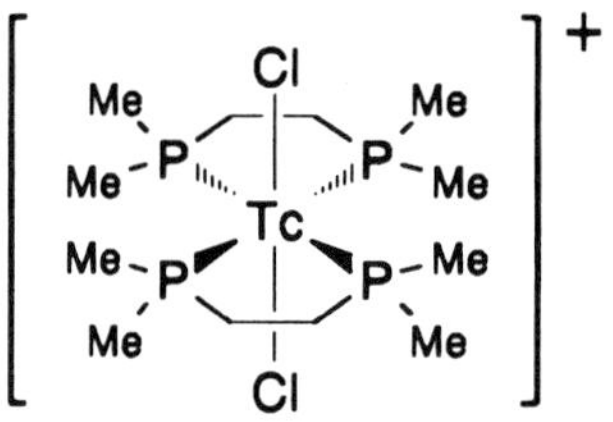

$Tc(III)Cl_2(DMPE)_2$

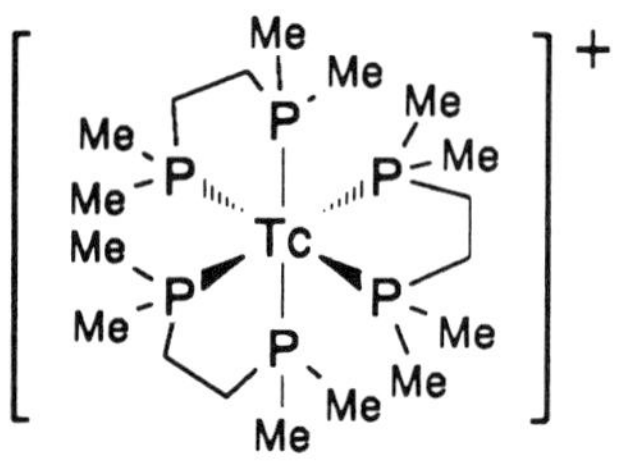

$Tc(I)(DMPE)_3$

Figure 1. The structures of technetium complexes of cyclam DMPE, and t-butylisonitrile.

oxidation state of technetium is lowered from + 7 by means of a chemical reductant (usually a stannous salt) incorporated in the formulation. In certain cases, excess ligand can also be the reductant.

Several factors will influence the resultant oxidation state of technetium following reduction of pertechnetate and complexation, including the nature of reductant and ligand, pH, and temperature. For example, reduction of TcO_4- with stannous ion in the presence of the tetradentate cyclam ligand provides a Tc(V) complex (Troutner *et al.*, 1980), while the same reductant with an alkyl isonitrile produces (with heating) a Tc(I) complex (Abrams *et al.*, 1983). The bidentate phosphine ligand, DMPE, provides a Tc(V) complex from TcO_4- at low pH/room temperature, a Tc(III) complex at low pH and an elevated temperature, and a Tc(I) complex at high pH/elevated temperatures (Vanderheyden *et al.*, 1984). The commercially-available renal imaging kit based on the ligand DMSA is formulated at a slightly acidic pH level; when the pH of complex formation is raised, a complex is formed with much reduced renal affinity, but with demonstrable soft tumor uptake (Yokoyama *et al.*, 1985; Ohta *et al.*, 1988).

The single most important factor influencing the oxidation state of technetium is the nature of the ligand atoms coordinated to this metal. Traditionally, ligands have been classified according to 'hardness' (Huheey, 1972). Hard ligands tend to be small atoms or groups, which retain the negative charge associated with them, while soft ligands are larger atoms or groups which are capable of sharing their negative charge or electron lone pairs.

The Tc(V) oxidation state is dominated by complexes which have either one or two oxygen atoms directly bonded to technetium, with four or five coordination sites available for binding to other ligands (Davison, 1983). These vacant sites can form complexes with selected members from both the hard and soft groups of ligands; as a rule of thumb, complexes with a dioxo core are preferred with hard ligands, while the monoxo core is more usually obtained with softer ligands.

Low oxidation state complexes of technetium (+ 1 and + 3) tend to be stabilised by the inclusion of pi-acceptor ligands in the coordination sphere, in common with other low oxidation state transition metals (Huheey, 1972). Examples of such ligands are phosphine, isonitrile, arenes, and nitrosyl.

The coordination chemistry of technetium is complicated by the ease with which it can move from one oxidation state to another (Deutsch *et al.*, 1983). Given any new ligand and/or new set of reduction/coordination conditions, it is often difficult to predict which oxidation state(s) of technetium will result.

3.2.3 Coordination Number and Geometry

A further complication which has an influence on the nature of complex formed is the coordination number (number of ligating atoms bound to technetium), and the geometry of those donor groups around the metal. Coordination numbers from 4 to 9 are recorded for technetium (Deutsch *et al.*, 1983), with several coordination numbers and/or geometries known within each oxidation state.

In the +5 state, the oxidation number most commonly encountered in technetium radiopharmaceuticals, coordination numbers range between five and seven. Usually one or two of those sites are bound to an oxygen atom (Davison, 1983; Steigman and Eckelman, 1992). By comparison, and with few exceptions, the +3 and +1 oxidation states tend to have coordination numbers of six, with ligands placed in an octahedral arrangement. Figure 1 shows technetium in the +5 oxidation state with two bonded oxygen atoms in the cyclam and DMPE chelates, and the octahedral +1 and +3 complexes of t-butylisonitrile and DMPE.

3.2.4 Complex Stability

The stability of complexes can be considered in one of two ways; thermodynamic or kinetic. The former is the equilibrium between free and complexed metal ion in a solution containing at least a molar equivalent of the ligand. An equilibrium constant, K, provides a measure of thermodynamic stability (Perrin, 1964). The rate at which complexes decompose is a measure of their kinetic stability. There is no direct relationship between these two parameters; it is not unusual for thermodynamically stable complexes to be kinetically labile, or for unstable complexes to decompose only very slowly (Perrin, 1964). Complex decomposition rate will be dependent upon the environment; stability (or lack of it) *in vivo* may not automatically be inferred from *in vitro* data.

Technetium complex stability can influence radiopharmaceutical performance in a number of ways. Instability *in vivo* could result in the transfer of metal from the administered ligand to some other site. This effect, termed ligand exchange, is one hypothesis for the renal retention of ^{99m}Tc complexes of gluconic and glucoheptonic acids.

For most radiopharmaceuticals, it is essential that no dissociation occurs *in vivo* for the period during which image acquisition is required. Increased background activity is a usual consequence of such dissociation. This is a particular issue in recent developments in ^{99m}Tc-labelling of monoclonal antibodies, when imaging several hours after radiopharmaceutical administration may be required (Fritzberg *et al.*, 1988).

In vitro complex stability will influence post-reconstitution shelf life. As will be described later, certain deficiencies in complex stability can be overcome through additives in cold kit formulation. With thermodynamically unstable complexes, such as gluconate and methylene diphosphonate, high (>100 mg) ligand concentrations are used in kit formulations to produce acceptable yields of these ^{99m}Tc complexes following kit reconstitution.

3.2.5 Metabolism

In the development of new radiopharmaceuticals, it has become increasingly important to gain some understanding of the *in vivo* biochemistry of the complex. The gamma camera cannot discriminate between the various chemical forms *in vivo*, and thus the image produced is generated by all of chemical forms of technetium in the field of view. The biolocalisation properties of the distinct chemical forms will be different, so that it will be necessary to have some understanding of the contribution of each form in order to achieve reliable image interpretation.

Instability of the chelate (as described in the previous section) is only one source of *in vivo* modification. Another is the case where the chelate remains intact, but peripheral groups on the ligand are chemically altered. Some examples are known (as described in section 3.4), but understanding metabolism will be a vital consideration in the coming generation of radiopharmaceuticals being developed as biochemical probes (Eckelman, 1991). Two recent examples of areas where new technetium complexes are being evaluated as 'biochemical probes' include receptor density imaging (Lever and Wagner, 1990) and the identification of tissue at risk from hypoxia (Di Rocco *et al.*, 1992a; Linder *et al.*, 1992).

3.2.6 Isomerism

While it has been known for many years that there can be striking differences in the pharmacological effect observed between two (or more) stereochemical forms of a drug, only recently have examples been found in the biodistribution of technetium complexes. Later in this chapter, descriptions of individual radiopharmaceuticals will include sections on some of the implications of stereochemistry specific to each compound. There are several other examples, which have been reviewed elsewhere (Volkert, 1990; Nowotnik and Jurisson, 1992).

3.3 TECHNETIUM COLD KIT COMPONENTS

While the ligand is the most important constituent of technetium cold kits, several other components may be present to ensure that the desired complex is consistently prepared in high yield. The kit must be dependable over a wide range of reconstitution conditions, and a vast amount of work is expended during kit development by the manufacturer to achieve a reliable formulation. The nature and purpose of these kit components are described in the following sections:

3.3.1 Reductant

A wide range of reductants are known to lower the oxidation state of pertechnetate. The list includes sodium borohydride (Smith, J.E. *et al.*, 1978; Deutsch *et al.*, 1980; Kung *et al.*, 1984), sodium dithionite, sodium bisulphite, formamidine sulphinic acid, and hydrazine (Fritzberg *et al.*, 1977; Jones *et al.*, 1980), hydrochloric acid (Eckelman *et al.*, 1972), tin foil (Ruddock, 1979; Grogg *et al.*, 1985), zinc metal (Kremer *et al.*, 1989) ferric ion and ascorbic acid (Stern *et al.*, 1965), and antimony (III) (Vilcek *et al.*, 1982), molybdenum (III) (Vilcek *et al.*, 1984) and tungsten (III) salts (Vilcek *et al.*, 1985). Electrolytic methods have also been employed to reduce technetium oxidation state (Steigman *et al.*, 1974; Russell and Speiser, 1980; Savio *et al.*, 1991). Certain ligands, such as phosphines and arsines (Deutsch *et al.*, 1981), pyridoxal (Baker *et al.*, 1975) and penicillamine (Tubis *et al.*, 1975) can also act as reductants, so eliminating the need for a separate reductant. However, in such cases, the ligand excess must be sufficient to minimise the formation of mixed complexes.

The nature of reductant employed in the formation of any technetium complex can have a significant effect on the biodistribution of the resultant complex (Baldas *et al.*, 1982). The choice of reductant can influence the oxidation state of technetium, and, if a mixture of complexes is formed, the proportion of the radioactive components of that mixture. The reductant may form an integral part of the radiopharmaceutical, demonstrated in the case of technetium phosphonate bone agents, when produced in the presence of stannous reductant (Steigman *et al.*, 1978), and use of reductants formamidine sulphinic acid (Baldas *et al.*, 1982) and hydrazine (Baldas *et al.*, 1982) and a tin-capped dioxime complex (Deutsch *et al.*, 1976).

For practical reasons (water solubility, stability, low toxicity, and effectiveness at room temperature; Salehi *et al.*, 1987), stannous salts are the preferred reductants for kit formulations, and without exception, all current commercially available cold kits contain a stannous salt as reductant.

Without the addition of a ligand, reduction of pertechnetate leads to the formation of the thermodynamically stable dioxide, $TcO_2.xH_2O$. Following intravenous administration, this species (often called 'reduced-hydrolysed technetium', 'tin colloid', or 'technetium colloid') is extracted by phagocytosis, so can provide images of liver and spleen (Lin *et al.*, 1971). Phagocytic labeling of isolated granulocytes with TcO_2 is a possible further application of this technetium compound, although cell labeling with this compound is less than ideal (Danpure *et al.*, 1985).

In the presence of a ligand, production of TcO_2 will compete with technetium complex formation. For this reason, TcO_2 will be present as an impurity in all technetium radiopharmaceuticals, and it is one of the major objectives in 'cold' kit development to minimise the formation of this impurity. The proportion of TcO_2 formed is dependent upon several factors, principally rate of complex formation, and complex stability.

3.3.2 Antioxidants

A common problem which limits the post reconstitution shelf life of technetium cold kits is the oxidation of complexed reduced technetium to pertechnetate. There are two sources of this problem.

When taking a patient dose from a reconstituted vial, it is normal practice to introduce a volume of air equal to the volume of solution removed, to maintain atmospheric pressure within the vial. The introduction of oxygen in the vial (previously containing nitrogen as the only gaseous component) will start to consume the stannous reductant, such that any reoxidation to pertechnetate cannot be reversed. A similar effect is achieved when patient doses are subdispensed, or held in syringes, for a significant period of time prior to patient administration. Stannous reductant may also be consumed by oxidants formed through self radiolysis within the vial, as will be described later in this chapter.

In cases where the technetium complex is kinetically inert, loss of reductant need not cause any practical problem in use of the radiopharmaceutical. However, kinetically labile complexes need to be stabilised to preserve radiopharmaceutical purity. While the employment of greater quantities of stannous salts might be one solution, this may, as in the case of phosphonate bone agents (Deutsch *et al.*, 1980) be deleterious to biological performance.

In such cases, antioxidants have been used to provide radiopharmaceuticals with greater stability. These materials are believed to compete with stannous salts in reaction with oxygen or oxidants, so conserving the reducing environment provided the reductant. Antioxidants which have been used in conjunction with technetium complexes include ascorbic acid (Tofe and Francis, 1976), gentisic acid (Tofe *et al.*, 1980) and p-aminobenzoic acid (Rimmer, 1982).

3.3.3 Buffers

There are numerous examples where the radiochemical purity of ^{99m}Tc complexes is highly pH dependent (for example, Yokoyama *et al.*, 1976; Troutner *et al.*, 1984); in addition, the predominant product of complex formation may vary with solution pH. The example of the ligand meso-dimercaptosuccinic acid (DMSA) giving a complex suitable for renal imaging at pH<6, and a soft tissue tumour avid-complex at pH>8 was described, earlier.

Given that the pH of technetium generator eluates may vary between generators from different suppliers, and the pH dependence of complex formation, buffers can be important components in cold kit formulations. However, it is not uncommon for the ligand to act as buffer in cold kits, so eliminating the need for further buffering additives. For example, PnAO (Troutner *et al.*, 1984) and similar ligands (Canning *et al.*, 1986) provide optimal yields of their technetium complexes at pH levels (8–10) where the amine atoms in the ligands are non-protonated. In these cases, cold kits are formulated with ligand in the form of free base, and excess ligand acts as 'buffer' to low pH generator eluates.

3.3.4 Other components

The miscellaneous other components in technetium cold kits may be classified as catalysts, accelerators, solubilising agents, and fillers.

'Catalyst' is the name frequently given to ligands, other than the one providing the final ^{99m}Tc complex, which are added to the cold kit formulation. The purpose of these additional ligands is to maximise the yield of the desired complex through the process of ligand exchange.

As described earlier, during reduction of pertechnetate, formation of reduced-hydrolysed technetium can compete with the production of the coordination complex. For certain ligands, the complex formation can be slow relative to formation of reduced-hydrolysed technetium, resulting in poor complex yields. However, yields of the desired complex may be improved if another ligand is present, one which rapidly forms a coordination complex, yet is able to give up the reduced metal to the primary ligand. Ligands which form weak technetium complexes, such as gluconate, DTPA, and citrate (Davison, 1983) are used for this purpose. Ligand exchange provides the basis of several methods recently described for the ^{99m}Tc labelling of monoclonal antibody fragments (for example, Reno and Bottino, 1987).

The term 'acclerator' was first used in technetium cold kit formulations by Tweedle (1983) in describing the effect of additives containing vicinal hydroxyl groups. Employing such additives with ligands such as DMPE improves the product radiochemical yield, and increases rate of formation (Tweedle, 1983). The mechanism of these effects is unclear.

Ligand and/or complex aqueous solubility was rarely a problem for developers of cold kit formulations prior to the early 1980s, as research concentrated on new hydrophilic complexes. However, in recent years, the major emphasis of commercial research was directed towards developing new lipophilic ^{99m}Tc tracers for cerebral and myocardial blood flow imaging. The use of lipophilic ligands, and formation of lipophilic complexes, has created new problems in kit formulation. Use of low ligand concentrations, as is the case with dl-HM-PAO (Neirinckx *et al.*, 1987), provides one solution, but this tactic may also result in a reduction in radiochemical purity of the product. The use of surfactants is an alternative strategy, as applied to initial formulations of the isonitrile heart agent MIBI (Bergstein and Subramanyam, 1986). Surfactants may also be used to prevent particle aggragation in cold kits for lung perfusion imaging (Lunghi, 1983). There are now a wide range of pharmaceutically acceptible solubilising agents which could be applied to meet the challenge of these problems.

In the preparation of a technetium radiopharmaceutical, it is essential that the solids within the vial dissolve the instant generator eluate is added to the vial. If solid dissolution were to be slow, then the chemistry occuring within the vitally important first few seconds of reconstitution would be unpredictable. Rapid solubilisation of vial contents is achieved through the control of particle size during the lyophilisation process in cold kit production. For the majority of cold kits, kit solids are seen as a fine 'plug'. The size of this plug, and particle size, are controlled by the freeze-dry cycle in kit production, and, if necessary, by the presence of inert fillers. Sodium chloride, added, for example, to dl-HM-PAO kits, and mannitol (in MIBI kits) are typical examples of fillers used in cold kits.

From the preceding sections, it can be seen that there are many variables in kit formulation, and all have to be explored by a manufacturer each time a new product is developed. Several other factors, such as shelf life and compatibility with all available technetium generators, must also be taken into consideration. Therefore, it may take a year or more to convert a newly discovered promising technetium complex into a form which is suitable for clinical trials, and ultimately routine clinical use.

3.4 TECHNETIUM COMPLEXES IN NUCLEAR MEDICINE

3.4.1 Products developed prior to 1980

Many of the kits developed prior to 1980 contained just

ligand and reductant. With these fomulations, formation of the desired technetium complex involves a few simple steps:

1. The radioactive concentration of generator eluate has to be calculated, and, if necessary, eluate is diluted with saline to achieve a radioactive concentration which meets both the manufacturer's guidelines, and the necessary number of patient doses.
2. An appropriate amount of technetium generator eluate is added to the cold kit via a syringe and needle.
3. The vial is inverted a few times to provide agitation to dissolve solids and mix the solution.

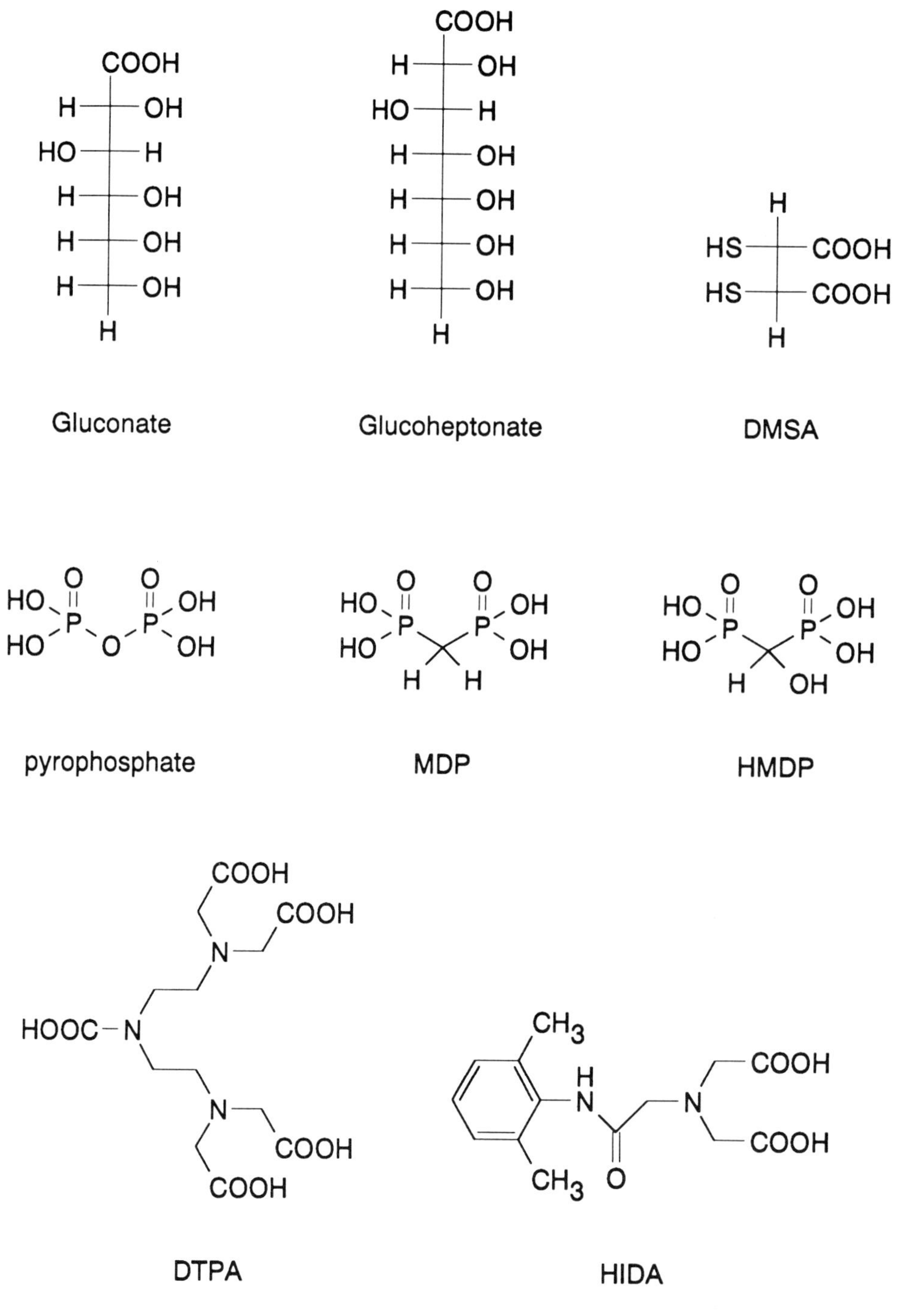

Figure 2. Structures of ligands in kits developed prior to 1980.

4. Incubation at room temperature for approximately one minute permits the chemical reactions of pertechnetate reduction and complexation to go to completion.

The earliest examples of the use of reduced technetium in nuclear medicine resulted from research using metal complexing compounds which were well established in chemistry. For example, ^{99m}Tc complexes of the carbohydrate acids, gluconate and glucoheptonate, and dimercaptosuccinic acid were found to localise in the kidneys; complexes of phosphonates provided the basis for bone imaging, and the complex of diethylenetriaminepentaacetic acid (DTPA) was found to clear through the kidneys by glomerular filtration, so could provide data on renal function (Marzilli *et al.*, 1983). The structures of these ligands are shown in Figure 2, and their applications are listed in Table 1.

Table 1
Applications of Kits Developed Prior to 1980.

Renal Imaging:	Gluconate, glucoheptonate, DMSA
Renal function:	DTPA (GFR); DADS
Hepatic function:	HIDA, EHIDA
Bone:	Flurophosphate, pyrophosphate, EHDP, MDP, HMDP, IDP, DPD
Labelled red cells:	pyrophosphate, MDP
Labelled particles:	liver: tin colloid, sulphur colloid lung: Macroaggregated albumin (MAA), Albumin microsheres

While these developments provided the foundation for the widespread use of technetium in nuclear medicine, little was known at that time of the nature of the complexes formed with such ligands. To extend the range of technetium radiopharmaceuticals, it was realised that new ligands would be required, and a better understanding of the chemistry of technetium was essential. This research resulted in the discovery and development of several new technetium complexes with applications in nuclear medicine, as described in the next section.

3.4.2 Some products developed after 1980

The main areas for the development of new technetium radiopharmaceuticals during the 1980s were cerebral perfusion, myocardial perfusion, kidney function, and liver function. Figure 3 displays the structures of ligands outlined in this section.

3.4.2.1 HM-PAO (Ceretec^{TM})

The commercial kit formulation for the formation of Tc-99m d,l-HM-PAO is shown below, with the structure of the complex.

d,l-HM-PAO	0.5 mg
Stannous chloride	7.6 μg
Sodium chloride	4.5 mg
pH	8.0

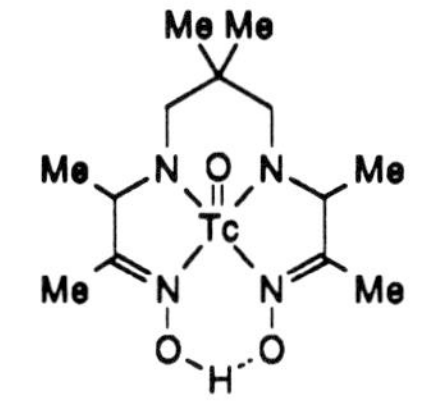

Ceretec ^{TM} was the first commercially-available technetium radiopharmaceutical for imaging cerebral blood flow (Nowotnik *et al.*, 1985). It was initially available in certain countries in 1985, and was rapidly approved in most of the major markets thereafter. While its initial intended use was for perfusion imaging, Ceretec's most widespread application appears to be in blood cell labeling (Kelly *et al.*, 1987; Srivastava and Straub, 1990).

The ability of this agent to perform both functions is thought to be related to its instability. The complex is neutral and lipophilic (log P is approximately 1, Neirinckx *et al.*, 1987). It is thought to be able to diffuse across cell membranes, then react rapidly with intra-cellular components to produce a hydrophilic complex, which cannot back diffuse across the membrane (Nowotnik *et al.*, 1985). In this way, technetium is trapped within the cell, be it in organ tissues following i.v. administration, or a blood cell following *in vitro* incubation. It has been proposed that intracellular glutathione is the primary reagent to effect this conversion (Neirinckx *et al.*, 1988), but, after a number of studies, there is no firm consensus for or against this hypothesis (Babich, 1991).

While rapid degradation of the complex *in vivo* (Nakamura *et al.*, 1989; Lucignani *et al.*, 1990) might be essential for efficacy, it is a nuisance in the kit. The initial RCP of the diffusible ('primary') complex is >90%, but it falls to >80% in 30 minutes. To ensure that complex formation and degradation are no worse than this, the manufacturer places severe restrictions on the volume, radioactive concentration, and age of the generator eluate. Eluate age and radioactive concentration influence the level of oxidants formed through radiolysis. As the amount of reductant in Ceretec^{TM} kits is low, very little of these oxidants can be tolerated. In addition, there is evidence that the primary complex is also susceptible to radiolysis (Tubergen *et al.*, 1991), which places a restriction on radioactive concentration. Some studies (Ponto, 1990; Millar, 1992) have indicated that there can be more flexibility in the eluate age than recommended, but use of eluate outside of the stated age limits is not without risk. It has also been proposed that aged generator eluate can be used with Ceretec^{TM} kits following the addition of iodide

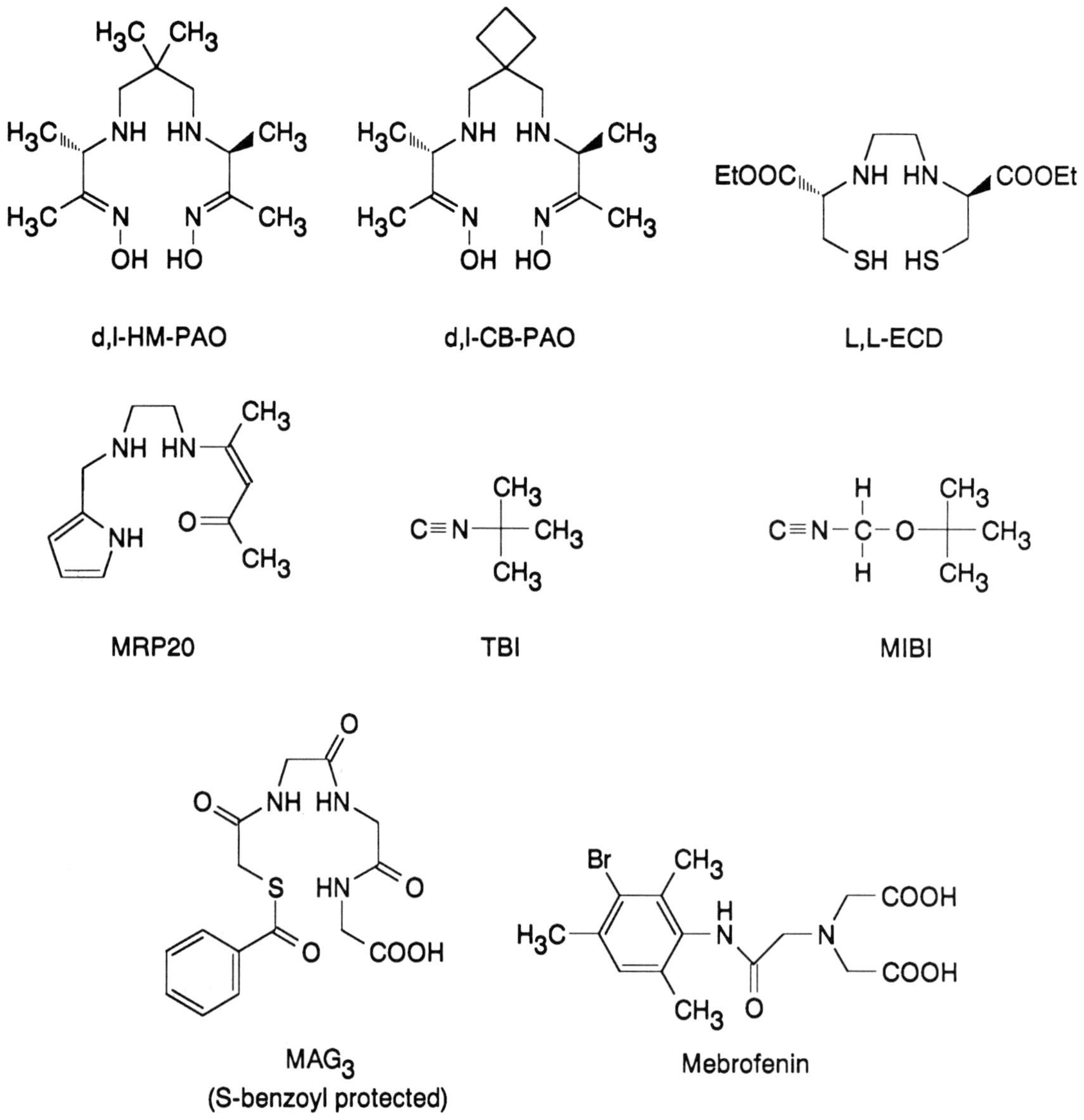

Figure 3. Structures of ligands in kits developed since 1980.

(Bayne *et al.*, 1989), but this suggestion has received little attention.

The low level of stannous in Ceretec™ kits is the primary reason for the eluate age and radioactive concentration restrictions. Such low levels are necessary as the rate of degradation of the primary complex to the so-called secondary complex (Neirinckx *et al.*, 1987) is directly related to concentration of stannous ion (Hung *et al.*, 1988). The restriction on reconstitution volume is a direct result of this relationship. Kit dilution after reconstitution appears to reduce the rate of complex conversion (Ballinger and Gulenchyn, 1991). Thus, stannous ion is required during reconstitution for the initial reduction of pertechnetate, but appears to be undesirable after complex formation. A patented method of stabilising the primary technetium complex of d,l-HM-PAO is based on this observation; good stability of the primary complex is claimed when hypochlorite is added immediately after reconstitution to oxidise the remaining stannous ion (Solanki, 1990).

There now appear to be several potential ways of stabilising the primary technetium complex of d,l-HM-PAO. Isolation of the technetium complex from other kits components (particularly if the isolated complex is stored in ether; Hung *et al.*, 1988) or dilution with ethanol (Ballinger and Gulenchyn, 1991; Billinghurst *et al.*, 1991) are effective, but impractical. The stability of Tc-99m d,l-HM-PAO appears to be improved by lowering pH to 7.4, with further improvements achieved by adding the anti-oxidant gentisic acid (Hung *et al.*, 1989). In addition, certain additives to the formulation are claimed to stabilise the primary HM-PAO complex (Anon., 1989; Lang *et al.*, 1989). These data indicate that a single-vial, or two-vial, reformulated kit for producing stable Tc-99m, d,l-HM-PAO is a distinct possibility. The introduction of such a kit will, no doubt be based upon market factors. For a further discussion see Chapter 7, Section 7.3.6.

An analogue of d,l-HM-PAO, called d,l-CB-PAO (see Figure 3), has been proposed as an alternative ligand system for technetium cerebral perfusion imaging (Deutsch, 1990). It is claimed that this ligand forms a complex with superior *in vitro* stability (Colombo *et al.*, 1990), although, when allowance is made for differences in formulation, Tc-99m d,l-CB-PAO is only marginally more stable than is Tc-99m d,l-HM-PAO (Nowotnik, 1992). The quality of cerebral perfusion images obtained with Tc-99m d,l-CB-PAO in man is inferior to those obtained with Tc-99m d,l-HM-PAO (Bacciottini *et al.*, 1990).

The initial radiochemical impurity in Ceretec^{TM} kits is the so-called secondary complex. Typically, the proportion of this complex rises as the primary complex degrades, until approximately two hours post reconstitution (Tubergen *et al.*, 1991). At this point, presumably the reductant is exhausted, and pertechnetate grows in, while the proportion of secondary complex remains essentially stable. Although some data suggests that the primary complex might degrade directly to pertechnetate (Hung *et al.*, 1989), it is more likely (given the stability of the primary complex to added oxidant; Solanki, 1990) that the degradation process proceeds from primary to secondary complex to pertechnetate.

There has been a certain amount of interest in the 'secondary complex' of Tc-99m d,l-HM-PAO. Published HPLC chromatograms show it as a single peak, suggesting that it is a single, well-defined complex (Neirinckx *et al.*, 1987; Hung *et al.*, 1988). However, this is far from the case. Analysis under certain reversed-phase HPLC conditions (Hung *et al.*, 1988), and normal phase HPLC (Nowotnik 1987) demonstrates that the 'secondary complex' is a mixture of unstable compounds (Figure 4) in which the 'fingerprint' of peaks is dependent upon reaction time and conditions (Pettit, unreported data). Studies of the biodistribution of the 'secondary complex' (Nakamura *et al.* 1989) have little meaning given the heterogeneous and variable nature of this species.

The HM-PAO ligand has two diastereoisomeric forms, meso and dl (Nowotnik *et al.* 1985). The technetium complexes of both these stereochemical forms have the ability to cross the blood-brain barrier, but the dl-diastereoisomer complex demonstrates far better brain retention (Neirinckx *et al.* 1987), and it is this form which is commercially available. The dl-diastereoisomer is composed of a racemic mixture of the d and l-enantiomers of this ligand,

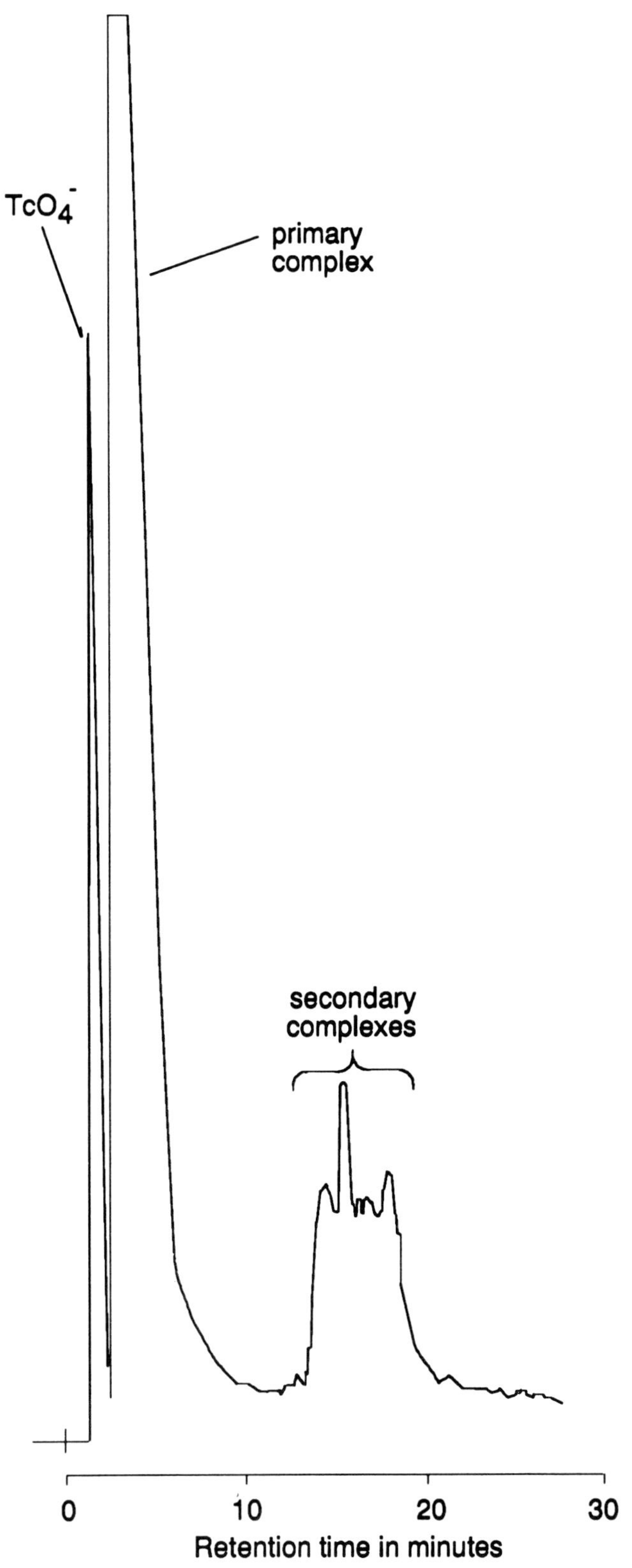

Figure 4. HPLC chromatogram of the secondary complexes of Tc-d,l-HM-PAO.

and there is certain evicence that the l-complex has superior brain retention to the d-form (Canning *et al.*, 1986; Neirinckx and Harrison, 1988; Hoffman *et al.*, 1992).

3.4.2.2 ECD (Neurolite[R])

Preliminary clinical trials of the cerebral perfusion tracer ECD were conducted with a two vial kit (Leveille *et al.*, 1989), as outlined, below:

Vial 1:	
Ethyl cysteinate dimer (ECD.2HCl)	**0.9 mg**
Stannous chloride	**72 µg**
disodium EDTA	**360 µg**
Mannitol	**24 mg**
Vial 2:	
pH 7.5 phosphate buffer	**1 mL**

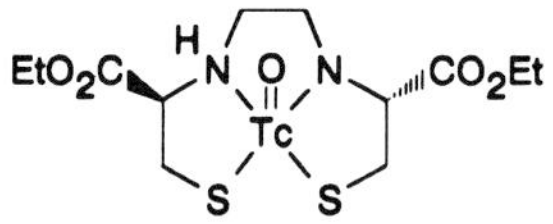

Formation of Tc-99m L,L-ECD involved reconstitution of vial 1 with 1.2ml of generator eluate, followed by addition of 1.0 ml of this solution to vial 2; 15 minutes after this transfer, the radiochemical purity of Tc-99m L,L-ECD was >95% (Leveille *et al.*, 1989). The chemistry involved in these steps has not been described, but, presumably, step one involves reduction of pertechnetate, and formation of an intermediate EDTA complex, which, on pH adjustment, undergoes ligand displacement by ECD to give the desired complex. In preparing this formulation, the ability of phosphate buffer to etch glass (giving a hazy solution) was overlooked, and, after an initial clinical study, this formulation was withdrawn from use.

Tc-99m L,L-ECD is a neutral, lipophilic complex which is thought to diffuse across cell membranes, and become trapped as a result of conversion to a less lipophilic form (Walovitch *et al.*, 1988, 1989). This conversion process is thought to be enzyme catalysed; it is stereospecific (Walovitch *et al.*, 1989; Harris *et al.*, 1992), species specific (Bormans *et al.*, 1990), and tissue specific (for example, unlike HM-PAO, Tc-99m L,L-ECD is not able to label blood cells; Verbruggen, 1990). *In vivo* metabolism of Tc-99m L,L-ECD proceeds via desterification to the mono- and di-acid (Van Nerom *et al.*, 1990; Verbruggen *et al.*, 1990). The metabolites are rapidly cleared via the kidneys; in fact, clearance of the diacid 'metabolite' is so rapid that it is being considered as an alternative to MAG3 for renal function imaging (Verbruggen *et al.*, 1992).

As the 'degradation' of Tc-99m L,L-ECD appears to be enzymatic rather than a simple chemical process (as is the case for Tc-99m d,l-HM-PAO), Tc-99m L,L-ECD appears to be stable in the kit form, so it should not have a similar time restriction to use as in the case of the first HM-PAO formulation. Clinical trials of Tc-99m L,L-ECD using a new formulation have begun (Walovitch *et al.*, 1992), but details of the new formulation are not available at the time of writing.

Like HM-PAO, the ECD ligand also has three stereochemical forms. The technetium complexes of all three can cross the blood-brain barrier, but cerebral retention of activity follows the series LL > DL > DD (Walovitch *et al.*, 1989; Harris *et al.*, 1992). These complexes also demonstrate marked species differences in brain uptake and retention, thought to reflect differences in rates of *in vivo* ester group hydrolysis (Harris *et al.*, 1992).

3.4.2.3 MRP20

MRP20 was the first (Bossuyt *et al.*, 1991) of a series of linear tetradentate ligands (Thornback *et al.*, 1990) consisting of a pyrrole, amine, imine, and ketone donor set (see Figure 3). This ligand forms a complex with technetium which appears to have similar properties to Tc-99m d,l-HM-PAO; the complex is neutral, moderately lipophilic, and degrades *in vitro* and *in vivo*. It is suggested that the complex crosses the blood-brain barrier after i.v. administration, then degrades to a non-lipophilic form which is trapped (like HM-PAO) giving a stable distribution within the brain which reflects blood flow (Morgan *et al.*, 1991). While initial clinical data suggests that this complex is capable of providing reasonable SPECT images of cerebral blood flow, it is unclear at this time whether this ligand (or a close analogue) will be developed into a commercial kit.

3.4.2.4 MIBI (Cardiolite[R])

The formulation of the MIBI kit, and the structure of the complex, are shown below:

$[Cu(I)(MIBI)_6]^+ BF_4^-$	1.0 mg
Stannous Chloride	75 µg
Sodium citrate	2.6 mg
L-Cysteine. HCl. H_2O	1.0 mg
Mannitol	20 mg
pH	5.5

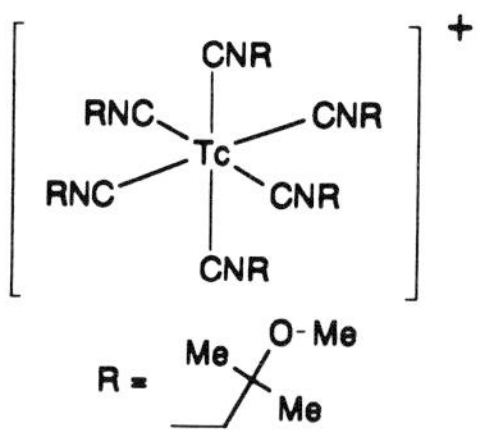

The development of Cardiolite[R] resulted from approximately 8 years of research into technetium isonitrile complexes. Unsubstituted alkylisonitriles were investigated initially; once the conditions for formation of the +1 oxidation state hexacoordinate complexes were determined (Jones *et al.*, 1983), a wide range of alkyl isonitriles were examined as potential heart perfusion agents (Jones *et al.*, 1984; Nowotnik, 1989). Of these, the t-butyl complex demonstrated optimum heart uptake. However, this complex suffered from high liver and lung background activity (Piwnica-Worms *et al.*, 1989). The ligands were then modified to incorporate metabolisable functions, in an attempt to solve the problem of background radioactivity. Esters were used initially (Kronauge, 1987), but the ester isonitriles, typified by the CPI ligand (Piwnica-Worms *et al.*, 1988), gave Tc-99m complexes which, when taken up by the myocardium were also cleared rapidly from heart as well as background tissues (researchers were seeking a complex with long retention in the heart). Tc-99m$(CPI)_6$ shows considerable species variation in heart uptake, which could be attributed to differences in ester hydrolysis in serum (Kronauge *et al.*, 1992b).

Using ethers instead of esters gave complexes which were retained in the heart, but showed improved background clearance compared to the alkylisonitrile complexes (Bergstein and Subramanyam, 1986; Wackers *et al.*, 1989). Why this improvement is achieved with ether derivatives is unclear, but there is evidence that ethers are metabolised in the liver to hydroxyl groups (Kronauge *et al.*, 1990). The hydroxyls may be further metabolised, for example, the formation of glucuronides. These processes reduce lipophilicity and should improve hepatic clearance of radioactivity. Of a series of ether-isonitriles, the complex of MIBI proved to have the best range of properties for myocardial scintigraphy (Bergstein and Subramanyam, 1986), although studies aimed at identifying superior ether-isonitrile ligands are continuing (Barbarics and Janoki, 1990; Verbruggen, 1991; Kronauge *et al.*, 1992a).

The properties of an isonitrile ligand present a major challenge in the development of a lyophilised kit; they are toxic, unstable, (generally) volatile, and possess a foul odour (Ramalingam, 1989). To overcome these difficulties, kits based on transition metal chelates were developed (Iqbal *et al.*, 1989; Sachdev *et al.*, 1990). These complexes stabilised the ligand, and reduced toxicity and odour. However, these complexes must be sufficiently labile to give up the ligand to technetium during complex formation, yet be sufficiently stable to prevent liberation of toxic free ligand *in vivo*, and to provide a robust kit with reasonable shelf life. The copper(I) complex appears to have these properties. While the function of individual components in the kit formulation of MIBI has not been described, it is assumed that citrate is present as a buffer, cysteine forms a temporary chelate with reduced technetium, and mannitol serves as a filler and 'accelerator' (Tweedle, 1983). Heating (to 100 °C) is required to lower the oxidation state of Tc to one, and to effect ligand exchange.

3.4.2.5 CDO-MeB (CardioTec^R)

Cyclohexanedione dioxime	2.0 mg
methylboronic acid	2.0 mg
Stannous chloride	60 μg
DTPA	2.0 mg
citric acid	9.0 mg
sodium chloride	100 mg
γ-cyclodextrn	50 mg
pH	3.7

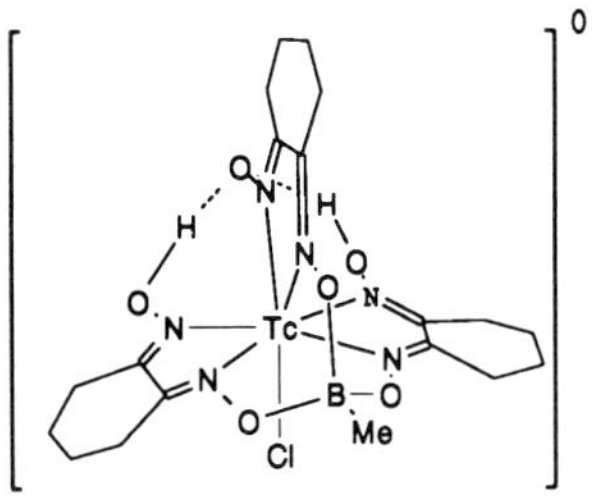

CardioTec^R is one of a series of technetium complexes termed as BATOs (Boronic Acid adducts of Technetium diOximes) which were discovered and developed at the Squibb Institute (Nunn *et al.*, 1987; Nunn, 1992). These complexes are unusual in so far as the ligand from which they are made is constructed during the labeling process from individual components in the kit (template synthesis). The only previous example of template synthesis of a technetium radiopharmaceutical was the series of Tc-99m pyridoxylidine amino acid hepatobiliary agents (Baker *et al.*, 1975). In the case of BATOs, the ligand is constructed from three vicinal dioximes, which are bound to technetium via their nitrogen atoms, and a boronic acid, which 'caps' the complex by attachment to three oxime groups. The BATOs are heptadentate; a monodentate chloride ligand occupies the remaining coordination site. A wide variety of BATOs were made and evaluated; from this investigation CDO-MeB (CardioTec^R) was selected as the complex with optimum properties for myocardial perfusion imaging (Nunn *et al.*, 1990).

CardioTec^R is formed in the kit by a reaction sequence involving several steps (see Figure 5; Linder *et al.*, 1990). Initial reduction of pertechnetate presumably gives rise to Tc(V)/Tc(IV) complexes ('held' by citric acid and DTPA), which are further reduced by heating and ligand exchange to give a tin-capped tris-dioxime complex. This complex looses its tin cap, and rearranges to give a parallel grouping of oximes around technetium. This 'tris' complex is then capped at one end by a boronic acid to give the BATO complex (Linder *et al.*, 1990). In other boron-capped transition metal dioxime complexes, capping of both ends of the molecule occurs (for example Zakrzewski *et al.*, 1971); mono-capping in the BATOs is attributed to the size of technetium and the coordination geometry associated with the heptacoordination of the metal (Jurisson *et al.*, 1991a). Simply, capping at one end requires the oximes at that end to be pulled inwards, forcing the oximes at the other end of the molecule apart, as seen in crystal structures of BATOs (Treher *et al.*, 1989). In spite of the complexity of the chemistry, a high (>95%) radiochemical yield is obtained consistently using the manufacturer's recommended protocol.

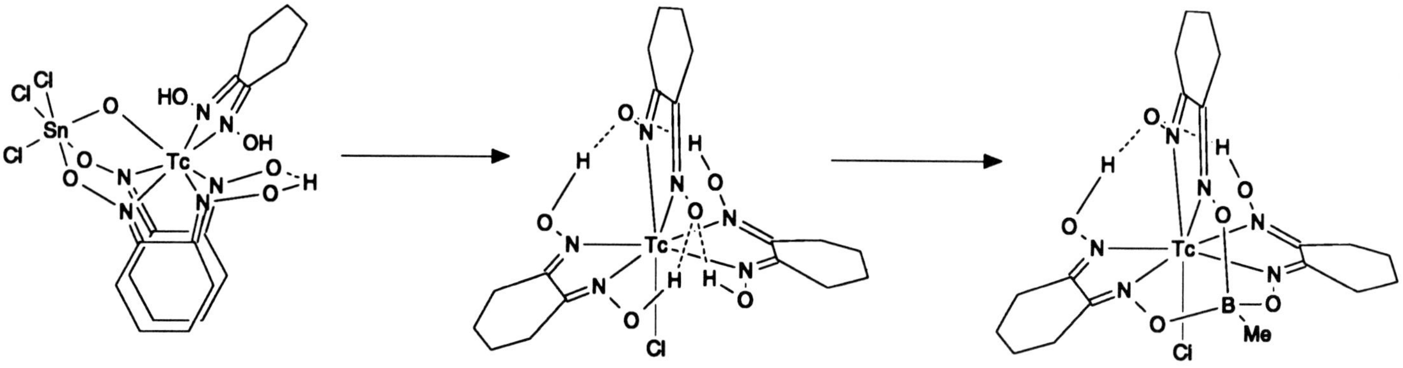

Figure 5. Steps in the formation of Tc-99m Cardiotec[R].

The monodentate chloride ligand in CardioTec[R] is labile to substitution under certain conditions; for example, raising pH to ≥5.5 causes the choro ligand to be displaced by a hydroxy group (Jurisson *et al.*, 1991b). The biodistribution profiles of chloro and hydroxy analogues of CDO-MeB are different (Jurisson *et al.*, 1991b), so it is important that this exchange is inhibited in the kit. While the raised chloride ion concentration in the kit ensures formation of the chloro complex, the low pH and presence of γ-cyclodextrin prevent conversion to the hydroxy form. γ-Cyclodextrin also ensures that the high lipophilic CardioTex[R] complex (Nunn *et al.*, 1990) remains in aqueous solution.

While the cationic heart perfusion tracers show modest heart extraction with long retention in the heart, CardioTec[R] has high extraction with rapid myocardial washout (Di Rocco *et al.*, 1992b). High extraction is important for good delineation of high and low flow regions. The rapid washout of CardioTec[R] places a restriction on the time of imaging post administration, but it does permit stress/rest studies to be completed in much less time than with the retained compounds (Nowotnik and Nunn, 1992). Also, study of the washout kinetics may provide additional diagnostic information (Nunn, 1991).

3.4.2.6 P53 (Myoview™)

Tetrofosmin	**0.23 mg**
Di-sodium sulphosalicylate	**0.32 mg**
D-gluconate	**1.0 mg**
Stannous chloride	**30 μg**

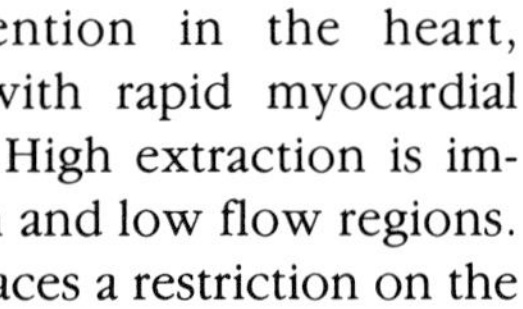

Scientists at Amersham produced and screened a large number of cationic technetium complexes as potential myocardial perfusion imaging agents (Kelly *et al.*, 1990). This study was based upon previous investigations, which involved a limited number of phosphine ligands (Deutsch *et al.*, 1987a). Those earlier studies had achieved some limited success in animals, but species differences coupled with high liver, lung, and blood retention prevented these compounds from becoming useful agents in man (Deutsch *et al.*, 1987a). The Amersham study involved the synthesis of a wide variety of new phosphine ligands (which contained additional functional groups) and the complexation of these ligands to various technetium cores (Kelly *et al.*, 1990). As had been the case in studies leading to Cardiolite, ligands containing ether moieties appeared to possess the best overall qualities. Three ether-phosphine ligand complexes were selected for clinical evaluation (Lahiri *et al.*, 1989). From clinical and radiopharmaceutical considerations, the ligand code-named P53 was selected as the agent of choice (Smith, F.W. *et al.*, 1991).

In Myoview™, the technetium core is $Tc(V)O_2$ (Forster *et al.*, 1992); the majority of technetium phosphine complexes examined previously as potential myocardial imaging agents have been in the Tc(III) or Tc(I) oxidation states (Nunn, 1990). The higher oxidation state of technetium in Myoview™ provides it with one advantage; heating is not required. However, the $TcO_2(P53)_2$ complex forms slowly at room temperature. Initial clinical studies were conducted with kits which required over 60 minutes room temperature incubation. The current formulation requires 15 minutes 'standing' at room temperature to achieve a radiochemical purity of 90% (Jain *et al.*, 1992). The presence of gluconate in the kit is necessary to 'hold' technetium in the +5 oxidation state after reduction, while, presumably, the sulphosalicyclic acid is present to 'accelerate' ligand exchange.

Phase II clinical trial results have been reported (Braat *et al.*, 1992; Jain *et al.*, 1992; Leclerq *et al.*, 1992; Ohtake *et al.*, 1992; Sridhara *et al.*, 1992). Heart uptake in man is low (1%), a reflection of the poor myocardial extraction of this compound (found in isolated rabbit hearts; Dahlberg *et al.*, 1992). Also in the isolated heart, the slope of the uptake vs flow graph for Myoview™ was found to be inferior to Cardiolite[R] (Dahlberg *et al.*, 1992). These data suggest that Myoview™ may be of limited value in myocardial perfusion studies when attempting to differentiate high and low flow regions.

3.4.2.7 Q12 (TechneCard[R])

TMPP	0.8 mg
Copper (I)	? **
Na ascorbate	2 - 5 mg
pH	9 - 9.5

** Only preliminary details of the kit formulation were available at the time of writing.

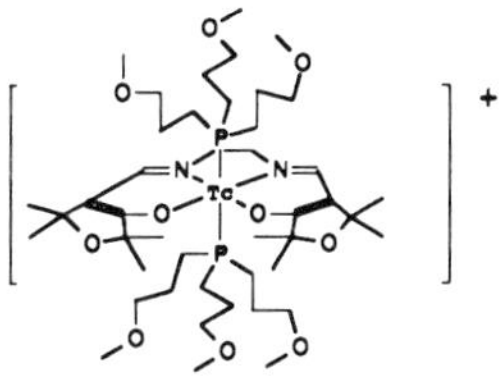

Like Myoview^{TM}, the development of the 'Q' series of complexes was based on the early studies of cationic technetium phosphine heart agents. Deutsch and Hirth (1987) proposed that the difference in performance observed for the $Tc(III)Cl_2(DMPE)_2$ complex in man and most other animal species (Deutsch *et al.*, 1989) was due to a selective reductive mechanism. According to this hypothesis, while the $TcCl_2(DMPE)_2$ complex is in the Tc(III) form, it is a cation, and will be retained in the myocardium. However, on reduction, a neutral Tc(II) complex is formed, which can be washed out of the heart. This reduction process is species dependent, and is prominant in the human myocardium (Deutsch and Hirth, 1987). Support for this hypothesis is provided in studies of $MCl_2(DMPE)_2$ complexes (M = Tc or Re, Deutsch *et al.*, 1987a). The rhenium complex is harder to reduce. The technetium and rhenium complexes have similar heart uptake, but myocardial washout of the rhenium complex is always less than that for technetium. Thus, Tc(III) cationic complexes were developed which are more difficult to reduce than $Tc(III)Cl_2(DMPE)_2$ (Deutsch *et al.*, 1987b). These were based on tetradentate Schiff base complexes which form complexes in the +5 oxidation state (Jurisson *et al.*, 1984b), but which can be reduced with an excess of monodentate phosphine ligands to give +3 complexes, with two phosphine ligands (Jurisson *et al.*, 1984a). A series of these complexes (varying the Schiff base ligand and the monodentate phosphine ligand; Deutsch *et al.*, 1987b) were examined. Generally, they displayed reasonable heart uptake in man, but had poor background clearance. As was the case for MIBI, and P53, phosphines with ether substituents showed superior background clearance, and one of these complexes, Q12 (in which the phosphine is tris(3-methoxy-1-propyl)phosphine; TMPP) was selected for further evaluation (Marmion *et al.*, 1991; Woulfe *et al.*, 1991).

Q12 was initially prepared in a 2-step process (forming first the Tc(V) Schiff base complex, then reacting with the TMPP to give Tc(III) Q12; Marmion *et al.*, 1991), but a 1-vial kit has been developed (available details of the formulation are shown, above; De Rosch *et al.*, 1992). Like MIBI, the kit of Q12 contains copper to chelate the phosphine ligand. The ratio of phosphine/copper has to be greater than 4 (De Rosch *et al.*, 1992). As excess phosphine is the reductant as well as ligand, presumably some phosphine has to be free for the initial reduction of pertechnetate. The presence of an antioxidant (ascorbate) is essential for a good RCP (De Rosch *et al.*, 1992). The pH of the 1-vial kit is midway between the two pH levels (approximately 11 and 8) reported (Marmion *et al.*, 1991) as optimum in the 2 step process.

3.4.2.8 Mebrofenin (Choletec[R])

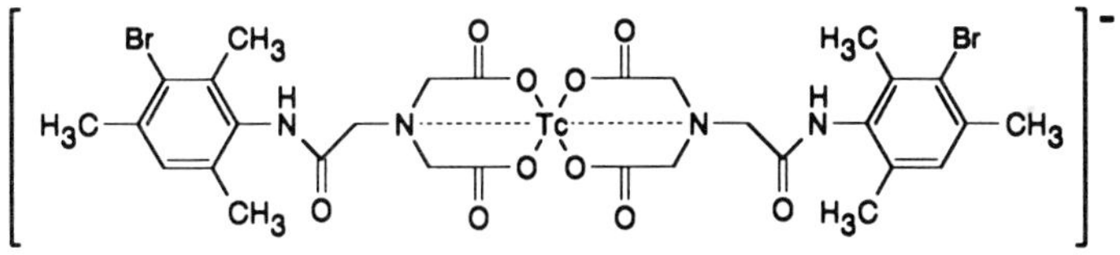

Mebrofenin	45 mg
Stannous fluoride dihydrate	540 µg
Methylparaben	5.2 mg
Propylparaben	0.58 mg
pH	5.0
Reconstitution:	RT/ 1 min

One of the first ligands designed specifically for use with technetium was the lipophilic iminodiacetic ligand termed 'HIDA' (hepatobiliary IDA), which provided a single technetium complex in the +3 oxidation state, and demonstrated rapid hepatic clearance following i.v. administration (Loberg *et al.*, 1976). In an extensive systematic study, varying the substituents on the phenyl ring of HIDA, a complex with much improved hepatic characteristics was obtained; Mebrofenin (3-bromo-2,4,6-trimethyl HIDA; see Figure 3; Nunn *et al.*, 1983). In addition to ligand and stannous reductant, the formulation of Choletec[R] contains a mixture of methyl and propylparaben, as bacteriostat and solubiliser, which allow the reconstituted kit to be used as a multi-dose vial for up to 24 hours after reconstitution.

3.4.2.9 MAG3^{TM}

	Formulation	
	European	U.S.
Betiatide	1 mg	1 mg
Disodium tartrate	16.9 mg	40 mg
Stannous chloride	40 µg	200 µg
Lactose	none	20 mg

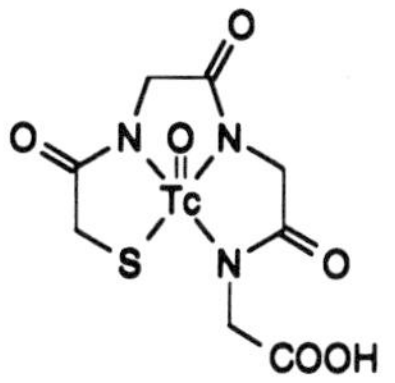

The development of a Tc-99m renal function agent has focussed on anionic Tc(V)O complexes of amide-thiol ligands; several compounds were examined prior to the discovery and subsequent commercialisation of MAG3^{TM} (Eshima *et al.*, 1990). Comparison of Tc-99m MAG3^{TM} with Hippuran suggests that it is not the ideal replacement for the latter (Prenen *et al.*, 1991), but it has found acceptance in many centres as an alternative tubular function agent.

There have been several reports of poor RCPs in the preparation of Tc-99m MAG3^{TM} (for example, Brandau *et al.*, 1988), such that HPLC purification of the radiopharmaceutical is required prior to administration. These problems appear to be related to the impurities in the ligand when this is prepared locally by the investigator. The manufacturers of the MAG3™ kit have examined the synthesis of Betiatide (S-benzoyl-mercaptoacetyl-triglycine, the ligand used in the commercial kit formulation) and eliminated the impurities which give rise to these extraneous complexes. Tc-99m MAG_3 produced from the commercial kit does not require purification (Nosco *et al.*, 1990).

The formulation of the MAG3™ kit available in Europe is not the same as that in the U.S.A. The U.S. kit has higher levels of stannous ion, which is deemed necessary to accommodate pertechnetate from all commercially-available generators in that country (Nosco *et al.*, 1992). Excess stannous ion appears to be detrimental to the stability of Tc-99m MAG_3 once formed, so excess stannous ion is oxidised by the addition of air to the vial after complex formation (Nosco *et al.*, 1990). Deliberate addition of air to the vial is not required in the European kit, because of the lower initial level of stannous ion. Both kits contain sodium tartrate to hold reduced technetium prior to the heating step, which causes ligand exchange resulting in Tc-99m MAG_3. The U.S. formulation also incorporates lactose as a filler.

Kit formulations containing the MAG_3 ligand without a benzoyl protecting group have been prepared and studied (Noll *et al.*, 1992). These appear to provide a high yield of the Tc-99m MAG_3 complex at high pH, suggesting that the heating step in the commercial kits is only required for deprotection of the ligand.

The MAG_3 ligand was developed as part of a program which investigated the potential of amide-thiol ligand as the basis for technetium renal function agents (Eshima *et al.*, 1990). One of the ligands which preceded MAG_3 was termed carboxy-DADS (Fritzberg *et al.*, 1982). This ligand had a chiral centre, which, on complexation with technetium gave two complexes. These could be separated by conventional HPLC (Fritzberg *et al.*, 1986). Two complexes were formed because the carboxyl substituent could be either syn- or anti- to the oxygen atom bound to technetium (Rao *et al.*, 1989). In fact, each of the isolated complexes is a mixture of enantiomers; when separated, the individual complexes had different biodistribution properties (Fritzberg *et al.*, 1986). MAG_3 was designed to fulfil the requirements for renal tubular excretion without the presence of a chiral center in the ligand (Fritzberg *et al.*, 1986). However, while the MAG_3 ligand is achiral, it forms two enantiomeric complexes, which show similar renal clearance characteristics in man, but are slightly different in baboons (Verbruggen *et al.*, 1989). A recently-published patent application claims a formulation which provides an enantiomeric excess of one of the Tc-99m MAG_3 steroisomers (Noll *et al.*, 1991).

3.5 THE PREPARATION OF TECHNETIUM RADIOPHARMACEUTICALS

3.5.1 Quality control of technetium radiopharmaceuticals

Following preparation, it is recommended that quality control (QC) of technetium radiopharmaceuticals is routinely carried out. Documentation accompanying cold kits will describe manufacturers recommended QC procedures. For hydrophilic complexes, this will generally involve paper or thin layer chromatography (instant thin layer chromatographic (ITLC) strips are frequently used for this purpose; Kowalsky and Creekmore, 1982). The majority of analyses involve the use of two strips; one developed in acetone, or methyl ethyl ketone (MEK), and the other with 0.9% aqueous sodium chloride (saline). Full technical details of quality testing are described in Chapter 9.

Several factors, such as sample size, drying (or not drying) the sample on the ITLC strip prior to elution, method of storage of chromatography strips (Kowalsky and Creekmore, 1982), and age of solvent in the development tank (these should be changed daily) can influence the result, and care in following the manufacturers recommenations is essential.

Column chromatography, particularly gel filtration (Eckelman *et al.*, 1972; Chervu *et al.*, 1977) and high performance liquid chromatography (HPLC: Fritzberg and Lewis, 1980; Fritzberg and Nunn, 1986; Zhou *et al.*, 1988) may also be used for technetium radiopharmaceutical QC. These techniques offer advantages in the research environment, as it may be possible to separate multiple technetium complexes, but are not as convenient as TLC or paper chromatography for routine use. However, the principles of column chromatography have been applied recently (though the use of Sep-pak cartridges) to produce some rapid methods for the quality control of technetium radiopharmaceuticals (Hammes *et al.*, 1991; Nosco *et al.*, 1992).

Two of the major reasons for poor radiopharmaceutical purity are described in the following section. However, there can be many other factors which have an adverse influence on purity, yet are identified only with great difficulty. For example, contamination of vial or syringe contents by isopropanol (Peterson *et al.*, 1985) or antiseptics (Fisher *et al.*, 1977) from antiseptic wipes can lower radioactive purity. For a fuller discussion see Chapter 10.

Even with confirmed high radiochemical purities immediately prior to administration, it is still possible to obtain patient scans which might indicate an impure radiopharmaceutical. In such cases, patient therapy should be investigated; there are many known examples of drugs and disease states which can alter radiopharmaceutical biodistribution (Shaw, 1985; see also Chapter 19).

3.6 THE IMPORTANCE OF SPECIFIC ACTIVITY AND RADIOLYSIS

The decay process $^{99}Mo \rightarrow {}^{99m}Tc \rightarrow {}^{99}Tc$ which occurs on the column of the $^{99}Mo/^{99m}Tc$ generator was described in the previous chapter. An outcome of this decay scheme is the production of ^{99}Tc; chemically identical to ^{99m}Tc, it appears in all eluents from the generator, and takes part in all chemical processes in the cold kit. ^{99}Tc is termed 'carrier' when considering reactions of ^{99m}Tc, and the quantity of this carrier can have an influence on the ^{99m}Tc radiopharmaceutical product performance. The amount of carrier present is a function of the quantity of ^{99}Mo on the generator column, and the time since previous elution of the generator. The amount of ^{99m}Tc (in mCi or MBq) in total technetium in generator eluate is termed the specific activity of that generator eluate.

In many cold kits, the amount of ligand and reductant present is in large excess over the highest amount of total technetium which could be added in unmodified generator eluate. In these situations, the amount of carrier technetium should have little influence on the nature of the product formed. However, in cold kits containing unusually low amounts of reductant, such as the kit for dl-HM-PAO, the amount of carrier technetium can have an adverse effect (Moore, 1984), particularly when other factors resulting in diminution of reductant are present.

While in general it is not necessary to know precisely the concentration of technetium, several methods have been developed to determine the total quantity of technetium in generator eluate (Deutsch *et al.*, 1982; Hetherington, 1983; Holland *et al.*, 1986).

A more significant problem for all technetium radiopharmaceuticals is that of radiolysis. It is well known that ionising radiation will decompose water molecules to give hydrogen perioxide and free radicals (Allan, 1961). Oxidants can accumulate on the columns of $^{99}Mo/^{99m}Tc$ generators, and be eluted with saline with ^{99m}Tc-pertechnetate (Molinski, 1982). This build-up of oxidants is particularly severe during the period between generator production and first elution, such that it is generally recommended that the first eluate obtained from a new generator should not be used for the preparation of technetium radiopharmaceuticals.

Oxidants also build up in the vial of generator eluate, and following kit reconstitution (Molinski, 1982). This can be a major source of loss of reductant. Once all the stannous ion has been consumed, then the technetium radiopharmaceutical is at risk from oxidation to pertechnetate. Thus, while the initial radiochemical purity of the radiopharmaceutical may be satisfactory, at an indeterminate time after preparation, rapid reoxidation of ^{99m}Tc to pertechnetate can start to lower radiopharmaceutical purity if the complex is kinetically labile.

Cold kit formulations may contain large excess quantities of reductant and/or antioxidants to consume oxidants as formed. Development testing under adverse conditions provides the data on which manufacturers base their recommendations on kit period of use post reconstitution. However, addition of air to the vial (when equilibrating pressure in the vial after removing patient doses), or sub-dispensing the radiopharmaceutical into syringes some time before use, can introduce other sources of oxidants and accelerate the loss of reductant. Therefore, care must be taken in following manufacturer's recommended protocols to ensure satisfactory performance of the radiopharmaceutical.

3.5 CONCLUSIONS

Through the use of commercially produced 'cold kits', the applications for ^{99m}Tc in nuclear medicine are broad based. The preparation of these complexes usually involves the simple addition of $^{99}Mo/^{99m}Tc$ generator eluate to the vial of the cold kit. In a few cases, an additional heating step is required to complete the complex formation reaction. Compliance with the manufacturer's recommendations should guarantee the formation of a high purity product, but quality control chromatographic procedures should be carried out routinely to confirm radiochemical purity.

While developments over the past decade have expanded the number of technetium complexes available to nuclear medicine, this period has also experienced an increase of effort in fundamental research into the chemistry of technetium. That research has improved approaches in the design of new radiopharmaceuticals, extended our understanding of how these complexes are formed, and provided the opportunity for further expansion of the applications of ^{99m}Tc in the next decade.

Recommended Reading

Deutsch E.A., Libson K., Jurisson S. and Lindoy L.F. (1983) *Technetium Chemistry and Technetium Radiopharmaceuticals. In* Progress in Inorganic Chemistry, vol 30, edited by S.J. Lipard, pp. 75–139, J. Wiley & Sons, Inc, New York.

Steigman J. and Eckelman W.C. (1992) *The Chemistry of Technetium in Medicine.* Published by National Academy Press, Washington, D.C.

Nunn A.D. (editor). (1992). *Radiopharmaceuticals: Chemistry and Pharmacology.* Published by Marcel Dekker, Inc, New York.

Verbruggen A.M. (1990) *Radiopharmaceuticals: State of the Art.* Eur. J. Nucl. Med., **17**, 346–364.

Nunn A.D. (1992) *New radiopharmaceuticals based on technetium. In* Progress in Radiopharmacy, edited by P.A. Schubiger and G. Westera, pp. 55–65. Kluwer Academic Publishers, Dordrecht, The Netherlands.

Nowotnik D.P. and Nunn A.D. (1992). *Technetium compounds for imaging myocardial and cerebral perfusion.* Drug News & Perspectives, **5**, 174–183.

Technetium in Chemistry and Nuclear Medicine 2, (1987) edited by M. Nicolini, G. Bandolini and U. Mazzi, Cortina International, Verona, Italy.

Technetium and Rhenium in Chemistry and Nuclear Medicine 3, (1990) edited by M. Nicolini, G. Bandoli and U. Mazzi, Cortina International, Verona, Italy.

Robbins P.J. (1984). *Chromatography of Technetium-99m Radiopharmaceuticals – A Practical Guide,* Society of Nuclear Medicine, New York.

Fritzberg A.R. and Nunn A.D. (1986). *Radio-HPLC: Application to organics and metal chelate chemistry. In* Analytical and chromatographic techniques in radiopharmaceutical chemistry. Edited by D.M. Wieland, M.C. Tobes and T.J. Mangner, Springer-Verlag, New York, 183–212.

References

Abrams M.J., Davison A., Jones A.G., Costello C.E. and Pang H. (1983). *Synthesis and characterization of hexakis(alkylisocyanide) complexes of technetium (I).* Inorg. Chem., **22**, 2798–2800.

Allan O.A. (1961). *The radiation chemistry of water and aqueous solutions.* Published by Van Norstrand, Princeton, NJ, USA.

Anon. (1989). *In vitro stabilization of technetium-99m exametazime (HM-PAO).* Res. Discl., **305**, 666.

Babich J.W. (1991). *Technetium-99m-HMPAO retention and the role of glutathione – the debate continues. Editorial.* J. Nucl. Med., **32**, 1681–1683.

Bacciottini L., Lunghi F., Pupi A., Bonino C., Formiconi A.R., Decristofaro M.T.R., Petti A.R.M. and Meldolesi U. (1990). *Evaluataion of technetium-99m cyclobutylpropylene amine oxime as a potential brain perfusion imaging agent for SPET.* Eur. J. Nucl. Med., **17**, 242–247.

Baker R.J., Bellen J.C. and Ronai P.M. (1975). *Technetium-99m pyridoxylideneglutamate: A new hepatobiliary radiopharmaceutical. 1. Experimental aspects.* J. Nucl. Med., **16**, 720–727.

Baldas J., Bonnyman J., Pojer P.M. and Williams G.A. (1982). *The influence of reducing agents on the composition of ^{99m}Tc-complexes: Implications for ^{99m}Tc-radiopharmaceutical preparation.* Eur. J. Nucl. Med., **7**, 187–189.

Ballinger J.R. and Gulenchyn K. (1991). *Alternative formulations of technetium-99m HMPAO.* Int. J. Appl. Radiat. Isotop., **42**, 315–316.

Barbarics E. and Janoki G.A. (1990). *Synthesis, characterization, biodistribution and metabolism of new technetium-99m etherisonitrile complexes.* Nuklearmedizin, **27**, 103–105.

Bayne V.J., Forster A.M. and Tyrell D.A. (1989). *Use of sodium iodide to overcome the eluate age restriction for Ceretec reconstitution.* Nucl. Med. Commun., **10**, 29–33.

Bergstein P.L. and Subramanyam V. (1986). *Ether isonitriles and radiolabeled complexes thereof.* Eur. Pat. Appl. 86117847.3.

Billinghurst M.W., Abrams D.N. and Lawson M.S. (1991). *Stabilization of [^{99m}Tc]HMPAO-1. Ethanolic preparation.* Int. J. Appl. Radiat. Isotop., **42**, 607–612.

Bormans G., Van Nerom C., De Beukelaer C., Hoogmartens M., De Roo M. and Verbruggen A. (1990). *Comparison of technetium-99m-ECD metabolism in organ homogenates of rat and baboon.* Nuklearmedizin, **26**, 90–92.

Bossuyt A., Morgan G.F., Deblaton M., Pirotte R., Chirico A., Clemens P., Vandenbroeck P. and Thornback J.R. (1991). *Technetium-99m-MRP20, a potential brain perfusion agent:* In vivo *biodistribution and SPECT studies in normal male volunteers.* J. Nucl. Med., **32**, 399–403.

Braat S.H., Lahiri A., Itti R. and Rigo P. (1992). *Comparison of defect size 5 and 240 minutes after injection of Tetrofosmin at peak exercise.* J. Nucl. Med., **33**, 874.

Brandau W., Bubeck B., Eisenhut M. and Taylor D.M. (1988). *Technetium-99m renal function and imaging agents: III Synthesis of Tc-99m MAG3 and biodistribution of by-products.* Int. J. Appl. Radioat. Isotop., **39**, 121–129.

Canning L.R., Nowotnik D.P., Neirinckx R.D. and Piper I.M. (1986). *Complexes of technetium-99m with propyleneamine oximes.* Eur. Pat. Appl. 194,843.

Chervu L.R., Vallabhajoshula S.R. and Blaufox M.D. (1977). *Quality control of technetium lung imaging agents.* Nucl. Med. Biol., **4**, 201–203.

Colombo F., Libson K., Jiang Z., Deleide G., Matarrese M., Bonino C., Belletire J., Lunghi F., Fazio F and Deutsch E. (1990). *Comparative chemical and biological properties of the rCBF agents and ^{99m}Tc-d,l-CB-PAO and ^{99m}Tc-d,l-HM-PAO. In* Technetium and rhenium in chemistry and nuclear medicine 3, edited by M. Nicolini, G. Bandoli and U. Mazzi, pp. 469–474. Cortina International, Verona, Italy.

Dahlberg S.T., Gilmore M.P. and Leppo J.A. (1992) *Effect of coronary blood flow on the 'uptake' of Tetrofosmin in the isolated rabbit heart.* J. Nucl. Med., **33**, 846.

Danpure H.J., Osman S., Saverymutta S.H., Forster A.M., Laidler J.B. and Lavender J.P. (1985). *Evaluation of Tc-99m tin colloid as a selective* in vitro *cell labelling agent for phagocytic cells in whole blood.* Brit. J. Radiol., **58**, 287.

Davison A. (1983). *The coordination chemistry of technetium. In* Technetium in Chemistry and Nuclear Medicine, edited by E. Deutsch, M. Nicolini and H.N. Wagner, pp. 3–14. Cortina International, Verona, Italy.

De Rosch M.A., Brodack J.W., Grommon G.D., Marmion M.E., Nosco D.L., Deutsch K.F. and Deutsch E. (1992). *Kit development for the Tc-99m myocardial imaging agent TechneCard™.* J. Nucl. Med., **33**, 850.

Deutsch E., Elder R.C., Lange B.A., Vaal M.J. and Lay D.G. (1976). *Structural characterization of a bridged Tc-99-Sn-dimethylglyoxime complex: Implications for the chemistry of Tc-99m radiopharmaceuticals prepared by Sn(II) reduction of pertechnetate.* Proc. Natl. Acad. Sci. USA, **73**, 4287–4289.

Deutsch E., Libson K., Becker C.B., Francis M.B., Tofe A.J., Ferguson D.L. and McCreary L.D. (1980). *Preparation and biological distribution of technetium diphosphonate radiotracers synthesized without stannous ion.* J. Nucl. Med., **21**, 859–866.

Deutsch E., Glavan K.A., Sodd V.J., Nishiyama H., Ferguson D.L. and Lukes S.J. (1981). *Cationic Tc-99m complexes as potential myocardial imaging agents.* J. Nucl. Med., **22**, 897–907.

Deutsch E.A., Heineman W.R., Zodda J.P., Gilbert W.T., and Williams C.C. (1982). *No-carrier added technetium complexes: Determination of the total technetium in generator eluents.* Int. J. Appl. Radiat. Isotop., **33**, 843–848.

Deutsch E., Libson K., Jurisson S., and Lindoy L.F. (1983). *Technetium chemistry and technetium radiopharmaceuticals. In* Progress in Inorganic Chemistry, edited by S.J. Lippard, pp. 75–139. J. Wiley & Sons, Inc, New York.

Deutsch E. and Hirth W. (1987). *In vivo inorganic chemistry of technetium cations.* J. Nucl. Med., **28**, 1491–1500.

Deutsch E., Libson K. and Vanderheyden J.L. (1987a). *Technetium-99m myocardial imaging agents. In* Technetium in Chemistry and Nuclear Medicine 2, edited by M. Nicolini,

G. Bandoli and U. Mazzi, pp. 161–168. Cortina International, Verona, Italy.

Deutsch E.A., Vanderheyden J.-L., Gerundini P., Libson K., Hirth W.W., Colombo F., Savi A., and Fazio F. (1987b). *Development of non-reducible technetium-99m(III) cations as myocardial perfusion imaging agents: Initial experience in humans.* J. Nucl. Med., **28**, 1870–1880.

Deutsch E.A., Ketring A.R., Libson K., Vanderheyden J.-L. and Hirth W.W. (1989). *The Noah's Ark experiment: Species dependent biodistributions of cationic ^{99m}Tc complexes.* Nucl. Med. Biol., **16**, 191–232.

Deutsch E.A. (1990). *Cyclo-substituted propyleneamine oxime and its use as a brain imaging agent.* U.S. Patent, 4,895,960.

Di Rocco R.J., Bauer A., Kuczynski B.L., Pirro J.P., Linder K.E., Narra R.K. and Nunn A.D. (1992a) *Imaging regional hypoxia with a new technetium-labeled imaging agent in rabbit myocardium after occlusion of the left anterior descending coronary artery.* J. Nucl. Med., **33**, 865.

Di Rocco R.J., Rumsey W.L., Kuczynski B.L., Linder K.E., Pirro J.P., Narra R.K. and Nunn A.D. (1992b). *Measurement of Myocardial Blood Flow Using a Co-injection Technique for Technetium-99m-Teboroxime, Technetium-96-Sestamibi and Thallium-201.* J. Nucl. Med., **33**, 1152–1159.

Eckelman W.C. (1991). *The status of radiopharmaceutical research.* Nucl. Med. Biol., **18**, (7), iii–vi.

Eckelman W.C., Meinken G. and Richards P. (1972). *The chemical state of ^{99m}Tc in biomedical products. II. The chelation of reduced technetium with DTPA.* J. Nucl. Med., **13**, 577–581.

Eshima D., Fritzberg A.R. and Taylor A. (1990). *^{99m}Tc Renal tubular function agents: Current Status.* Semin. Nucl. Med., **20**, 28–40.

Fisher S.M., Brown R.G. and Greyson N.D. (1977). *Unbinding of Tc-99m by iodinated antiseptics.* J. Nucl. Med., **18**, 1139–1140.

Forster A.M., Storey A.E., Archer C.M., Nagle K.R., Booker F.S., Edwards B., Gill H.K., Kelly J.D. and McPartlin M. (1992). *Structural characterisation of the new myocardial imaging agent technetium-99m Tetrofosmin (^{99m}Tc-P53).* J. Nucl. Med., **33**, 850–851.

Fritzberg A.R. and Lewis D. (1980). *HPLC analysis of Tc-99m iminodiacetate hepatobiliary agents and a question of multiple peaks: Concise communications.* J. Nucl. Med., **21**, 1180–1184.

Fritzberg A.R. and Nunn A.D. (1986) *Radio-HPLC: Applications to organics and metal chelate chemistry. In* Analytical and Chromatographic techniques in radiopharmaceutical chemistry, edited by D.M. Wieland, M.C. Tobes and T.J. Mangner, pp. 183–212. Springer-Verlag, New York.

Fritzberg A.R., Lyster D.M. and Dolphin D.H. (1977). *Evaluation of formamidine sulphinic acid and other reducing agents for use in the preparation of Tc-99m labeled radiopharmaceuticals.* J. Nucl. Med., **18**, 553–557.

Fritzberg A.R., Kuni C.C., *et al.* (1982). *Synthesis and biological evaluation of Tc-99m N,N'-bis(mercaptoacetyl)-2,3-diaminopropionate: A potential replacement for I-131-o-iodohippurate.* J. Nucl. Med., **23**, 223–229.

Fritzberg A.R., Kasina S., Eshima D. and Johnson D.L. (1986). *Synthesis and biological evaluation of technetium-99m MAG_3 as a Hippuran replacement.* J. Nucl. Med., **27**, 111–116.

Fritzberg A.R., Berninger R.W., Hadley S.W. and Wester D.W. (1988). *Approaches to radiolabeling of antibodies for diagnosis and therapy of cancer.* Pharmaceut. Res., **5**, 325–334.

Grogg T.W., Bugaj J.E. and Bates P.E. (1985). *Dry powder imaging kit production by addition of tin metal to stabiliser solution.* U.S. Patent, 4,510,125.

Hammes R., Kies S., Koblenski D. and Julin C. (1991). *A better method of quality control for technetium-99m-sestamibi.* J. Nucl. Med. Tech., **19**, 232–235.

Harris T.D., Edwards D.S. and Platts S.H. (1992). *Synthesis and brain imaging characteristics of isomers L,L, D,D, and D,L of Tc-99m-ECD in monkeys.* J. Nucl. Med., **33**, 979–980.

Hetherington E.L.R. (1983) *Calculation of ^{99}Tc in generator produced ^{99m}Tc.* Int. J. Appl. Radiat. Isotop., **34**, 1638–1639.

Hoffman T.J., Corlija M., Reitz R., Volkert W.A. and Holmes R.A. (1992). *Biological evaluation of the Tc-99m complexes of the d and l isomers of HMPAO.* J. Nucl. Med., **33**, 1032.

Holland M.E., Deutsch E., Heineman W.R. and Holland E.M. (1986). *Studies on commercially available ^{99}Mo/^{99m}Tc radionuclide generators. I. Comparison of five analytical procedures for the determination of total technetium in generator eluents.* Int. J. Appl. Radiat. Isotop., **37**, 165–171.

Huggins D.K. and Kaesz H.D. (1964). *Carbonyl-stretching absorptions in the pentacarbonyl hydrides of manganese, technetium, and rhenium.* J. Amer. Chem. Soc., **86**, 2734–2736.

Huheey J.E. (1972) *Inorganic Chemistry: Principles of structure and reactivity.* Published by Harper and Row, Inc, New York.

Hung J.C., Corlija M., Volkert W.A. and Holmes R.A. (1988) *Kinetic analysis of technetium-99m d,l-HM-PAO decomposition in aqueous media.* J. Nucl. Med., **29**, 1568–1576.

Hung J.C., Volkert W.A. and Holmes R.A. (1989). *Stabilization of technetium-99m-d,l-hexamethylpropyleneamine oxime (^{99m}Tc-d,l-HM-PAO) using gentisic acid.* Nucl. Med. Biol., **16**, 675–680.

Iqbal T., Cain J.H. and Slosky J.J. (1989). *Tris(isonitrile)copper(I) adducts for preparing radionuclide complexes for scintigraphy.* PCT Int. Appl. WO 89,02,433.

Jain D., Mattera J.A., Sinusas A., McMahon M., Zaret B.L. and Wackers F.J.T. (1992). *Biokinetics of Tc-99m Tetrofosmin, a new myocardial perfusion imaging agent: implications for a one day imaging protocol.* J. Nucl. Med., **33**, 874.

Jones A.G., Orvig C., Trop H.S., Davison A. and Davis M.A. (1980). *A survey of reducing agents for the synthesis of $[Ph_4As][TcO(SCH_2CH_2S)_2]$ from [Tc-99]-pertechnetate in aqueous solution.* J. Nucl. Med., **21**, 279–281.

Jones A.G., Davison A. and Abrams M.J. (1983). *Isonitrile radionuclide complexes for labeling and imaging agents.* PCT Int. Appl. WO 83 03,761.

Jones A.G., Abrams M.J., Davison A., Brodack J.W., Toothaker A.K., Adelstein S.J. and Kassis A.I. (1984). *Biological studies of a new class of technetium complexes: the hexakis(alkylisontrile)-technetium(I) cations.* Nucl. Med. Biol., **11**, 225–234.

Jurisson S., Dancey K., McPartlin M., Tasker P.A. and Deutsch E. (1984a). *Synthesis, characterization, and electrochemical properties of technetium complexes containing both tetradentate Schiff base and monodentate tertiary phosphine ligands: single-crystal structure of trans-(N,N'-ethylenebis(acetylacetone-iminato))bis-(triphenylphosphine) technetium(III) hexafluorophosphate.* Inorg. Chem., **23**, 4743–4749.

Jurisson S., Lindoy L.F., Dancey K.P., McPartlin M., Tasker P.A., Uppal D.K. and Deutsch E.A. (1984b). *New oxotechnetium (V) complexes of N,N'-ethylenebis(acetylacetone imine), N,N'-ethylene(salcylideneamine), and o-phenylenebis(salicylidene-amine). X-ray structures of the complexes of N,N'-ethylene-bis(acetylacetone imine) and N,N'-ethylenebis(salicylidine amine).* Inorg. Chem., **23**, 227–231.

Jurisson S., Francesconi L., Linder K.E., Treher E.H., Malley M.F., Gougoutas J.Z. and Nunn A.D. (1991a) *Syntheses, characterization, and reactivity of manganese and rhenium dioxime complexes. X-ray crystal structures of $Mn^{II}(CDO)(CDOH)_2$*

$(BPh(OCH_3))_2$, an unusual pseudoclathrochelate complex, and $Re^{III}Cl(CDO)(CDOH)_2BPh$. Inorg. Chem., **30**, 1820–1827.

Jurisson S., Hirth W., Linder K., Di Rocco R.J., Narra R.K., Nowotnik D.P. and Nunn A.D. (1991b). Chloro→hydroxy substitution on technetium BATO ($TcCl(dioxime)_3BR$) complexes. Nucl. Med. Biol., **18**, 735–744.

Kelly J.D., Neirinckx R.D. and Nowotnik D.P. (1987). *Labelling blood cells with technetium propyleneamine oxime complexes.* Eur. Pat. Appl. 229,718.

Kelly J.D., HIgley B., Archer C.M., Canning L.R., Chiu K.W., Edwards B., Forster A.M., Gill H.K., Latham I.M., Pickett R.D., Webbon P., Edwards P.G., Imran A., Griffiths D.V., York D.C., Mahoney P.M., Tonkinson D.J., Dilworth J.R. and Lahiri A. (1990). *Technetium-99m complexes of functionalised diphosphines for myocardial imaging. In* Technetium and rhenium in chemistry and nuclear medicine 3, edited by M. Nicolini, G. Bandoli and U. Mazzi, pp. 405–412. Cortina International, Verona, Italy.

Kowalsky R.J. and Creekmore J.R. (1982). *Technical artifacts in chromatographic analysis of Tc-99m radiopharmaceuticals.* J. Nucl. Med. Tech., **10**, 15–19.

Kremer C., Leon A., Gambino D., Cartesio S., Ures C., Savio E., Campos E. and Kramer E. (1989). *Solid phase reduction of [99mTcO₄] with zinc. A method for the preapration of difficult ^{99m}Tc complexes* J. Lab. Cmpds. Radiopharm., **27**, 1331–1340.

Kronauge J.F. (1987). *Functionalized isonitrile complexes of technetium as radiopharmaceuticals.* PhD Thesis, Massachesetts Institute of Technology.

Kronauge J.F., Kawamura M., Lepisto E., Holman B.L., Davison A., Jones A.G., Costello C.E. and Zeng C.H. (1990). *Metabolic studies of the myocardial perfusion agent Tc-MIBI. In* Technetium and rhenium in chemistry and nuclear medicine 3, edited by M. Nicolini, G. Bandoli and U. Mazzi, pp. 677–681. Cortina International, Verona, Italy.

Kronauge J.F., Barbarics E., Chiu M.L., Davison A., Holman B.L., Jones A.G. and Piwnica-Worms D. (1992a). *Structure-function relationships for some cationic technetium complexes exhibiting myocardial tissue uptake.* J. Nucl. Med. **33**, 1033.

Kronauge J.F., Noska M.A., Davison A., Holman B.L. and Jones A.G. (1992b). *Interspecies variation in biodistribution of technetium (2-carbomethoxy-2-methyl isocyanopropane)$_6^+$.* J. Nucl. Med., **33**, 1357–1365.

Kung H.F., Molnar M., Billings J., Wicks R. and Blau M. (1984). *Synthesis and biodistribution of neutral lipid-soluble Tc-99m complexes that cross the blood-brain-barrier.* J. Nucl. Med., **25**, 326–332.

Lahiri A., Highley B., Crawley J.C.W., Chui K.W., Edwards B., Smith T., Griffiths D.V., Archer C.M., Latham I.A. and Kelly J.D. (1989) *Novel functionalised diphosphine complexes of Tc-99m for myocardial imaging in man.* J. Nucl. Med., **30**, 818.

Lang J., Barbarics E., Lazar J., Janoki G.A., Papos M. and Csernay L. (1989). *Effects of labeling conditions and formulation of kit on* in vitro *stability of 99mTc-d,l-HM-PAO.* Eur. J. Nucl. Med., **15**, 424.

Leclerq B., Larock M.P., Braat S., Lahiri A., Itti R. and Rigo P. (1992). *Clinical efficacy of Tetrofosmin, a new Tc-99m labelled myocardial imaging agent.* J. Nucl. Med., **33**, 874.

Leveille J., Demonceau G., De Roo M., Rigo P., Taillefer R., Morgan R.A., Kupranick D., and Walovitch R.C. (1989). *Characterization of Tc-99m-L,L-ECD for brain perfusion imaging, part 2: Biodistribution and brain imaging in humans.* J. Nucl. Med. **30**, 1902–1910.

Lever S.Z. and Wagner H.N. (1990). *The status and future of technetium-99m radiopharmaceuticals. In* Technetium and rhenium in chemistry and nuclear medicine 3, edited by M. Nicolini, G. Bandoli and U. Mazzi, pp. 649–659. Cortina International, Verona, Italy.

Lin M.S., Winchell H.S. and Shipley B. (1971). *Method for rapid preparation of technetium-tin(II)-albumin colloid and macroaggregate and a study of their properties.* J. Nucl. Med., **12**, 377–378.

Linder K.E., Malley M.F., Gougoutas J.Z., Unger S.E. and Nunn A.D. (1990). *Neutral, seven-coordinate dioxime complexes of technetium(III): synthesis and characterization.* Inorg. Chem., **29**, 2428–2434.

Linder K.E., Cyr J., Chan Y.W., Raju N., Ramalingam K., Nowotnik D.P. and Nunn A.D. (1992). *Chemistry of a Tc-PnAo-nitro-imidazole complex that localizes in hypoxic tissue.* J. Nucl. Med., **33**, 919.

Loberg M.D., Cooper M. and Harvey E. (1976). *Development of new radiopharmaceuticals based on N-substitution of iminodiacetic acid.* J. Nucl. Med., **17**, 633–638.

Lucignani G., Rossetti C., Ferrario P., Zecca L., Gilardi M.C. Zito F., Perani D., Lenzi G.L. and Fazio F. (1990). *In vivo metabolism and kinetics of technetium-99m-HMPAO.* Eur. J. Nucl. Med., **16**, 249–255.

Lunghi F. (1983). *^{99m}Tc-Radiopharmaceuticals: Development, production, and quality control at industrial level. In* Technetium in Chemistry and Nuclear Medicine, edited E. Deutsch, M. Nicholini and H.N. Wagner, pp. 99–107. Cortina International, Verona, Italy.

Marmion M., Kwiatkowski M., Nosco D., Woufe S., Neumann W., Grummon G., MacDonald J., Chang L.S., Deutsch K., Colombo F., Rossetti C., Fazio F. and Deutsch E. (1991). *Chemistry of a new class of 99m-Tc myocardial perfusion agents with optimized imaging properties.* J. Nucl. Med., **32**, 925.

Marzilli L.G., Kramer A.V., Burns H.D. and Epps L.A. (1983) *Design of technetium radiopharmaceuticals. In* Technetium in chemistry and nuclear medicine, edited by E. Deutsch, M. Nicolini and H.N. Wagner, pp. 63–72. Cortina International, Verona, Italy.

Millar A.M. (1992). *Preparation of $^{99}Tc^m$-exametazime: effect of generator eluate age on radiochemical purity.* Nucl. Med. Commun., **13**, 230.

Molinski V.J. (1982). *A review of ^{99m}Tc generator technology.* Int. J. Appl. Radiat. Isotop., **33**, 811–820.

Moore P.W. (1984). *Technetium-99 in generator systems.* J. Nucl. Med., **25**, 499–502.

Morgan G.F., Deblaton M., Clemens P., Van Den Broeck P., Bossuyt A. and Thornback J.R. (1991). *Technetium-99m-MRP20, a potential brain perfusion agent:* In vivo *biodistribution and SPECT studies in non-primate animals.* J. Nucl. Med., **32**, 500–505.

Nakamura K., Tukatani Y., Kubo A., Hashimoto S., Terayama Y., Amano T. and Goto F. (1989) *The behavior of ^{99m}Tc-hexa-methylpropyleneamineoxime (^{99m}Tc-HM-PAO) in blood and brain.* Eur. J. Nucl. Med., **15**, 100–107.

Neirinckx R.D. and Harrison R.C. (1988). *Method for localization of glutathione involving propylene amine oxime complexes which are retained in cells after reaction mediated by glutathione.* Eur. Pat. Appl., EP 277,754.

Neirinckx R.D., Canning L.R., Piper I.M., Nowotnik D.P., Pickett R.D., Holmes R.A., Volkert W.A., Forster A.M., Weisner P.S., Marriott J.A. and Chaplin S.B. (1987). *Technetium-99m d,l-HM-PAO: A new radiopharmaceutical for SPECT imaging of regional cerebral blood perfusion.* J. Nucl. Med., **28**, 191–207.

Neirinckx R.D., Burke J.F., Harrison R.C., Forster A.M., Andersen A.M. and Lassen N.A. (1988). *The retention mechanism of technetium-99m-labelled HM-PAO: intracellular reaction with glutathione.* J. Cerebral Blood Flow Metab., **8**, S4-S12.

Noll B., Johannsen B., Muenze R. and Spies H. (1991). *Two component kit with nonradioactive precursor for the preparation of an enantiometic form of the kidney function diagnostic agent, technetium-99m-labeled mercaptoacetyltriglycine.* Eur. Pat. Appl. EP 427,360.

Noll B., Johannsen B., May K. and Spies H. (1992). *Preparation of the renal function and imaging agent ^{99m}Tc-MAG$_3$ starting from S-unprotected mercaptoacetyltriglycine.* Int. J. Appl. Radiat. Isotop., **43**, 7.

Nosco D.L., Tofe A.J., Dunn T.J., Lyle L.R., Wolfangel R.G., Bushman M.J., Grummon G.D., Helling D.E., Marmion M.E., Miller K.M., Pipes D.W., Strubel T.W. and Wester D.W. (1990). *New developments in radiopharmaceuticals at Mallinckrodt. In* Technetium and rhenium in chemistry and nuclear medicine 3, edited by M. Nicolini, G. Bandoli and U. Mazzi, pp. 381–392. Cortina International, Verona, Italy.

Nosco D., Wolfgangel R.G., Bushman M., Grummon G. and Marmion M. (1992). *Technetium MAG3 – Labeling conditions and QC.* J. Nucl. Med., **33**, 1033–1034.

Nowotnik D.P., Canning L.R., Cummings S.A., Harrison R.C., Higley B., Nechvatal G., Pickett R.D., Piper I.M., Bayne V.J., Forster A.M., Weisner P.S., Neirinckx, R.D., Volkert W.A., Troutner D.E. and Holmes R.A. (1985). *Development of a Tc-99m-labelled radiopharmaceutical for cerebral blood flow imaging.* Nucl. Med. Commun., **6**, 499–506.

Nowotnik D.P. (1987). *Development of tracers for imaging cerebral blood flow.* Presented at the 194th National Meeting of the American Chemical Society, New Orleans.

Nowotnik D.P. (1989). *Quantitative structure-distribution relationships (QSDRs) of radiopharmaceuticals. In* Radiopharmaceuticals: Using radioactive compounds in Pharmaceutics and Medicine, edited by A.E. Theobald, pp. 28–56. Ellis Horwood Ltd., Chichester.

Nowotnik D.P. (1992). *Technetium-based brain-perfusion agents. In* Radiopharmaceuticals: Chemistry and Pharmacology, edited by A.D. Nunn, pp. 37–95. Marcel Dekker, Inc, New York.

Nowotnik D.P. and Jurisson S. (1992). *Structure and stereochemistry in technetium coordination complexes. In* The Chemistry of Technetium in Medicine, edited by J. Steigman and W.C. Eckelman, pp. 111–130. National Academy Press, Washington, D.C.

Nowotnik D.P. and Nunn A.D. (1992). *Technetium compounds for imaging myocardial and cerebral perfusion.* Drug News & Perspectives, **5**, 174–183.

Nunn A.D., Loberg M.D. and Conley R.A. (1983). *A structure-distribution-relationship approach leading to the development of Tc-99m mebrofenin: an improved cholescintigraphic agent.* J. Nucl. Med., **24**, 423–430.

Nunn A.D., Feld T.A. and Treher E.N. (1987). *Boronic acid adducts of technetium-99m dioxime complexes.* U.S. Patent, 4,705,849.

Nunn A.D. (1990). *Radiopharmaceuticals for imaging myocardial perfusion.* Semin. Nucl. Med., **20**, 111–118.

Nunn A.D., Feld T. and Narra R.K. (1990). *Quantitative structure distribution relationships (QSDRs) of BATOs. In* Technetium and rhenium in chemistry and nuclear medicine 3, edited by M. Nicolini, G. Bandoli and U. Mazzi, pp. 399–404. Cortina International, Verona, Italy.

Nunn A.D. (1991). *Is There Additional Useful Information in the Myocardial Washout Characteristics of Teboroxime? – Editorial.* J. Nucl. Med., **32**, 1988–1991.

Nunn A.D. (1992). *Single Photon Radiopharmaceuticals for imaging myocardial perfusion. In* Radiopharmaceuticals: Chemistry and Pharmacology, edited by A.D. Nunn, pp. 97–139. Marcel Dekker, Inc, New York.

Ohta H., Ento K., Frujita K., Konishi J., Torizuka K., Horiuchi K. and Yokoyama A. (1988). *Clinical evaluation of tumor imaging using $^{99}Tc(V)^m$ dimercaptosuccinic acid, a new tumor-seeking agent.* J. Nucl. Med., **9**, 105–116.

Ohtake T., Kubo A., Bunko H., Nishimura T. and Tamaki N. (1992). *Clinical evaluation of myocardial SPECT using a new technetium-99m diphosphine agent (PNN.1011).* J. Nucl. Med., **33**, 875.

Perrin D.D. (1964). *Organic complexing reagents: Structure, behaviour and application to inorganic analysis.* Published by Interscience, New York.

Peterson E.M., Ryan J.W. and Martin W.B. (1985). *Isopropyl alcohol is a cause of stomach activity on oxidronate bone scans.* Nucl. Med. Biol., **12**, 295–298.

Piwnica-Worms D., Kronauge J.F., Holman B.L., Lister-James J., Davison A. and Jones A.G. (1988). *Hexakis(carbomethoxyisopropylisonitrile) technetium(I), a new myocardial perfusion imaging agent: binding characteristics in cultured chick heart cells.* J. Nucl. Med., **29**, 55–61.

Piwnica-Worms D., Kronauge J.F., Holman B.L., Davidson A. and Jones A.G. (1989). *Comparative myocardial uptake characteristics of hexakis(alkylisonitrile) technetium(I) complexes: Effect of lipophilicity.* Invest. Radiol., **24**, 25–29.

Ponto J.A. (1990). *Effect of pertechnetate source and age on the radiochemical purity of technetium Tc-99m exametazime.* Am. J. Hosp. Pharm., **47**, 2511–2513.

Prenen J.A.C., Deklerk J.M.H., Schip A.D.V. and Vanrijk P.P. (1991). *Technetium-99m-MAG3 Versus Iodine-123-OIH – Renal Clearance and Distribution Volume as Measured by a Constant Infusion Technique.* J. Nucl. Med., **32**, 2057–2060.

Ramalingman K. (1989). *Facile synthesis of 2-methoxyisobutylisonitrile.* Synth. Commun., **21**, 511–514.

Rao T.N., Wester D., Vanderheyden J.L., Kasina S., Adhikesvalu D., Camerman A. and Fritzberg A.R. (1989). *Structures, stereochemistry, and liquid chromatography properties of technetium and rhenium diamide dimercaptide complexes.* J. Lab. Cmpds. Radiopharm., **26**, 44–46.

Reno J.M. and Bottino B.J. (1987). *Improved radionuclide antibody coupling.* Eur. Pat. Appl. 0 237 150 A2.

Rimmer J. (1982). *Radiopharmaceutical composition based on technetium-99m and the reagent for making it.* Eur. Pat. Appl. EP 78,642.

Ruddock C.F. (1979). *Container and methods for producing a diagnostic scanning agent.* Ger. Offen 2,907,880.

Russell C.D. and Speiser A.G. (1980). *Complexes of technetium with hydroxycarboxylic acids: gluconic, glucoheptonic, tartaric, and citric.* J. Nucl. Med., **21**, 1086–1090.

Sachdev S.S., Ramamoorthy N., Nayak U.N., Patel R.B., Ramanathan P., Srivastava S., Lal R., Raghavan S.V., Shah K.B. and Desai C.N. (1990). *Preparation and evaluation of ^{99m}Tc-t-butylisonitrile (^{99m}Tc-TBI) for myocardial imaging: a kit for hospital radiopharmacy.* Nucl. Med. Biol., **17**, 543–552.

Salehi N., Lichtenstein M. and Pojer P.M. (1987). *Technetium-99m radiopharmaceutical preparation by surface absorbed stannous ions.* J. Nucl. Med., **28**, 1041–1046.

Savio E., Kremer C., Gambino D., Kremer E. and Leon A. (1991). *Electrolytic Tc-99mO_4^- Reduction – A Different Pathway to Obtain Tc-99m-Labelled Compounds.* Int. J. Appl. Radiat. Isot., **42**, 669–672.

Shaw S.M. (1985). *Drugs and diseases that may alter the biodistribution or pharmacokinetics of radiopharmaceuticals.* Pharm. Int., 293–298.

Smith J.E., Byrne E.F., Cotton F.A. and Sekutowski J.C. (1978). *A thiol complex of technetium pertinent to radiopharmaceutical use of ^{99m}Tc.* J. Amer. Chem. Soc., **100**, 5571–5572.

Smith F.W., Smith T., Gemmell H., DasGupta P., Archer C., Davidson J., Hinge D., Gvozdanovic D., Forster A., Higley B.,

Nagel K. and Lahiri A. (1991). *Phase I study of Tc-99m diphosphine (P53) for myocardial imaging.* J. Nucl. Med., **32**, 967.

Solanki K.K. (1990). *Stabilization of radioelement complexes in clinical diagnosis. Brit. Pat. Appl.* GB 2,231,267.

Sridhara B.S., Itti R., Braat S., Rigo P., Cload P., Raval U., Hinge D. and Lahiri A. (1992). *Myocardial imaging characteristics of technetium-99m Tetrofosmin for evaluation of coronary heart disease.* J. Nucl. Med., **33**, 875.

Srivastava S.C. and Straub R.F. (1990). *Blood cell labeling with ^{99m}Tc: Progress and perspectives.* Semin. Nucl. Med., **20**, 41–51.

Steigman J., Eckelman W.C., Meinken G., Isaacs H.S. and Richards P. (1974). *The chemistry of technetium labeling of radiopharmaceuticals by electrolysis.* J. Nucl. Med., **15**, 75–80.

Steigman J., Meinken A. and Richards P. (1978). *The reduction of pertechnetate-99 by stannous chloride. The stoichiometry of the reaction in aqueous solutions of several phosphorus(V) compounds.* Int. J. Appl. Radiat. Isotop., **29**, 653.

Steigman J. and Eckelman W.C. (1992) *The Chemistry of Technetium in Medicine.* Published by National Academy Press, Washington, D.C.

Stern H.S., Zolle J. and McAfee J.G. (1965). *Preparation of technetium (Tc^{99m})- labeled serum albumin.* Int. J. Appl. Radiat. Isotop., **16**, 283–288.

Thornback J.R., Deblaton M. and Morgan G.F. (1990). *Preparation of alkylenediamine compounds and complexes especially useful in medical imaging* Eur. Pat. Appl. EP 394,126.

Tofe A. and Francis M. (1976). In vitro *stabilization of a low tin bone imaging kit.* J. Nucl. Med., **16**, 414–422.

Tofe A.J., Bevan J.A., Fawzi M.B., Francis M.D., Silberstein E.B., Alexander G.A., Gunderson D.E. and Blair K. (1980). *Gentisic acid: A new stabilizer for low tin skeletal imaging agents: concise communication.* J. Nucl. Med., **21**, 366–370.

Treher E.N., Francesconi L.C., Gougoutas J.Z., Malley M.F. and Nunn A.D. (1989). *Monocapped tris(dioxime) complexes of technetium(III): Synthesis and structural characterization of $TcX(dioxime)_3B$-R (X = Cl,Br; dioxime = dimethylglyoxime, cyclohexanedione dioxime; R = CH_3, C_4H_9).* Inorg. Chem. **28**, 3411–3416.

Troutner D.E., Simon J., Ketring A.R., Volkert W.A. and Holmes R.A. (1980). *Complexing of Tc-99m with cyclam: Concise communication.* J. Nucl. Med., **21**, 443–448.

Troutner D.E., Volkert W.A., Hoffman T.J. and Holmes R.A. (1984). *A neutral lipophilic complex of ^{99m}Tc with a multidentate amine oxime.* Int. J. Appl. Radiat. Isotop., **35**, 467–470.

Tubergen K., Corlija M., Volkert W.A. and Holmes R.A. (1991). *Sensitivity of Technetium-99m-d,l-HMPAO to Radiolysis in Aqueous Solutions.* J. Nucl. Med., **32**, 111–115.

Tubis M., Krishnamurthy G.T., Endow J.S. and Blahd W.H. (1975). *^{99m}Tc-Penicillamine complexes. In* Radiopharmaceuticals, edited by G. Subramanian, B.A. Rhodes, J.F. Cooper and V.J. Sodd, pp. 55–62. The Society of Nuclear Medicine, New York.

Tweedle M.F. (1983). *Accelerators for forming cationic technetium complexes useful as radiodiagnostic agents.* PCT Int. Appl., 83,02,615.

Vanderheyden J.L., Ketring A.R., Libson K., Heeg M.J., Roecker L., Motz P., Whittle R., Elder R.C. and Deutsch E. (1984). *Synthesis and characterization of cationic technetium complexes of 1,2-(dimethylphosphino)ethane (DMPE). Structure determinations of trans-$[TcV(DMPE)_2(OH)(O)](F_3CSO_3)_2$, trans-$[TcIII(DMPE)_2Cl_2]F_3CSO_3)_2$, and $[TcI(DMPE)_3]^+$ using x-ray diffraction, EXAFS, and technetium-99 NMR.* Inorg. Chem., **23**, 3184–3191.

Van Nerom C., Bormans G., De Beukelaer C., De Roo M. and Verbruggen A. (1990). *Metabolism of technetium-99m-ECD in organ homogenates of baboon.* Nuklearmedizin, **26**, 87–89.

Verbruggen A., Bormans G., Cleyhens B., Hoogmartens M., Vandecruys A. and De Roo M. (1989). *Separation of the enantiomers of technetium-99m-MAG3 and their renal exretion in baboons and a volunteer.* Nuklearmedizin, **25**, 436–439.

Vebruggen A.M. (1990). *Radiopharmaceuticals: state of the art.* Eur. J. Nucl. Med., **17**, 346–364.

Verbruggen A., Bormans G., Van Nerom C., Cleynhens B., Crombez D. and De Roo M. (1990). *Isolation of the mono-ester mono-acid derivatives of ^{99m}Tc-ECD and their distribution in mice. In* Technetium and rhenium in chemistry and nuclear medicine 3, edited by M. Nicolini, G. Bandoli and U. Mazzi, pp. 445–452. Cortina International, Verona, Italy.

Verbruggen A.M. (1991). *Radiopharmaceutical metal-radionuclide complex comprising isonitrile ligands.* PCT Int. Appl. WO 91 19,516.

Verbruggen A.M., Nosco D.L., Vannerom C.G., Bormans G.M., Adriaens P.J. and De Roo M.J. (1992). *Technetium-99m-L,L-Ethylenedicysteine – A Renal Imaging Agent. 1. Labeling and Evaluation in Animals.* J. Nucl. Med., **33**, 551–557.

Vilek S., Machan V. and Kalincak M. (1982). *Technetium-99m-labelled compounds prepared with antimony(III) as reducing agent.* Radiobiol. Radiother., **23**, 333–338.

Vilcek S., Machan V. and Kalincak M. (1984). *Technetium-99m-labelled compounds prepared with molybdenum(III) as reducing agent.* Int. J. Appl. Radiat Isot., **35**, 228–230.

Vilcek S., Kalincak M. and Machan V. (1985). *Technetium-99m-labelled compounds prepared with tungsten(III) as reducing agent.* J. Radional. Nucl. Chem., **88**, 359–367.

Volkert W.A. (1990). *Stereorcactivity of ^{99m}Tc-chelates at chemical and physiological levels. In* Technetium and rhenium in chemistry and nuclear medicine 3, edited by M. Nicolini, G. Bandoli, U. Mazzi, pp. 343–352. Cortina International, Verona, Italy.

Wackers F.J.T., Berman D.S., Maddahi J., Watson D.D., Beller G.A., Strauss H.W., Boucher C.A., Picard M., Holman B.L., Fridrich R., Inglese E., Delaloye B., Bischof-Delaoye A., Camin L. and McKusik K. (1989). *Technetium-99m hexakis 2-methoxyisobutylisonitrile: Human biodistribution, dosimetry, safety, and preliminary comparison with thallium-201 perfusion imaging.* J. Nucl. Med., **30**, 301–311.

Walovitch R., Makuch J., Garrity S., Burgess B., Morgan R., Williams S., Leveille J., Douesnard J., Rigo P., Demonceau G., Cantineau R. and De Roo M. (1988). *Neuropharmacological characterization of Tc-99m ECD in human and nonhuman primates.* Neurology, **38**, 363.

Walovitch R.C., Hill T.C., Garrity S.T., Cheesman E.H., Burgess B.A., O'Leary D.H., Watson A.D., Ganey M.V., Morgan R.A. and Williams S.J. (1989). *Characterization of technetium-99m-L,L-ECD for brain perfusion imaging, part 1: Pharmacology of Tc-99m ECD in nonhuman primates.* J. Nucl. Med., **30**, 1892–1901.

Walovitch R.C., Sakowski R., Hall K., Woodin M., Biegel J., Hua T. and LaFrance N. (1992). *Neurolite^R as an aid in the diagnosis and localization of stroke.* J. Nucl. Med., **33**, 878.

Woulfe S.R., Dunn T.J., Marmion M.E., MacDonald J.R., Rogic M.M. and Deutsch E. (1991). *The synthesis of analogous N_2O_2, N_2OS and N_2S_2 Schiff base ligands for use in radiopharmaceutical imaging agents.* J. Nucl. Med., **32**, 1101.

Yokoyama A., Saji H., Tanaka H., Odori T., Mori T. and Torizuka K. (1976). *Preparation of a chemically characterized ^{99m}Tc-penicillamine complex.* J. Nucl. Med., **17**, 810–815.

Yokoyama A., Hata N., Horiuchi K., Matsuda H., Saji H., Ohta H. *et al.* (1985). *The design of a pentavalent 99mTc-dimercapto-succinate complex as a tumor imaging agent.* J. Nucl. Med., **12**, 273–279.

Zakrzewksi G.A., Ghilardi C.A. and Lingafelter E.D. (1971). *Structure of the cobalt(III) and cobalt(II) complexes of the cage ligand 1,8-bis(fluoroboro)-2,7,9,14,15,20-hexaoxa-3,6,10,13,16,19-hexaaza-4,5,11,12,17,18-hexamethylbicyclo[6.6.6]eicosa-3,5,10,12,16,18-hexaene.* J. Amer. Chem. Soc., **93**, 4411–4415.

Zhou T.Z., Hirth W., Heineman W.R., and Deutsch E. (1988). *Quantitative HPLC determination of ^{99m}Tc-pertechnetate in radiopharmaceuticals and biological samples. I. Technique development.* Nucl. Med. Biol., **15**, 493–498.

Zuckman S.A., Freeman G.M., Troutner D.E. Volkert W.A., Holmes R.A., Van Derveer D.G., and Barefield E.K. (1981). *Preparation and x-ray structure of trans-dioxo(1,4,8,11-tetraazacyclotetradecane)technetium(V) perchlorate hydrate.* Inorg. Chem., **20**, 2386–2389.

Chapter 4

Design of Hospital Radiopharmacy Laboratories

C.R. Lazarus

4.1 INTRODUCTION

The practice of radiopharmacy is now well established in most countries where nuclear medicine is a routine clinical investigation. Radiopharmaceuticals are supplied for use from the radiopharmacy in a form ready to be administered to the patient. A trend now exists in the U.K., Europe and particularly in the USA where radiopharmaceuticals are supplied from one unit to one or more nuclear medicine departments in other hospitals – the so-called 'centralised radiopharmacies'. The radiopharmacy may be defined as 'a laboratory' suite in which radiopharmaceuticals are assembled and supplied in a form suitable for administration to humans'. 'Suitable' means that the person receiving the radiopharmaceutical will not be harmed by it as a result of any handling processes; and it will achieve the purpose for which it is intended. To fulfill this objective the radiopharmacy must perform several functions, but at the same time it must be capable of providing radiopharmaceuticals to the required standard, as well as being a safe place in which to work. This chapter will discuss a number of aspects to be considered in the setting up of a radiopharmacy laboratory. Detailed design considerations are outside the remit of this chapter because local factors such as space, financial budget and scope of work will greatly influence the design of the unit.

4.2 AIMS OF RADIOPHARMACY DESIGN

When setting out to design a radiopharmacy, including its contained equipment, several aims must be borne in mind, which can be summarised in the single word – "PROTECTION" (see Table 1). It is of paramount importance to protect the product from airborne contamination i.e. dust and other particulates which may be present in the environment. These contaminants can be shed from surfaces in the laboratory, carried into dispensing areas from outside in the air, and derive from operators themselves. The Guide to Good Pharmaceutical Manufacturing Practice (1983) (GGPMP) states 'operators and their garments are, potentially, the most significant sources of microbial and particulate contaminate'. It is also imperative to prevent the spread of contamination whether radioactive or of microbial origin, from one product to another by a combination of adequate design of facilities, operation of equipment and satisfactory technique. A radiopharmacy in a busy nuclear medicine department with a heavy patient workload will handle large quantities of radioactivity (up to 100 GBq or more of Tc-99m). It is essential that the operator should be protected from the hazards associated with the radioactivity which include gamma-ray and beta-particle emissions. Other hazards include radioactive aerosols which are created as a result of spillages and careless withdrawal of needles from rubber-capped multidose vials. Radiolabelling of red blood cells, white blood cells and platelets is now routine and often involves 'open' procedures. Such procedures expose the product to the environment at some stage with the potential for ingress of contaminants into the product as well as release of radioactivity to the environment. There is an additional risk here to the operator that the blood sample being labelled may be infected, for example with Hepatitis B virus. The operator must be protected from this hazard. Finally it is necessary to protect the environment from radioactive and microbial contamination in order to reduce the chances of contamination of other products, and reduce the risk to personnel. Sensitive radioactivity measuring equipment (such

Table 1
Aims of Radiopharmacy Design

- To protect the PRODUCT from the ENVIRONMENT, OPERATOR and OTHER PRODUCTS.
- To protect the OPERATOR from radioactivity and PATHOGENIC ORGANISMS.
- To protect the ENIVORNMENT, including EQUIPMENT from RADIOACTIVE and MICROBIAL CONTAMINATION.

as isotope dose calibrators, counting chambers and gamma cameras) must be shielded and protected from stray radiations.

The three aims discussed above are crucial to the design of the radiopharmacy and to ignore or inadequately consider any of them will place products, patients, operators, other personnel and equipment at risk.

4.3 FACTORS TO BE CONSIDERED IN RADIOPHARMACY DESIGN

The radiopharmacy is a laboatory suite in which two basic functions are undertaken:

(i) the handling of radioactivity which is not a sealed source, and
(ii) the preparation of pharmaceuticals, the majority of which will be administered to patients by the parenteral route, and must be sterile and free from pyrogens.

The successful design of a radiopharmacy is a complex process involving many factors. In the early phases of design these factors must be considered together with current regulations, codes of practice and guidelines for the types of work to be undertaken. Different countries will have their own national regulations and guidelines which will incorporate and refer to international recommendations. In the UK relevant regulations are laid down in The Ionising Radiations Regulations 1985 (IRR) and its Approved Code of Practice, The Protection of Persons Against Ionising Radiation arising from any Work Activity, The Ionising Radiations Regulations 1985. General guidance on good practice is given in the Guidance Notes for the Protection of Persons Against Ionising Radiations arising from Medical and Dental Use, 1988. For a more detailed discussion on regulations see Chapter 11. Guidance on the design of facilities can be obtained from the GGPMP. The radiopharmacy should be designed in consultation with the Radiation Protection Adviser (RPA) and others associated with the work and running of the laboratory. The factors to be taken into consideration are shown in Table 2.

Table 2
Factors to be Considered in Radiopharmacy Design

- Radiactivity
- Functions
  - Preparation procedures
  - Quality control
  - Storage
  - Office
  - Research and development
  - Centralized radiopharmacies
- Locations
- Size
- Layout
- Budget

4.3.1 Radioactivity

Nearly all radioactivity handled in the radiopharmacy will be unsealed and the handling areas will be either controlled or supervised depending on the combination of radionuclides and activities used (regulation 8. IRR). A controlled area is any area in which trhe instantaneous dose rate exceeds 7.5 μSvh^{-1} or is likely to exceed this level. Thus a radiopharmacy which handles more than 30 GBq of Tc-99m, 10 MBq of 1-131, 2 GBq of In-111, 3 GBq of Ga-67 or 6 GBq of TI-201 will need to be designated as a controlled area.

A supervised area is one where the surfaces of the room, benches, tables and seats are smooth, non-absorbent and can be cleaned and easily decontaminated. Bench surfaces should be coved to the walls and lipped at the edges. Floor coverings should be a continuous sheet and also coved to the walls. Floors and working benches should be strong enough to support the weight of shielding which it is planned to use. The increased weight of generator shielding with increased generator activity must also be considered. Any work which is liable to cause airborne radioactive contamination should be performed under conditions which contain the radioactivity, and do not present a hazard to the surroundings and personnel. This may involve the inclusion of ventilation exhaust systems in the design, or the use of contained workstations (see later). Wash-hand basins, fitted with knee, foot or elbow taps should be provided at the exit to the rooms.

A controlled area will contain the above features, but in addition other aspects associated with radiopharmaceutical dispensing must also be considered. The size of the controlled area may depend upon the level and type of work. In general it may be easiest to classify the whole room as a controlled area, but the area can be as small as a bench or fume cupboard.

4.3.2 Functions of the Radiopharmacy

The design of the radiopharmacy and the facilities provided will reflect the purposes for which the radiopharmacy is required. A large teaching hospital with a busy nuclear medicine department may wish to incorporate features allowing to perform extensive quality control, research and development, as well as radiopharmaceutical preparation. On the other hand a smaller District General Hospital operating with one gamma camera may require only the simplest of facilities.

4.3.2.1 Preparation Procedures

Unless a nuclear medicine department obtains its radiopharmaceuticals on a daily basis from another institution, it will need to store and use its own Tc-99m generator. Increasing workloads over the years have necessitated generators to be loaded with increasing quantities of radioactivity. These generators are supplied commercially to the radiopharmacy as sterile, pyrogen-free columns shielded with lead or depleted uranium. It is, therefore, necessary to store and elute the generator in such a way that its sterility and apyrogenicity is maintained throughout its period of use. At the same time personnel must be protected from radioactive emissions including release of radioactive droplets which can occur during elution of the generator. Although the evidence that generator columns can be contaminated with microorganisms if stored and eluted on an open bench is inconclusive, it is advisable to locate them in a workstation, where some degree of protection from radiation hazards can be provided. In the UK it is now generally accepted that radiopharmaceuticals should be prepared in accordance with guidance issued by the Department of Health and Social Security (DHSS, 1982) (also see Chapter 11).

The recommendation is that generators should be stored and eluted in a contained workstation, which complies with British Standard BS5295 (1989) for air, quality and BS5726 (1979) for protection of the operator.

Most radiopharmaceuticals are prepared by the simple addition of Tc-99m eluted from a generator and transferred to a kit vial, shaking the vial, or occasionally boiling may be required, followed by a short cooling period. A kit can be regarded as a prepacked set of sterile reagents or ingredients designed for the preparation of a specific radiopharmaceutical. The requirements are that the transfer of radioactivity should be performed aseptically, and that the operator, environment and other personnel should be protected from gamma rays and radioactive aerosols. The use of a kit is to be recommended wherever possible because, as an example of a 'closed' procedure, the radiopharmaceutical can be prepared by the transfer of sterile ingredients from one closed container to another, via a system closed to the atmosphere. The recommendations for this type of work are that the manipulations should be performed in a contained workstation provided with air complying with the requirements of BS 5295. Adequate operator protection conforming to BS 5726 should also be provided. In order to achieve the Class F environment required within the workstation it is necessary that the workstation should be located within a room with a good standard of hygiene, preferably with air filtered to Class K (BS 5295) or Class M (BS 5295) or a Controlled Area (BS 5295).

Few radiopharmaceuticals are prepared by open procedures whereby the ingredients at some stage in the preparation come into contact with the atmosphere. In addition to the increased risk of microbial contamination of the product, there is also an increased radiation hazard due to the possibility of spillage and also the increased preparation time. These procedures should be carried out in a workstation supplied with air conforming to BS 5295. To ensure this standard is maintained the workstation should be sited in a Clean Room of Class F of BS 5295. These facilities will require a two or three stage changing room through which personnel can enter the clean room and where normal clothing can be exchanged for garments appropriate for this standard of facility.

Radiolabelling of autologous blood cells is regarded as an open procedure, although a few workers have described techniques of radiolabelling using closed procedures. Autologous blood carries the potential hazard of viral contamination with, for example, Hepatitis B virus. In order to avoid the risk of cross contamination blood samples should ideally be handled in a separate facility to other work, but under the same conditions as for open procedures. Blood samples should also be handled consecutively with adequate disinfection of workstations between samples.

The oral route has been used for many years for administering radioactive drinks, e.g. I-131. It is now also used to administer a variety of radioactive meals for studying the structure and functioning of the gastrointestinal tract. Although these preparations are not required to be sterile, they must be prepared under hygienic conditions as described in Section 4 of the GGPMP, 1983. However, when handling radioactive materials which are potentially volatile, such as I-131 solutions, it is necesary to use a facility which ensures protectionof the operator from radioactive volatile material. In these examples of open procedures the radiation protection requirements should take precedence over the pharmaceutical requirements.

It is apparent therefore that the design of the radiopharmacy and its facilities depend upon the dispensing procedures to be undertaken. In some cases the need to maintain sterility is most important, whereas in others the radiation protection requirements predominate.

4.3.2.2 Quality Control

A separate room will usually be required for all but the simplest of in-process quality testing of radiopharmaceuticals. It is necesaary to locate larger pieces of equipment, such as radiochromatogram scanners and well counters, in separate areas from those where handling of large quantities of radioactivity may interfere with their performance. Sterility testing should be performed in an area specially designed for this type of work and not in the radiopharmacy. Radioimmunoassays need to be performed in an area separate from radiopharmaceutical manipulation so that the larger quantities of radioactivity associated with radiopharmaceuticals do not interfere with the counting of tracer, quantities of radioactivity handled in the assays.

4.3.2.3 Storage

Adequate storage space should be provided in the clean areas of the radiopharmacy so that equipment used can be kept there, thus minimising the risk of spreading radioactive contamination to other areas, as well as introducing microbial contamination into the radiopharmacy. All other moveable items such as non-radioactive kits, syringes, labels and paperwork should be stored outside the area used for preparation. Materials for dispensing of a radiopharmaceutical should be introduced into the preparation area before the session begins via a suitable hatch. Therefore adequate provision for storage is required outside the dispensing area. In a centralised radiopharmacy provision must be made for the storage of packaging materials and the dispatch of radiopharmaceuticals at sites which are separate from the dispensing area. An area should be provided for receipt and unpacking of all packages, including those containing radioactivity, where the packaging materials cannot compromise the conditions in the dispensing area.

In complying with Regulation 20 (IRR, 1985) it is necessary to provide a secure and shielded store for radioactive substances. This will mainly apply to materials with a longer physical half-life such as TI-201, Ga-67, In-111, Cr-51, and I-131 where there may be an interval of several days between their receipt and use. This storage area can be a room, separate space outside the working area, or a lead-lined safe within the working area. Further information on the amount of shielding required, and design of radioactive substance stores is given in Chapter 14 of the Guidance Notes for the Protection of Persons against Ionising Radiations arising from Medical and Dental use. In addition a lockable, shielded temporary store will be required for solid radioactive waste such as contaminated needles, syringes and vials. It may also be necessary to store used Tc-99m generators for a period of decay prior to their disposal.

4.3.2.4 Office Space

Documentation is an essential and integral function of the radiopharmacy so that records are available of the quality and efficacy of the final product. The achievement of this end results in the generation of quantities of paperwork describing all facets of operating the radiopharmacy. Documentation should not be stored in the dispensing area, but located elsewhere preferably at a readily available position, but also away from radioactive storage areas. Larger radiopharmacies may find that, space permitting, the inclusion of a small office in the design of the radiopharmacy would be of benefit.

4.3.2.5 Research and Development

Progressive nuclear medicine departments will be involved in the research, development and assessment of new radiopharmaceuticals. Depending on the techniques and procedures used a specially equipped laboratory may be required. The housing and use of animals must be in a facility completely separate from the radiopharmacy. Animals, excreta and body samples should not be taken into the areas where radiopharmaceuticals for patients are being prepared. This will elminate the risk of contamination from bacteria, animal hairs and excreta.

4.3.2.6 Centralised Radiopharmacies

In the UK it is now becoming common practice for hospitals which are setting up a nuclear medicine service to obtain their radiopharmaceuticals from an established centralised radiopharmacy. There are several advantages to this arrangement: the centralised radiopharmacy will be staffed by full-time personnel committed to radiopharmacy, and the economical preparation of radiopharmaceuticals with respect to staff, materials and facilities will be ensured. When designing a radiopharmacy with the intention of offering a centralised service, it will be necessary to include provision for extra equipment, radiation protection and personnel. An area separate from the preparation area, and isolated from it, must be set aside for storage of packaging materials and packing.

4.3.3 Location of the Radiopharmacy

The radiopharmacy should ideally be located within the nuclear medicine department to reduce the amount of radioactivity which needs to be transported around the hospital site. Within the nuclear medicine department a site for the radiopharmacy should be chosen such that it is conventient for the injection room, and does not require transportation of radioactivity through areas where patients, secretarial and other personnel may be working. The radiopharmacy must not be located adjacent to areas where radioactivity can affect stored film, gamma cameras and counters, and where low activity measurements are performed. Access to the radiopharmacy for deliveries should ideally be direct from outside the building to facilitate the save transportation of highly radioactive materials, and avoiding complicated routes and patient waiting areas. A site should also be chosen which is not adjacent to areas used for personnel over long periods of time, such as offices, waiting areas and busy corridors. Finally, the site should be inaccessible to unauthorised personnel.

4.3.4 Size of the Radiopharmacy

The radiopharmacy should provide sufficient space for the needs of the functions to be carried out and allow an efficient flow of work. It is advisable to bear in mind that the types of work procedures, as discussed in section 9.3.2.1 may change or increase in the future. For example a small nuclear medicine department may require only the kit preparation of radiopharmaceuticals. At a later date there may be the requirement for the radiolabelling of blood cells. An additional facility would therefore be needed, and the radiopharmacy should be designed with these future developments in mind.

There should be sufficient space within the radiopharmacy to allow the number of occupants to work comfortably and in safety. Space should also be provided for an entry lobby to the laboratory. In this area protective clothing can be donned and stored when not in use.

4.3.5 Layout of the Radiopharmacy

The layout of the rooms within the radiopharmacy suite will depend upon many of the factors already discussed. There are several points, however, which should be emphasised here. It is important to adopt a smooth orderly flow of work within the laboratory, avoiding accidents and confusion in procedural steps. Rooms within the suite should be positioned such that personnel and radioactivity can pass in an orderly way from one to another as the preparation work develops. Where different procedures are to be performed, e.g. kit dispensing, blood labelling, and quality control, they should be carried out in well separated areas and ideally in separate rooms. All clean room areas should be entered via the changing lobby where washing and drying facilities will also be provided. A typical layout for a radiopharmacy is shown in Figure 1.

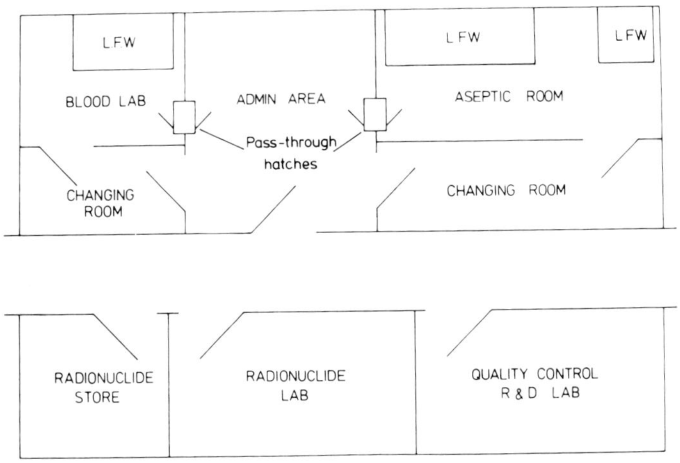

Figure 1. A typical layout for a radiopharmacy.

Guidance on the layout of controlled spaces is given in BS 5295: Part 2: 1989. The standard gives guidance on relevant matters such as access to the controlled space, changing rooms, windows, design concepts, construction, air filtration systems, air movement and ventilation, environmental control, provision of services and commissioning. Radiopharmacies employing clean rooms should have a changing room with three distinct sections; a 'black' area giving direct access to the external environment, a 'grey' area which acts as a transition zone between the 'black' area and the 'white' area from which access can be gained to the clean room. The environmental requirements increase from the 'black' to the 'white' areas such that the latter is maintained at, or near, the level of environmental cleanliness in the controlled space.

4.3.6 Budget

When a decision has been made to build a radiopharmacy, the cost of the project must be considered at a very early stage. The costs will include the building of the site, installation of equipment, running costs and maintenance charges.

If the radiopharmacy is to be built starting with a 'greenfield site' the cost is going to be very large depending on the number of rooms and the complexity of the layout involved. Existing areas can be converted and upgraded which will save considerably on the costings. However, this should be done carefully with considerable thought given to the layout of the rooms, their relationships to each other, and the positions of fans and ducting for air processing. The finishes on the floors, walls and ceilings must be considered. The budget must also allow for the high cost of maintaining the facilities at the high standards requried e.g. air ventilation and cleanliness, humidity, heating and lighting. Service contracts for the equipment such as the microbiological safety cabinets must be taken into account. The cost of staffing the radiopharmacy is, of course, a major budgetary item.

It is a mistake to try to design a radiopharmacy cheaply, yet expect it to be capable of serving all the radiopharmacy functions. This will inevitably lead to a falling of standards resulting in potential hazards to patient, staff and other personnel. It is far safer to consider what is to be demanded of the radiopharmacy, and then design and build within an adequate budget. An increasingly popular alternaive to clean rooms for the radiopharmacy is the purpose-built high integrity enclosure. The use of this 'glove-box' type of unit is considered in more detail in section 9.4. They have an advantage that more than one can be installed in an existing room when space is at a premium. These units may not be cheaper than the construction of clean rooms, (depending on the amount of building work to be done), but they require less space and are probably cheaper to run.

4.4 RECOMMENDATIONS

The radiopharmacy should provide a facility for the preparation of radiopharmaceuticals which satisfies both radiation safety and pharmaceutical quality requirements. The pharmaceutical requirements are described in the GGPMP, 1983, and in other publications (see section 11), and in guidance notes issued by the DHSS, 1982. These requirements have been discussed for the various radiopharmaceutical dispensing procedures in section 9.3.2.1. The guidance given in the above publications is advisory and it is the standards laid down in these publications to which one should aim when designing a radiopharmacy.

The required standards of air cleanliness in the laboratory are those described in BS 5295 which describes twelve classes of environment by the numbers and sizes of particles permitted in each. Part 1 of the standard compares the classes of environment in BS 5295, 1989 with those in the 1976 edition. The requirements of the twelve environmental classes are described. The description of a 'controlled area' is BS 5295 (1976) which was recommended as a suitable environment for the location of a work station used to prepare radiopharmaceuticals from kits, has been replaced by a new class M in the 1989 edition. Class M does have some specifications with regard to the maximum permitted number of particles per cubic metre. Part 2 of the Standard gives guidance on the construction and installation of clean rooms and workstations, and Part 3 the operational procedures in these environments. Part 4 of BS 5295 (1989) is a new part which specifies minimum requirements for monitoring clean rooms and clean air devices to provide continued compliance with Part 1 of the Standard. These British Standards do not have any statutory force, but are invaluable in understanding and discussing the levels required.

In order to provide the aseptic conditions necessary for dispensing radiopharmaceuticals, it is not necessary to have a clean room. A contained workstation within a class M area (BS 5295) is perfectly satisfactory, provided the recommended standard can be demonstrated within the workstation during its operation. The most useful type of workstations are Microbiological Safety Cabinets which are described in the British Standard on Microbiological Safety Cabinets, BS 5726 (1979). There are three classes of cabinet offering protection to the operator, the product and the environment. A Class 1 cabinet is similar to a fume cupboard and it is a requirement to have an efficient mechanical exhaust system to prevent spread of contamination into the working area. These cabinets should not be sited next to a door or window or any place which is subject to cross-draughts. More suitable in the radiopharmacy, however, is a Class II cabinet which is a contained workstation. In this type of cabinet the work area is flushed with a unidirectional downflow of filtered air which can be recycled. A balanced exhaust system is necessary to prevent the air passing from the cabinet into the room through the front opening. A Class II cabinet is suitable for the preparation of radiopharmaceuticals from kits, and for the radiolabelling of autologous blood components. Class III cabinets are of the 'glove-box' design, and are fitted with an exhaust fan which ducts air to outside the building. Air is drawn into the cabinet via a HEPA filter and is exhausted through a HEPA filter. The environment within the cabinet is completely isolated from the room in which the cabinet is situated, and the cabinet is, therefore, suitable for procedures involving volatile or gaseous radioisotopes e.g. radioiodination techniques. As with other British Standards, BS 5726 does not have any statutory force, but is offered for guidance.

The use of a workstation alone does not guarantee the required standard of environment. It is often necessary to locate the workstation in a room which is supplied with filtered air to a level of cleanliness which ensures the required standard within the workstation. Maintenance and operation of such a facility is complex and requires a high degree of skill from operators if the conditions are to be maintained. Entrance to the dispensing area via a lobby, and changing into clean room garments are pre-requisites. This inconvenience is apparent when it is necessary to enter the radiopharmacy to prepare a single dose of radiopharmaceutical which is required for, perhaps, an emergency patient study. In order to avoid many of the problems associated with clean rooms, workstations and changing areas, 'contained enclosures' have been introduced which combine operator safety and product protection with low running costs. An attraction with these enclosures is that they can be installed easily in an existing room and because of their totally enclosed nature, it is not necessary to have a changing area or wear clean garments when operating them. However, recommendations in 'The Rules Governing Medicinal Products in the European Community. Volume IV. Guide to

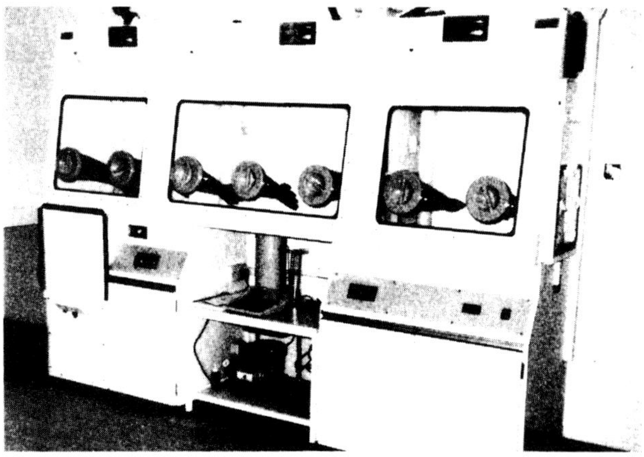

Figure 2. An Amercare™ high integrity glove box containment suite for the storage of technetium generators and reconstitution of scanning agents. (Reproduced with permission of Amercare Ltd).

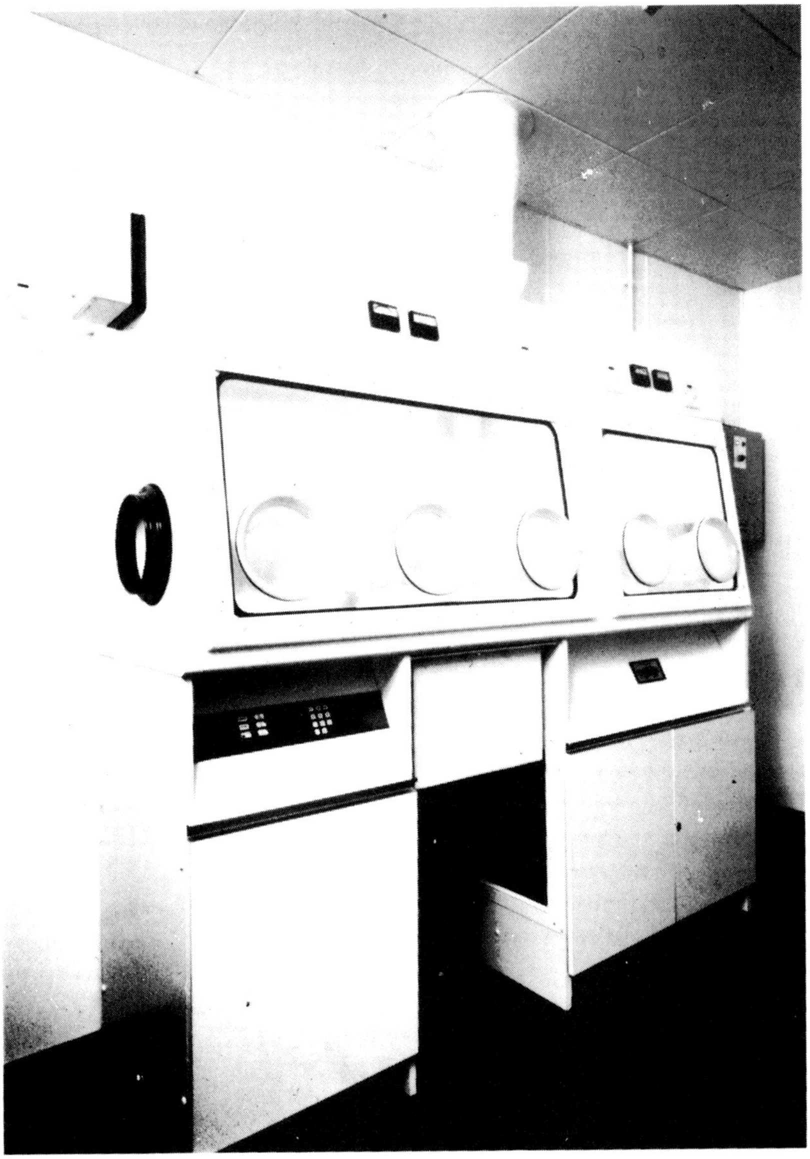

Figure 3. An Amercare™ high integrity glove box containment suite for radio-labelling of blood components. (Reproduced with the permission of Amercare Ltd).

Good Manufacturing Practice for Medicinal Products 'Draft Supplementary Guidelines for the Manufacture of Radiopharmaceuticals' 1992,' state that containment work-stations should be in an 'environment conforming to the equivalent of at least Class K, BS 5295 (1989)'. Such enclosures are offered by Amercare Ltd in their range of Amercare (Trademark) Containment Enclosures (Figure 2 and 3). The range includes a technetium dispensing suite, blood labelling suite, compact blood labelling suite and a volatile products suite. They provide complete containment with a very clean working environment with more than 150 air changes per hour.; Full operator protection is provided using controlled negative pressures within the cabinets. Integral lead shielding is provided for storage of technetium generators, and air is exhausted to outside the building. All equipment necessary for dispensing, including centrifuges and radioisotope calibrators can be included within the enclosure.

In addition to the guidance given in various Guidance Notes by the National Radiological Protection Board; DHSS (1982), and GGPMP 1983, several other publications have produced recommendations for the hospital production of radiopharmaceuticals. These publications tend to recommend the standards given in the official guidelines. The first publication on laboratory design was produced by the British Institute of Radiology (1975, revised 1979). An unofficial report was published by the Hospital Physicist's Association in 1976, and was followed by a technical report written by Kristensen (1979) and published by the International Atomic Energy Agency (I.A.E.A.). This latter report has no official status in the UK, but is officially recommended by the National Health Service of Denmark for use in that Country. Recommendations in a report 'Facilities for the Hospital Production of Radiopharmaceuticals' (1980) were compiled by a group of practicing UK Radiopharmacists and are based on the guidelines in the GGPMP.

The most recent publication Hospital Radiopharmacy Principles and Practice' is an update of the Hospital Physicist's Association report of 1976 and much useful information on laboratory design will be found in that publication.

4.5 CONCLUSIONS

The successful design and establishment of a radiopharmacy requires a careful consideration of many factors, as discussed in the preceeding sections. The design should combine the expertise of a team of experts including radiopharmacists, physicists, architects and others when their current speciality is required. Reference should be made to current regulations and guidelines when producing the design. It should at all times be borne in mind that the aim is to produce a facility capable of supplying radiopharmaceuticals which are safe and efficient to administer to patients, whilst at the same time minimising the hazard to those associated with their supply.

FURTHER READING

Approved Code of Practice, *The Protection of Persons Against Ionising Radiations Arising From Any Work Activity.* The Ionising Radiations Regulations 1985. London HMSO.

British Standards Institution (1989) *Environmental Cleanliness in Enclosed Spaces, Parts 0, 1, 2, 3, & 4.* BS5295, London.

British Standards Institution (1979) *Specification for Microbiological Safety Cabinets.* BS5726, London.

British Institution of Radiology, Special Report No. 11, (1975 revised 1979) *Guidelines for the Preparation of Radiopharmaceuticals in Hospitals.* London: British Institute of Radiology.

Department of Health and Social Security (1982) *Guidance Notes for Hospitals, Premises and Environment for the Preparation of Radiopharmaceuticals.* London HMSO.

Department of Health and Social Security (1983) *Guide to Good Pharmaceutical Manufacturing Practice.* 3rd Edition London HMSO.

Department of Health and Social Security (1977) *Guide to Good Pharmaceutical Manufacturing Practice.* 2nd Edition London HMSO.

Facilities for the Hospital Preparation of Radiopharmaceuticals (1980). Nucl. Med. Commun. 1.54.

Hospital Physicists' Association. Scientific Report Series – 16 (1976) *The Hospital Preparation of Radiopharmaceuticals.*

Kristensen K. (1986). Preparation and Control of Radiopharmaceuticals in Hospitals. International Atomic Energy Agency. Technical Reports Series No. 195 (Vienna: I.A.E.A.).

Medicines Act (1968) London HMSO.

National Radiological Protection Board (1988). *Guidance Notes for the Protection of Persons Against Ionising Radiations Arising from Medical and Dental Use.* NRPB. Oxford.

The Ionising Radiations Regulations (1985) (SI 1985 No 1333) London HMSO.

Institute of Physical Sciences in Medicine (1988) *Hospital Radiopharmacy Principles and Practice,* eds. M. Frier, S.R. Hesslewood, and R, Lawrence. IPSM Report No. 56.

Chapter 5

Techniques for Dispensing of Radiopharmaceuticals

C.R. Lazarus

5.1 INTRODUCTION

Radiopharmaceuticals as prepared in a radiopharmacy are unsealed radioactive substances which will be administered to humans for diagnosis, treatment for research. A radiation hazard may exist with the use of these materials either through external irradiation of the body, or by entry into the body by ingestion, inhalation, or absorption through the skin. The majority of radiopharmaceuticals are administered by the parenteral route, usually intravenously, and they must be sterile and free from pyrogens. It is necessary, therefore, to design protocols and adopt dispensing techniques which will enable radiopharmaceuticals to be prepared in such a way that they are safe to administer to a patient whilst minimizing the hazard to operatives handling the radioactivity, and to other personnel. When labelling autologous blood cells it is also necessary to take precautions against the possible hazard to the operative of handling blood contaminated with a virus.

The design of a hospital radiopharmacy laboratory is discussed in Chapter 4, where current guideline and recommendations are considered with the intention of providing an environment which assures the required quality of the radiopharmaceutical, and minimises the radiation hazard to the operative. The provision of a radiopharmacy conforming to all guidelines, recommendations and regulations does not, however, guarantee the desired quality or protection from radiation hazards. This can only be achieved by an awareness of the hazards, proper training in the use of protocols and dispensing techniques and the use and proper maintenance of equipment in the radiopharmacy.

This chapter aims to give some indication of general working procedures in the radiopharmacy and also describes some currently used dispensing techniques. For a more detailed discussion on operator safety Chapter 4 should be sought.

5.2 GENERAL WORKING PROCEDURES

Internal irradiation occurs when the environment has been contaminated with radioactivity due either to release of radioactive gas, vapours, aerosols or spillage of solutions. Radioactivity can then enter the body by inhalation, ingestion or absorption through the skin. The main aim of working procedures is to prevent the escape of radioactivity during handling, and to protect the product from the environment at the same time. When new procedures are to be introduced, or major changes to existing procedures are to be made, the advice of the Radiation Protection Adviser (RPA) should be sought.

Protective clothing as described in Chapter 14 will reduce the risk of absorption of radioactivity and provide protection for the.product. However, it is important that any cut or other skin damage be properly covered before the workers enter an area where unsealed sources are to be handled. Any cuts sustained during working with radioactivity should be treated immediately and the Radiation Protection Supervisor (RPS) informed. Protective clothing should be put on before entering the working area, and removed on leaving. Unless disposable the clothing should be monitored before removal and placed in appropriate containers if contaminated. Hands should be subsequently washed and monitored together with clothing and the rest of the body. Soap and disposable towels or hot air dryers should be provided.

To avoid ingestion of radioactivity no food or drink should be consumed in the laboratory. Cosmetics should not be applied and smoking must be banned. Foodstuffs should not be stored in refrigerators where radioactive sources are kept. Pipetting should not be done by mouth.

To protect operatives against hazards associated with inhalation of radioactivity it is important that the correct facility should be used. Radioactive gases and solutions releasing radioactivity as vapour e.g. I-131 should be handled in a fume cupboard or workstation where the exhaust from the working area is ducted to the outside of the building, and not allowed to recirculate into the laboratory or other occupied areas. Other manipulative procedures should be performed in appropriate workstations where the chances of inhaling of ingesting radioactivity are reduced, and where the need for aseptic handling can be coped with where necessary. The use of 'closed' manipulative dispensing techniques (see section 5.3) will help to reduce radiation hazards to operatives. Adherence to correct and safe working procedures will also ensure that the radiopharmacy is a safe place in which to work, as well as providing an environment where preparations can be prepared safely.

The working area should be kept tidy and free from articles which will not be immediately required for the work in hand. A cleaning schedule should be in operation for the radiopharmacy, together with procedures for monitoring for radioactive and microbiological contamination (see Chapter 12). The total radioactivity handled and or stored in the radiopharmacy should not exceed the level for which the laboratory has been designed. All radioactive sources, including prepared radiopharmaceuticals should be clearly labelled with the radionuclide, activity, chemical form, reference time and date, and batch number where appropriate. Relevant tests of the quality of generators, radionuclides and prepared radiopharmaceuticals should be performed (see Chapter 9). Radioactive waste and disposal should comply with local rules and guidelines.

5.3 'OPEN' AND 'CLOSED' PROCEDURES

A 'closed' procedure has been defined as 'a procedure whereby a sterile radiopharmaceutical is prepared by the addition of sterile ingredients to a pre-sterilised closed container via a system closed to the atmosphere'. (DHSS, 1982) The use of a solution from an ampoule, whilst strictly not a 'closed' procedure may be considered as such provided the ampoule is opened within a contained workstation, only one withdrawal is made and the contents are added immediately to the closed container. The same reference also defines an 'open' procedure as 'a procedure during which an ingredient or semi-finished product is at some stage after sterilisation open to the atmosphere (i.e. not closed in a vial, syringe, generator or other sealed container). The hazards associated with the use of open procedures are more significant, both to the operatives and to the products. The advantages and disadvantages associated with both types of procedures are summarised in Table 1.

Open procedures should be avoided whenever possible, and are usually used in centres where new radiopharmaceuticals are being developed and commercially prepared products, such as kits (see Section 5.5.2) are not available. The use of open procedures exposes the ingredients to the atmosphere. This means that the product cannot be regarded as sterile and a terminal sterilisation step will be necessary. It also means that there is an increased risk to the operative from radioactivity, although the labelling protocol should emphasise that the radionuclide is added as late in the procedure as possible. If blood is being radiolabelled there is the additional potential hazard in that it may be contaminated with a virus. Closed procedures using sterile ingredients and aseptic techniques are less risky both to the operative and the product in that the ingredients are not exposed to the atmosphere, and there is less risk of spillage. Open procedures, therefore, require more stringent techniques, and cleaner facilities than closed procedures. They may also require additional equipment and a longer preparation time than closed procedures.

The Department of Health and Social Security has, in addition to defining 'open' and 'closed' procedures given recommendations on the standard of facility required for each of those procedures (DHSS, 1982). Radiopharmaceuticals which are to be prepared by open procedures and then terminally sterilised should be assembled in a clean room supplied with air filtered to the requirements of Class J of BS 5295 (1989), and entered via a changing room with hand washing facilities. If the radiopharmaceutical is neither to be terminally sterilised nor prepared by a closed procedure, then an aseptic room with air filtered to the requirements of Class F of BS 5295 (1989) must be used, and the manipulations carried out in a contained workstation. Preparatory work prior to aseptic procedures should be performed in

Table 1
Advantages and Disadvantages of Procedures Involving the Use of 'Closed' and 'Open' Procedures

Closed procedures	*Open procedures*
Ingredients not exposed to atmosphere	Exposure of ingredients to atmosphere
Less risk of spillage	Increased risk of spillage
Less stringent conditions may be used for handling	Full aseptic conditions are necessary
Procedures are rapid and short	Procedures are lengthy
Aseptic technique used	Sterlisation step necessary
Minimum of equipment required	More equipment may be required
Minimum radiation hazard to operatives	Radiation hazard may be higher

Table 2
Summary of the Preparation Conditions Required for Various Dispensing procedures

Procedure	*Preparation conditions*
Generator storage and elution	Contained workstation with air to BS 5295, and BS 5726 for protection.
Kit preparations	Closed procedure performed within a contained workstation with air to BS 5295 Class F, and conforming to BS 5726. The workstation should be within a room with air filtered to BS 5295 Class M or Class K.
In-house preparations e.g. non-kit preparations and monoclonal antibodies to be used same day	For open procedures a clean room supplied with air to BS 5295 Class J if preparation is to be terminally sterilised. For open procedures which are not terminally sterilised an aseptic room with air to BS5295 Class F, and a contained workstation, are required. Preparatory work prior to aseptic procedure should be performed in an adjacent clean room supplied with air to BS 5295 Class J, with connection to the aseptic room via an airlocked hatchway.
radiopharmaceuticals labelled with longlived radionuclides and not used within same day	For closed and open procedures the conditions above for open procedures and not terminally sterilised should be used.
Gases and volatile radionuclides	The workstation should provide adequate protection to the operative and environment.
Blood component labelling	Workstation with air to BS 5295, and Class II or III BS 5726 for protection.
Oral products	Hygienic conditions conforming to BS 5726 for protection for volatile radionuclides.

The above preparation conditions are taken from Guidance Notes for Hospitals, Premises and Environment for the Preparation of Radiopharmaceuticals, DHSS, 1982.

an adjacent clean room supplied with air filtered to Class J of BS 5295 (1989). For open procedure work a changing room must be available so that appropriate protective clothing can be exchanged for normal clothing immediately before entry into the clean rooms. Manipulations performed by closed procedures can be undertaken in less stringent conditions. Manipulations should be performed in a contained workstation complying with the requirements of BS 5295. Class F conditions should be maintained in the working zone of the workstation which should be sited in a room with a good standard of hygiene supplied with air filtered to the requirements of a Class M or Class K Area of BS 5295. These requirements and standards of facility are summarised in Table 2, together with the requirements for other working procedures.

5.4 DISPENSING PROCEDURES

Radiopharmaceuticals will be supplied for use within a nuclear medicine department after preparation by one or more of the dispensing procedures shown in Table 2.

5.4.1 Generators

All radiopharmacies involved in the supply of Tc-99m labelled radiopharmaceuticals will store and use a generator. Several commercial generators are available all consisting of the Mo-99 adsorbed onto a sterile aluminium oxide column. The Tc-99m0_4^- (pertechnetate) is eluted from the column with sterile 0.9% w/v sodium chloride solution (see Chapter 2).

The generator is a sterile system which will be used over a period of one to two weeks, although the pertechnetate will be used for not more than one working day. Generators are now supplied with large quantities of Mo-99 loaded onto the column to supply the increasing demand for Tc-99m and its radiopharmaceuticals.

The storage and elution of the generator should be under conditions which will maintain the sterility of the column and also protect operatives from radiation and radioactivity released from the system as aerosol droplets. These conditions require the use of a contained workstation complying with BS 5295 (1989), inlcuding an unidirectional vertical flow of filtered air, and with BS 5726 (1979) standard of protection to the operative.

An alternative to the contained workstation which is becoming widely accepted is the high integrity glove box containment suite for the storage of technetium generators and reconstitution of scanning agents (e.g. Amercare™ enclosures, see Chapter 4). A separate workstation should be used only for the storage and elution of the generator.

Table 3
Procedures Involved in the Use of Tc-99m Generators

Receipt	Check for damage to casing and generator itself. Check labelling for activity, reference date and time, presence of all components and accessories.
Siting	Generator may require swabbing with antiseptic before location at desired site. Requirements of BS 5295 (1989) and BS 5726 (1979) must observed. Adequate radiation shielding must be provided. A site remote from gamma-cameras, sensitive counting equipment and personnel areas is required.
Elution	Strictly according to manufacturers' instructions. Disinfect with swabs provided. Use vials and eluting solvent provided. Collect eluate in a prelabelled vial, measure activity and volume in vial. Label with activity, volume, time, date and batch number.
Quality tests	Should be performed on at least the first elution of each generator. The final elution should be tested for sterility (see Chapter 9).
Documentation	Record all relevant data on installation, elution and quality testing (see Chapter 11).
Dismantling	Dismantle and store or return according to manufacturer's instructions.

Generator systems are examples of closed systems, and in order to maintain the sterility and integrity of the system they should be eluted strictly in accordance with the manufacturer's instructions using the eluting solvent and collection vials provided. Although the column is shielded with lead or depleted uranium, it may be necessary to use secondary shielding to reduce radiation to desirable levels.

A generator when new will provide Tc-99m in a radioactive concentration which is probably too high for patient use. It will be necessary to dilute to the required concentration using 0.9% w/v sodium chloride solution. The quantity of eluted and dispensed Tc-99m should be measured in a suitable radioisotope ionisation chamber. Other tests of quality should be carried out as described in Chapter 9. The necessary steps involved in the installation, storage and use of Tc-99m generators are described in Table 3. Similar steps will apply to generators of other radionuclides.

5.4.2 Kit Preparation

A kit can be defined as 'prepacked set of sterile ingredients designed for the preparation of a specific radiopharmaceutical' (DHSS 1982). It may be prepared in a hospital pharmacy, but more commonly by a commercial company. The reconstitution of a kit is an example of a closed procedure, but in addition to the advantages listed in Table 1 there are other good reasons why the use of kits should be the preparation procedure of choice whenever possible (see Table 4). Preparation of the radiopharmaceutical is rapid and involves the transfer of the required quantity of Tc-99m in an appropriate volume from the generator elution vial to the kit vial. Subsequent agitation with a short period of standing is then all that is required to form the final product. Boiling may be required for some colloids and other products.

Table 4
Advantages of Kits in Preparing Radiopharmaceuticals

Closed procedure
Rapid and easy preparation of product
Low radiation hazard to operative
Sterile and pyrogen-free product
Stable and diagnostically effective product
Reproducible and reliable product
Long shelf-life of unreconstituted kit
Fully quality-controlled by manufacturer
Readily available
Economic cost patient dose

The radiolabelling is performed in lead or tungsten vial shields, and transfer of radioactivity is by shielded syringe. The radiation hazard to the operative is kept to a minimum because the procedure is rapid and easy to perform. Provided the manufacturers' instruction are strictly adhered to, particularly with regard to maximum activity and volumes of Tc-99m which should be transferred, the final product is sterile, pyrogen-free, reproducible and reliable, supplying a diagnostically effective product. Reconstituted kits are usually stable for six to eight hours, although some can be very much shorter. The kits themselves, as supplied by the manufacturer, have a long shelf-life, usually in excess of one year. They are fully tested before release to ensure their stability, apyrogenicity, efficient radiolabelling and compatibility with eluates from different commercial generators.

Quality testing should be performed on the final product at frequent intervals (see Chapter 9). Although the kits may be expensive to buy, several patient doses can often be drawn from a single vial, and this, together with advantageous prices due to commercial competition, makes them economical in use.

The steps involved in the kit preparation of radiopharmaceuticals are described in Table 5.

Table 5
Procedure Involved in the Preparation of a Radiopharmaceutical Using a Kit.

- Select kit appropriate for study required.
- Calculate amount of Tc-99m and volume required for number of patient studies.
- Gather together kit, radioactivity, syringes, needles, vial and syringe shields, swabs etc.
- Place in workstation following working procedures.
- Reconstitute kit strictly according to manufacturer's instructions.
- Assay vial for radioactivity and label with activity, time, date, volume, batch number, name of product, expiry date, and any other instructions e.g. a warning to shake the vial for particulate preparations.
- Perform quality tests where required (see Chapter 9).
- Release vial for use according to release procedures.
- Record all necessary documentation (see Chapter 11).
- Store the final product according to the manufacturer's instructions.

5.4.3 'In-House' Preparations

Whereas the preparation of a radiopharmaceutical using a kit is an example of a 'closed' procedure, preparations made using 'in-house' formulations involve 'open' procedures. The steps involve the weighing of ingredients, the preparation of solutions, radiolabelling and sterilisation. In-process quality testing is an essential part of this type of procedure. In addition the product should be tested for radiochemical purity, pH, particle size and other parameters where necessary, before administration to the patient.

The disadvantages of the use of 'in-house' procedures are summarised in Table 6. A greater level of protection, both of the product and the operator, is required. Full aseptic conditions are necessary to cope with the increased exposure of the ingredients to the atmosphere associated with lengthier procedures. There is a hazard to the operative from higher radiation doses resulting from increased handling of the radioactivity, particularly with the sterilisation steps and, for example, column chromatographic procedures used in purification of some radiolabelled preparations such as monoclonal antibodies.

Table 6
Disadvantages of the Use of 'In-House' Procedures for the Preparation of Radiopharmaceuticals

Exposure of the contents to the atmosphere.
Procedures can be lengthy.
Higher radiation dose to the operative is possible.
Full aseptic conditions for preparation are necessary.
Sterilisation step is necessary.
Quality testing must be performed before administration of final product to patient.
More equipment may be required.

Most radiopharmacies should avoid the use of 'in-house' preparations in favour of kits. These more hazardous procedures tend to be used in centres developing new radiopharmaceuticals where kits are not available. The procedures involved in the preparations of a radiopharmaceutical by 'in-house' methods are shown in Table 7.

Table 7
Procedures Involved in the Preparation of a Radiopharmaceutical Using 'In-House' Methods

Preparation of master formula.
Acquisition and testing of raw materials, including radionuclides.
Selection and preparation of facilities and equipment.
Preparation of solutions of ingredients.
Calculation and dispensing of radionuclide.
Assembling of radiopharmaceutical from ingredients.
In-process testing where possible.
Purification step where required.
Sterilisation.
Quality testing of final product (see Chapter 9).
Assay for radioactivity and label.
Complete documentation (see Chapter 11).
Release preparation for use according to release procedures.
Store final product appropriately.

5.4.4 Dilution and Subdivision

The situation sometimes arises when a radiopharmaceutical, usually labelled with a radionuclide with a longer $t_{1/2}$ than Tc-99m, e.g. Cr-51, Ga-67, is received and repeated doses are required to be drawn on separate occasions, perhaps several days apart. These preparations often do not contain a preservative. Successive doses can be removed under aseptic conditions, and the remainder returned to stock after resterilisation when possible. Occasionally the volume required to provide an individual dose can be very small. This can occur when the radioactive concentration is high, and also when removing paediatric doses. Examples when these situations can arise are with Cr-51 EDTA for glomerular filtration rate determination when the dose administered must be known accurately; and the use of sodium Cr-51 chromate for red blood cell labelling.

A proven method of dealing with the above situations is to dilute the radiopharmaceutical to the required concentration. The diluted solution can then be dispensed as individual patient doses in separate sterile containers. These can then be removed for use when required.

Several precautions must be taken before dilution. The diluent must be appropriate for the radiopharmaceutical. If in doubt about the compatibility of a diluent, a check should be made with the manufacturer of the radiopharmaceutical. The diluent should be of the desired quality, either if purchased or prepared within the hospital. Preparation of diluents within the hospital is best done by the hospital pharmacy sterile production department. If the radiopharmaceutical contains a preservative this may be diluted to below its effective concentration in the final product. The inclusion of a preservative in the diluent should be considered. Dilution and dispensing into individual patient sterile containers should be done under BS 5295 Class F air conditions. If possible the product should be resterilised before storage. It may be possible to sterilise by aseptic transfer through a sterilising membrane filter into the final container. Appropriate quality testing including radioassay should be performed before release. A sample should always be sent for sterility testing.

5.4.5 Predispensed Products

These radiopharmaceuticals are purchased ready for use. No pharmaceutical manipulations are required before administration to the patient. It is necessary, however, to verify that the details on the manufacturer's label, including radioactivity and reference date, are correct. These preparations can be single dose or multidose depending on the delivery date with respect to the reference date. The contents of the vial should be used on one occasion and the residue discarded if there is no preservative or no possibility of resterilisation. Examples in this category are Tl-201 thallous chloride and In-111-DTPA for cisternography.

5.4.6 Aerosol and Gases

Ventilation studies of the lungs can be carried out with radioactive gases e.g. Kr-81m and Xe-133. However, Kr-81m is available only at infrequent intervals and Xe-133 is limited by the problem of disposal of exhaled air contaminated with the isotope ($t_{1/2}$ = 5.3 days). To improve availability, and take advantage of the ideal properties of Tc-99m, radioactive aerosols of technetium have been developed.

A generator is available for the supply of Kr-81m, and is readily eluted with moist air. The short $t_{1/2}$ of 13 seconds does not present a waste disposal problem, but the generator must be sited next to the gamma camera so that the Kr-81m laden air can be passed directly from the generator to the face mask of the patient via narrow-bore tubing. Extra shielding around the generator may be required. The generator is only available for a single day due to the short $t_{1/2}$ of Rb-81 (4.6 hours), the parent radionuclide of Kr-81m. Xe-133 can be kept in stock for use when required. However, its administration is rather more complex requiring complicated apparatus. It is also necessary to trap the exhaled air. Recently, radioactive aerosols have been labelled with Tc-99m. The radiopharmaceutical is prepared from a kit as a concentrated solution of, for example, Tc-99m-DTPA, and then transferred to a nebuliser. Equipment for the generation of aerosols is available from several commercial suppliers. After loading the Tc-99m-DTPA into the nebuliser, air under pressure is passed through the solution. The generated radioactive aerosol droplets are inhaled into the patient's lungs through the mouthpiece. Droplets larger than those required for the ventilation study settle in the reservoir bag. Exhaled radioactivity is trapped by a filter. One-way flap valves ensure the unidirectional flow of the aerosol. All parts of the system are disposable and it is recommended that they should be replaced at the end of the working day. The mouthpiece should be changed for each patient. The whole system is enclosed in lead shielding, with access for loading and air entry, and administration to the patient.

The use of aerosols is sometimes associated with practical limitations which can interfere with the diagnostic quality of ventilation lung images. The formation of radioactive droplets of a larger than desirable size can produce the appearance of localised hot spots on an image. A newer development in the preparation of a Tc-99m radiopharmaceutical for ventilation imaging is the introduction of 'Technegas'. The preparation is a structured ultra-fine dispersion of Tc-99m-labelled carbon, and is generated by heating Tc-99mO^{-4} in a graphite crucible at 2500°C in an atmosphere of pure argon using dedicated commercially available equipment.

5.4.7 Oral Preparations

Oral preparations can often be used for administering radiopharmaceuticals for diagnosis or therapy. The commonest examples I-131-sodium iodide, or the I-123 equivalent as a solution in water or fruit juice. The required dose is dispensed from the purchased vial and diluted to the required volume, usually 10 ml. The product is administered to the patient via a drinking straw. The dilution and dispensing procedure is anothere example of an 'open' procedure. The radiation hazard to the operative and other personnel from spillage is considerable, particularly at the time of administration to the patient. This hazard can now be reduced b the use of capsules containing an adsorbent material laden with the radionuclide. Capsules are useful for the administration of, for example, large therapeutic quantities of I-131.

Studies of gastric emptying hepatobiliary reflux, transit time and oesophageal reflux are popular in many centres. A variety of recipes have been reported in the literature for each of these studies. The radiolabel in these radiopharmaceuticals is attached to a solid or liquid phase depending on the study to be undertaken. It is possible to use different radionuclides on the two phases at the same time in a dual label study. Bran, ion-exchange resin, scrambled eggs and chicken liver are a few examples of solid materials, and milk and fruit juice as liquid markers. It is important that the solid phase remains as a solid throughout the study or the results may be misinterpreted. The radionuclide should also remain attached to the phase to ensure that it is the food material which is being imaged and not dissociated radionuclide.

Oral preparations are not required to be sterile, but should be prepared under hygienic conditions. Where the radionuclide is volatile, e.g. I-131, a workstation should be used setting the appropriate standards for operator protection (BS 5726) or a fume cupboard.

5.4.8 Blood Labelling

It is common practice in nuclear medicine departments to radiolabel autologous blood cells such as red cells, white cells and platelets. Red cells are labelled with Tc-99m for cardiac and other blood pool imaging. Two techniques are available for radiolabelling, both based on the reduction of pertechnetate within pre-tinned cells. The *in vitro* method involves the removal of a sample of the patient's blood and separation of the red cells. After incubation with tin and addition of pertechnetate the cells are ready for reinjection. The removal of blood from the patient can be avoided using the *in vivo* technique when the tin is administered intravenously into the patient followed by the pertechnetate about 30 minutes later. In addition there is a need to protect the blood from the environment during labelling and to protect the operative from radioactivity and from potentially contaminated blood e.g. Hepatitis B virus. This need is, of course, avoided with the *in vivo* technique.

It is recommended that blood labelling should be performed in a separate area to avoid cross-contamination with other products. Closed procedures should be used wherever possible. Manipulations should be performed in a workstation providing air filtered to Class F BS 5295 and also complying with the requirements of a Class II or III microbiological safety cabinet (BS 5726) (DHSS, 1982). In addition, the radiolabelling should be carried out in a tray of sufficient size to contain spillage. The workstation should be reserved for handling blood samples only, and no other products should be exposed or handled in the room at the same time as the blood samples. After working, gloves, syringes and other apparatus should be assumed to be contaminated and disinfected or disposed of accordingly. Disinfectants must be suitable for use in the presence of blood cells. Centrifugation is a necessary step in the separation of blood cells, and hazards can arise from the production of aerosols of blood during this process. The centrifuge should have a wind shield or sealable buckets so that any aerosols are confined and not released into the radiopharmacy.

The radiolabelling of white cells and platelets with In-111 or Tc-99m present similar hazards to the operative and products. Generally there are more steps involved with labelling these cells than red cells, and there is, therefore, an increased risk. The conditions for radiolabelling are the same as those described above for the *in vitro* labelling of red cells.

The techniques for the radiolabelling of blood cells are described fully in Chapter 7. Several factors to be considered when radiolabelling cells are described in Table 8.

Table 8
Some Factors to be Considered when Radiolabelling Autologous Blood Cells

Need to protect cells from environment.
Need to protect operative from radioactivity and infectious material in patient blood sample e.g. Hepatitis B
Many procedures are open and multi-step. Centrifugation can generate aerosols of hazardous radioactive droplets.
Techniques must provide the necessary protection, and prevent cross contamination with other blood products and other radiopharmaceuticals.
Consider use of kits and adoption of closed procedures whenever possible.
Radiolabel in an isolated area, in a workstation reserved for cell labelling or, ideally, in a workstation in a separate room if the workload is heavy.
Class F of BS 5295 air is required with the protection of a Class II or III microbiological safety cabinet (BS 5726).
Contained enclosures (Amercare) are suitable as described in Chapter 4.

On completion of the cell labelling procedure it is essential to disinfect all equipment which may have come into contact, or have been contaminated by the blood cells. This includes all internal surfaces of the workstation, lead pots and screens, test-tube racks, centrifuge bowl and buckets. Disinfection if necessary to prevent possible cross contamination of subsequent blood samples radiolabelled in the workstation, and transfer of microbiological contamination to other equipment and areas in the radiopharmacy. Recommendations on disinfectants for laboratory use are given in the Code of Practice for the Prevention of Infection in Clinical Laboratories and Post-mortem Rooms (1978) (Appendix 8), but local policy on the use of disinfectants should be followed. In general clear phenolics should not be used for blood and viruses, and although hypochlorites are suitable for small amounts of blood and viruses, they attack metals to varying degrees and should not be used for centrifuges or metal surfaces. Aldehydes such as glutaraldehyde do not readily penetrate organic matter and should be used only on clean surfaces. It is useful for disinfecting centrifuges, but instructions on its use should be carefully followed. Formaldehyde gas can be used to disinfect cabinets and workstations, but equipment manufacturers' directions should be carefully followed.

5.4.9 Monoclonal Antibodies

Recent years have witnessed a surge of activity, both commercially and within hospitals and research institutions, in the development of radiolabelled monoclonal antibodies. This development is an attempt to produce a radiopharmaceutical specific for a certain type of tumour. Mixed success in their development and use, both diagnostically and therapeutically, has been reported in the literature. The production of antibodies is a costly and complex process, beyond the means of most nuclear medicine departments.

Radiolabelling of the antibody is, however, well within the scope of the radiopharmacy. Excellent reviews of technique for labelling with I-123, I-131, In-111 and Tc-99m appear in the literature (Mather, 1985; Mather 1986), and are also covered in Chapter 8.

Although some commercial kits are now available, and can be considered as closed procedures, most radiolabelling of antibodies is by open procedure techniques. This must, therefore, be done under BS 5295 Class F air conditions. It is necessary to protect the operative from radiation hazards, but the volatile nature of some radioiodine solutions must be considered. The recirculating type of workstation is not suitable for the handling of volatile radionuclides unless they have a facility for dumping the exhaust to the outside atmosphere. A suitable type of workstation would be a microbiological safety cabinet, BS 5726 Class III, which is a totally enclosed unit operated through gloved ports. Air is filtered before entry into the cabinet providing the required standard of cleanliness, and then dumped to the outside via another filter to trap any volatile radionuclides. The Amercare enclosure system (see Chapter 4) also provides a suitable facility for labelling antibodies with radioiodine and other radionuclides.

5.4.10 Manipulation of Radioactive Liquids

The techniques used for manipulation of radioactive liquids should minimise the risk of spillage or release of radioactive droplets and aerosols. It should be borne in mind that a single 10 microlitre drop of Tc-99m-pertechnetate from a new generator could contain as much as 50 MBq of radioactivity, and even more in certain circumstances. The inadvertent release of one drop of such a solution would, therefore, constitute a major spill.

In addition to working in trays, the adoption of appropriate techniques in the use of hypodermic syringes and needles can help to minimise release of radioactivity. In the radiopharmacy problems mainly occur with the transfer of radioactive solutions from one vial to another in a closed system e.g. the transfer of Tc-99m-pertechnetate from the elution vial to a kit during reconstitution of the kit. Although carried out less frequently the transfer of radioactive iodine is hazardous and the consequences of a spill can be considerably more serious because of the nature and half-lives of some radioiodine isotopes e.g. I-131.

When withdrawing Tc-99m-pertechnetate from an elution vial an increasing vacuum inside the vial will be created. Some workers cope with the difficulty of subsequent withdrawals against the vacuum. Others prefer to allow air into the vial to relieve the vacuum. This can be achieved with an air-bleed such as 25G needle with an attached sub-micron filter. However, care should be taken when inverting the vial that radioactive solution does not drip from the needle or wet the filter, which will then fail to allow the passage of air. Transferring Tc-99m-pertechnetate to a kit vial will create a positive pressure within the vial. This cannot be allowed to exist, since the next penetration of the rubber septum will cause the sudden release of the overpressure, with expulsion of radioactive droplets. The use of an air-bleed to solve this problem may, in itself, create other problems. The air-bleed will allow air into the kit vial, not only threatening the sterility of the contents, but some Tc-99m-labelled radiopharmaceuticals are unstable in the presence of oxygen in the air. A suitable technique for transferring radioactive solution in a syringe to a closed vial is, after penetration of the septum, to pass some of the solution into the vial, and withdraw an equivalent volume of the the atmosphere in the vial into the syringe. This process can be repeated several times, the actual number depending on the volume to the transferred, until all the radioactive solution in the syringe has been exchanged for atmosphere from the vial. Before withdrawing the needle from the septum a check should be made that the volume of atmosphere in the syringe is that same as the volume of radioactive solution, which has been transferred. This technique will help to ensure that the pressure within the vial is now atmospheric, and will not cause problems with subsequent penetrations.

It is advisable to penetrate a rubber septum with the vial firmly resting on the bench, and needle and syringe approaching vertically downwards. Similarly removal of a needle and syringe should take place with the vial firmly on the bench, and the needle removed in a vertical direction. Needles should always be removed slowly and carefully in order to avoid the creation and release of aerosols of radioactive droplets. Subsequent removals from a vial of a radiopharmaceutical which is sensitive to oxygen will be against increasing vacuum, as air cannot be allowed to enter the vial. Each time a rubber septum is penetrated with a needle a fresh hole should be made to avoid the risk of coring the septum or producing a large hole, which will not close adequately. Particular care should be exercised in the transfer of I-131 solutions so as not to release droplets, or allow drops of radioactive solution to fall from the tip of the needle.

As a matter of good practice it is advisable to aim to use a syringe, which is at least twice the volume of the solution to be manipulated. This technique will increase the distance between the radioactive solution and fingers, thus reducing the radiation dose to the fingers, The use of lead or tungsten syringe shields will also help to reduce the finger dose (see 6.3.7).

5.5 USE AND MAINTENANCE OF CONTAINED WORKSTATIONS

A contained workstation can be defined as a work bench or small working enclosure which has its own filtered air supply and which normally has unidirectional air flow (BS 5295, Part 2, 1989). Such workstations should comply with BS 5295 filtered air, and with BS 5726 for standard of protection to the operator. It should be noted that horizontal air flow workstations provide very little, if any, protection to the operative, and should not be used for the preparation and handling of radioactive materials. The use of workstations does not guarantee the protection of the product or the operative against poor technique. The correct use, location and maintenance of these units will provide the best chance of reaching the levels of protection required.

Written procedures for the operation and maintenance of the workstation should be available. These procedures should cover entry of material into the workstation, manipulation techniques and the exit of the finished product and waste disposed. All items should be appropriately disinfected before entry with recommended disinfectants. The laminar flow of air in these workstations can be disturbed by objects, movements and heating sources within the workstation. The resulting turbulence can create a risk of contamination of the product, and increase the hazard to the operative.

The workstation should be switched on a least 15 minutes before work begins. The 'night door' must always be closed when the workstation is not in use, and then removed at the time the unit is switched on. If an openable viewing panel is provided, this must not be raised when the unit is in use. Apparatus and material in the workstation must be kept to a minimum. All manipulations should be performed within the unit and the work viewed through a lead glass screen. A hand-cleaning procedure before work begins should be in operation, and the appropriate garments donned. Turbulence within the cabinet can be further minimised by using slow hand movements during the dispensing manipulations.

Workstations should be washed down before and after use with a suitable disinfectant e.g. industrial methylated spirits. Formaldehyde disinfection of the cabinet should be carried out according to the manufacturers' instructions. The working surface and inside panels of the workstation should be disinfected with cleaning materials that do not shed particles. If blood spillage occurs within the unit it must be immediately swabbed with a disinfectant which is not inactivated in the presence of organic material e.g. glutaraldehyde 2 per cent solution (e,g, Cidex).

The performance of workstations must be regularly checked. Air-flow indicators should be checked daily, and airflow tested weekly with a vane anemometer. The cabinet must not be used if the airflow is less than 0.75 metres per second at any point on the working face. If the airflow does fall below this level, indicating that the filters may be blocked, then the filters should be changed. Changing of filters must be by designated personnel or the manufacturer's service engineer (BS 5726, 1979). British Standard BS 5295, 1989 part 3, describes the frequency of monitoring and sampling techniques for particulate contamination within the workstation.

Workstations should be tested and serviced by a suitably trained qualified service engineer (i.e. one trained by the manufacturer) at intervals of not more than six months. Fans and electrical components such a lighting should also be checked. Certificates of compliance with the required standards should be provided by the service engineer.

5.6 CONCLUSIONS

To provide the necessary protection of the product and operative written protocols should be prepared and adhered to when preparing radiopharmaceuticals. The appropriate dispensing procedures should be adopted using closed kit preparations wherever possible. Operatives should be made aware of the sources of hazards from radiation and microbiological contamination. They should be trained in techniques which reduce these hazards to an acceptable minimum. The correct techniques for dispensing, use and maintenance of equipment should be an integral part of the training.

Further Reading

K. Kristensen. *Preparation and Control of Radiopharmaceuticals in Hospitals* (1979). Technical Reports Series No. 194. I.A.E.A. Vienna.

Code of Practice for the Prevention of Infection in Clinical Laboratories and post Mortem Rooms (1978). Department of Health and Social Security. HMSO London.

Guide to Good Pharmaceutical Manufacturing Practice (1983). Department of Health and Social Security. HMSO London.

British Standards Institution (1989). *Environmental Cleanliness in Enclosed Spaces.* Parts 0, 1, 2, 3, and 4. BS 5295 London.

British Standards Institution (1979). *Specification for Microbiological Safety Cabinets.* BS 5726 London.

D.H.S.S. (1982). Department of Health and Social Security *Guidance Notes for Hospitals. Premises and Environment for the Preparation of Radiopharmaceuticals.* London D.H.S.S.

References

Mather S.J. (1985). *Immunoscintigraphy. In* Radiopharmacy and Radiopharmaceuticals. Ed. A.E. Theobold. Taylor and Francis, London pp. 29–50.

Mather S.J. (1986). *Radiolabelled Antibodies as Radiopharmaceuticals. In:* Progress in Radiopharmacy. Eds. P.H. Cox, S.J. Mather, C.B. Sampson and C.R. Lazarus. Martinus Nijhoff, Dordrecht, Netherlands. pp. 512–529.

Trott N.G. (1985). *In* Radiopharmacy and Radiopharmaceuticals. Edited by A.E. Theobald, pp. 113–123. London: Taylor and Francis.

Chapter 6

Radiolabelling of Blood Cells – Theory

H.J. Danpure and S. Osman

6.1 INTRODUCTION

Red blood cells (RBC), granulocytes, mixtures of leucocytes, lymphocytes and platelets can be radiolabelled with a variety of radiopharmaceuticals for clinical investigations. Today the most widely used radionuclides are gamma emitters such as chromium-51, technetium-99m and indium-111, although positron emitters such as fluorine-18, cobalt-55 and iron-52 may be used for studies on the positron camera in the near future.

Generally blood cells are radiolabelled *in vitro* then reinjected into the patient where they migrate to various organs of the body depending on the type of cells that are labelled and the health of the patient. For example, labelled granulocytes migrate to the spleen, bone marrow, and liver in a healthy individual, whereas in a patient with a site of inflammation such as an abscess, inflammation in the bowel or inflammation following hip surgery, they also migrate to these sites where they are detected using a gamma camera.

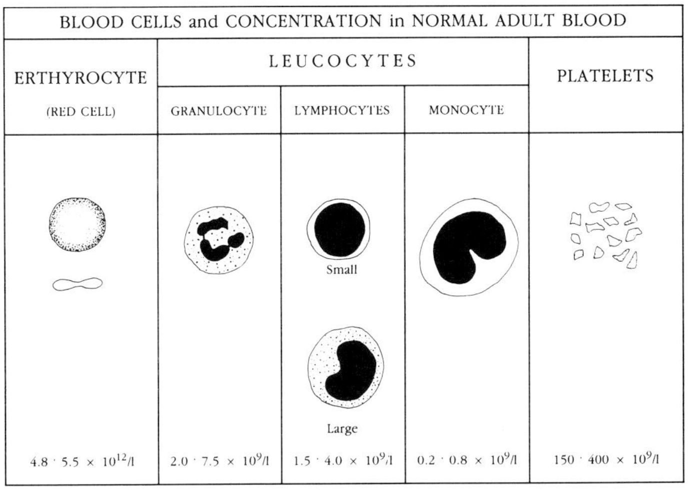

Figure 1. Schematic representation of the types of cell in blood and their concentration in a normal adult.

Thus labelled cells are a non-invasive method of detecting abnormalities in the body. They can also be used for cell kinetic studies.

In order to fully understand the theory and clinical utility of labelled cells a summary of the main blood cell types will first be given. Blood contains several types of cells as shown in Figure 1. Red cells or erythrocytes are non-nucleated biconcave discs with a diameter of 8.5μm which are produced in the bon-marrow at a rate of approximately 200 thousand million per day. They transport oxygen from the lung alveoli to the tissues of the body and transport carbon dioxide back to the lungs using the protein haemoglobin, which is present in the red cells in high concentration (14–15 +/– 2.5 g/dl). A mature erythrocyte is present in the circulation for about 120 days before being destroyed in the spleen.

Granulocytes are highly differentiated non-dividing cells which are produced in the bone-marrow before being released into the blood stream. They are 12–14μm in diameter, i.e. nearly twice the size of the red cells, and are so called because of the granules in their cytoplasm. They are also called polymorphonuclear leucocytes (PMN's) because of their multilobed nuclei. Granulocytes are the most numerous of the white cells (leucocytes) representing up to 75% of the leucocytes in the blood. Granulocytes are subdivided into three groups, neutrophils, eosinophils and basophils, based on their staining properties and in a normal individual more than 90% of the granulocytes are neutrophils. Granulocytes have a half-life in the blood of 6–7 hours and remain in the circulation for about 10 hours before passing through the endothelial blood vessel walls into the tissues of the reticulo-endothelial system (RES), namely the spleen, liver and bone-marrow. They also migrate to sites of infection and inflammation such as abscesses and active inflammatory bowel disease where they ingest particulate matter and micro-organisms by a process called phagocytosis. If the granulocytes are radiolabelled with a gamma-emitting compound their accumulation in the RES tissues and inflammatory sites can be detected as a 'hot' spots on a gamma-camera image (Peters *et al.*, 1983). Although labelled granulocytes are required for studies of inflammatory lesions, such as abscesses, a mixed leucocyte preparation, containing predominantly granulocytes, but also lymphocytes and monocytes and a few platelets, is often used as a source of granulocytes as they are easier to prepare than pure granulocytes.

Granulocytes leave the circulation randomly i.e. irrespective of age, resulting in an exponential disappearance curve if sequential blood samples are counted after injection of labelled cells. Once in the tissues the granulocytes do not return to the circulation but remain in the tissues for about 4 days before being destroyed in the tissues of the RES.

Platelets are non-nucleated cells approximately 3 μm long which are formed by fragmentation of megakaryocytes produced in the bone-marrow. They remain in the blood from 7.3 to 9.5 days (International Committee for Standardisation in Haematology, 1988) before being cleared from the circulation by cells of the RES. Unlike the granulocytes, platelets disappear from the circulation as they get old resulting in a linear curve if sequential blood samples are taken. In addition, if the walls of a blood vessel are damaged the platelets adhere to the damaged area forming a plug or clot to prevent bleeding. This property of platelets has been successfully used to detect thromboses (Knight *et al.*, 1978). In addition, labelled platelets are used to measure platelet life-span (Peters and Lavender, 1983) and monitor the success of kidney transplants (Smith *et al.*, 1979).

In summary radiolabelled blood cells can be used for three types of investigation:

(a) to detect abnormalities in the body.
(b) to monitor response to treatment.
(c) for cell kinetic studies.

6.2 PROPERTIES OF AN IDEAL CELL LABELLING AGENT

Although there are many useful applications of radiolabelled blood cells, finding appropriate methods of radiolabelling them are often difficult as there are several conditions which must be fulfilled. First, the labelled cells must behave the same as unlabelled cells, as it is the normal migratory properties of the cells which are being used to target the radioactivity to specific sites in the body. It is therefore essential that the cells are not modified or damaged during the labelling process. Secondly, the radionuclide used to label the cells must have a suitable energy for detection by a gamma-camera and a half-life which is long enough to allow the clinical study to be completed, but not so long that the patient and the people around them receive a high radiation dose. Finally, the radionuclide should remain on or in the cells throughout the study as any activity released from the labelled cells is likely to hamper interpretation of the images. This problem will be discussed later in the section on labelling leucocytes with Tc-99m HM-PAO (also known as Exametazine, see section 7.3).

6.3 CHELATING AGENTS USED IN CELL LABELLING

Except for F-18, all the radionuclides suggested so far as suitable for labelling cells are metallic elements. Unfortunately, as cells will not incorporate a radio-metal in the form of an inorganic salt, such as In-111Cl_3, other methods are required. The approach that has been successfully used is to form a lipophilic complex between a metal salt and a chelating agent. The complex passes into the cell by passive diffusion. Figure 2 gives the structures of three chelating agents, or ligands, which have been successfully used to label granulocytes and platelets, they are oxine and tropolone which form lipophilic complexes with indium-111 and hexamethyl propylene amine oxime (HM-PAO) which complexes with technetium-99m. The main drawback with this approach is that these lipophilic complexes are non-selective and will diffuse into *any* cells. Therefore if added to whole blood *all* the cells will become labelled. In practice, as the number of red cells in whole blood is 1000 times greater than the number of leucocytes and 10 times greater than the number of platelets, (see Figure 1), nearly all the radioactivity is incorporated into the red cells (Osman and Danpure 1987). To label other cells, such as granulocytes, it is necessary to isolate the required cells from whole blood prior to adding the radioactive cell labelling complex. Thus most of the techniques given in Chapter 7 involve the *separation* and *labelling* of blood cells. In fact the separation procedures are the more time-consuming and need the greater skill in contrast to the cell labelling which is very straightforward and much quicker.

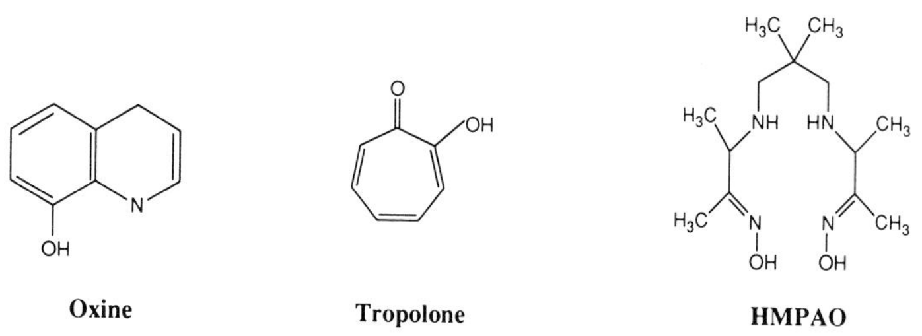

Figure 2. Structure of some cell chelating agents.

6.4 CHOICE OF RADIONUCLIDE

As mentioned above the choice of radionuclide is very important. Currently all clinical studies detect the location of the labelled cells in the patient's body using a gamma-camera and therefore require the cells to be labelled with a gamma-emitting radionuclide. The two most widely used gamma-emitting radionuclides for these studies are In-111 and Tc-99m. They both have half-lives and gamma energies which are suitable for detection on a gamma-camera (see Table 1, Chapter 7).

In general the maximum imaging time should be no longer than three to four times the half-life of the radionuclide. The optimum time to image patients receiving labelled granulocytes or mixed leucocytes is between 1 and 5 hours after administration, occasionally a 24 hour image is also required. These studies can therefore be performed using In-111 or Tc-99m. But for measuring platelet life-span only In-111, with its longer half-life, is suitable as the patient may have to be imaged at 24 hours and blood samples are required for about 5 days.

However, with the increasing use of positron-emission tomography (PET), positron-labelled blood cells may soon be required. For these studies the cells could be labelled with radionuclides such as fluorine-18 (F-18, half-life 110 minutes); iron-52 (Fe-52, half-life 8.3. hours) or cobalt-55 (Co-55, half-life 17.5 hours). Carbon-11 (C-11, half-life 20 min) and oxygen-15 (O-15, half-life 2 min), which are the most widely used radionuclides for PET studies, would not be appropriate for cell labelling studies as their half-lives are too short.

6.4.1 Indium

Indium is a metallic transition element with a valency of three. The radionuclide of indium used for labelling blood cells is indium-111, which has a half-life of 67.9 hours and is produced on a cyclotron by bombardment of a cadmium target with protons (Brown and Beets, 1972). In-111 decays to stable cadmium by electron capture producing two gamma-rays in cascade at 171 and 245 keV plus internal conversion electrons, X-rays and Auger electrons (Table of Isotopes, 1978). The In-111 preparation also contains trace amounts, $<0.08\%$ at reference time, of the longer lived indium isotope In-114m, which has a half-life of 49.5 days. The In-111 used to label cells (from Amersham International) has a high specific activity of >1.85 GBq/μg and is 'no carrier added', which means that no stable indium has been added to the preparation. Although the In-111 preparation contains $<2\,\mu$g/ml indium it contains about ten times more cadmium than indium as cadmium is both the target and the decay product of In-111.

Indium salts are stable at low pH, but hydrolysed above pH 3.5 to produce a precipitate of indium hydroxide or trioxide. Therefore to keep the In-111 in solution In-111 is supplied in 0.04 M hydrochloric acid and should any dilution be necessary the In-111 must be diluted in the same concentration of acid. If it is diluted in water or saline the In-111 comes out of solution and sticks firmly to the wall of the vessel in which it is contained. Indium will however remain in solution above pH 3.5 if it is complexed with a weak chelating agent such as sodium acetate or sodium citrate to form indium acetate or indium citrate. Unfortunately, if indium, in the form of the chloride, acetate or citrate, is administered to the patient intravenously or added to a sample of blood it binds to the plasma proteins, predominantly tansferrin (Hosein *et al.*, 1969) and does not label any cells. Indium, as the chloride, acetate or citrate will however rapidly form lipophilic complexes with many chelating agents (Brady *et al.*, 1985). Two that have been found suitable for radiolabelling blood cells with In-111 are 8-hydroxy quinoline (oxine) and 2-hydroxy-2,4,6, cycloheptatrienone (tropolone). Their structures are shown in Figure 2.

6.4.2 Technetium

All isotopes of the metallic element technetium are radioactive, the one used for labelling cells is technetium-99m which has a half-life of 6 hours and decays by isomeric transition to Tc-99 (half-life 2.1×10^5 years) giving a single gamma ray at an energy of 140 keV. It is produced as a decay product of Mo-99 from a Mo-99/Tc-99m commercial generator. The Tc-99m is separated from the Mo-99 using isotonic saline in the form of sodium pertechnetate ($NaTc\text{-}99mO_4^-$).

In the form of sodium pertechnetate, technetium has a valency of +7 and as such will not label cells nor form complexes with chelating agents. If it is reduced to a valency of +5 with stannous ions it will form an uncharged complex with dl 4,8-diaza-3,6,6,9-tetramethyl-undecane-2,10-dione bisoxime, called hexamethyl propylene amine oxime or HM-PAO (Exametazine) which labels cells (Peters *et al.*, 1987). The structure is shown in Figure 2.

6.5 PARAMETERS REQUIRED FOR SUCCESSFUL CELL LABELLING

Before describing these parameters it is necessary to define the term Labelling Efficiency (LE) as this measurement is used to quantitate the amount of radioactivity incorporated into the cells. To measure the LE the labelled cells should be separated from the medium in which they are labelled by centrifugation. The amount of radioactivity in the cells and the medium is measured and the percent LE is calculated using the following formula:

$$\% LE = \frac{\text{activity in cells} \times 100}{\text{activity in cells} + \text{activity remaining in the labelling medium}}$$

The parameters which affect the amount of a cell labelling agent that is taken up by a cell i.e. the labelling efficiency are:

1. the concentration of chelating agent or ligand present when the cells are radiolabelled;
2. the concentration of plasma in the labelling medium;
3. the cell concentration;
4. the type of cells being labelled;
5. the incubation time and temperature;
6. the pH of the labelling medium.

In general the aim should be to incorporate as much of the added radioactivity as possible i.e. obtain a high LE provided that in so doing the viability of the cells is not adversely affected.

6.5.1 Amount of In-111 or Tc-99m and Chelating Agent Added to Cells

The In-111 and Tc-99m compounds used to label cells are formed by adding 18.5 MBq In-111 or 450 MBq Tc-99m to 50 μg tropolone (0.4×10^{-6} moles) or 500 μg HM-PAO (1.8×10^{-16} moles) respectively. But 18.5 MBq of In-111 contains only 10×10^{-12} moles indium and 450 MBq Tc-99m contains only 25×10^{-12} moles technetium, therefore when these metals react with the ligand only picomole (10^{-12} mole) amounts of the radioactive complex are formed. Therefore almost all of the million fold excess of tropolone or HM-PAO added to the In-111 or Tc-99m does not complex with the radiometal nor is it separated from the complex before it is added to the cells. Some of this non-complexed ligand will react with contaminating stable metal impurities in the radioactive solutions, however most will remain uncomplexed. The concentration of the 'free' ligand affects the amount of the radionuclide which is incorporated into the cells possibly by ensuring that the indium remains complexed to the ligand rather than dissociating. Each cell labelling agent has its optimum concentration of 'free' chelating agent for labeling cells and concentrations above and below result in a lower uptake of the radioactive complex by the cells. This applies even if the amount of radionuclide varies. For example the optimum concentration of tropolone for labelling all types of blood cells with In-111 tropolonate in a plasma-free medium is 4×10^{-5} M (Danpure and Osman 1988a). This increases ten fold when the cells are labelled in a medium containing 90% plasma, (the effect of plasma will be discussed in section 6.5.2 below).

The optimum ligand concentrations for eight different indium-chelating agents have been determined (Brady *et al.*, 1985). Eighty μg/ml HM-PAO was chosen as the optimum concentration for labelling mixed leucocytes (Danpure *et al.*, 1988) and platelets (Danpure and Osman 1988b), as there was insufficient HM-PAO in the commercial kit from Amersham plc to determine the effect at higher concentrations.

6.5.2 Plasma Concentration

Blood cells in the circulation are suspended in plasma, a pale straw-coloured liquid rich in proteins. When leucocytes and platelets were labelled with In-111 oxine it was found that In-111 oxine was not incorporated into cells in the presence of plasma (Thakur *et al.*, 1977). This occurred because In-111 from the In-111 oxine bound to plasma proteins rather than being incorporated into cells. Therefore the cells were washed with saline to remove the plasma and resuspended in saline for labelling. Deleterious effects on the viability of the leucocytes were observed when the cells were removed from plasma (Saverymuttu *et al.*, 1983). Nowadays one of the criteria for any new cell labelling agent is that it should label cells in plasma. Our studies showed that the labelling medium only needs to contain 10% plasma to have a protective effect on cell viability (Roddie *et al.*, 1988).

The amount of any In-111 or Tc-99m complex incorporated into a fixed number of cells decreases as the plasma concentration increases, this is due to competition between cells and plasma proteins for the In-111 or Tc-99m from the metal complexes, (Danpure and Osman 1988a and Danpure *et al.*, 1988).

6.5.3 Effect of Cell Concentration

When cells are labelled in *plasma* with an excess of a cell labelling agent, the amount of In-111 or Tc-99m incorporated into the cells is proportional to the *cell concentation*. For example when 10^8 granulocytes were labelled with In-111 tropolonate in 1 ml 90% plasma a LE of 89% was observed. However, if the same number of cells were labelled in 10 ml plasma i.e. at a cell concentration of 10^7/ml the LE decreased to 30% (Danpure and Osman 1988a). This was due to competition between the cells and the plasma for the In-111 tropolonate.

In the *absence of plasma* there is no competition between the cells and the plasma for In-111 or Tc-99m, and the amount of cell labelling agent incorporated is determined by the *number of cells*, rather than their concentration. The greater the number of cells the more compound is taken up provided there is excess compound, for example, 10^8 granulocytes incorporate more In-111 tropolonate than 10^7 cells when labelled in a plasma-free medium.

6.5.4 Effect of Different Cell Types in Cell Sample

As stated earlier, the In-111 and Tc-99m complexes used to label cells are non-selective and will label all types of cells, but the amount incorporated depends on the type of cell. Larger cells take up more than smaller cells i.e. granulocytes incorporate more than red cells which incoroporate more than platelets. But uptake is not proportional to cell volume. The volume of a granulocyte, a red cell and a platelet are 450, 86, and 10–20 μm^3 respectively (Documenta Geigy, Scientific Tables, 1970). When mixtures containing equal numbers of granulocytes and red cells were labelled nine times more In-111 tropolonate was incorporated into the granulocytes (Danpure and Osman, 1988a) than the red cells, but a granulocyte is only five times bigger than a red cell. Similarly, when equal numbers of platelets and red cells were labelled together, about a third of the In-111 was incorporated into the platelets (Danpure *et al.*, 1990), much more than would be predicted on the basis of the relative volumes of platelets to red cells.

6.5.5 Incubation Temperature

Cells are usually labelled with the In-111 or Tc-99m complexes at room temperature (16–25 °C). Labelling can however be performed at 37 °C but this does not guarantee that an increased uptake will occur. Labelling cells at 4 °C results in a slower rate of uptake.

6.5.6 pH of the Labelling Medium

Cells should be labelled at a pH which ensures maximum viability of the cells even if it results in a lower uptake of the cell labelling complex. The normal pH of blood is 7.4, but the pH of plasma used to label granulocytes and mixed leucocytes is lowered to 7.2 by addition to the anti-coagulant, acid-citrate-dextrose. When labelling platelets the pH of the labelling medium is deliberately reduced even further to a pH of 6.5 to inhibit the spontaneous aggregation of the platelets which occurs at higher pHs.

6.6 HEALTH AND SAFETY ASPECTS IN WORKING WITH BLOOD CELLS

Health and safety aspects of any study involving human blood are very important with the known risks of contracting hepatitis and acquired immune deficiency syndrome (AIDS). It is therefore essential that all personnel who work with blood are fully aware of the dangers and are carefully instructed in the safe handling and disposal of blood samples. It is equally important that they learn the correct procedures for handling and disposal of radioactive substances. Laboratories where *in vitro* cell labelling procedures are performed should contain a laminar flow safety cabinet where the majority of the manipulations take place. The cabinet should only be used for handling blood. Alternatively, an isolator can be used (see Chapter 5). The blood should be spun in a centrifuge with buckets that have sealed caps. Although the provision of suitable laboratory facilities are very important the success or failure of the methods depends on the care and competence of the people who are preparing the labelled cells. This is especially crucial with leucocytes and platelets. It is therefore essential that they receive good instructions preferably from someone who is familiar with the methods. Further information on facilities and quality control procedures have already been published (Danpure and Osman, 1987).

References

Brown L.C. and Beets A.L. (1972). *Cyclotron produced carrier-free In-111.* Int. J. Appl. Rad. Isotopes, **23**, 57–59.

Brady F. *et al.* (1985). *Chelates of In-111 for granulocyte labelling. In:* Radiolabelled cellular blood elements, Pathophysiology, Techniques and Scintigraphic applications. Ed. M.L. Thakur. pp. 427–429. NATO ASI Series, Life Sciences 88, Plenum Press, New York.

Danpure H.J. and Osman S. (1987). *Specificiations and quality control methods for labelled cells. In* Safety and Efficacy of Radiopharmaceuticals 1987, edited by K. Kristensen and E. Norbygaard, pp. 161–184. Dordrecht, Martinus Nijhoff.

Danpure H.J. and Osman S. (1988a). *Optimum conditions for radiolabelling human granulocytes and mixed leukocytes with ^{111}In tropolonate.* Eur. J. Nucl. Med., **13**, 537–542.

Danpure H.J. and Osman S. (1988b). *Investigations to determine the optimum conditions for radiolabelling human platelets with ^{99m}Tc-hexamethyl propylene amine oxime (^{99m}Tc-HM-PAO).* Nucl. Med. Commun., **9**, 267–272.

Danpure H.J. *et al.* (1988). *The development of a clinical protocol for radiolabelling mixed leucocytes with ^{99m}Tc-hexamethyl propylene amine oxime. Nucl. Med. Commun.*, **9**, 465–475.

Danpure H.J. *et al.* (1990). *Labelling autologous platelets with ^{111}In tropolonate for platelet kinetic studies: limitations imposed by thrombocytopaenia.* Eur. J. Haematology, **45**, 223–230.

Documenta Geigy, Scientific Tables, 7th Edition (1970). Edited by K. Diem and C. Lentner, Geigy Pharmaceuticals, Macclesfield.

Hosein E. *et al.* (1969). *Binding of trace amounts of ionic indium-113m to plasma transferrin.* Clin. Chim. Acta, **24**, 69–75.

International Committee for Standardization in Hematology (ICSH) (1988). *Recommended method for indium 111 platelet survival studies.* J. Nucl. Med., **29**, 564–566.

Knight L. C., *et al.* (1978). *Comparison of In-111 labelled platelets and iodinated fibrinogen for the detection of deep vein thrombosis.* J. Nuc. Med., **19**, 891–894.

Osman S. and Danpure H.J. (1987). *A simple* in vitro *method of labelling human erythrocytes in whole blood with ^{113m}In-tropolonate.* Eur. J. Hematol, **39**, 125–127.

Peters A.M. *et al.* (1983). *Imaging inflammation with In-111 tropolonate labelled leucocytes.* J. Nucl. Med., **24**, 39–44.

Peters A.M. and Lavender J.P. (1983). *Platelet kinetics with In-111 platelets: comparison with chromium-51 platelets.* Seminars in Thrombosis and Heamostasis, **9**, 100–114.

Peters A.M. *et al.* (1987). *Tc-99m-HM-PAO for labelling leucocytes in infection.* Lancet **I**, 44.

Roddie M.E. *et al.* (1988). *Imaging inflammation with Tc-99m hexamethyl propylene amine oxime (HM-PAO) labelled leucocytes.* Radiology, **166**, 767–772.

Saverymuttu S.H., *et al.* (1983). *Lung transit of Indium-111-labelled granulocytes. Relationship to labelling techniques.* Scand. J. Haematol., **30**, 151–160.

Smith N. *et al.* (1979). *Indium labelled autologous platelets as a diagnostic aid after renal transplantation.* Lancet, **2**, 1241–1242.

Table of Isotopes (1978). Edited by C.M. Lederer and V.S. Shirley: Chichester, Wiley.

Thakur M.L. *et al.* (1977). *Indium-111 labelled leucocytes for the localisation of abscesses: preparation, analysis, tissue distribution and comparison with gallium-67 citrate in dogs.* Lab. Clin. Med., **89**, 217–228.

Chapter 7

Radiolabelling of Blood Cells – Methodology

H.J. Danpure and S. Osman

7.1 INTRODUCTION

The simplest method of labelling cells would be to give the patient an intravenous injection of a radiolabelled cell-labelling agent to label the cells *in vivo*. The problem with this approach is to ensure that the radio-pharmaceutical reaches the cells and labels them before it is metabolised and excreted. *In vivo* cell labelling has been successfully used to label red cells (see section 7.2.2.2) with Tc-99m pertechnetate and platelets with a platelet-specific monoclonal antibody, P256 (Stuttle *et al.*, 1988), but has not been so successful at labelling granulocytes (see section 7.3).

The approach which has been most widely used for radio-labelling granulocytes, platelets and erythrocytes is to take a fresh sample of venous blood from the patient, label the cells *in vitro* then reinject the labelled cells into the patient. This procedure labels cells of different ages, random labelling, rather than cells of the same age, cohort labelling. Although it is more accurate to measure the life-span of cells of the same age, labelling cohorts of cells takes several days and it cannot be done using the short-lived radionuclides, In-111 and Tc-99m, that are currently preferred for cell labelling. In contrast *in vitro* cell labelling takes up to two hours depending on the type of cells that are being labelled. It requires trained personnel and specialist laboratories for handling the blood, but one of the advantages of this method is that the patient receives only labelled cells and as the methods only involve the removal and reinjection of a sample of blood the technique can be used in very sick patients. This method, unlike any *in vivo* method, can also be used to give quantitative information.

The way that granulocytes and platelets are isolated and the conditions under which they are radiolabelled have a profound affect on the integrity of the cells and amount of the cell labelling agent incorporated into them. Unfortunately there are many different publications describing methods of isolating and labelling granulocytes and mixed leucocytes and therefore it is difficult for someone new to the subject to decide which method to use. There is however a definitive method for labelling platelets (ICSH 1988).

The procedures described in this chapter for labelling granulocytes, mixed leucocytes and platelets are ones that we have developed as a result of extensive *in vitro* experimentation and clinical study.

7.2 RADIOLABELLING ERYTHROCYTES

There are several methods of labelling erythrocytes, some involve labelling red cells *in vitro*, others *in vivo* and a third where a combination of the two is used. Some of these procedures have been published by the International Committee for Standardisation in Haematology (ICSH, 1980a and b). All the isotopes listed in Table 1 are used for labelling red cells though Tc-99m is the most popular. The choice of radionuclide and labelling method will depend on the length of the clinical study and whether the patient has to be imaged. For example, gastrointestinal (GI) bleeding can be detected by administering Cr-51-labelled RBC or Tc-99m-labelled RBC. Chromium-51 cannot be satisfactorily imaged on the gamma-camera but Cr-51 in the faeces will indicate that the patient is bleeding. If it is important to identify the site of bleeding Tc-99m RBC should be used because Tc-99m gives excellent images on the gamma-camera. Although chromium-51 cannot be satisfactorily imaged on the gamma-camera, its gamma-ray can be detected with a probe counter, for example it is used to determine the site of destruction of Cr-51 labelled RBCs. Examples of the clinical uses of

Table 1
Principal Radionuclides Used to Label Blood Cells

Radionuclide	*Half-life*	*Principal emissions (KeV)*
^{111}In	67.9 h	171, 245
^{113m}In	99.5 min	392
^{99m}Tc	6 h	141
^{51}Cr	27.7. d	320

Table 2
Parameters for Clinical Studies with Radiolabelled Red Cells

Clinical use	*Radionuclide*	*Labelling method*	*Relevant section in text*
Blood volume and red cell volume	^{51}Cr	chromate	57.2.1
	^{99m}Tc	*in vitro* or	7.2.2.1
		in vivo/in vitro	7.2.2.3
Red cell life-span	^{51}Cr	chromate	7.2.1
Site of RBC destruction	^{51}Cr	chromate	7.2.1
GI bleeding	^{51}Cr	chromate	7.2.1
	^{99m}Tc	*in vivo*	7.2.2.2
		in vivo/in vitro	7.2.2.3
	^{111}In	oxine/tropolonate	7.2.3.1/3
Spleen function	^{99m}Tc	tin *in vivo*	7.2.2.2
		heat damage and label *in vitro*	7.2.4
Cardiac and vascular imaging	^{99m}Tc	*in vivo*	7.2.2.2
	^{99m}Tc	*in vivo/in vitro*	7.2.2.3
	^{113m}In	tropolonate	7.2.3.2
	^{111}In	tropolonate/oxine	7.2.3.3/1
Compatibility testing	^{113m}In	tropolonate	7.2.3.2
	^{51}Cr	chromate	7.2.1

labelled red cells are given in Table 2 together with the recommended radionuclide, labelling method and its relevant section in the text.

7.2.1 *In vitro* Red Cell Labelling with Chromium 51

Although Cr-51 does not have ideal physical characteristics, with its long half-life of 27.7 days and energetic, low-abundance gamma ray, it is still widely used in non-imaging studies if the investigations include the measurement of RBC life-span which is 120 days in normal individuals. Chromium-51 in the form of sodium chromote enters the red cell where it is reduced from the hexavalent to the trivalent state and binds to the beta-chain of haemoglobin. Chromium is toxic to red cells; the maximum permissible concentration is 2 μg per ml packed red cells. Cr-51 sodium chromate is supplied at a specific activity of 9.25–18.5 MBq/μg (250–500 μCi/μg) and at a concentration of 37 MBq/ml (1 μCi/ml) at reference time (Amersham International). The stock solution should be diluted in saline as required.

Method

1. Collect 8.5 ml blood into a syringe containing 1.5 ml acid-citrate-dextrose (ACD, NIH formula A).
2. Centrifuge the blood at 1200–1500 g for 5 min.
3. Discard the plasma and white buffy coat which sits on top of the red cells and contains the leucocytes and platelets.
4. Slowly, with continuous mixing, add the $Na_2{}^{51}Cr_2O_4$ in at least 0.2 ml saline. The activities required for different investigations are given in Table 3.

Table 3
Maximum Permissible Activity Per Test for Radiolabelled Red Cells Used in Adult Investigations[a]

Investigation	*Radionuclide*	*Maximum activity per test (MBq)*
Red cell volume	^{51}Cr	0.8
	^{99m}Tc	2
	^{111}In	3.7–7.4
	^{113m}In	3.7
Life-span	^{51}Cr	2
Site of RBC destruction	^{51}Cr	4
GI bleeding	^{51}Cr	4
	^{99m}Tc	400
	^{111}In	18.5
Spleen imaging	^{51}Cr	4
	^{99m}Tc	100
	^{113m}In	9.25
Cardiac and vascular imaging	^{99m}Tc	800
Compatibility testing	^{113m}In	1
	^{51}Cr	0.74

[a]Activities for ^{99m}Tc and ^{51}Cr are those recommended by the UK Administration of Radioactive Substances Advisory Committee (ARSAC).

Table 4
Imaging and Post-Injection Samples Times for Clinical Studies with Labelled Red Cells

Clinical study	*Post-injection samples*[a]	*Imaging times*
Blood volume	10, 20 and 60[b] min	–
Life-span	10 min, 24 h, 48 h, 7 d and twice per week until activity in the blood is halved	–
Site of RBC destruction	–	probe counting over heart, spleen and liver at 30–60 min then daily for 14 d
GI bleeding	daily faecal collection (^{51}Cr)	–
	–	with ^{99m}Tc image every 30 min to 2 h then hourly for as long as possible
Spleen function	3, 8, 13, 18, 23, 28 and 60 min	20 min
Spleen size	–	20 min
Cardiac imaging	–	5–30 min gated acquisition
Compatibility testing	3, 10, and 60 min	–

[a]5–10 ml blood anticoagulated with EDTA unless stated otherwise.
[b]Only necessary if mixing time is likely to be long e.g. in patients with splenomegaly, cardiac failure or shock.

5. Leave the blood to incubate at room termperature for 15 min.
6. After radiolabelling, wash the cells with 4–5 volumes of saline. If it is known that the red cells are osmotically fragile, e.g. in patients with hereditary spherocytosis, the red cells should be washed with hypertonic saline at 205 mM (12g/l).
7. Resuspend the cells in 11–12 ml saline. Take up 10 ml into a weighed syringe and reinject into the patient as soon as possible. Note the time and reweigh the syringe. Details of the post-injection samples required for the different clinical uses are given in Table 4.

CALCULATION OF RED CELL AND BLOOD VOLUME

The volume of blood injected is calculated from the following formula:

$$\text{volume injected (ml)} = \frac{\text{weight of suspension injected (g)}}{\text{density of suspension (g/ml)}}$$

where the density of the suspension

$$= 1.000 + \frac{\text{Haemoglobin conc. of suspension (g/1)} \times 0.097}{340}$$

This assumes that the packed red cells have a mean cell haemoglobin concentration (MCHC) of 340 g/l and a density of 1.097 g/ml.

Measure the packed cell volume (PVC) of samples of blood taken at 10, 20 and if necessary 60 min, as described by Dacie and Lewis (1984). Lyse the remained with a detergent such as saponin and measure the radioactivity in 2 or 3 ml aliquots. Prepare a standard from the remaining original sample by diluting it 1/100 in water and measure the radioactivity in 2 or 3 ml samples.

Red cell volume (RCV) = [radioactivity of standard (cpm/ml) × dilution of standard × volume injected (ml)]/[radioactivity of post-injection sample (cpm/ml)].

The blood volume can be calculated from the RCV using the following equation:

$$\text{Blood volume (BV)} = \frac{\text{RCV}}{\text{whole body PCV}}$$

where the whole body PCV or haematocrit is approximately 0.9 times the PCV measured on the venous blood (ICSH, 1980b).

7.2.2 Red Cell Labelling with Technetium-99m

All the methods of labelling red cells with Tc-99m outlined below involve treating the red cells with a reducing agent, usually stannous tin in the form of chloride, fluoride, pyrophosphate, citrate or DTPA followed by administration of the technetium in the form of pertechnetate (Tc-99m-O_4^-), the labelling may be done *in vivo* or *in vitro*. The stannous tin is necessary because pertechnetate freely diffuses in and out of cells, whereas if it is reduced within the cells it becomes bound to the beta-chain of haemoglobin and is retained by the cell. It is also important to remove any surplus extracellular stannous ions before the Tc-99m pertechnetate is added, because it could reduce the (Tc-99m O_4^-) to a form which is unable to penetrate the cells with the result that the porportion of the technetium which becomes cell-associated, will be reduced. The amount of Tc-99m incorporated by the cells is called the labelling efficiency.

Labelling efficiency (LE) =

$$\frac{\text{amount of technetium-99 m incorporated by cells}}{\text{total amount of technetium-99 m added to cells}} \times 100\%$$

It is not possible to get rid of excess stannous ions or measure the LE if the cells are labelled *in vivo*, so in this situation it is important to ensure that the amount of tin is kept low. Although methods vary, 10–20 μg stannous ions per kilogram should be satisfactory. Using this amount of tin Popescu *et al.*, (1984) found that 5 minutes after injection of the Tc-99m pertechnetate 96% of the technetium was bound to the red cells and it remained at this level for 60 mins. But there have been several reports that in the presence of heparin low labelling efficiences have been obtained Rao *et al.* (1986). With the *in vitro* or *in vivo/in vitro* methods the amount of stannous ions used is not so important because any excess can be washed from the cells before the Tc-99mO_4^- is added.

Unfortunately stannous salts are unstable in solution and are readily oxidised to stannic salts which are not transported across the red cell membrane. The solutions of stannous salts therefore have to be prepared just before use.

7.2.2.1 *In vitro* Red Cell Labelling with Technetium-99m

The method of labelling red cells with Tc-99m given below is that of Jones and Mollison (1978): is is also given by Dacie and Lewis (1984). Using this method most of the Tc-99m remains cell-associated, but about 5% of the Tc-99m is released or eluted from the cells per hour. This method is only used for the estimation of red cell and blood volume.

Method

1. Collect 10 ml blood into a syringe containing 200 International Units (IU) of heparin, add 20 ml sterile saline, centrifuge at 1200–1500 g for 5 min, remove and discard as much of the plasma/saline supernatant and buffy coat as possible.
2. Weigh out 2 mg of stannous chloride ($SnCl_2.H_2O$) and dissolve it in 20 ml isotonic saline. Sterlise the solution by passing it through a 0.22 μm Millipore filter. Add 0.2 ml of this solution to 100 ml saline to give a solution containing 0.2 μg/ml stannous chloride and approximately 0.1 μg/ml stannous ions. Using a 1 ml syringe add 0.3 ml (0.03 μg tin) to the packed red cells (about 5 ml) to give an approximate final concentration of 0.006 μg tin/ml red cells. As the stannous chloride is readily oxidised it is very important that the time between preparing the solution of stannous chloride and adding it to the red cells does not exceed 10 min.
3. Incubate the blood with the tin for 5 min at room temperature (RT). Using this low tin concentration it is not necesary to wash the cells.
4. Add 2 MBq Tc-99m-O_4^- in 0.2 ml saline, freshly eluted from the generator, and incubate for 5 min at RT.
5. Add about 10 ml ice-cold saline to the cells and centrifuge at 1200–1500 g for 5 min. Discard the supernatant and resuspend the cells in 25 ml of the same ice-cold saline for injection. Store the labelled cells on ice until they are ready to be injected. The method for calculating red cell volume is the same as that given for Cr-51 in section 7.2.1.

7.2.2.2 *In vivo* Red Cell Labelling with Technetium-99m

Although the *in vitro* method of labelling red cells gives satisfactory results the procedure is time-consuming and requires a sterile environment in which to manipulate the cells. To overcome these difficulties a method which radiolabels the red cells *in vivo* was published by Pavel *et al.* (1977). The method simply involved injecting two solutions, first a solution of stannous tin followed later by Tc-99m pertechnetate i.e. the red cells incorporated the tin *in vivo* so that when the pertechnetate was subsequently injected it was taken up by the red cells, reduced by the tin and retained by the cells. The problem with this method is that the labelling efficiency (LE) was found to be variable. This method is not quantitative and cannot be used for the measurement of red cell volume. It is however useful for detecting GI bleeding and studying cardiac function.

Method

1. Reconstitute the Amerscan stannous agent (Amersham International) which contains 4 mg stannous fluoride (3 mg of tin) and 6.8 mg sodium medronate with 6 ml saline and inject 0.03 ml per kg body weight (equivalent to 15 μg/kg tin).
2. After a lag of 20–40 mins to allow thorough mixing with the blood intravenously inject the amount of pertechnetate required for the clinical study as given in Table 3.

7.2.2.3 *In vivo/in vitro* Red Cell Labelling with Technetium-99m

A combination of the *in vitro* and *in vivo* methods has also been developed to produce a simple yet quantitiative method for radiolabelling red cells, Callahan *et al.* (1982), and Bauer *et al.* (1983). This procedure can be used for several clinical applications (Table 2). The red cells are tinned *in vivo* but labelled *in vitro* to allow accurate measurement of labelling efficiency and to enable any unincorporated technetium to be washed from the cells before they are reinjected into the patient. This method also prevents pertechnetate distributing in the extracellular fluid compartment. There are minor differences in the published methods, the one outlined below is that given by Dacie and Lewis (1984).

Method

1. Reconstitute the Amerscans stannous agent (Amersham International) with 6 ml sterile saline and intravenously inject 0.03 ml/kg as above.
2. After 15–30 minutes collect 10 ml of the *in vivo* tinned blood into a syringe rinsed with heparin. Add 5 ml sterile saline and centriuge at 500 g for 5 mins to separate the cells from the plasma. Remove the plasma and buffy coat and repeat the washing step once more. This ensures that any extracellular stannous ions have been removed from the cells before addition of the pertechnetate.
3. To 2 ml of washed, packed cells add the appropriate amount of Tc-99m pertechnetate (see Table 3).
4. Mix on a roller for 5 mins.
5. Add 20 ml saline and centrifuge for 5 mins at 1200–1500 g. Measure the amount of Tc-99m in the supernatant and red cell pellet to determine the labelling efficiency.
6. Resuspend the cells in 5–10 ml isotonic saline and inject the labelled red cells ino the patient.

7.2.3 Radiolabelling Red Cells with Indium-111 and Indium-113m

Red cells can also be labelled with two isotopes of indium, In-111 (half-life 67.9 h) and the generator-produced radionuclide In-113 m (half-life 99.5 min). These isotopes have the advantage that they are more firmly held by the erythrocytes than Tc-99 m. The indium is administered to the cell in the form of a lipophilic complex which rapidly passes across the cell membrane by passive diffusion and is subsequently retained within the cell. Three chelating agents which form complexes with In-111 or In-113 m have been used to radiolabel erythrocytes, 8-hydroxyquinoline (oxine) Ferrant *et al.* (1980), acetylacetone (acac) Radia *et al.* (1981) and tropolone (Osman and Danpure, 1987). These same agents are also used to label leucocytes and platelets as described in later sections. The methods of labelling red cells with In-111 or In-113 m are as follows:

7.2.3.1 Method Using Indium-111 Oxine

1. Prepare red cells from 20 ml blood as described in section 7.2.1 and wash them twice with 20 ml saline.
2. Resuspend about 2 ml of packed red cells in 5 ml of 0.9% w/v saline and add the appropriate amount of In-111 oxine (Amersham International) from Table 3.
3. Incubate the RBC for 15 minutes at room temperature. Wash off any unincorporated activity from the cells with 10 ml saline and resuspend the cell pellet in 10 ml saline and reinject into the patient.

7.2.3.2 Method Using Indium-113m Tropolonate

(from Osman and Danpure, 1987)

1. Collect 8.5 ml blood into a syringe containing 1.5 ml ACD and transfer the blood to a Universal tube.
2. Elute a sterile Sn-113/In-113m generator (Amersham International) with 6 ml elute containing 0.04 M HCI and 0.1% chlorocresol. Increase the osmolarity to isotonicity by adding 0.1 ml of 1.5 M (90 g/l) saline to each ml of eluant to prevent haemolysis of the erythrocytes. If necessary the eluants should be diluted in 0.04 M HCl containing saline as described above.
3. Mix the required amount of In-113m-Cl_3 in 2 ml 0.04 M HCI with 1 ml tropolone at 1.3 mM in 20 mM Hepes-saline buffer pH 7.6 and add it to the 10 ml blood. No more than 2 ml In-113m-Cl_3 should be used per 10 ml blood or it will reduce the pH of the blood and reduce the labelling efficiency.
4. Incubate the blood for 3 minutes at room temperature, add 10 ml saline, spin at 1200–1500 g for 5 min. Carefully remove and discard the plasma and buffy coat which contains the platelets and leucocytes. Resuspend the labelled red cells in 10 ml saline for reinjection into the patient.

7.2.3.3 Method With Indium-111 Tropolonate

The method given below has been adapted from the one given in section 7.2.3.2 for use with Indium-113 m.

1. Collect 8.5 ml blood as described for In-113 m tropolonate.
2. Mix the required amount of In-111-Cl_3 in 2 ml 0.04 M HCI with 1 ml tropolone at 1.3 mM in 20 mM Hepes, 0.8% w/v saline buffer pH 7.6 and add it to the 10 ml of anticoagulated blood. No more than 2 ml In-111-Cl_3 must be added to 10 ml blood for the reason given above.
3. Incubate, wash and reinject as given above for In-113 m.

7.2.4 Preparation of Heat-Damaged Erythrocytes

To measure spleen function the red cells have to be damaged by heating. The method given below gives the procedure for red cells that are to be labelled with Tc-99m, if the heat-damaged cells are to be labelled with In-113m the method is the same except that the initial pretinning is not required.

Method

1. Pre-tin the red cells *in vivo* as given in section 7.2.2.3 and collect 5 ml blood into a syringe rinsed with heparin. Wash the blood twice with 20 ml saline and discard the supernatants.
2. Transfer 2 ml of the packed red cells to a GLASS container and heat at 49.5°C for exactly 20 mins, mixing every 5 mins. Wash the heat-damaged cells twice with 20 ml saline.
3. The cells are now ready to be labelled with the appropriate amount of Tc-99m-O_4^- (or In-113m tropolonate) as given in Table 3 and described in other sections.

7.2.5 Compatibility Testing of Blood for Transfusions

To determine whether blood is suitable for transfusion about 1 ml of blood can be radiolabelled with 7.4 MBq Cr-51 or 1 MBq In-113m tropolonate *in vitro* as described as section 7.2.3.2. After reinjection into the patient blood samples should be taken at 3, 10 and 60 min post injection from a different vein from the one used for injecting the blood. If the blood is compatible the radioactivity in the 60 min sample will be about 99% of that in the 3 min sample. (ICSH, 1980a).

7.3 RADIOLABELLING LEUCOCYTES

Granulocytes and mixed leucocytes are labelled with gamma-emitting radionuclides for the study and detection of inflammation and infection. The types of investigations using these cells are given in Table 5 and by Peters *et al.* (1986). All make use of the normal migratory properties of leucocytes, in particular granulocytes.

Radiolabelled mixed leucocytes became widely used in nuclear medicine following the introduction of In-111 oxine in 1976 by McAfee and Thakur. Other radiopharmaceuticals with better properties such as In-111 tropolonate (Danpure *et al.*, 1982) and Tc-99m HM-PAO (Peters *et al.*, 1987) have subsequently been introduced. Although ^{99m}Tc HM-PAO gives excellent gamma-camera images, the stability of Tc-99m HM-PAO in blood cells is lower than In-111 and this results in some loss of Tc-99m from the labelled leucocytes after they have been reinjected into the patient. This eluted Tc-99m accumulates in the kidneys, bladder, gall bladder and bowel (Roddie *et al.*, 1988) and may impair interpretation of the images.

Unfortunately, the established methods of radiolabelling leucocytes involve using non-selective cell-labelling agents which indiscriminantly label all types of blood cells. To label a particular type of blood cell it is therefore essential to isolate it from whole blood before it can be labelled. To study inflammation or infection it is necessary to radiolabel granulocytes or mixtures of leucocytes as a source of granulocytes. Thus, the first task is to master the procedures for preparing 'mixed' leucocytes and 'pure' granulocytes.

Table 5
Investigations Using Radiolabelled Granulocytes and Mixed Leucocytes

Localisation of sepsis[a]	(i)	abdominal abscesses
	(ii)	lung infection
	(iii)	arterial reconstructive surgery infections
	(iv)	osteomyelitis and infections after hip surgery
Inflammatory bowel disease (IBD)[b]		
Granulocyte kinetics[c]		

[a]Both mixed leucocytes and granulocytes can be used.
[b]For quantitative studies granulocytes labelled with ^{111}In are required, but for non-quantitative studies mixed leucocytes or granulocytes labelled with ^{111}In or ^{99m}Tc can be used.
[c]For these studies the granulocytes must be labelled with ^{111}In.

Although the procedures given below with the non-selective complexes will radiolabel lymphocytes, studies (see review by Peters *et al.*, 1986) have shown that these cells are very radiation sensitive. To obtain lymphocytes, which show a normal biodistribution, the radiation level for In-111 should not exceed 0.74–1.48 MBq per 10^8 lymphocytes.

Monocytes have not been radiolabelled with the ^{111}In and Tc-99m complexes because of the difficulty of separating them from whole blood. They have however been labelled with radioactive colloids such as Tc-99m tin colloid which are phagocytosed by granulocytes and monocytes (Hanna and Lomas, 1986) when added to a sample of blood.

All procedures are carried out on the patients' own blood using aseptic techniques, sterile equipment and sterile, pyrogen-free solutions. Unless there is any statement to the contrary, all saline solutions are isotonic i.e. at 150 mM (9 g/l). It is recommended that any samples of labelled blood that are required are taken from a different vein from the one used to administer the labelled cells or cell-labelling agent to ensure that there is no contamination of the blood samples by any radioactivity remaining in the injection site.

7.3.1 Separation of Mixed Leucocytes from Whole Blood

The method is illustrated in Figure 1.

1. Dispense 9 ml aliquots ACD into two 60 ml polystyrene syringes.

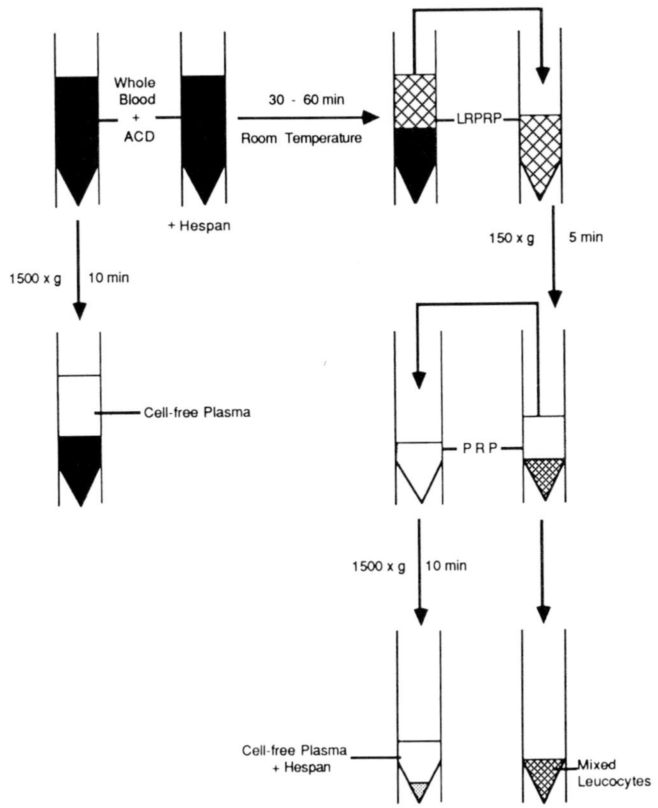

Figure 1. Method of separation of mixed leucocytes from whole blood. ACD = acid-citrate-dextrose, LRPRP = leucocyte-rich platelet-rich plasma and PRP = platelet-rich plasma.

2. Collect 51 ml of fresh venous blood into each syringe using a 19 G butterfly needle.
3. Dispense 20 ml of blood into a sterile Universal tube (Sterilin) if mixed leucocytes are to be prepared, but 40 ml into 2 tubes if 'pure' granulocytes are to be prepared. Centrifuge the blood at 1500 g for 10 minutes to give cell-free plasma containing ACD, pH approximately 7, and discard the cells. This plasma is used for:
   (i) Percoll/plasma gradients (if granulocytes are to be prepared)
   (ii) suspending cells for labelling
   (iii) suspending labelled cells for reinjection into the patient.
4. Dispense the remaining 80 or 100 ml blood into 4 or 5 Universals each containing 2 ml aliquots of Hespan (6% w/v hydroxyethyl starch, Dupont).
5. Mix and leave the blood for 30–60 minutes at room temperature to sediment the red cells.
6. Sample the supernatant containing the leucocytes and platelets (usually referred to as leucocyte-rich platelet-rich plasma, LRPRP), using a sterile syringe without a needle and dispense 15 ml aliquots into Universal tubes.
7. Centrifuge the LRPRP at 150 g for 5 minutes to pellet the mixed leucocytes.
8. Remove and save the supernatant platelet-rich plasma (PRP).
9. Resuspend the mixed leucocytes in either:
   (a) 1 ml of cell-free plasma prepared in step 3 if the cells are to be labelled as mixed leucocytes;
   or
   (b) 4 ml PRP from step 8 if 'pure' granulocytes are to be prepared.
10. Centrifuge the remaining PRP (from step 8) at 1500 g for 10 minutes to give cell-free plasma containing Hespan for washing the labelled cells.
11. In paediatric studies use only 10–50 ml blood, omit step 3 and prepare cell-free plasma from PRP containing Hespan.

7.3.2 Separation of Pure Granulocytes from Mixed Leucocytes Using 3-Step Discontinuous Percoll-Plasma Gradients

For an illustration of the gradients see Danpure (1985).

1. Prepare iso-osmotic Percoll (IOP = 100%) by mixing 9 volumes of Percoll (specific gravity 1.13 g/ml, Pharmacia) with 1 volume of 1.5 M sodium chloride (90 g/l).
2. Dilute IOP with the patient's cell-free ACD-plasma, prepared from step 3 above, to obtain 65%, 60% and 50% v/v solutions of Percoll in plasma.
3. Prepare two 3-step discontinuous density-gradient by carefully layering 2 ml of each solution in order of decreasing density into a serile 10 ml polystyrene centrifuge tube. One gradient is needed for the mixed leucocytes from 50 ml blood.
4. Gently overlay about 2 ml of mixed leucocytes in plasma on to each gradient.
5. Centrifuge the gradients at 150 g for 5 minutes.
6. Discard the plasma and the cells (platelets and mononuclear cells) at the plasma/50% interface and sample the granulocytes from the 50/60% interface.
7. Wash the granulocytes free of Percoll by adding 10 ml of cell-free plasma containing Hespan from step 10 above and centrifuging the cells at 150 g for 5 minutes.
8. Discard all of the supernatant.
9. Resuspend the granulocyte pellet in ACD-plasma without Hespan so that the volume of cells and plasma is 1 ml.

7.3.3 Preparation of Technetium-99m HM-PAO and Labelling of Mixed Leucocytes

Details have been published, Danpure *et al.* (1988).

The procedure is shown in Figure 2. It can also be used to label 'pure' granulocytes if they are suspended in 1 ml plasma.

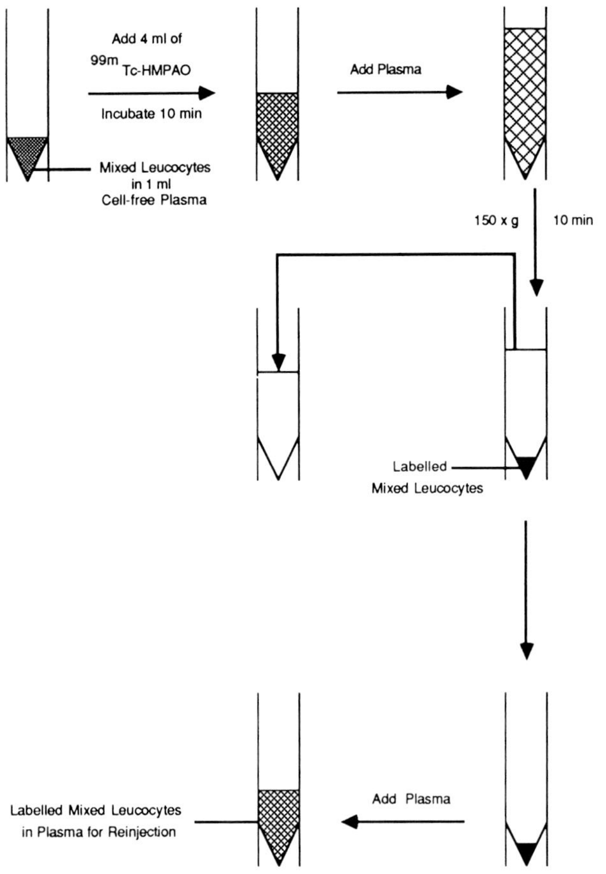

Figure 2. Method of labelling mixed leucocytes with ^{99m}Tc-HM-PAO.

1. Add 5 ml Tc-99m pertechnetate containing 450 MBq Tc-99m to a vial of Ceretec (Amersham International) which contains 0.5 mg hexamethyl propylene amine oxime (HM-PAO), 7.6 μg stannous chloride dihydrate and 4.5 mg sodium chloride sealed under nitrogen. Shake for 10 sec to dissolve the HM-PAO and
   (a) *immediately* add 4 ml to the mixed leucocytes in 1 ml ACD-plasma. (This results in a plasma concentration of 20% and a HM-PAO concentration of 80 μg/ml).
   (b) *immediately* measure the amount of lipophilic Tc-99m-HM-PAO complex formed using the 3 chromatography systems given in the Ceretec pamphlet.
2. Incubate cells with Tc-99m-HM-PAO for 10 minutes at room temperature.
3. Add about 15 ml cell-free plasma (from step 10 of the procedure for the separation of mixed leucocytes) and spin at 150 g for 5 minutes.
4. Remove and save all of the supernatant and resuspend the cell pellet in about 5 ml cell-free plasma without Hespan.
5. To calculate the percentage labelling efficiency (LE) i.e. percentage of total activity bound to the cells, measure the radioactivity on the cells and in the supernatant plasma (from step 4).
6. Transfer the labelled cells to a 10 ml syringe, measure the activity and inject a maximum of 185 MBq of Tc-99m-labelled mixed leucocytes into a the patient as soon as possible.
7. Image the patient at 1 h and 3–4 h post-injection. For patients with osteomyelitis, infection or equivocal results further images may be required between 18 and 24 h.

7.3.4 Labelling of Mixed Leucocytes and Pure Granulocytes with Indium-111-Tropolonate

1. Prepare the In-111 tropolonate by mixing approximately 11 MBq (300 μCi) In-111-Cl_3 in less than 50 μl of 0.04 HCl, with 0.1 ml tropolone at 4.4 mM in Hepes-saline buffer, pH 7.6 just before addition ot the cells.
2. Add the cells in 1 ml plasma. This will give a final tropolone concentration of 0.4 mM which is the optimum concentration for labelling leucocytes.
3. Incubate the cells for 5 minutes at room temperature.
4. Add 5 ml of cell-free plasma containing ACD.
5. Centrifuge the cells at 150 g for 5 minutes.
6. Remove all the supernatant and resuspend the cell pellet in 5 ml cell-free plasma containing ACD.
7. Calculate the percentage labelling efficiency (LE) as described in section 7.3.3.
8. Transfer the cells to a 10 ml syringe, measure the activity in the syringe and reinject the labelled cells into the patient as soon as possible.

A method of obtaining pure neutrophils from whole blood was recently described by Sampson and Solanki (1992) which does not require the prior collection of mixed leucocytes. Briefly, 15 ml whole blood are layered onto a double gradient consisting of 8.5 ml of 1.119 g/ml and 7.5 ml of 1.077 g/ml. The suspension is spun at 750 g for 15 minutes. The neutrophils separate out as a distinct layer above the sedimented red cells. The purity is 96% ±3 (n = 10).

Critical Points to Obtain a Good Labelling Efficiency with Indium-111 Tropolonate in Plasma

(This does not apply to the labelling of red cells with In-111 tropolonate given in section 7.2.3.3.)

1. The cells (mixed leucocytes, granulocytes or platelets) should be labelled in plasma containing 0.4 mM tropolone as this is the optimum concentration for labelling blood cells in 90% plasma containing ACD,

(Danpure *et al.* (1982) and Danpure and Osman (1988a).
2. $In\text{-}111\text{-}Cl_3$ is supplied in 0.04 M HCl at a specific activity of > 1.85 GBq/μg (> 50 mCi/μg) and a radioactive concentration of 370 MBq/ml (10 mCi/ml) at reference. If necessary it *must* be diluted in 0.04 M HCl not water or saline as an insoluble colloid will be formed.
3. Fifty μl is the maximum volume of $In\text{-}111\text{-}Cl_3$ that should be added to 0.1 ml tropolone at 4.4 mM (in Hepes-saline buffer) for labelling cells in 1 ml ACD-plasma. If more than 50μl of $In\text{-}111\text{-}Cl_3$ is used:
   (a) the In-111 and tropolone will not completely react to form In-111 tropolonate,
   (b) when the mixture of $In\text{-}111\text{-}Cl_3$ and tropolone is added to the plasma the pH of the plasma will be lowered.

   Both effects will result in a reduction in labelling efficiency (LE). If it is necessary to use more than 50 μl of $In\text{-}111\text{-}Cl_3$, the volume of tropolone and plasma used to label cells must be proportionately increased.
4. It is important to use a high cell concentration. For 'pure' granulocytes a cell concentration exceeding 2×10^7 cells/ml and for platelets a cell concentration exceeding 5×10^8/ml should be used. If only low numbers of cells are available they should either be labelled at a high cell concentration in 0.5 ml 90% plasma or in 1 ml 50% plasma.
5. In paediatric studies use 10–50 ml of blood and add 1.85–3.7 MBq (50–100 μCi) of $In\text{-}111\text{-}Cl_3$. In these studies mixed leucocytes can be used instead of 'pure' granulocytes.
6. Do not use heparin to anticoagulate blood, or plasma containing heparin to label the granulocytes or platelets as it significantly reduces the amount of In-111 tropolonate incorporated by the cells (see Danpure and Osman 1986).

7.3.5 Radiolabelling Lymphocytes

Lymphocyte scintigraphy could be potentially useful for evaluation of disease involving chronic inflammation and, possibly, disorders of lymphocyte proliferation (Wagstaff *et al.*, 1981a; Wagstaff *et al.*, 1981b). A number of workers have been able to radiolabel lymphocytes with indium but these techniques have not found favour with clinicians because of evidence that chromosomal damage may occur in lymphocytes labelled with that radionuclide (ten Berge and Natarajan, 1983; Sparshott *et al.*, 1981). An alternative to indium has been sought and a number of workers have proposed technetium as a suitable label. Although technetium has been reported to be radiotoxic to lymphocytes (Schmidt *et al.*, 1990; Mertz *et al.*, 1986), cell damage is considerably less than that with indium and it is likely that technetium labelled lymphocytes will become clinically acceptable in the future.

One of the main difficulties in using labelled lymphocytes in nuclear medicine is the problem of getting a satisfactory imaging dose of technetium on the small number of cells available for labelling. Lymphocytes account for only 20–30% of the total leucocyte count; 100 ml of blood are therefore needed to obtain sufficient cells for labelling. Sampson and Goffin (1991) have developed a method which has been used in clinical practice. Briefly, two 50 ml portions of blood are collected from the patient anticoagulated with acid-citrate-dextrose solution. The blood is transferred to 50 ml Falcon tubes each containing 10 ml Hespan. The blood is sedimented for 45 minutes and the supernatants collected and centrifuged at 100 g for 7 minutes. The supernatants are removed to produce cell free plasma for final dilution. The two plugs of mixed leucocytes are mixed together and made up to 4 mls with cell-free plasma. The cell suspension is layered onto 3 ml 'Lymphoprep' (Nycomed Laboratories) and spun at 400 g for 40 minutes. After centrifugation the first band containing lymphocytes (and monocytes) is removed. The cells are washed with cell-free plasma and labelled according to the method described later (Sampson *et al.*, 1991).

A more recent development has been described in which lymphocytes can be obtained from whole blood (Sampson1992). Briefly, 90 mls of anticoagulated blood are distributed into three 'Accuspin' tubes (Sigma) which have been pre-filled with Hypaque of density 1.077 g/ml. The tubes are spun at 1000 g for 30–40 minutes. The main advantage of the technique is that a prior step to remove mixed leucocytes is not necessary and that the purity of the lymphocyte/monocyte fraction is greater than 90%.

7.3.6. Recent Developments in the Use of Tc-99m Exametazime for Leucocyte Labelling

Exametazime is now firmly established as the 'gold standard' for technetium leucocyte chelators. Once incorporated into the cell little is eluted from the cell over a period of 4–5 hours and phagocytic activity is not impaired. However, technetium-99m exametazime is inherently unstable due to rapid oxidation of the small amount (7.6 μg) of stannous chloride present in the freeze-dried kit. Because of its instability the manufacturer recommends that the reconstituted material should be used within 30 minutes and that the contents of a vial should be used for only one dose of labelled cells. These constraints render the radiopharmaceutical comparatively uneconomic and quite a large group of workers have attempted to improve the stability. Cryopreservation slows down the oxidative process and several researchers have used this principle together with sub-division of a vial to obtain several doses of exametazime over a period of days, weeks or even months. Piera *et al.* (1990) was able to use exametazime over a period of two weeks by subdivision and storage at − 20 °C and Ballinger (1992) was able to use the reconstituted material for up to a month if stored at − 10 °C and nitrogen purged vials were used during subdivision. Sampson *et al.* (1991) advocated the use of small volumes and a high concentration of exametazime together with cryopreservation. Briefly, a vial of exametazime is made up to 1.5 mls with saline. 0.25 ml is removed, added to the pertechnetate in a small volume and incubated with the cell plug. The advantage of the technique is that labelling efficiency is increased and only 50 ml blood are needed from the patient. Also, if the reconstituted exametazime is cryopreserved at − 20 °C several doses may be withdrawn over a period of several days. A recent approach is based on the premise that tin lost by oxidation should be replaced by further amounts in order to maintain a stoichimetric balance. In this technique (Solanki *et al.*, 1993) small volumes of tin solution containing 20 μg/ml stannous chloride are added to 0.3 ml aliquots of exametazime solution. If the material is cryopreserved up to 15 doses may be obtained over a period of up to 6 months.

At this point it should be emphasised that any deviation from a manufacturer's recommended procedure transfers the onus of liability from the manufacturer to the user. However, it must be borne in mind that new and improved methods do become available from time to time, and provided that rigid controls are established throughout the process there can be no objection to the use of these development (see Hewat and Sampson, 1992).

7.4 RADIOLABELLING PLATELETS

Radiolabelled platelets are used for a variety of investigations which make use of their role in haemostasis as outlined in Table 6 and given in the reviews by Peters *et al.* (1986) and Peters (1988). The recommended method for Indium-111 platelet survival studies is given by the ICSH (1988).

Table 6
Investigations Using Radiolabelled Platelets

Imaging	(i) deep vein thrombosis
	(ii) chronic arterial disease
	(iii) renal transplantation rejection
	(iv) prosthetic arterial grafts
	(v) imaging the heart
Platelet kinetics[a]	

[a]For these studies the platelets must be labelled with In-III.

Platelets are labelled with the non-selective In-111 and Tc-99m complexes, In-111 oxine, In-111 tropolonate and Tc-99 HM-PAO, and therefore have to be isolated from whole blood before labelling in a similar manner to the leucocytes. Platelets are very sensitive to the manipulations that are required for these procedures and readily aggregate and become irreversibly damaged unless measures are taken to prevent it. The usual method of inhibiting spontaneous aggregation is to acidify the platelet-rich-plasma with ACD before they are centrifuged. The same effect can be achieved by using anti-aggregating prostaglandins, Peters *et al.* (1986).

7.4.1 Isolation of Platelets from Whole Blood

The Method is illustrated in Figure 3.

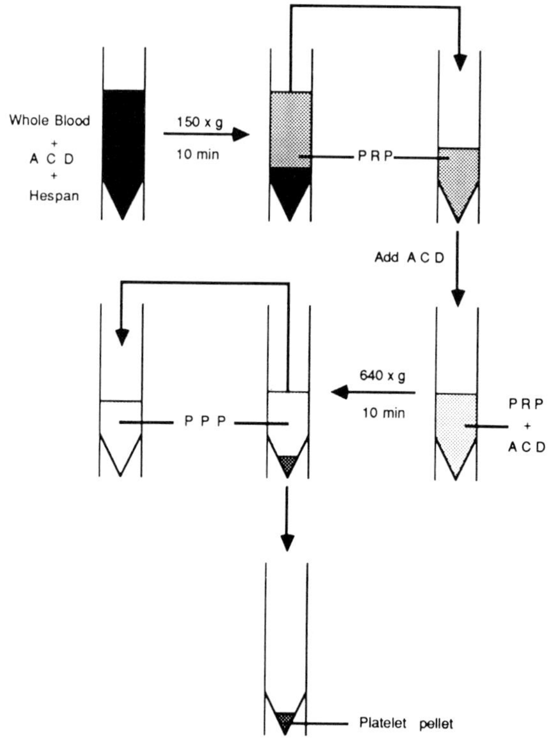

Figure 3. Method of isolating platelets from whole blood. ACD = acid-citrate-dextrose, PRP = platelet-rich-plasma and PPP = platelet-poor-plasma.

1. Dispense 9 ml of ACD into a 60 ml polystyrene syringe and collect 51 ml of fresh venous blood using a 19 G needle.
2. Remove the needle and dispense the 60 ml of blood into 3 Universals each containing 2 ml of Hespan.
3. Mix and immediately centrifuge the blood at 150 g for 10 minutes to give a pellet of leucocytes and erythrocytes and a supernatant of platelet-rich-plasma (PRP).
4. Remove the PRP using a syringe without a needle. *Acidify the PRP by adding 1 volume of ACD to 10 volumes of PRP.* This acidification step is very important, if it is not carried out the platelets will aggregate when centrifuged.

5. If the PRP contains a lot of red cells a second centrifugation at 150 g for 5 minutes can be performed to remove the red cells. Otherwise, centrifuge the PRP at 640 g for 10 minutes to pellet the platelets.
6. Remove and save the supernatant of platelet-poor-plasma (PPP, pH 6.5) and use 1 ml for resuspending the platelet pellet for labelling. This plasma is also used for washing and resuspending the labelled cells.

7.4.2 Labelling Platelets with Technetium-99m HM-PAO

Details of the development of the method are given by Danpure and Osman (1988b).

1. Prepare the Tc-99m-HM-PAO as described above and immediately add 4 ml to the platelets in 1 ml PPP, pH 6.5.
2. Incubate the platelets with Tc-99m-HM-PAO for *30 minutes* at room temperature.
3. Add 10 ml PPP containing ACD, pH 6.5, and centrifuge at 640 g for 10 minutes.
4. Remove all the supernatant and resuspend the cell pellet in about 5 ml PPP.
5. Calculate the percentage labelling efficiency, and reinject a maximum of 185 MBq of labelled platelets as described above for mixed leucocytes.
6. Image the patient at 3–4 h and again at 18–24 h post injection.

7.4.4 Labelling Platelets with Indium-111 Tropolonate

The critical points given in section 7.3.4 also apply to the labelling of platelets. Further details are given by Danpure *et al.* (1982).

1. Prepare the In-111 tropolonate by mixing approximately 11 MBq (300 μCi) In-111-Cl_3 in less than 50 μl of 0.04 M HCl, with 0.1 ml tropolone at 4.4 mM in Hepes-saline buffer, pH 7.6, just before addition to the platelets.
2. Add the platelets in 1 ml PPP pH 6.5, this will give a final tropolone concentration of 0.4 mM.
3. Incubate the cells for 5 minutes at room temperature.
4. Add 5 ml of PPP, (pH 6.5).
5. Centrifuge the platelets at 640 g for 10 min.
6. Remove all the supernatant and resuspend the platelets in 5 ml PPP, (pH 6.5). Measure the activity in the cells and supernatant to calculate the LE.
7. Transfer the platelets into a 10 ml syringe, measure the activity in the syringe and reinject the labelled platelets into the patient as soon as possible.
8. For the measurement of platelet life-span image at 40 min then take blood samples daily until no labelled platelets are detectable in the circulation. For the detection of thrombosis image at 3–4 h and 18–24 h. For further details see Peters *et al.* (1986).

7.5 CONCLUSIONS

There is widespread use of the methods given in this chapter despite the fact that the procedures, especially those for preparing and labelling leucocytes and platelets, required skilled personnel, expensive laboratory facilities and are time-consuming to perform. To increase the use of radiolabelled blood cells research studies are in progress to develop new methods of radiolabelling leucocytes and platelets which will be quicker and easier to perform. The main approach is in the development of selective agents which will radiolabel specific populations of cells when added to a sample of whole blood or injected into the patient. An example of the former is the use of radiolabelled colloids which may be phagocytosed by granulocytes and monocytes. Studies have shown that Tc-99m tin colloid will radiolabel these cells when added to a sample of whole blood but in some instances the incorporation of the radiocolloid damaged the cells. A recent modification by Hanna and Lomas (1986) of the method of Schroth *et al.* (1989). It does however require care in the preparation of the colloid and is consequently not widely used.

The other new approach is to selectively label leucocytes and platelets with radiolabelled cell-specific monoclonal antibodies (MABS). Studies with radio-labelled anti-granulocyte MABS have shown that they will label granulocytes *in vivo* but the proportion of the labelled MAB on the cells is less than 30% (Seybold, 1988, and Joseph *et al.*, 1988) and *in vivo* data is different from that obtained when granulocytes are labelled *in vitro* with the In-111 or Tc-99m complexes. The reason for the disparity is not known. In contrast, studies with the anti-platelet MAB, P256 (Stuttle *et al.* (1988) are similar to those obtained with platelets labelled with In-111 tropolonate.

There is also interest in radiolabelling granulocytes and platelets with positron-emitting radionuclides for investigations where the patient is imaged on a positron camera.

Although the methods given in this chapter for radiolabelling blood cells with gamma-emitting radionuclides for imaging on the gamma-camera will continue to be used, the search for new selective cell labelling agents which will simplify the procedures indicate that an exciting future is in prospect for cell labelling.

ACKNOWLEDGEMENTS

The authors would like to thank M. Deenmamode, A.M. Peters, C. Sampson and B. Henderson for their help in preparing this manuscript.

REFERENCES

Ballinger J. (1990). *Preparation of Tc-99m HMPAO.* J. Nucl. Med., **3126**, -31.

Bauer R. *et al.* (1983). In vivo/in vitro *labelling of red blood cells with* ^{99m}*Tc.* Eur. J. Nucl. Med., **8**, 218–222.

Callahan R.J. *et al.* (1982). *Modified method for the* in vivo *labelling of blood cells with* ^{99m}*Tc: Concise communication.* J. Nucl. Med., **23**, 315–318.

Dacie J.V. and Lewis S.M. (1984). Practical Haematology, 6th edn. London: Churchill Livingstone.

Danpure H.J. (1985). *Cell labelling with* ^{111}*In complexes. In* Radiopharmacy and Radiopharmaceuticals, edited by A.E. Theobald, pp. 51–85. London: Taylor and Francis.

Danpure H.J. and Osman S. (1986). *The importance of radiolabelling human granulocytes with* ^{111}*In tropolonate or* ^{111}*In 2-mercaptopyridine-N-oxide in plasma containing acid-citrate-dextrose.* British J. Radiology, **59**, 907–910.

Danpure H.J. *et al.* (1982). *The labelling of blood cells in plasma with* ^{111}*In tropolonate.* British J. Radiology, **55**, 247–249.

Danpure H.J. and Osman S. (1988a).

Danpure H.J. and Osman S. (1986).

Danpure H.J. *et al.* (1988).

Ferrant A. *et al.* (1980). *Scintigraphy with* ^{111}*Indium-labelled red cells in intermittent gastrointestinal bleeding.* J. Nucl. Med., **21**, 844–845.

Hanna R.W. and Lomas F.E. (1986). *Identification of factors affecting technetium 99m leukocyte labelling by phagocytic engulfment and development of an optimal technique.* Eur. J. Nucl. Med., **12**, 159–162.

Hewat C.D.R. and Sampson C.B. (1992). *Reconstitution protocol for Ceretec, comment and response.* Nucl. Med. Commun., **13**, 121–122.

International Committee for Standardization in Hematology (ICSH) (1980a). *Recommended method for radioisotope red cell survival studies.* British J. of Hematology, **45**, 659–666.

International Committee for Standardization in Hematology (ICSH) (1980b). *Recommended methods for measurement of red cell and plasma volume.* J. Nucl. Med., **21**, 793–800.

International Committee for Standardization in Hematology (ICSH) (1988). *Recommended method for indium 111 platelet survival studies.* J. Nucl. Med., **29**, 564–566.

Jones J. and Mollison P.L. (1978). *A simple and efficient method of labelling red cells with* ^{99m}*Tc for the determination of red cell volume.* British J. of Hematology, **38**, 141–148.

Joseph K. *et al.* (1988). *Imaging inflammation with granulocytes labelled* in vivo. Nucl. Med. Commun., **9**, 763–769.

McAfee J.G. *et al.* (1991). *The localisation of In-111-leucocytes, gallium-67-polyclonal IgG and other radioactive agents in acute focal inflammatory lesions.* J. Nucl. Med., **32**, 2126–2131.

McAfee J.G. and Thakur M.L. (1976). *Survey of radioactive agents for* in vitro *labelling of phagocytic lencocytes. I. Soluble agents.* J. Nucl. Med. **17**, 480–487.

Mertz T. *et al.* (1986). *Technetium-99m labeled lymphocytes: a radiotoxicity study.* J. Nucl. Med. **27**, 105–110.

Osman S. and Danpure H.J. (1987). *A simple* in vitro *method of labelling human erythrocytes in whole blood with* ^{113m}*In-tropolonate.* Eur. J. Hematol., **39**, 125–127.

Pavel D.G. *et al.* (1977). In vivo *labelling of red blood cells with* ^{99m}*Tc: a new approach to blood pool visualisation.* J. Nucl. Med., **18**, 305–308.

Peters A.M. (1988). *Review of platelet labeling and kinetics.* Nucl. Med. Commun., **9**, 803–808.

Peters A.M. *et al.* (1986). *Cell labelling. In* Methods in Hematology, volume 14, Radionuclides in Hematology, edited by S.M. Lewis and R.J. Bayly, pp. 79–109. Edinburgh: Churchill Livingstone.

Peters A.M. *et al.* (1987). *Tc-99m HM-PAO for labelling leucocytes in infection.* Lancet, **1**, 44.

Piera C., *et al.* (1990). *Preparation of Tc-99m HM-PAO.* J. Nucl. Med., **31**, 127–128.

Popescu H.J. *et al.* (1984). In vivo *labelling of RBC with* ^{99m}*Tc for blood pool imaging using different stannous radiopharmaceuticals.* Eur. J. Nucl. Med., **9**, 295–299.

Radia R. *et al.* (1981). *Measurement of red cell volume and splenic red cell pool using* ^{113m}*Indium.* British J. of Hematology, **49**, 567–591.

Rao S.A. *et al.* (1986). *Effect of Sn(II) ion concentration and heparin on technetium 99m red blood cell labelling.* J. Nucl. Med., **27**, 1202–1206.

Roddie M.E., *et al.* (1988). *Imaging inflammation with Tc-99m hexamethyl propylene amine oxime (HM-PAO) labelled leucocytes.* Radiology, **166**, 767–772.

Sampson C.B. and Goffin E. (1991). *Technetium-labelled autologous lymphocytes: clinical protocol for radiolabelling using a high concentration and low volume of Tc-99m exametazime,* Nucl. Med. Commun. **12**, 875–878.

Sampson C.B., *et al.* (1991). *Tc-99m exametazime labelled leucocytes; effect of volume and concentration of exametazime on labelling efficiency and clinical protocol for high-efficiency multi-dose radiolabelling.* Nucl. Med. Commun. (1991) **12**, 719–723.

Sampson C.B. (1992). *Separation and radiolabelling of lymphocytes: a plain man's guide.* Nucl. Med. Commun.

Sampson C.B. and Solanki (1992). *Separation and technetium labelling of pure neutrophils: development of a simple and rapid clinical protocol.* Nucl. Med. Commun., **13**, 210 (abstract).

Schmidt K.G., *et al.* (1990). *In* Radiolabelled Cellular Blood Elements. Wiley-Liss, USA, pp. 209–218.

Schroth H.J. *et al.* (1981). *Cell labelling with colloidal substances in whole blood.* Eur. J. Nucl. Med., **6**, 469–472.

Seybold K. (1988). In vivo *labelling of granulocytes using* ^{123}*I-tagged anti-granulocyte antibodies.* Nucl. Med. Commun., **9**, 745–752.

Solanki C., *et al.* (1992). *Stabilisation of exametazime for leucocyte labelling: a new approach using tin enhancement.* Revista Espanola Medicina Nuclear XI, **141**.

Sparshott S.M., *et al.* (1981). *Factors influencing the fate of indium-111 labelled lymphocytes after transfer to syngenic rats.* J. Immunol. Methods, **41**, 303–320.

Stuttle A.W.J. *et al.* (1988). *Use of anti-platelet mono- clonal antibody F(ab')$_2$ for imaging thrombus.* Nucl. Med. Commun., **9**, 647–655.

ten Berge R.Y.M. and Natarajan A.T. (1983). *Labelling with indium-111 has detrimental effects on human lymphocytes: concise communication.* J. Nucl. Med., **24**, 615–619.

Wagstaff J., *et al.* (1981a). *Human lymphocyte traffic assessed by indium oxine labelling in clinical observations.* Clin. Exp. Immunol., **43**, 443–446.

Wagstaff J., *et al.* (1981b). *A method for human lymphocyte traffic using indium oxine.* Clin. Exp. Immunol., **43**, 435–436.

Chapter 8

Radiolabelled Antibodies as Radiopharmaceuticals

S.J. Mather

8.1 INTRODUCTION

Antibodies are a part of the defence services mobilised by the body's immune system in response to attack by micro-organisms. When an invading bacterium enters any body fluids, it encounters an array of lymphocytes each bearing on its surface a recognition molecule capable of binding to a particular molecular structure. If the bacterium carries any of these structures on its surface, then it combines with a complimentary lymphocyte(s) and initiates the first stage in the host's specific immune response. One result of this response is a clonal proliferation of the lymphocytes which produce large amounts of antibody with the same binding specificities as the original lymphocytes. These antibodies bind to the invading bacteria and invoke secondary immune mechanisms such as complement fixation. Thus antibodies have two main functions (i) to recognise and bind to a specific target (antigen) on the bacterium and (ii) to invoke attack on the microorganism by secondary forces such as complement and phagocytic macrophages. These two functions are quite independant and a performed by different parts of the antibody molecule.

The basic antibody molecule consists of two pairs of two protein chains, called heavy and light chains, held together by disulphide bonds (see Figure 1). Each chain has a number of domains, lights chains having two – called VL and CL – and heavy chains having four – VH, CH1, CH2 and CH3. VL and VH domains have highly **variable** amino-acid sequences so that the variable domains of different antibodies will be quite different. CL and CH domains have relatively **constant** sequences and will be the same for antibodies with different specificities. These domains are combined in the antibody molecule to produce a variable region which is responsible for the antigen recognition function of the molecule and a constant region which mediates the secondary biological functions of the antibody.

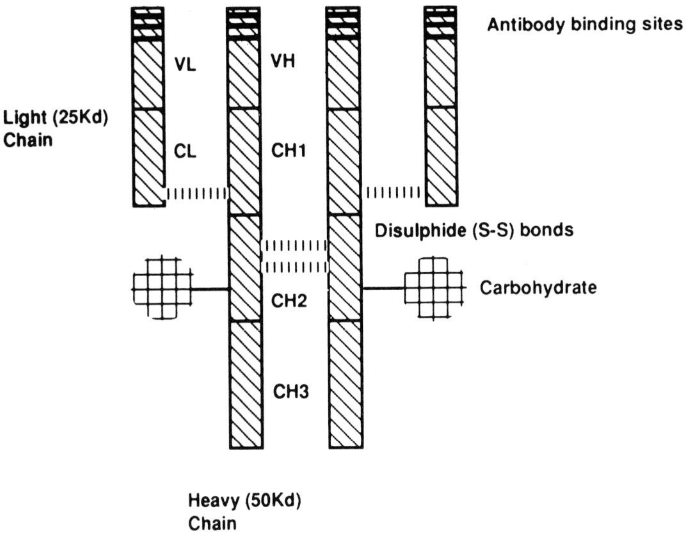

Figure 1. Structural diagram of immunoglobulin molecule.

Different microorganisms have different structures and the body needs to make a great variety of different antibodies capable of recognising these different molecules. This is done by a process of combining approximately 700 different genes in such a way as to create several million different combinatorial possibilities. It has been estimated that as many as 10^8 different antibodies circulate in normal serum each with a different molecular specificity.

While the vasty majority of this diversity resides in the variable domains of the molecule responsible for antigen recognition, antibodies may posses a number of different constant domains and consequently different biological functions. These antibodies are described as having different isotypes called IgG, IgA, IgE, IgD and IgM.

Thus nature has divised a way in which molecules can be generated which recognise specific molecular sequences. In addition to the 'natural' process of antibody production as a result of infection. Antibodies can also be 'artificially' induced by the injection of any foreign antigen into a host and antibodies can be generated against any molecular structure desired.

8.2 TUMOUR ANTIGENS

Although tumours originate from normal cells, the process that induces malignancy results in changes on the surface of the cell such that a tumour cell can be recognised as different from a normal cell. The expression of tumour-specific markers on cancer cells raises the possibility that antibodies can be generated which can distinguish between the malignant cells and their normal counterparts. In fact, most of these differences are not due to the appearance of entirely novel antigens on the tumour cells but to the altered expression of normal cellular constituents. Thus, for example, a protein which in normal cells is intracellular may appear on the surface of tumour cells, a normal protein may be glycosylated aberrantly during its passage through to the surface of a tumour cells or alternatively, a protein which is normally only expressed during a certain phase development such as embryogenesis may reappear after malignant transformation. Most tumour markers are therefore not entirely tumour 'specific' but should be regarded as tumour 'associated.

8.3 ANTIBODY PRODUCTION

8.3.1 Polyclonal Antibodies

Antibodies are traditionally produced from hyperimmune serum. A suitable animal undergoes a programme of injections with an immunogen designed to boost the levels of antibody present in the blood. The animal is then bled and the antibodies can be purified from the many other blood constituents. This process has a number of disadvantages: the purification process is long and laborious and results only in a limited amount of the antibody. In addition to the antibodies which recognise the immunogen, the animal will also possess its native repertoire of antibodies and these will contaminate the end product. Moreover, the animal responds to the immunisation with a polyclonal antibody response. Thus not just one, but a variety of different antibodies having different isotypes and different affinities and directed against different parts of the immunogen will be produced. The end-product is therefore not one antibody but a heterogeneous mixture of immunoglobulins.

8.3.2 Monoclonal Antibodies

The first step in monoclonal antibody production is identical. The animal, normally a mouse but alternatively any small mammal, is injected several times with the immunogen in order to boost the immune response. Instead of harvesting the serum, however, the animal is killed and the spleen, which contains the majority of the lymphocytes responsible for antibody production, is dissected and separated into a cell suspension. The lymphocytes present in the cell suspension will grow and produce antibody for a short time in tissue culture, but after a few days will normally die. In order to immortalize the cells, they are fused with tumour cells – normally myeloma cells – by using polyethylene glycol which destabilises the cell membranes. The result of the fusion process are 'hybridoma' cells which have both the antibody-producing properties of the lymphocyte and the immortality of the tumour cell. They can thus be grown in tissue culture indefinitely. At this stage, the cell population is still heterogeneous consisting of a number of different hybridomas producing different antibodies. The cells can now be 'cloned' in order to separate them into 'monoclonal' populations of cells each producing a single antibody (Figure 2).

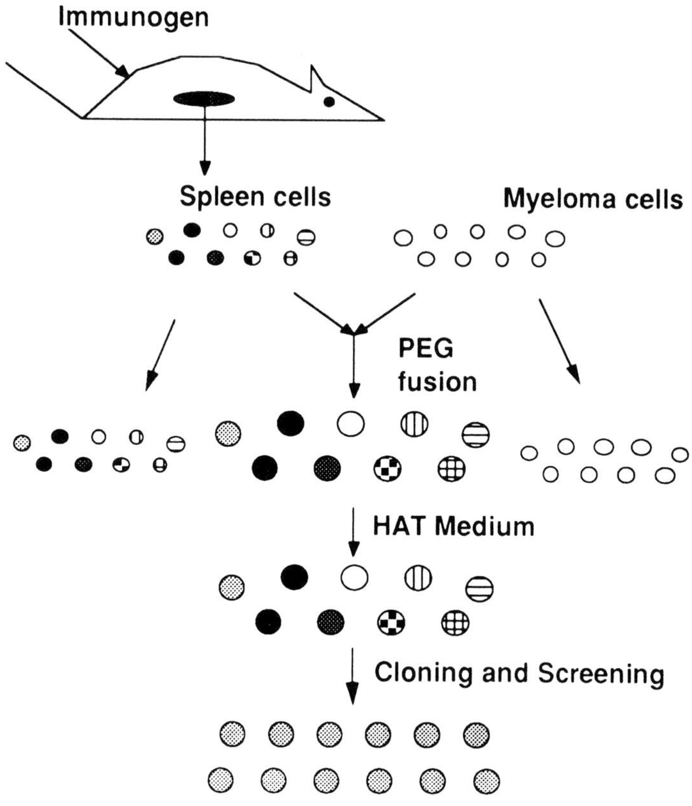

Figure 2. Initial steps in monoclonal antibody production.

This process therefore overcomes the disadvantage of polyclonal antibody production. It results in the production of a potentially infinite batch of a single homogeneous antibody preparation. It has the added advantage that material produced by tissue culture is much more suitable for clinical application than that harvested directly from animals. Antibody preparations intended for clinical use must comply with the appropriate standards of quality such as measures of purity and freedom from contaminating microorganisms including bacteria, mycoplasma and virus. Suitable standards for application in both academic studies and commercially produced antibody preparations have been published (Report 1, 1986; Report 2, 1988).

8.4 CHARACTERISATION OF ANTIBODIES

Soon after, if not during, production, antibodies need to be characterised to see if they are suitable for their intended purpose. Checks need to be made to ensure that the antibody still binds to the antigen. It is also wise to confirm regularly that the cell culture is truly 'monoclonal' since the hybridi-domas undergo spontaneous mutation at a high rate and can alter after the nature of the antibody binds to any normal tissues. This is done by immunohistochemistry on a panel of normal tissues such as liver, spleen, bone marrow etc. The differential between staining of tumour tissues and normal tissues is a measure of the degree of tumour 'specificity' of the antibody. It is normal to find some weak staining of normal tissues which are related to the cancer type, so that antibodies which bind strongly to colorectal tumours, for example, may show a degree of reactivity with the normal gastrointestinal tract. The significance of this cross reactivity is by no means certain. In a therapeutic application, one has to be careful of potential side-effects of the therapy in these normal tissues and, in a diagnostic modality, uptake in normal tissues may complicate the interpretation of the images. However, the appearance of cross-reactivity on a microscope slide does not necessarily mean that the antibody will bind to these tissues *in vivo*. In order to bind to antigen, the antibody must have physical access to it. In normal tissues, antigens are often hidden behind cellular barriers such as basement membrane and are inaccessible to circulating antibody. In a tumour, the normal architectural conformation of tissues is destroyed and antigens which are normally hidden behind cellular barriers such as basement membrane and are inaccessible to circulating antibody. In a tumour, the normal architectural conformation of tissues is destroyed and antigens which are normally hidden become exposed. Care must therefore be taken when relating immunohistochemical results to the *in vivo* situation.

Other important antibody parameters which need to be characterised are the isotype and the antigen binding affinity.

8.5 RADIOLABELLED ANTIBODIES

A variety of antibody conjugates have been used in drug targeting. Monoclonal antibodies have been attached to cytotoxic drugs, plant and bacterial toxins, cytokines and enzymes in attempts to treat cancer. In nuclear medicine we are concerned with using radiolabelled antibodies to either treat or diagnose the disease. The choice of radionuclide will depend upon the application envisaged. Table 1 lists the isotopes most commonly used for this purpose.

Table 1
Radionuclides of Interest for Antibody Labelling

Radionuclide	*Half life*	*Decay characteristics*
Imaging		
Iodine-131	8 days	364 keV γ, + β
Iodine-123	13 hours	159 keV γ
Indium-111	2.8 days	245, 171 keV γ
Technetium-99m	6 hours	141 keV γ
Therapy		
Iodine-131	8 days	364 keV γ, 0.6 MeV β
Yttrium-90	64 hours	2.3 MeV β
Rhenium-186	90 hours	1.1 MeV β
Rhenium-188	17 hours	2.1 MeV β
Copper-67	61 hours	0.4–0.6 MeV β
Samarium-153	1.95 days	0.8 MeV β
Phosphorus-32	14.3 days	1.7 MeV β
Astatine-211	7 hours	7.5/5.9 MrV α
Lead/bismuth-211	36 mins/2 mins	6.6 MeV α

8.5.1 Iodine Labelled Antibodies

Iodine was the first isotope to be used for radiolabelling studies. I-125 and I-131 have the advantages of cheapness and wide availability and although neither is ideal for either diagnostic or therapeutic use, the same iodination methods can be used for I-123.

Electrophilic substitution is by far the most widely practised method of labelling proteins with iodine. The labelling is mediated by oxidation of the iodide ion to the positively charged iodous ion which labels the phenolic ring of the tyrosine amino acid side chain in the ortho- and para-positions as shown in figure 3. Many oxidising systems have been used for this purpose, but the most popular are Chloramine-T and Iodogen™. Chloramine-T (Hunter and Greenwood, 1962) is a powerful oxidant and if exposed to the antibody for long periods of time may oxidise the side chains of its constituent amino acids. For this reason, after a brief exposure to the Chloramine-T, the reaction is stopped by the addition of sodium metabisulphite. For laboratory work, this method has the advantage of flexibility. The concentrations of the reagents can be adjusted in order to optimise the labelling for different proteins. When labelling for clinical application, however, the need to prepare fresh reagents for each labelling and the difficulties in ensuring sterility of the process argue against the use of this method. The Iodogen method (Fraker and Speck, 1978) is much more suitable for clinical application. Iodogen tubes are first prepared by dispensing a solution of the oxidant in dichloromethane into sterile glass of polypropylene tubes and allowing the solvent to evaporate under aseptic conditions. The resulting iodogen coated tubes can be stored

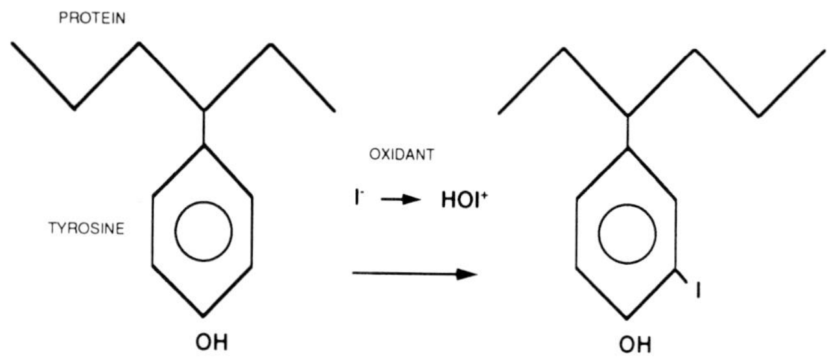

Figure 3. Mechanism of radioiodination by electrophilic substitution.

in a freezer for many months and used as required. Radiolabelling is performed by the addition of the protein and the radiolabel to the tube and incubation for 5—10 minutes. At the end of this time a labelling efficiency of 70—80% will be achieved, and the free iodine can be removed by either gel-filtration or ion-exchange chromatography.

These methods may need modification when used with I-123. This isotope has a much higher specific activity that either I-125 or I-131, and the chemical amounts of iodine present in the radioiodine solutions will be correspondingly much smaller. In the presence of a very low iodide concentrations, these methods are not very efficient, but labelling efficiency can be improved by adding small amounts of carrier iodide in the form of 'cold' potassium iodide.

A detailed method for labelling antibodies with Iodine-123 using Iodogen is described in Appendix I.

When labelling antibodies for *in-vivo* targetting, it is essential that the labelling process does not damage the antigen-binding ability of the antibody. For most antibodies, the Iodogen and Chloramine-T methods will preserve the antibodies immunoreactivity unchanged. On occasion, however an antibody may be encountered in which these methods result in a fall in binding ability, in which case it will be

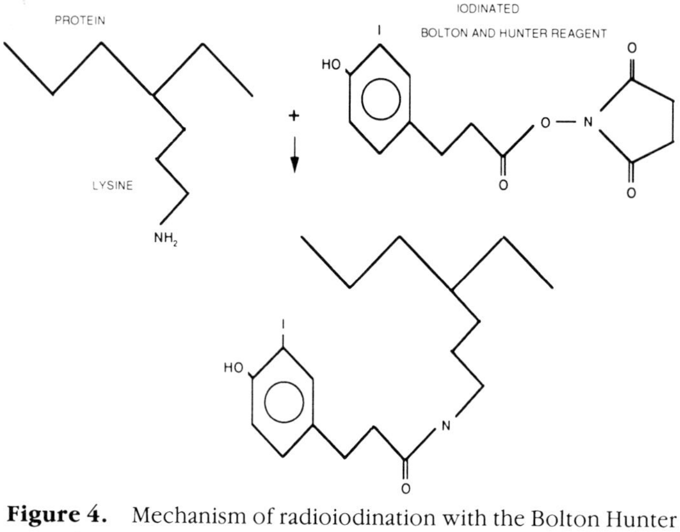

Figure 4. Mechanism of radioiodination with the Bolton Hunter reagent.

necessary to adopt a different methodology. Two approaches may be considered: (a) to use an oxidant which provides more gentle labelling conditions in order to avoid damaging the antibody. For this option the method of choice is probably an enzymic method based on lactoperoxidase or glucose oxidase. In the presence of hydrogen peroxide, these generate very mild oxidising conditions but normally give poorer labelling efficiences than Iodogen. The second alternative (b) is to use a chemistry which attaches the iodine to a different amino-acid. The most widely practised of these methods uses the Bolton and Hunter reagent (N-succimidyl 3-(4-hydroxyphenyl) propionate (Bolton and Hunter, 1973) (Figure 4). The molecule is first labelled with iodine using Chloramine-T and the labelled compound is then conjugated to amino groups on lysine amino-acid side chains. This multi-stage method is much more cumbersome and less efficient than Iodogen and has not generally been used for clinical studies.

8.5.2 Indium labelled antibodies

Indium-111 has the advantage of wider availability than Iodine-123. Its longer half-life also means that images may be taken for a longer period of time after injection. Antibodies cannot be directly labelled with Indium and a multi-stage approach using a bifunctional chelating agent (BFC) is required. A BFC consists of a chelating agent with a chemically reactive group capable of covalently binding to the protein. Any suitable chelator combined with a variety of reactive groups may be used, but the most popular have been based upon diethylene triamine penta acetic acid (DTPA) and ethylenediamine tetra acetic acid (EDTA). These polycarboxylic acid compounds has been widely used in radiopharmacy and form stable chelates with indium and other trivalent metals such as gallium and yttrium. Two main approaches have been taken towards the synthesis of these compounds. The simplest approach starts with the chelator itself and modifies one of the carboxylic acid groups in order to produce a suitable means of attachment to the antibody as shown in Figure 5. The most widely used BFC is the bicyclic dianhydride of DTPA which is commercially available (Hnatowich *et al*, 1983). A consequence of this approach is that one of the carboxyl groups of the DTPA, normally used to chelate the metal is now used for antibody attachment and is no longer available for chelation. This may result in a less stable conjugate. Accordingly the second, more synthetically difficult approach is to place the point of antibody attachment on the backbone of the chelator, thereby leaving all the carboxylic acid groups available for chelation (Esteban *et al*, 1987) (Figure 6). Even more stable conjugates may be produced by the use of macrocyclic chelating agents such as 'DOTA' which provide a closed 'cage' in which the metal ion is contained conferring a greater degree of thermodynamic stability (Broan *et al*, 1991).

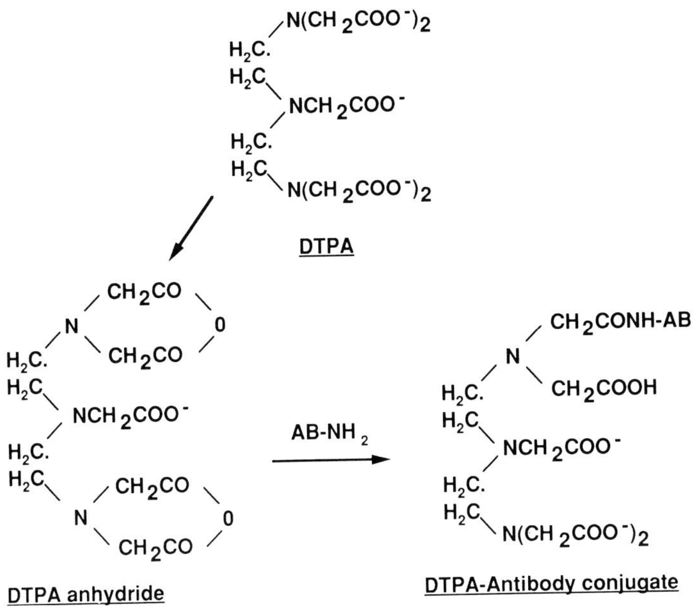

Figure 5. DTPA conjungation using the cyclic anhydride.

Thermodynamic stability, normally expressed in terms of association and dissociation constants are not the only important measure of stability for BFC's. Ka and Kd relate to conditions of equilibrium between chelate and free metal in a particular buffer at a particular pH. After IV administration of the conjugate, the equilibrium is lost and the metal will tend to dissociate from the chelate. However the rate at which this happens will vary greatly. It may happen within microseconds, or it may take days. Practical experience suggests that the rate of dissociation of the DTPA conjugates is very low and that despite a thermodynamic instability, the kinetic stability is sufficient for imaging investigations occuring over a period of a few days.

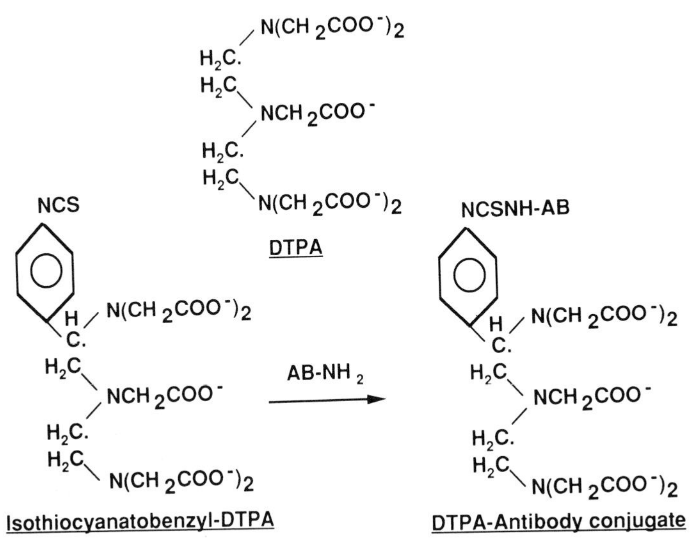

Figure 6. DTPA conjugation using a backbone substituted bifunctional chelating agent isothiocynatobenzyl DTPA.

The choice of chemically reactive group for the BFC depends upon the desired point of attachment on the antibody. The three most favoured sites are the amino groups of lysine, the thiol groups of cysteine and the carbohydrate side chains. The thiol and carbohydrate groups have the potential advantage that they are distant from antigen-binding part of the immunoglobulin. Thus the substitution of the chelating agent in this area is unlikely to affect antigen-binding. However the favoured site of attachment remains the lysine residues through reaction with anhydrides, active esters or isothiocyanates.

In practical terms, indium-labelling is a three-stage process:

1. Derivatisation in which the antibody is reacted in bulk with the BFC.
2. Purification in which unreacted chelating agent is removed, the solvent is changed and the antibody divided into patient-sized aliquots and
3. Radiolabelling in which the radioindium is attached to the protein-bound chelator.

A detailed method for labelling antibodies with Indium-111 using DTPA anhydride is described in Appendix II.

While developed initially for labelling with Indium-111 many of these methods may also be used for other trivalent metals such as yttrium and gallium (Mather *et al*, 1987). The stability of the resultant radioconjugate will, however vary considerable from metal to metal.

8.5.3 Technetium-labelled Antibodies

For many years it was believed that technetium was an unsuitable radiolabel for antibodies since the short half-life prevents imaging later than 24 hours after injection while the slow blood clearance of antibodies means that the best tumour: background ratios may not be obtained until after a delay of several days. Experience has now shown, however, that the superior imaging properties of technetium outweigh this disadvantage and Tc-99m is now the isotope of choice for immunoscintigraphy.

The direct labelling methods used for labelling albumin with Tc-99m for blood pool studies are unsuitable for antibodies since the label is unstable *in-vivo* and dissociates from the antibody during the imaging period. Two approaches have been followed to produce a stable technetium labelled antibody:

8.5.3.1 Reduction Mediated Labelling

Technetium forms stable complexes with sulphur-containing compounds and can bind to the sulphur containing amino-acids in the immunoglobulin. Normally these thiol groups are in the oxidised, disulphide form and are unavailable for labelling. However, in the presence of mild reducing conditions, free thiols can be exposed in order to form a stable complex with technetium (Mather and Ellison, 1990). The most popular reducing agents are either stannous ions or sulphur-containing compounds such as mercaptoethanol. After a reduction in bulk, the reducing agent is removed and the antibody divided into patient-size aliquots. At this stage the reduced thiols are prone to re-oxidation to disulphides and this must be prevented by removing oxygen from solvents and storing the reduced antibody either in a frozen or lyophilised form. The antibody is labelled by the addition of technetium, stannous ion and a weak complexing agent such as methylene diphosphonate. This ensures that any labelling of the protein occurs via the exposed thiol groups and not at other, low-affinity, binding sites in the protein. Labelling efficiencies of at least 95% can be routinely achieved preventing the need for any further purification of the radiopharmaceutical. (A detailed method for labelling antibodies with technetium-99m using a 2-mercaptoethanol reduction is described in Appendix III)).

8.5.3.2 Technetium Labelling with Bifunctional Chelating Agents

The method of labelling antibodies with BFC's as used for indium-111 cannot be directly used for technetium labelling. The problem arises during the labelling step when the technetium may bypass the chelator and bind directly to the protein from whence it dissociates when administered *in-vivo*. An alternative approach is to label the BFC first before attachment to the antibody, thus ensuring that all of the technetium is bound via the chelating agent. An example of this method was developed by Fritzberg and co-workers (Kasina *et al*, 1991) and is shown in Figure 7. These methods are necessarily more time consuming than the reduction methods and invariably result in a much lower labelling efficiency. However, the stability of the resulting complex is likely to be greater and these methods can be used for proteins other than immunoglobulins which may lack the disulphide bridges necessary for the reduction-mediated approach.

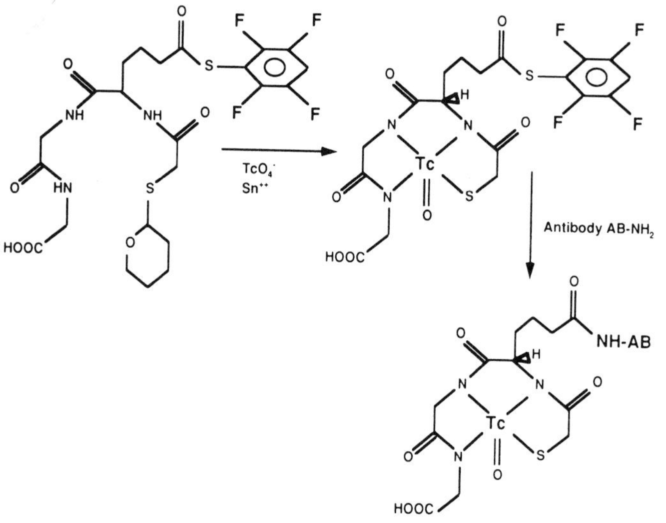

Figure 7. Technetium labelling using a pre-labelled bifunctional chelate (from Kasin *et al.*, 1991).

8.6 ANTIBODY ANALYSIS AND QUALITY CONTROL

8.6.1 Immunoreactivity

The term 'immunoreactivity' has two interpretations, either (a) the antigen binding ability of the radiolabelled antibody compared to the unlabelled starting material or (b) a measure of the proportion of the radiolabelled antibody preparation able to bind to antigen. More accurate descriptive terms might therefore be (a) Relative immunoreactivity and (b) immunoreactive fraction.

Both parameters are useful measures of the antibodies ability to bind to antigen, however it is important to appreciate that they are actually different and each has its own place in antibody targetting.

8.6.2 Relative Immunoreactivity

This is a useful way of finding if a particular process has damaged the antigen binding of an antibody preparation. It is effectively a 'before' and 'after' comparison normally performed as an Enyme Linked Immunosorbent Assay (ELISA) on a multi well plate (Figure 8).

A source of the antigen, either in a purified form or as a tumour cell line is first bound to the surface of the wells in a 96 well plate. Each well therefore contains a constant amount of antigen. Serial 1 in 10 dilutions of the two antibody preparations to be compared, ranging from undiluted,

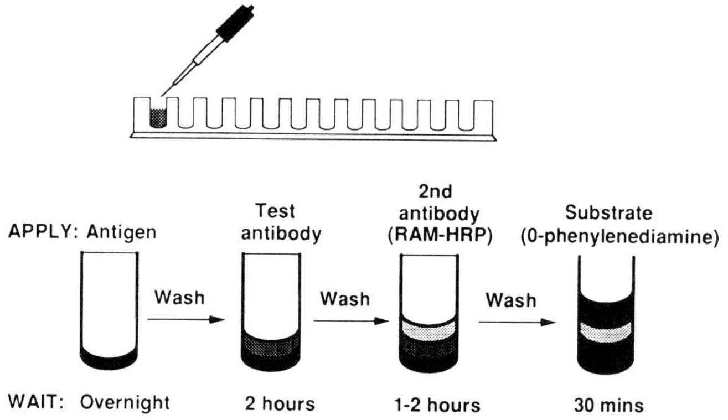

Figure 8. Steps in immunoreactivity by enzyme-linked immunosorbent assay (ELISA).

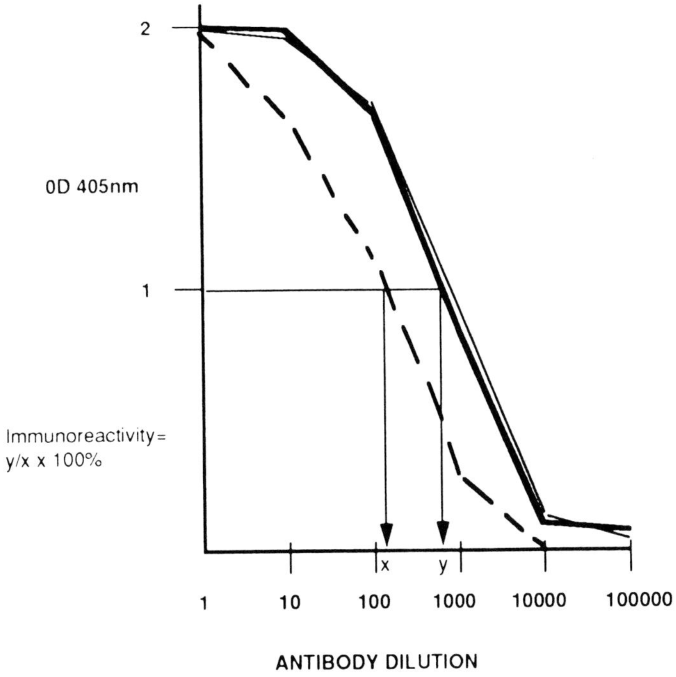

Figure 9. Example of immunoreactivity determination by ELISA. See text for details.

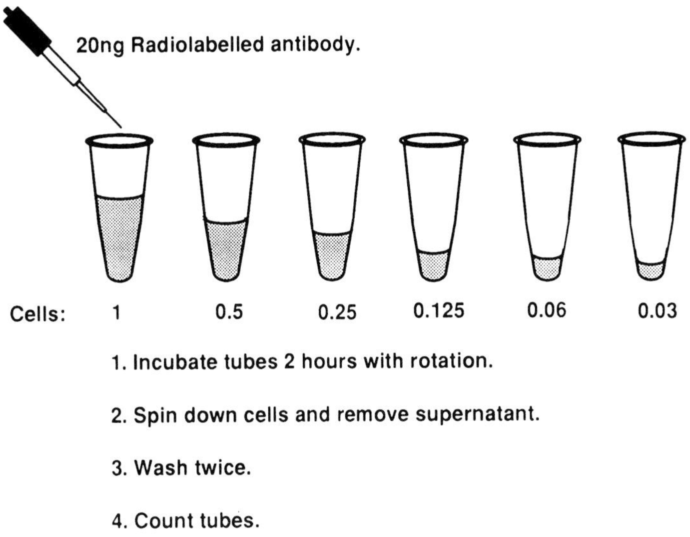

Figure 10. Steps in immunoreactivity determination by radioimmunoassay (RIA).

to 1 in 100,000 are made. 50µl of each dilution are added, in duplicate or triplicate, to the wells and the plate is incubated for 1—2 hours to allow the antibodies to bind to the antigen. The amount of antibody that binds at any particular dilution will depend upon the affinity of that antibody preparation. Thereafter, any unbound antibody is removed by aspirating the solution from the wells and washing the plate. In order to measure the amount of antigen-bound antibody, a second antibody, capable of binding to the test antibodies is used. This is normally an anti-species antibody such as, for example, a 'rabbit anti-mouse' antibody which will bind to all immunoglobulins derived from mice. This second antibody can be bought in a form in which an enzyme such as horseradish peroxidase is conjugated to it. The enzyme-conjugated-rabbit-anti-mouse antibody is diluted 1 in 500 and 50µl added to each well on the plate where it binds to the test antibodies bound to antigen. Any unbound second antibody is then, once again, washed away. 100µl of a solution of a chromogenic peroxidase substitute, such as o-phenylene diamine, is then added. This substrate turns yellow in the presence of the peroxidase and the intensity of the colour can be read in a spectrophotometer. Thus the amount of yellow colour produced is proportional to the amount of test monoclonal antibody binding to the plate.

A graph can be plotted of absorbance (intensity of yellow) versus antibody dilution giving a result as shown in Figure 9. The thickest line shows the results obtained with the standard unprocessed antibody preparation. This thin unbroken line indicates the type of result that would be obtained with a processed antibody for which the antigen binding ability was unaffected. The dotted line, on the other hand indicates a significant loss in antigen binding as a result of the processing. The results are normally quantified by comparing the concentrations of antibody giving an absorbance of 50% of the maximum.

The advantage of this technique is that you do not have to radiolabel the antibody to do the assay and the effect of any process on immunoreactivity can be determined. The assay has two disadvantages however. The first is that the result is only relative. It does not give an absolute measure of the actual ability of the antibody preparation to bind to antigen. The other problem relates to heterogeneity within the antibody preparation. When an antibody is radiolabelled with a high specific radionuclide such as technetium-99m, only a proportion of the antibody molecules will be radioactive. The actual proportion will depend upon the specific activity of the preparation, but it may well be less than 10%. If a result of the radiolabelling process is an absolute loss of immunoreactivity, then all the radioactive molecules will be unable to bind to antigen, but the unlabelled molecules will. The ELISA is unable to distinguish between 'hot' and 'cold' antibody and the binding of the 90% of unlabelled antibody will mask the effect of the radiolabelling.

8.6.3 Immunoreactive Fraction

A 'direct' binding assay overcomes these disadvantages. Firstly, it measures only the binding ability of the radioactive antibody molecules and secondly it gives an absolute measure of immunoreactivity. This assay normally uses tumour cells as its source of antigen. A series of 1 in 2 dilutions of cells is prepared in test tubes ranging from undiluted to 1 in 32 (Figure 10). To each tube is added a constant small amount of radiolabelled antibody. The tubes are incubated for 1—2 hours to allow the antibody to bind, and unbound radioactivity is then removed by centrifuging and washing the cells. The amount of antibody binding to each cell preparation can then be calculated by counting the tubes and comparing the counts bound with the counts initially added. A graph is then plotted of [total counts added]/[counts bound] versus cell dilution and a straight line is obtained as shown in Figure 11. The reciprocal of the intercept of the line on the y axis is a measure of the proportion of the radiolabelled antibody that would bind in the presence of an infinite amount of antigen. In other words, the proportion of radioactive antibody molecules that have the ability to bind to antigen, otherwise known as the immunoreactive fraction. Details of the methodology and mathematics of this and other direct binding technique can be found in the paper by Badger *et al.* (1987).

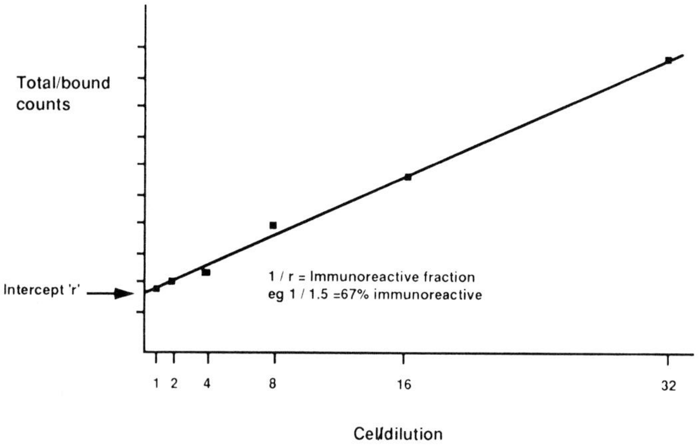

Figure 11. Example of determination of immunoreactive fraction by RIA. See text for details.

8.6.4 Chemical Purity

Two issues are of importance in relation to the purity of the antibody 1) freedom from other contaminating proteins 2) the molecular forms of the antibody itself.

8.6.4.1 SDS-PAGE

The first parameter is normally measured by polyacrylamide gel electrophoresis (PAGE). The antibody sample is loaded onto the top of a gel contained between glass plates. Under the influence of an electric potential difference, the protein passes into the gel and migrates at a rate determined by the

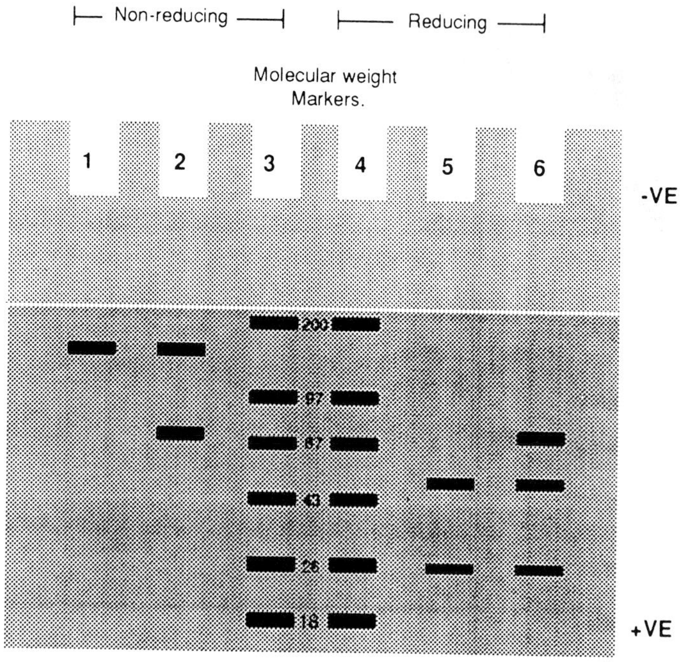

Figure 12. Example of SDS-Polyacrylamide gel electrophoresis. See text for details.

size and shape of the molecule. Effects of the electrical charge borne by the protein are nullified by the addition of a detergent – sodium dodecyl sulphate (SDS) – which gives everything an equal negative charge. The separation may be run in one of two modes; either reducing, in which the disulphide bonds holding the antibody together are cleaved, and non-reducing, in which the antibody migrates as a single molecule. After separation, the protein bands in the gel can be visualised by staining with a dye such as Coomassie Blue. An example is shown in Figure 12. Antibody preparations have been applied to tracks number 1, 2, 5 and 6 in a gel. Standards consisting of proteins of known molecular weights have been applied to tracks 3 and 4, the numbers indicate the molecular weights in kD. Tracks 1—3 have been run in a non-reducing mode and tracks 4—6 under reducing conditions. Track 1 shows a pure, non-reduced antibody preparation with a molecular weight of approx. 150,000 while track 2 shows a contaminating band of protein with a molecular weight of approx 67kD. Tracks 5 and 6 show the corresponding antibody preparations after reduction. The antibody has been separated into its constituent heavy and light chains with molecular weights of 50 and 25 kD respectively while the molecular weight of the contaminant remains unaltered.

8.6.4.2 Gel filtration

Immunoglobulins have a tendency to aggregate and, under certain circumstances can fragment into their constituent

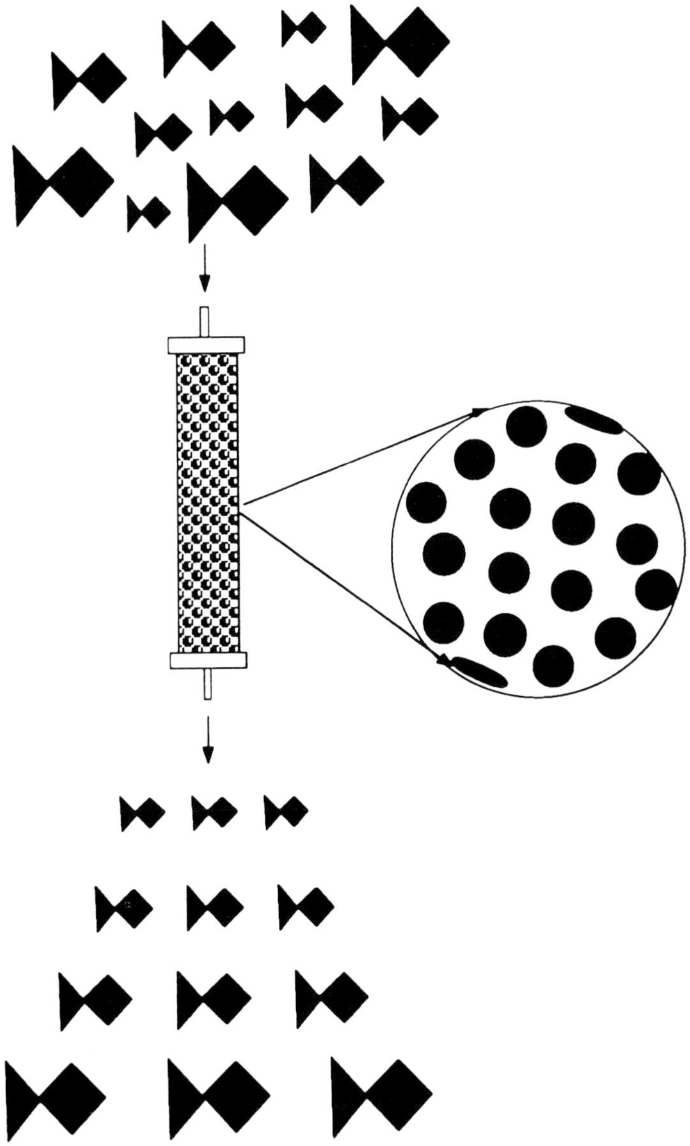

Figure 13. Principle of gel filtration showing sorting of molecules on the basis of size.

protein chains. Because the conditions prevailing in SDS-PAGE tend to dissociate these aggregates, a method which separates the proteins under more physiological conditions is often useful. Gel-filtration is the technique most commonly used. The antibody preparation is passed down a column comprised of microscopic beads containing small pores. Small molecules in the preparation are able to enter these pores while larger molecules are excluded from the beads and pass around them. As the mixture of molecules pass down the column, the flight path of the smaller molecules becomes gradually longer and longer resulting in a gradual separation of the molecules on the basis of their size (Figure 13). As the proteins pass out of the end of the column their presence can be detected by UV absorption. This method is widely used both for purification and analysis of protein mixtures. Radiolabelled proteins can also be analysed in this way by monitoring the radioactivity of the outflow from the column. Gel-filtration can be practised in a very simple manner by packing the beads into a hypodermic syringe and manually eluting the proteins with a suitable buffer. At the other end of the technological spectrum, gel-filtration can be practised in an HPLC mode in which all operations are automated. Much more efficient separations can be achieved by using pre-packed HPLC columns than are possible using open-column techniques although the resolution of this technique is not as great as that of SDS—PAGE.

8.6.5 Radiochemical purity

Simple chromatographic techniques can be used to measure the radiochemical purity of radiolabelled antibodies. Instant thin-layer chromatography strips (ITLC) are most commonly used for the solid phase and either 0.9% saline or 85% methanol as mobile phase. Under these conditions, labelled antibodies have an Rf = 0 and unbound radioisotope species such as free iodide and pertechnetate migrate with the solvent front. A disadvantage of this technique is that the labelled protein does not migrate from the origin and it is not easy to distinguish this species from any radioactive colloids which may be formed. This is particularly important in relation to indium-labelled antibodies since indium has a tendency to form colloidal hydroxides which also remain at the origin of the chromatogram.

A less simple but useful technique is cellulose acetate electrophoresis which has the ability to separate labelled protein from any colloidal contaminants while the most comprehensive method for measurement of RCP is probably HPLC gel-filtration (see example, Figure 14).

8.7 ANIMAL MODELS FOR RADIOLABELLED ANTIBODIES

Newly developed radiopharmaceuticals are normally investigated by performing biodistribution studies in suitable animals. A difficulty arises in relation to monoclonal antibodies in that the antibodies normally recognise antigens carried on the surface of human cancers but not on animal cancers. It is possible to raise antibodies against animal tumours and these can be useful in performing basic studies which help us to understand the behaviour of these radiotracers. However, in order to perform tumour targetting studies on antibodies intended for human use an alternative strategy must be employed. The most common approach is

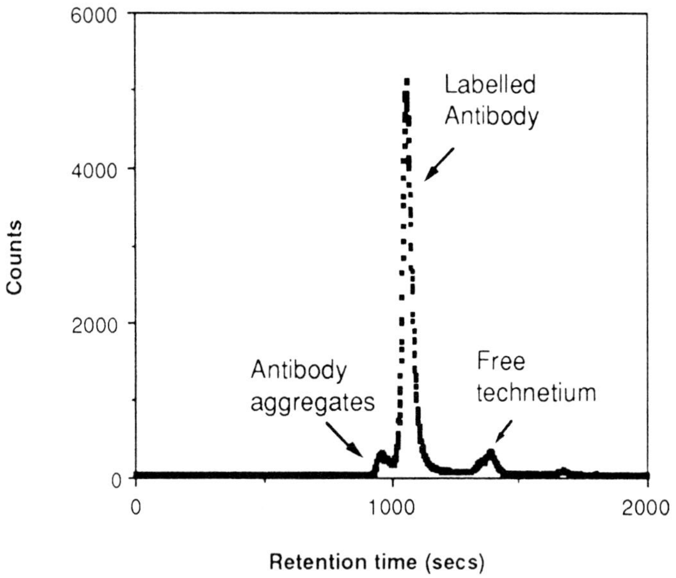

Figure 14. Example of radioactive trace from HPLC gel filtration of technetium labelled antibody.

to use the nude mouse model. The nude mouse congenitally lacks a thymus gland and is therefore unable to manufacture mature T-cells. Its immune system is therefore severly compromised, in particular, its ability to reject transplanted tissue grafts. Human tumour cells appropriate for the antibody under consideration can be grown in tissue culture and injected into the flanks of these animals. After a few weeks, the tumours will grow into discrete tumours a few millimeters in diameter. These tumours bear the antigen recognised by the antibody and biodistribution studies can therefore be performed using the radiolabelled immunoglobulin to determine its tumour targetting *in vivo*. Care must be taken in interpreting the results of these experiments for the following reasons: (i) Most monoclonal antibodies are of mouse origin. Biodistribution studies performed in mice will not therefore reproduce any foreign protein recognition systems which might be present in man. An indication of this factor is the difference in the plasma half-times of injected antibodies. In mice, radioiodinated antibodies have clearance half-times of the order of 3–7 days while in man, these are reduced to 1-2 days due to accelerated clearance of the foreign protein. (ii) In man, the tumour-associated antigens recognised by the antibody are often carried on normal tissues as well as in the tumour. Although the level of expression on normal tissues may be many orders of magnitude less than in tumour, the much larger bulk of normal tissue means that the total levels of antigen borne by normal and malignant tissues may be comparable. In the nude-mouse/xenograft model the antigens are carried only by the tumour and targetting may therefore be more efficient in this model. (iii) The weight of the mouse, the weight of the tumour and the pathology of the xenograft are quite different to the same parameters in actual patients. The proportion of an injected dose of radiolabelled antibody accumulated by both normal tissues and the tumour in the nude-mouse are orders of magnitude different to the results obtained in man. For example, an injection of a radiotracer uniformly distributed in a 20 gramme mouse would give a mean uptake of 5% of the injected dose per gramme of tissue. In a 70 kilogramme man, the equivalent figure would be $100/70{,}000 = 0.0014\%$ per gramme. It is usual to obtain figures of approximately 20% of the injected dose per gramme of tumour in the nude mouse. In man, the tumour uptake is very much less than this (see below).

Despite these considerations, useful results can be obtained from animal experiments provided these are designed and interpreted correctly. In particular, results of comparisons obtained in animals are normally also valid in man. Thus a comparison of one antibody preparation with another, or one labelling method with another will normally produce results which can be directly extrapolated to the human situation.

8.8 PHARMACOKINETIC ASPECTS OF RADIOLABELLED ANTIBODIES

As with all radiotracers, it is important to remember that the tissue distribution of the radioactivity observed is not necessarily the distribution of the intact radiopharmaceutical but may result from metabolism of the starting material. Radiolabelled antibodies are not exception to this rule and the biodistribution of these materials depends to a very large degree on the radioisotope being used and the method of radiolabelling employed. The pharmacology of these tracers is complex and by no means fully understood. In this chapter it is not possible to include more than a general overview of the results obtained from a decade of the clinical use of these materials.

After intravenous injection all radiolabelled antibodies undergo a phase of relatively rapid distribution with plasma half-lives of a few hours during which the protein equilibrates with the extracellular fluid. After equilibration, the tracer follows a phase of much slower metabolism and clearance with plasma half-lives ranging from 12–48 hours. The actual rate of clearance varies not only from antibody to antibody but also from patient to patient. Accelerated clearance rates are seen in patients who have pre-existing antibodies to mouse proteins. These bind to the radiolabelled antibody, forming immune complexes which are rapidly cleared by the reticuloendithelial system.

Studies on the serum stability of radiolabelled antibodies suggest that very little breakdown occurs in the blood. Some studies have suggested that indium may transchelate to circulating transferrin which is present in great excess. However this occurs very slowly and does not influence the biodistribution a great deal.

Although the mean rate of blood clearance of antibodies labelled with different radionuclides is not dramatically different, there are great differences in the subsequent metabolism of these materials. The liver appears to be the main site of antibody metabolism and all radiolabelled antibodies show initial high levels of hepatic uptake. The liver uptake is not due to recognition of the antibody either as 'foreign' or as 'damaged due to the labelling process' since even biosynthetically labelled antibodies in mice exhibit this phenomenon. The mechanism of this uptake has been much discussed but not unequivocably identified.

Within the liver, the antibodies undergo metabolism and radiolabelled catabolites are produced. The use of radioiodinated antibodies results in the release of radioiodide and iodotyramine which are secreted back into the bloodstream from whence they undergo rapid renal excretion. This results in a gradual diminution of the levels of radioactivity in the liver. Approximately 30% of the injected dose of radioiodine is excreted in the first 24 hours after injection provided that the thyroid gland is effectively blocked. It is believed that a large proportion of this iodine is released by the action of iodotransferase enzymes since the *o*- and *p*-iodinated phenolic side chain of tyrosine bears a structural resemblance to the thyroid hormones. In order to try and overcome this instability it is possible to produce reagents in which the iodine is contained in a non-phenolic ring. These can be conjugated to antibodies in a manner similar to the Bolton and Hunter reagent. Studies in animals have shown that these conjugates undergo much less dehalogenation than occurs with antibodies labelled by electrophilic substitution (Wilbur *et al*, 1989).

When indium-labelled antibodies are used, the catabolic process results in metabolites which remain trapped within the liver. Hepatic uptake of indium remains high and may even increase with time. The identity of the indium-labelled metabolites has not been proven. Evidence indicates, however, that the indium remains chelated and presumably attached to small peptides. A small amount (3-5%) of radioindium is excreted in the urine and a few percent is excreted via the gastrointestinal tract. The large majority of the radionuclide, however, remains in the body and the whole body clearance rate is very similar to the physical rate of decay of the isotope.

Technetium labelled antibodies show a hepatic uptake intermediate between that of indium and iodine with a large degree of interpatient variation. In addition technetium shows some uptake in the kidney, presumably as a result of transchelation of the isotope to renal metalloproteins.

In non-malignant tissues, therefore, the picture is one of slow blood clearance, early uptake into the liver which is either transient or persistant, and some uptake into kidney, spleen, bone-marrow and bowel depending upon the radiolabel used.

Tumour uptake occurs quite early and is probably maximal by about 24 hours after injection although tumour to non-tumour ratios will continue to increase thereafter as normal tissue activity declines. The amount of injected antibody taken up by the tumour is small – ranging from 0.001 to 0.02% of the injected does per gramme of tumour with a mean of approx. 0.005%. Thus a 100g tumour will take up about 0.5% of the injected dose. There is evidence that the antibody can undergo metabolism in the tumour and that the picture seen in the liver is reproduced to a certain extent. Tumour-uptake of iodine labelled antibodies may therefore be more transient that of indium. Microscopic studies of the intratumoural distribution of the radioactivity show that this is normally confined to the most highly perfused areas of the tumour – the periphery and the areas surrounding the blood vessels.

The major factor limiting antibody uptake by the tumour appears to be physical access. While tumours require a blood supply for growth, they do not possess lymphatic vessels. A consequence of this is that hydrostatic pressures rise within the tumour as it grows, inhibiting access of materials to the centre of the mass. Molecules are transported into the tumour either by blood flow or by diffusion, the larger the molecule, the more important becomes blood flow and the less significant diffusion. Antibodies are relatively large molecules and are thus entirely dependent upon blood flow for access to the tumour. A result of high interstitial pressure and poor blood flow is therefore low tumour uptake of radiolabelled antibodies. Attempts have been made to overcome this problem by using smaller molecules. Immunoglobulins undergo proteolytic digestion to produce smaller fragments which retain their ability to bind to antigen. F(ab')2 and Fab fragments do show better penetration into tumours than intact antibodies. However, the total amount of radiotracer taken up is actually reduced in comparison to whole antibody as a result of the more rapid blood clearance of these fragments. Fab and F(ab')2 fragments are still large molecules compared to the majority of radiopharmaceuticals, having molecular weights of 50,000 and 100,000 daltons respectively. Using genetic engineering techniques smaller antigen binding molecules still can be created. It is hoped that these will improve the tumour access of these materials still further.

Genetic engineering may also help to overcome a problem associated with the repeated use of radiolabelled antibodies. Since most monoclonal antibodies are of mouse origin, the human immune system recognises them as foreign molecules and generates Human Anti-Mouse Antibodies against them. The severity of the HAMA response depends upon the number of administrations and the amount of antibody injected. A consequence of HAMA is the formation of immune complexes in the serum. These are rapidly cleared by the reticuloendothelial system preventing tumour uptake of the antibody. Recombinant DNA techniques can generate 'chimeric' or 'humanised' antibodies which are more human-like and induce a much weaker immune response.

8.9 CLINICAL USES OF RADIOLABELLED ANTIBODIES

The low absolute amounts of antibody taken up by tumours has not prevented the successful application of this technique in imaging cancer. Better results have been obtained in certain types of cancer eg ovarian and colorectal tumours than in others such as breast cancer. The reasons for this relate in part to the anatomical locations of the disease in relation to major blood vessels for example and also to the pathology of the tumour – its structure and vascularity.

Experience has also confirmed what every student of nuclear medicine should already know – that technetium-99m produces better quality images – and hence better diagnostic results – than other isotopes. Using the labelling and analytical techniques described above in conjunction with appropriate tumour-associated antibodies, imaging sensitivities of greater than 90% can be achieved. Some examples of images obtained in colorectal and ovarian cancer are shown in Figures 15 and 16.

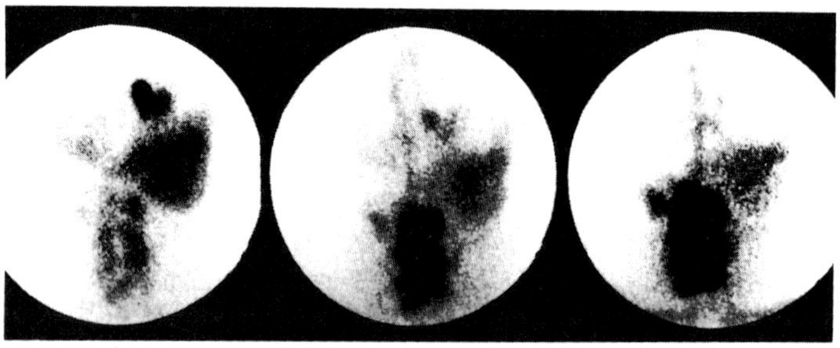

Figure 15. Images of a patient with poorly differentiated adenocarcinoma of the transverse colon injected with 99m-Tc-PR1A3. The figure shows anterior views of the chest taken 5 minutes, 6 hours and 22 hours after injection. Note the decreasing activity in the heart and the increasing uptake in the tumour (just below the liver) with time.

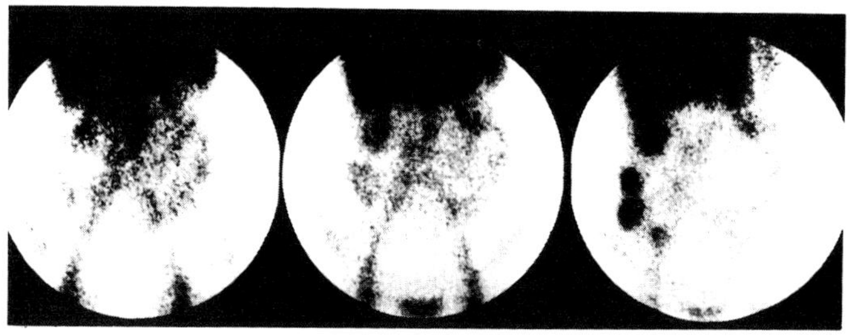

Figure 16. Images of a patient with recurrent ovarian carcinoma injected with 99m Tc-HMFG1. The figure shows anterior views of the pelvis 10 minutes, 6 hours and 22 hours after injection. Focal uptake in two tumour sites in the right pelvis are seen on the 22 hour image. Note the relatively high uptake in the liver and slight uptake in the kidneys (see text). (Reproduced from Britton and Granowska, 1991).

The improvements resulting from the use of technetium labelled antibodies means that immunoscintigraphy now has the potential to become a routine part of nuclear medicine. Technetium labelling of antibodies is a relatively recent development and has only become widely practised in the last two years or so. At the time of writing no such product is commercially available and the delays imposed by regulatory considerations mean that no such preparation is likely to become widely available for some years to come. For the time being, therefore, the use of these materials will be confined to institutions with the facilities to produce their own antibodies and label them appropriately.

For imaging tumours, it is sufficient if a small proportion of the tumour cells take up sufficient of the radioactivity to enable the observer to distinguish a focus of activity from the background. The therapeutic application of these materials requires a jump of several orders of magnitude in targetting efficiency. At the present time, successes in radioimmunotherapy are somewhat anecdotal and no large degree of efficacy has yet been demonstrated. It is possible that the improvements in antibody design and labelling technology currently under development will enable the leap from diagnostics to therapeutics to be made. Only time will tell.

8.10 CONCLUSION

Monoclonal antibodies have been developed which can differentiate between normal and malignant cells. These can be produced in large amounts by tissue culture to the required standards for pharmaceutical application. Techniques have been developed for radiolabelling these antibodies with a variety of radionuclides in such a way that their ability to bind to specific antigen remains undiminished. When administered to patients, radiolabelled antibodies show specific uptake in tumours bearing the relevant antigens as well as in a number of normal organs, notably the liver. Tumour imaging has ben most successful using technetium-99m labelled antibodies in ovarian and colorectal cancer.

Appendix 1: Iodination of Monoclonal Antibodies with I-123 using Iodogen™

1. In a fume cupboard set up a gel-filtration column (see Figure 17): Remove the barrel from a 20 ml syringe. On a melolin dressing pack mark a circle with a diameter equal to that of the inside of the syringe. Cut out the circle, remove the paper wrapping and place the dressing in the bottom of the syringe. Clamp the syringe vertically. Close the bottom with a blind hub. Shake a bottle of swollen Sephadex-G50 (2 gramme

in 30 mls of water). Pour into the syringe right to the top. Allow a few minutes to settle. Remove the blind hub and allow the liquid to run into a suitable waste container. When all the supernatant has run through, gently add phosphate buffered saline (PBS) containing 1% Human serum albumin (HSA) to the top of the column taking care not to disturb the gel. Continue to do this until threee column volumes of PBS/HSA have run through the column. Recap the syringe when approx 1 ml of liquid remains above the gel. Stir up the top 1 cm of the gel with hypodermic needle and allow it to settle.

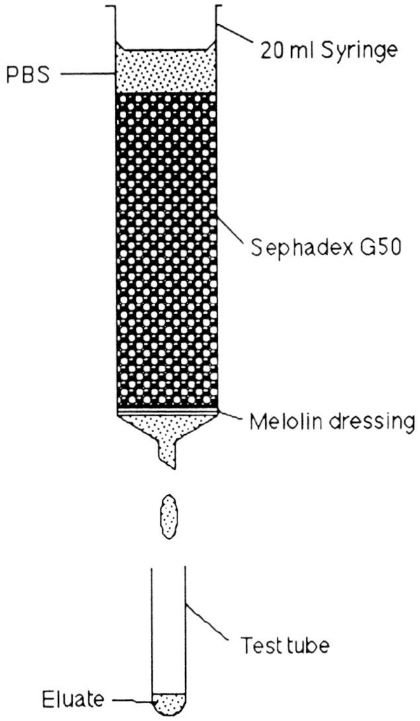

Figure 17. Sephadex Gel filtration column made from hypodermic syringe.

2. Prepare a solution of potassium iodide 5mg in 100ml of water for injection.
3. In rapid succession pipette 500 μg of antibody solution*, the required activity of I-123 and 5 μl of potassium iodide solution into an iodogen tube. Mix well and incubate for 10 minutes at room temperature.
4. Transfer the solution from the iodogen tube to a fresh test tube. Measure the labelling efficiency by ITLC-SG chromatography using 85% methanol as mobile phase. Labelled protein has Rf = 0.
5. Purify the labelled protein by gel-filtration: Remove the blind hub from the syringe and allow the supernatant to run through leaving a flat top to the gel. GENTLY layer the labelled antibody mixture onto the gel and allow to run into the column. Gently add 12 consecutive 1ml aliquots of PBS/1% HSA to the top of the column and collect 1ml factions from the bottom of the syringe. Cap the tubes containing the fractions as they come off. Measure the activity in the tubes in an ionisation chamber and the activity remaining on the column. Calculate the labelling efficiency from the proportions of radioactivity in the two peaks.
6. Pool the fractions containing the labelled protein and measure the radiochemical purity of the labelled antibody using ITLC chromatography.

*The iodination has a pH optimum between pH 7 and 8. The antibody solution should have a concentration of at least 1mg/ml in a buffer at a neutral pH.

Appendix II: 111-Indium Labelling of antibodies

NOTE: All reagents and materials should be as free of metal ion contamination as is practically possible. The highest analytical grade of chemicals, and in particular water, should be used. Disposable plastic containers are preferable to glassware which, if unavoidable, should be of borosilicate glass, washed with IM hydrochloric acid and rinsed with de-ionised water until neutral to litmus.

Derivatisation

1. The antibody should be obtained in a suitable buffer (eg Hepes, phosphate, bicarbonate) at a pH compatible with the biological properties of the antibody, but designed to optimise the reaction (pH 8-8.5). Protein concentration (measurable by optical density at 280nm) should be high – >5 mgs per ml.
2. Cyclic DTPA anhydride (CDTPAA, Sigma chemicals) is dissolved in dry DMSO to a concentration of 2—10 mgs per ml. (DMSO is hygroscopic, anhydrous material should be purchased and stored over a molecular sieve.
3. Sufficient CDTPAA solution to give an anhydride : antibody molar ratio of 2–4:1 is added dropwise to the stirred antibody solution. The mixture is then stirred for a further five minutes.
4. At this stage an estimation of the success of the derivatisation procedure is useful. This can be performed as follows:-

   Adjust the pH of a small sample of the reaction mixture to pH 5-6 by the addition of 1M acetate buffer pH 5. Add a trace amount (approx 1MBq) of 111-In-acetate and incubate for 5 minutes. Separate the protein bound and unbound forms of indium either on a short gel-filtration column (eg Sephadex) or by an appropriate TLC method (eg ITLC paper developed with 0.1M citrate buffer). The proportion of activity associated with the protein should be at least 35%.

Purification

The unbound DTPA is now separated from protein-bound DTPA by passage down a suitable chromatographic column. Ideally this should be a plastic-based HPLC column such as the FPLC Superose columns (Pharmacia). Alternatively a 30—60 cm Sephacryl or Sephadex column may be used. (The FPLC or Sephacryl columns will remove antibody aggregates formed during the derivatisation reaction, Sephadex columns will not).

The column should be first equilibrated and the sample then eluted with 0.1M acetate (or citrate) buffer pH 5—6. Fractions containing the monomeric antibody peak should be collected and pooled. After measurement of the protein concentration, the derivatised antibody can be aliquotted into suitably sized patient doses and frozen for future use.

Radiolabelling

To a vial of 111-In-chloride is added sufficient 5M acetate buffer pH5.5 to produce a final concentration of 0.5M acetate. A vial of antibody is thawed and added dropwise to the indium acetate solution. The mixture is incubated for 10–30 minutes. The radiochemical purity of the preparation can be measured by a suitable TLC method (e.g. ITLC paper developed in 0.5M acetate buffer pH6 containing 1 mg per ml EDTA or DTPA). If further purification is required, this can be performed on a Sephadex or HPLC column.

Appendix III: 99m-technetium Labelling of Antibodies

Antibody reduction:

1. Purge a 100ml bottle of phosphate buffered saline (PBS) with nitrogen. Keep on ice.
2. If necessary, concentrate the MoAb to a concentration of 5—10mg/ml.
3. Calculate the volume of 2-mercaptoethanol that must be added to the MoAb to give a molar ratio of 2000:1 (2-ME:MoAb) NB. MWt MoAb = 150,000, MWt 2-ME = 78, density of 2-ME = 1.114.
4. Draw up the required volume, add to the MoAb, cap the tube and mix well. [NB 2-mercaptoethanol emits a foul odour – do this quickly!]
5. Leave the tube to incubate at room temperature for 30 minutes.
6. Prepare a gel filtration column (See figure 17): Remove the barrel from a 20 ml syringe. On a melolin dressing pack mark a circle with a diameter equal to that of the inside of the syringe. Cut out the circle, remove the paper wrapping and place the dressing in the bottom of the syringe. Clamp the syringe vertically. Close the bottom with a blind hub. Shake a bottle of swollen Sephadex-G50 (2 gramme in 30 mls water). Pour into the syringe right to the top. Allow a few minutes to settle. Remove the blind hub and all the liquid to run into a suitable waste container. When all the supernatant has run through, gently add cold N_2 purged PBS to the top of the column taking care not to disturb the gel. Continue to do this until three column volumes of PBS have run through the column. Reclose the syringe when approx 1ml of liquid remains above the gel. Stir up the top 1cm of the gel with a hypodermic needle and allow it to settle.
7. When the 30 minute incubation period is complete, remove the blind hub and allow the supernatant to run through leaving a flat top to the gel. GENTLY layer the antibody onto the gel and allow to run into the column. Gently add 12 consecutive 1ml aliquots of PBS to the top of the column and collect 1ml factions from the bottom of the syringe. Cap the tubes containing the fractions, and keep them on ice when they come off.
8. Measure the OD 280nm of each fraction on a UV spectrophotometer. Pool all fractions with a concentration >1mg/ml. (Absorbance of 1mg/ml solution of IgG = 1.4/cm light path). Measure the concentration of the pooled antibody. Cap the tube and keep on ice. Divide into 500μg aliquots and freeze at the lowest temperature available.

Antibody labelling:

1. Reconstitute an Amersham MDP kit with 5mls of 0.9% sodium chloride injection. Add 40μl to 500μg of the reduced antibody. Mix. Add 740 MBq of sodium [Tc^{99m}] pertechnetate. Mix and wait 10 minutes.
2. Measure the labelling efficiency of the preparations by chromatography using ITLC-SG and 0.9% saline as mobile phase. [Labelled antibody has an Rf = O].

References

Badger C.C., Krohn K.A. and Bernstein I.D. (1987). *In-vitro measurement of avidity of radioionated antibodies.* Nucl. Med. Biol. **14**, 605–610.

Bolton A.E. and Hunter W.M. (1973). *The labelling of proteins to high specific activities by conjugation to an I–125 containing acylating agent.* Biochemical J. **133**, 529.

Britton K.E. and Granowska M. (1991). *The role of radiolabelled antibodies in cancer diagnosis. In "Monoclonal Antibodies. Applications in Clinical Oncology".* Ed. A. Epenetos. Chapman and Hall, London.

Broan C.J., Cox J.P.L., Craig A.S., Kataki R., Parker D., Harrison A., Randall A.M. and Ferguson G. (1991). *Structure and solution stability of indium and gallium complexes of 1,4,7-triazacyclononanetriacetic acid and of yttrium complexes of 1,4,7,10-tetraazacyclododecanetetraacetate and related ligands.* J. Chem. Soc. Perkin Trans. **2**, 87–99.

Esteban J.M., Schlom J., Gansow O.A., Atcher R.W., Brechbiel M.W., Simpson D.E. and Colcher D. (1987). *New method for the chelation of indium-111 to monoclonal antibodies: Biodistribution and imaging of athymic mice bearing human colon carcinoma xenografts.* J. Nucl. Med. **28**, 861–870.

Fraker P.J. and Speck J.C. (1978). *Protein and cell membrane iodinations with a sparingly soluble chloroamide 1,3,4,6-tetrachloro, 3a, 6a diphenylglycoluril.* Biochem. Biophys Res. Comm. **80**, 849.

Hnatowitch D.J., Childs R.L., Lanteigne D and Najafi A. (1983). *DTPA-coupled antibodies radiolabelled with metallic radionuclides: an improved method.* J. Immunological methods. **65**, 147–157.

Hunter W.M. and Greenwood F.C. (1962). *Preparation of Iodine-131 labelled human growth hormone of high specific activity.* Nature. 194–495.

Kasina S., Rao T.N., Srinivasan A., Sanderson J.A., Fitzner J.N., Reno J.M., Beaumier, P.L. and Fritzberg, A.R., (1991). *Development and biologic evaluation of a kit for preformed chelate technetium-99m radiolabelling of an antibody Fab fragment using a diamide dimercaptide chelating agent.* J. Nucl. Med. **32**, 1445–1451.

Mather S.J. and Ellison D. (1990). *Reduction Mediated Technetium-99m Labelling of Monboclonal Antibodies.* J. Nucl. Med. **31**, 692–697.

Mather S.J., Tolley D., White G.W. (1989). *Labelling Monoclonal Antibodies with Yttrium-90.* Eur. J. Med. **15**, 307–312.

Meares C.F., McCall M.J., Reardan D.T., Goodwin D.A., Diamanti C.I. and McTigue M. (1984). *Conjugation of antibodies with bifunctional chelating agents: Isothiocyanate and bromoacetamide reagents, methods of analysis and subsequent addition of metal ions.* Analytical Biochemistry. **142**, 68–78.

Report 1. (1986). *Operation Manual for control of production, preclinical toxicology and phase 1 trials of anti-tumour antibodies and drug antibody conjugates.* British Journal of Cancer. **54**, 557–568.

Report 2. (1988). *Guidelines on the production and quality control of monoclonal antibodies of murine origin intended for use in man.* Tibtech. **6**, G5–G8.

Wilbur D.S., Hadley S.W., Hylarides M.D., Abrams P.G., Beaumier P.A., Morgan A.C., Reno J.M. and Fritzberg A.R. (1989). *Development of a stable radioiodinating reagent to label monoclonal antibodies for radiotherapy of cancer.* J. Nucl. Med. **30**, 216–226.

Recommended Further Reading

Antibodies in Radiodiagnosis and therapy. M.R. Zalutsky. CRC press (1989).

Essential Immunology. I. Roitt. Blackwell Scientific Publications (1991).

Radioiodination techniques. Reviewed 18. Amersham International plc.

An introduction to radioimmunassay and related techniques. Chard, T. Laboratory techniques in Biochemistry and molecular biology Vol 6. Elsevier Science Publishers. (1990).

Chapter 9

Quality Control of Radiopharmaceuticals

A.E. Theobald

9.1 INTRODUCTION

Radiopharmaceuticals are usually formulated as sterile, apyrogenic injections and are administered to patients for diagnostic or therapeutic purposes. In this respect they are no different to conventional parenteral medicines in their requirements of purity or efficacy. Standards of quality and purity must be divised for these materials and dispensed products should tested to. ensure compliance with those standards.

The main difference between radiopharmaceuticals and conventional medicines lies in the (sometimes) very short usable life of the radioactive product (often measured in hours) compared with conventional injectable pharmaceuticals (measured in months or years). Table 1 shows the characteristics of all the radionuclides presently included in the BP 1988 and its Addenda. Unlike standard parenteral

Table 1
BP Radionuclides

Radionuclide	$T_{1/2}$	*Most prominent gamma photons*	*Radionuclidic impurities*
^{32}P	14.3 d	B_{max} = 1.71 MeV	None listed
^{51}Cr	27.7 d	0.320 MeV	Non listed
^{57}Co	271 d	0.122 MeV	nmt 0.1% ^{56}Co and ^{57}Co
^{58}Co	70.8 d	0.511, 0.811 MeV	^{57}Co, ^{60}Co (nmt 1%), nmt 2% total
^{59}Fe	44.6 d	1.10, 1.29	Not listed, ^{55}Fe not normally detected
^{67}Ga	3.26 d	0.093, 0.185, 0.30	nmt 0.2% ^{66}Ga (9.4h, 1.039 MeV)
^{75}Se	118.5 d	0.136, 0.265	Non listed
^{99}Tc^{m}	6.02 h	0.140	^{99}Mo, nmt 1×10^{-1}%
			^{131}I*, nmt 5×10^{-3}%
			^{103}Ru*, nmt 5×10^{-3}%
			^{89}Sr*, nmt 6×10^{-5}%
			^{90}Sr*, nmt 6×10^{-4}%
			α-emitters*, nmt 1×10^{-7}%
			*fission-derived only
^{111}In	2.8 d	0.173, 0.247	^{114m}In, nmt 0.2% (49.5 d, 0.190 MeV)
^{123}I	13 h	0.027, 0.160	^{124}I, nmt 2% (4.2d, 0.603 MeV)
			^{125}I, and ^{126}I, nmt 2%
^{125}I	60.1 d	0.027	^{126}I (13.0 d, 0.388, 0.666)
^{131}I	8.04 d	0.365	Non listed
^{133}Xe	5.29 d	0.081, 0.03–0.035	^{133}Xe^{m} (2.19 d, 0.233 MeV)
^{198}Au	2.70 d	0.412 MeV	^{199}Au (0.158 MeV)
^{201}Tl	73 h	0.068, 0.083	^{200}Tl, (1.09 d, 0.368, 0.579, 0.828, 1.206 MeV)
			^{202}Tl* (12.2 d, 0.440 MeV)
			^{201}Pb (9.4 h, 0.331 MeV)
			^{203}Pb (2.17d, 0.279 MeV)
			*nmt 2% of total, nlt 97% ^{201}Tl
Other radionuclides			
^{113}In^{m}	104m	0.390	

pharmaceuticals, radiopharmaceuticals cannot be manufactured, tested and quarantined until the test results (e.g. sterility) are available as most (if not all) of the radioactivity will have decayed to non-useful levels. In contrast to ordinary pharmaceuticals many radiopharmaceuticals have to be manufactured, quality tested, and then administered to the patient within a short period of time, often within the same working day.

Under these circumstances the radiopharmacist has often adopted a set of quick, efficient discriminative tests which can be applied to the dispensed materials before they are released for use in the nuclear medicine clinic. These quality control tests are the subject of this chapter. By themselves they do not and cannot guarantee the quality of the radiopharmaceutical. Alongside these tests lies another set of controls such as operator training and performance testing, environmental monitoring, etc which are the subjects of other chapters in this volume.

Radiopharmaceutical quality control testing involves the application of a set of well defined and validated test procedures to samples of the dispensed or manufactured product. All quality control laboratories will apply the principles of good laboratory practice, among which is the provision and use of Standard Operating Procedures (SOP's). Throughout this chapter, test methods are illustrated by the inclusion of SOPs in the hope that the reader can adopt similar procedures, suitably modified for local conditions and equipment.

9.2 QUALITY CONTROL PARAMETERS

There are a number of parameters which are routinely measured as indicators of quality.

9.2.1 Radioactivity

Radioactivity is defined in the BP 1988 as 'the number of nuclear transformations per unit time in a given amount of the [radioactive] preparation.' Radioactivity is measured in units of the Becquerel (Bq), equivalent to an average transformation rate of one per second. The Becquerel is an inconveniently small unit for radiopharmaceutical work and the multiples kBq (10^3 Bq), MBq (10^6 Bq), and GBq (10^9Bq) are used in are used in practice. The older units of the Curie (Ci, equivalent to 37 GBq), and its submultiples mCi (37MBq) and μCi (37kBq) are still used in the USA and in many other countries.

Absolute measurement of radioactivity is difficult and time consuming: it requires equipment and techniques available only in specialist laboratories such as the National Physical Laboratory. The BP sets limits of +/− 10% (or 15% in some cases) for the radioactivity of most official radiopharmaceuticals and in the radiopharmacy there is a requirement to measure the radioactivities of dispensed radiopharmaceuticals to a precision of about 2 – 5%.

9.2.1.2 Ionisation Chambers

Radioactivities in the high kBq and MBq range (i.e. the normal radioactive doses given to patients) are measured with ionisation chambers or radionuclide calibrators. In these instruments the current flowing between a charged cylindrical electrode and ground depends on the radioactivity of a sample placed in a re-entrant chamber. Although the magnitude of this current is small, about 1–10 pA (10^{-12} A), it is easily measured with modern electrometric instruments. The ionisation current (i) depends on the radioactivity (A) and ionising ability (k) of a particular radionuclide

$$i \ (pA) = k(pA\,MBq^{-1}) \times A\,(MBq)$$

Different radionuclides have specific ionising factors (k) and commercial ionisation chambers have built-in scaling factors for commonly used radionuclides which give a direct read out in appropriate units (kBq or MBq, or mCi). More advanced instruments can print the measurements on a label or a quality control record sheet.

These instruments will give measurements of adequate precision for the radiopharmacy as long as they are regularly checked with standard calibrated radioactive sources.

9.2.1.3 Calibration

Checking the calibration of an ionisation chamber or radionuclide calibrators involves three separate measurements:

(a) the *calibration factor*: Calibration factors are checked by using standard sources, either sealed solid, or liquid, obtained from a national testing and calibration agency such as the National Physical Laboratory in the UK, or by comparing measurements on samples previously measured in a Secondary Standard (271 + 671) Radionuclide Calibrator. In either case a correction for radioactive decay is essential to compensate for the loss of radioactivity in the time between initial standard calibration and local calibration measurements.

Standardised sources of short-lived radionuclides are expensive, of limited availability, and impracticable. Radiopharmacies use secondary standards containing long-lived radionuclides of similar gamma energy. Table 2 details some of these standards.

(b) the *sample geometry factor:* All ionisation chambers are sensitive to changes in the geometry of the radioactive sample and for reliable measurements the calibration standard sources should have the same geometry as the radioactive sample (i.e. same volume in the same size injection vial).

Table 2
Secondary Calibration Standards

Radionuclide to be assayed	$^{99}Tc^{m}$	$^{113}In^{m}$
Secondary standard	^{57}Co	^{113}Sn/^{113}In^{m}
Half life	270 d	115 d

Calibration problems can arise when measurements are made on small volumes (less than 5 ml) contained in 20 ml vials, and with single doses pre-packed in disposable syringes because the calibration factor will vary according to sample volume and shape. It is good practice to recalibrate the instrument for use with syringes pre-loaded with radiopharmaceuticals and the small volume, high radioactivity bolus injections.

The effect of variations in sample geometry should be assessed initially, then at yearly intervals over a range of sample volumes, vial sizes, and radionuclides expected to be used.

(c) the *dynamic range accuracy:* All measuring and readout devices used with ionisation chambers have a number of different ranges or scales, and it is essential to check that the range factors are correct and provide a continuous linear scale over the full measuring range of the instrument.

The simplest method of checking is to take a high activity sample of a short-lived radionuclide and to measure its radioactivity frequently and repeatedly over the full range of the instrument. Assuming the initial reading is correct, a semilogarithmic plot of measured and calculated radioactivities against time will quickly show any errors in the range factors and linearity of instrument response. A detailed procedure is given in Hauser and Caudle (1977) and a typical operating procedure is illustrated in SOP 1. A quicker procedure is to use a set of commercially available lead shields of different wall thickness (and hence attenuation). The highly active sample is placed inside each shield and the apparent radioactivity recorded. The observations can be plotted against the known attenuation factor of the shields and the linearity and slope of the line compared with standard readings.

It is standard practice to check the radioactivity of all preparations leaving the radiopharmacy for the nuclear medicine clinic or satellite departments, and for the radioactivity to be re-checked on receipt and before administration to the patient. Separate measuring instruments will be used in these locations and it is a wise precaution to check that all instruments remain in calibration by measuring the same standardised sample on each of them, correcting for decay if necessary.

9.2.2 Radionuclide Identity

The British and European Pharmacopoeias describe tests for establishing the identity of the radionuclide. These may be a determination of the half-life, measurement of the energy of the radiations emitted, or a combination of both. Determination of the half-life of most medical radionuclides can be done in the radiopharmacy, by a modification of the method suggested for checking the linearity of the ionisation chambers described in section 9.2.1 and in SOP (Standard Operating Procedure) 1. The BP gives some general guidance on the preparation of sources and the frequency and number of activity determinations needed to ensure a reliable result. Measurements at intervals of about half the expected half-life which extend over a period of three half-lives (i.e. 6 measurements) are considered satisfactory. The readings are converted to their logarithms and plotted against the time of measurement. The slope of the plot gives the decay constant, λ defined by the relation:

$$\ln(A_t) = \ln(A_o) - \lambda t$$

from which the half-life is calculated from the expression:

$$T_{1/2} = \ln(2)/\lambda$$

Determination of the energy spectrum of the radionuclide requires equipment that may not be available in the radiopharmacy. In most cases the gamma spectrum is required. The gamma spectrum of a radionuclide that emits gamma and/or X rays is unique and characteristic and can be used as an identity test. The spectrum is best obtained with a Ge(Li) semiconductor detector which gives narrow photopeaks (ca. 2 keV) coupled to a multichannel analyser. The NaI(Tl) scintillation detector can be used for gamma spectroscopy, but suffers from a much lower intrinsic resolution (ca. 50 keV) which may obscure photopeaks of any impurities. Both spectrometer systems needs to be calibrated by determining the relationship between the photopeak channel number and standard sources of known gamma energy for identification of radionuclides.

The spectrometer system must also be calibrated for detection efficiency when used to determine radioactivities and levels of radionuclidic impurities. Standard sources of known radioactivity and gamma energy are required. These measurements are normally considered to be outside the activities of the radiopharmaceutical control laboratory.

Identification of pure beta emitters is sometimes performed in the radiopharmacy. The BP and EP method consists of determining the count rate of a sample and standard source when attenuated by a series of aluminium screens of increasing thickness and comparing their beta absorption curves. SOP 2 illustrates a typical procedure for this test.

9.2.3 Radionuclidic Purity

The term 'radionuclidic purity' is defined in the BP 1988 as 'The ratio, expressed as a percentage, of the radioactivity

Table 3
Standards for BP Radiopharmaceuticals

Preparation	*Limits*	*Radionuclidic purity*	*Radiochemical purity*	*Details of method*
Iodinated [^{125}I] Albumin Injection	85.0 to 115.0%	nmt 1% ^{126}I	nlt 95% HSA	ep on paper at 500V for 60 min using barbitone + acetate + octanoate +
Chromium [^{51}Cr] Edetate injection	90.0 to 110.0%	gamma spectrum same as std ^{51}Cr	nlt 95% Cr edetate	ep on paper at 30 V/cm for 30 min using barbitone + nitrate buffer
Cyanocobalamin [^{57}Co] Solution	85.0 to 115.0%	nmt 0.1% due to ^{56}Co, ^{58}Co, and other radionuclides	nlt 90% activity in the form of cyanocoabalamin	hplc on C-8 silica with phosphate methanol pH3.5 at a flow rate of 1ml/min, uv detection at 361 nm and radiation detection of ^{57}Co.
Cyanocobalamin [^{57}Co] Capsule	90.0 to 110.0%	nmt 0.1% due to ^{56}Co, ^{58}Co and other radionuclide impurities	nlt 95% activity in the form of Cyanocobalmin	hplc on C-8 silica with phosphate methanol pH3.5 at a flow rate of 1ml/min, uv detection at 361nm and radiation detection of ^{57}Co.
Cyanocobalamin [^{58}Co] Solution	90.0 to 110.0%	nmt 1% ^{60}Co and nmt 2% total radionuclide imp. nmt 1% due to ^{60}Co nmt 2% due to ^{60}Co + ^{57}Co + others	as above	as above
Ferric Citrate [^{59}Fe] Solution	90.0 to 110.0%	gamma spectrum same as std ^{59}Fe specific activity nlt 37MBq/mg Fe	no test specified	complies with limit test for iron 1ppm
Dried Iodinated [^{125}I] Fibrinogen	85.0 to 115.0%	nmt 1% ^{126}I	nlt 95% as protein bound activity	paper electrophoresis in PBS pH 6.4 on 20 cm strip at 200 V for 60 min. Free iodide moves 7 cm towards anode iodinated fibrinogen remains near origin
Gallium [^{67}Ga] Citrate Injection	90.0 to 110.0%	nmt 0.2% ^{66}Ga	no test specified	limit test for zinc (5 ppm)
Colloidal Gold [^{198}Au] Injection	90.0 to 110.0%	gamma spectrum same as ^{198}Au except that up to 10% ^{199}Au may be present	nlt 98% colloidal Au	ascending pc using acetone: water:HCl (70:20:10); colloidal Au stays at origin $R_f = 0$; soluble Au moves to sf and visualised by Sn(II) iodide spray.
Indium [^{111}In] Pentate Injection	90.0 to 110.0%	nmt 0.2% ^{114}In	nlt 95% as pentetate	activated ITLC-SG using 0.9% saline over 10–15 cm in 10 min. Complex migrates at $R_f = 0.0 - 1.0$.
L-Selenomethionine [^{75}Se] Injection	90.0 to 110.0%	gamma spectrum same as std ^{75}Se specific activity nlt 37MBq/mg	nlt 90% in the principal spot	descending pc using butanol: water:glacial acetic acid (60:25:15); add L-methionine as carrier
Sodium Chromate [^{51}Cr] Sterile Solution	90.0 to 110.0%	gamma spectrum same as std ^{51}Cr	nlt 90%	ascending pc using water:ethanol: 10 M ammonia (125:50: 25) for 2.5 hr. Cr(III) ions remain at origin

Table 3 *(cont)*
Standards for BP Radiopharmaceuticals

Preparation	*Limits*	*Radionuclidic purity*	*Radiochemical purity*	*Details of method*
Sodium Iodide [^{123}] Solution	90.0 to 110.0%	nmt 2% ^{124}I by gamma spectrometry specific activity nlt 185 GBq/mq I^- mnt 2% total impurity; specific activity nlt 185GBq/mg I^-	nlt 95% as iodide with R_f within 5% of std spot	ascending pc using methanol: ater (75:25) and stds of 1% I^- and 2% IO_3^- for 2 hrs; stds visualised; acid and a mixture of 2-iodobenzoic acetic + IO_3^- or I^- papers
Sodium Iodide [^{131}I] Solution	90.0 to 110.0%	gamma spectrum same as std ^{131}I specific activity nlt 185 GBq/mg I^-	nlt 95% as iodide with R_f within 5% of std spot	ascending pc using methanol: water (75:25) and stds of 1% I^- and 2% IO_3^- for 2 hrs; stds visualised
Sodium Iodohipurate [^{123}I] Injection	90.0 to 110.0%	nmt 2% as ^{124}I nmt 2% as ^{125}I both by gamma spectrometry nmt 2% total imp.	nlt 96% as 2-iodohippuric acid nmt 2% as 2-iodobenzoic acid and/or iodide	tlc on silicagel GF254 using toluene:butanol:glacial acetic acid:water (80:20:4:1) for 75 min or 12 cm and stds of 2-iodohip-puric acid and 2-iodobenzoic acid
Sodium Iodohippurate [^{131}I] Injection	90.0 to 110.0%	gamma spectrum same as std ^{131}I	nlt 96% as 2-iodohippuric acid nmt 2% as 2-iodobenzoic acid and/or iodide	tlc on silicagel GF254 using toluene:butanol:glacial acetic acid:water (80:20:4:1) for 75 min or 12 cm and stds of 2-iodohippuric
Sodium Pertechnetate [^{99m}Tc] Injection (Fission)	90.0 to 110.0%	^{99}Mo nmt 1×10^{-1}% ^{131}I nmt 5×10^{-3}% ^{103}Ru nmt 5×10^{-3}% ^{89}Sr nmt 6×10^{-5}% ^{90}Sr nmt 6×10^{-6}% other gamma emitters nmt $1 \times 10^{-2\%}$ alpha emitters nmt 1×10^{-7}%	nlt 95%	descending pc using methanol: water (80:20) for 2 hrs. $Tc0_4^-$ has R_f about 0.6
Sodium Pertechnetate [^{99m}Tc] Injection (Non-Fission]	90.0 to 11.0%	^{99}Mo nmt 0.1% nmt 0.01% other radionuclides	nlt 95%	descending pc as above
Sodium Phosphate [^{32}P] Injection	90.0 to 110.0%	beta spectrum same as standard ^{32}P solution specific activity nlt 11.1MBq ^{32}P/mg orthosphosphate	nlt 95% nmt 0.0033% PO_4^- per 37 MBq	ascending pc using propanol: water: (75:25) with trichloracetic acid and ammonia for 16 hrs with orthophosphoric acid as carrier, visualise carrier with pechloric acid followed by ammonium molybdate and exposure to H_2S to give a blue spot
Thallous [^{201}] Chloride Injection	90.0 to 110.0%	nmt 2% ^{202}Tl nlt 97% ^{201}Tl specific gravity nlt 3.7 GBq/mg Tl	nlt 95% as Thallium(I)	cellulose acetate electrophoresis with 1.86% disodium edetate at 17 V per cm for 30 min. nlt 95% activity migrates towards the cathode

of the radionuclide concerned to the total radioactivity of the source.' Standards for radionuclide impurities are given in the BP and EP monographs on all radiopharmaceuticals. Table 3 shows the impurity limits specified by the BP 1988.

The principle underlying the control of radionuclidic impurities is protection of the patient from unnecessary radiation. Tight limits must be placed on all alpha emitters and long-lived radio-nuclides which also have a long biological half-life.

No radionuclide sample is completely free of other radioactive species. The nature of the contaminants will depend on the method of radionuclide production, the impurity profile of the target or other starting material, and the production process employed. Sometimes the contaminants are radioisotopes and these cannot, of course, be removed by chemical treatment. In these situations the only means of quality control lies in the method of production of the radionuclide which is outside the province and control of the radiopharmacist.

The specified radionuclidic impurity limits reflect the radiological hazard associated with the impurity, the clinical use of the radiopharmaceutical, and the practicality of achieving tighter standards. For example, the BP 1988 specifies a limit of 1.0% I–126 in I–125 Iodinated Human Albumin and a similar limit for Co–60 in Co–58 Cyanocobalamin. In both examples the radionuclidic impurities have longer half-lives than the principal radionuclide so that the proportion of the radionuclidic impurity increases with time due to the differential decay rates of principal and impurity radionuclides. Another important consequence is that the BP radionuclidic impurity limit also effectively defines a shelf life for these materials.

A higher impurity level is seen with Colloidal Gold [Au–198] Injection where up to 10% of the slightly longer-lived Au–199 isotope ($T_{1/2}$ = 3.14 d, E_{gamma} = 0.158 MeV) is permitted with the principal isotope Au–198 ($T_{1/2}$ = 2.70 d, E_{gamma} = 0.412 MeV, E_{beta} = 0.96 MeV).

A more complex set of radionuclidic impurity specifications is given for the most popular diagnostic radionuclide $^{99}Tc^{m}$. The radionuclidic purity specification of Sodium Pertechnetate [$^{99}Tc^{m}$] Injection depends on the source of the parent ^{99}Mo. In the case of Non-Fission Pertechnetate (^{99}Mo produced by neutron bombardment of ^{98}Mo) not more than 0.1% of the total radioactivity is due to the parent ^{99}Mo, and not more than 0.01% of all other radionuclidic impurities. With Fission Sodium Pertechnetate (where the ^{99}Mo is extracted from uranium fission products) the radionuclidic purity specification is much more stringent. Six different impurities are controlled–^{99}Mo (0.1%), I–131 (0.005%), Ru 103 (0.005%), Sr–89 (0.00006%), Sr–90 (0.000006%), and alpha emitting impurities (0.0000007%). In both sources of $^{99}Tc^{m}$ an unspecified quantity of the long-lived isotope ^{99}Tc resulting from decay of the ^{99} is permitted.

However, it should be noted that high levels of ^{99}Tc can interfere with the labelling efficiency of a number of newer $^{99}Tc^{m}$ radiopharmaceuticals through isotopic dilution and competition for binding sites on the ligands. Manufacturers may specify a maximum regrowth time for $^{99}Tc^{m}$ in a generator (i.e. maximum time between elutions) to limit the build up and subsequent eluant content of this isotope and thus maintain the apparent efficiency of radiolabelling.

The method for determining radionuclidic impurity is usually the technique of gamma spectroscopy described above. In many cases the Pharmacopoeias control radionuclidic impurities by specifying that the sample spectrum (beta or gamma) does not differ significantly from that of a standardised solution, so that the limit for impurities is effectively that of the standard solution for which no details are provided. In other cases the characteristics of the impurities are listed so that they may be identified in the spectrum.

Sometimes a detailed method is provided in the BP. For example the limit of ^{126}I in Iodinated [^{125}I] Albumin Injection is controlled by measuring the gamma spectra of the sample and standardised solutions of ^{125}I and ^{137}Cs. The gamma energies of ^{126}I (0.666 MeV) and ^{137}Cs (0.662 MeV) are very similar so that the detector sensitivity for the impurity and Cs standard will be almost identical, and the latter can be used as a reference or standard as long as a correction is made for the different abundances of photons emitted (86% for ^{137}Cs and 33% for ^{126}I, leading to a correction factor of 30/86 = 0.349).

For Sodium Pertechnetate [$^{99}Tc^{m}$] Injection several radionuclidic impurity tests are described. As discussed above the standards are different for the injection derived from fission-produced ^{99}Mo parent and reactor (non-fission) produced ^{99}Mo, the standard being more stringent in the first case. An approximate method of parent ^{99}Mo estimation is described which can be performed before clinical use of the material. The gamma spectrum of a 37 MBq sample is obtained through a 6 mm thick lead shield which acts as a selective filter by absorbing virtually all the 0.140 MeV photons from $^{99}Tc^{m}$, but only 50% of the higher energy 0.740 MeV photons from the parent ^{99}Mo. The resulting spectrum is that of the attenuated ^{99}Mo, and comparison with a ^{99}Mo standard allows a rapid estimation of the parent radionuclide contamination level.

Even this method is time-consuming, and most radiopharmacies perform a 'molybdenum breakthrough test' on their radionuclide calibrator or ionisation chamber by placing the freshly eluted sample of Sodium Pertechnetate Injection in a 6 mm wall lead container, measuring the ionisation current and comparing this value with the current expected from the maximum permitted level of ^{99}Mo. Some commercial chambers give a direct readout of the ^{99}Mo content, thus further simplifying a measurement which must be done at the busiest period of the radiopharmacist's working day. A typical method is outlined in SOP 3.

The BP definitive test requires the accurate measurement on a decayed sample of a number of radionuclides by specific tests. The parent ^{99}Mo is determined by gamma ray spectroscopy and comparison with a standard source solution. The impurities ^{131}I and ^{103}Ru are determined similarly and other gamma-emitting impurities are detected from the spectrum. All alpha emitting impurities must be identified. The beta-emitting impurities ^{89}Sr and ^{90}Sr are first chemically separated from the sample, then identified and estimated through a technically complex series of beta absorption and radionuclide parent-daughter separations.

A 'breakthrough' test cannot be applied to the ^{113}Sn/$^{113}In^m$ generator system because the daughter $^{113}In^m$ emits higher energy (390 keV) photons than the parent ^{113}Sn (30 keV). In this, and similar cases, the generator eluate is left for a time sufficient to allow all the shorter-lived daughter to decay, thus leaving any co-eluted parent ^{113}Sn or other radionuclide easily detected from the residual radioactivity seen once secular equilibrium is re-established.

9.3 RADIOCHEMICAL PURITY DETERMINATIONS

9.3.1 Introduction

Radiochemical purity is defined in the BP 1988 as 'The ratio, expressed as a percentage, of the radioactivity of the radionuclide concerned that is present in the source in the chemical form declared to the total radioactivity of that radionuclide present in the source.' Alternatively, radiochemical purity may be defined as the proportion of the total radioactivity in the sample associated with the desired radiolabelled species.

For most diagnostic radiopharmaceuticals a purity of above 95% is desirable (although not always achievable!) since the radiochemical impurities will almost certainly have a different biodistribution which may distort the scintigraphic image and so invalidate a clinical diagnosis based on the scintigram. Radiochemical purities of radiopharmaceuticals described in the BP 1988 vary from 98% (Colloidal Gold [^{198}Au] Injection) to 90% (e.g. Cyanocobalamin ^{57}Co] Solution) but most are specified to have a minimum radiochemical purity of 95%.

Radiochemical purity (or labelling yield) determinations are carried out in all radiopharmacies, either to check the quality of a standard formulation or kit, or to establish standards for an in-house preparation. Some form of physicochemical separation technique msut be used in order to separate the various radioactive species in the sample prior to measurement of their radioactivities and subsequent calculation of their porportion in the sample.

Although extraction and phase separation methods are coming into use, chromatographic separation methods are universally employed in radiochemical purity determinations, planar techniques and electrophoresis being the most popular. Their main advantage over column and other elution methods is that all the applied radioactivity remains on the developed chromatoplate or electrophoretogram which can then be examined and quantitated by a number of techniques (e.g. scanned, autoradiographed, cut into regions or strips and the radioactivity associated with each area measured under identical conditions.

The BP 1988 specifies planar separation methods in all the radiochemical purity tests described. These range from descending paper chromatography through thin layers to paper electrophoresis. More recently, ITLC methods have been included for a number of ^{99m}Tc- labelled radopharmaceuticals. Table 4 gives some details.

Whatever separation technique is used, the method of calculation is identical. The radioactivity in each spot, sample, or other sector is measured, corrected for background, and the percentage activity in each piece is calculated from the formula:

$$\% \text{ component} = 100 \frac{(\text{count for component})}{(\text{total counts})}$$

The method is described on page 131–133. Chromatographic and other separation techniques for radiochemical purity determinations are extensively reviewed in Wieland, *et al.* (1986).

Insoluble radioactive species (colloids or highly lipophilic materials) are measured along with all other radioactive species in planar separations. Elutive techniques (i.e. column methods) invariably retain these species on the column making their quantitation or estimation more difficult. Even so, the radioactivity associated with insoluble species must be distinguished from that due to lipophilic or slowly moving species by using a combination of separative methods. This problem has been known for many years, being addressed by Eckelmann in an editorial for the Journal of Nuclear Medicine in 1976.

Many conventional radiochromatographic systems are unsatisfactory because only the impurity migrates and the principal component remains at the point of application, Systems must be developed which ensure that *all* potentially soluble components migrate. It is good analytical practice to employ three different stationary/mobile phase combinations to demonstrate the homogeneity of the spots or peaks for the components being measured.

Calibration and validation

Whichever separation technique is employed it is essential to calibrate the measuring or counting equipment and to validate the proposed counting or assay procedure. In most cases this will take the form of an assessment of the sensitivity

Table 4
Standards for BP Technetium Radiopharmaceuticals

Preparation	*Radiochemical purity method*	*Other tests*
Technetium [^{99m}Tc] Albumin Injection	Activated ITLC-SG using butan-2-one for 10–15 cm in 10 min; labelled albumin remains at origin, TcO_4^- migrates behind solvent front. HPLC-SEC on silicagel FC with phosphate azide buffer at 0.6 mL/min. Multiple peaks eluted but nlt 80% of activity associated with albun fractions II, III, IV and V.	Albumin: by colorimetry; tin; by colorimetry; physiological distribution: nmt 15% in liver, nlt 3.5% in blood in 2/3 rats.
Technetium [^{99m}Tc] Colloidal Antimony Sulphide Injection	Activated ITLC-SG using 0.9% NaCl over 10–15 cm in 10 min. Colloid remains at origin, pertechnetate migrates with Rf = 0.95–1.0. nlt 95% as colloid	Physiological distribution: nmt 5% in lungs, nlt 80% in liver & spleen of 3/3 mice. Antinomy: ±10% of label claim by UV.
Technetium [^{99m}Tc] Colloidal Sulphur Injection	Ascending PC using 0.9% NaCl over 10–15 cm. Colloid remains at origin, pertechnetate migrates with Rf = 0.6. Other ^{99m}Tc impurities with Rf =0.8–0.9. nlt 92% as colloid.	Physiological distribution: nmt 5% in lungs, nlt 80% in liver and spleen of 3/3 mice.
Technetium [^{99m}Tc] Colloidal Tin Injection	Activated ITLC-SG using N_2 purged 0.9% saline for 10–15 cm over 10 min; colloid at origin, TcO_4^- at front. nlt 95% activity as colloid	Tin: nmt 1 mg/mL yb colorimetry physiological distrubition: nlt 80% liver and spleen, nmt 5% in lungs of 2/3 mice.
Technetium [^{99m}Tc] Etifen Injection	Activated ITLC-SA using 0.9% saline for 10–15 cm in 10 min; colloid at origin, complex at Rf = 0.5, TcO_4^- with solvent front. nlt 95% as complex.	Identification: HPLC on RP-silica using pH 2.5 phosphate-methanol as mobile phase; etifen EPCRS used as reference. Physiological distribution: nlt 80% in gall bladder + intestines, nmt 3% in liver, nmt 2% in kidneys in 2/3 mice.
Technetium [^{99m}Tc] Macrosalb Injection	Non-filterable radioactivity: by 3 μm polycarbonate filter retention, nlt 90%.	Particle size: nmt 10/5000 > 100 μm none > 150 μm. Aggregated albumin: bu UV nlt 37 MBq ^{99m}Tc per mg albumin. Tin: nmt 3 mg/mL by colorimetry physiological distribution: nlt 80% in lungs, nmt 5% in liver and spleen in 2/3 rats.
Technetium [^{99m}Tc] Microspheres Injection	Non-filterable radioactivity: by 3 μm polycarbonate filter retention, nlt 95%.	Particle size: nmt 10/5000 > 100 μm none > 100 μm. Number of particles: by counting in haemocytometer nlt 185 MBq ^{99m}Tc/10^6 particles. Tin: nmt 3 mg/mL by colorimetry physiological distribution: nmt 5% in liver and spleen, nlt 80% in lungs of 2/3 rats.
Technetium [^{99m}Tc] Medronate injection	Activated ITLC-SG using butan-2-one for 10–15 cm in 10 min; medronate and colloid at origin, nmt 2% TCO_4^- at solvent front. Repeat using 13.6% sodium acetate; colloids at origin, complex and TcO_4^- at front. From both chromatograms nmt 5% total impurities.	Tin: nmt 3 mg/mL by colorimetry physiological distribution: nlt 2.5% in femurs, nmt 1% in liver; femur to muscle ratio nlt 100, femur to blood ratio nlt 40.

Table 4 *(cont)*
Standards for BP Technetium Radiopharmaceuticals

Preparation	*Radiochemical purity method*	*Other tests*
Technetium [^{99m}Tc] Pentetate Injection	Activated ITLC-SG using butan-2-one for 10 15 cm in 10 min; TcO_4^- moves behind solvent front, complex and colloid at origin. Repeat using 0.9% sodium chloride; colloid at origin, complex and TcO_4^- at front. From both chromatograms nmt 5% total impurities.	Tin: nmt 1 mg/mL by colorimetry.
Technetium [^{99m}Tc] Succimer Injection	Activated ITLC-SG using butan-2-one for 10–15 cm in 10 min; complex at origin, TcO_4^- at solvent front. nmt 2% TcO_4^-; nlt 95% complex.	Tin: nmt 1 mg/mL by colorimetry physiological distribution: nlt 40% in kidneys, nmt 10% in liver, nmt 2% in stomach, nmt 5% in lungs of 2/3 rats.
Technetium [^{99m}Tc] Tin Pyrophosphate Injection	Activated ITLC-SG using butan-2-one over 10–15 cm in 10 min. Complex remains at origin, TcO_4^- migrates with Rf = 0.95–1.0. Test repeated using 1M sodium acetate as mobile phase; both complex and TcO_4^- migrate with Rf = 0.9–1.0, colloid remains at origin; nmt 10% impurity.	Sodium pyrophosphate: 1 to 50 mg/mL by colorimetry. Tin: nmt 3 mg/mL by colorimetry.

and linearity of the counting or measuring system. The thallium-activated sodium iodide scintillation detector is preferred for radiopharmaceutical gamma counting because of its sensitivity and ease of operation. All counting systems can show deviation from linearity at high count rates due to paralysis, co-incidence, or pulse pileup. The correct working conditions (detector voltage and threshold settings) and the range over which linearity is maintained must be determined by experiment. Measuring conditions must then be adjusted to maintain count rates within the linear region.

It is easy to paralyse the detector by applying too large a quantity of radioactivity in the sample. For example, a single drop of a 100 MBq mL^{-1} $^{99}Tc^{m}$ radiopharmaceutical will contain about 2 MBq, an amount more than sufficient to cause paralysis of most detectors. In these situations the inverse square law can be used to advantage by placing samples for counting on a rigid jig held a suitable distance from the detector (after performing systems suitability tests).

Typical SOPs for optimising operating conditions and detector linearity checks are illustrated in SOP 4 and SOP 5.

9.3.2 Planar Chromatography

Planar chromatography includes paper, thin layer, and high performance thin layer chromatography. The techniques are similar in that a sample is applied to the stationary medium and developed with a suitable mobile phase.

9.3.2.1 Paper Chromatography

Paper chromatography is now largely replaced by TLC methods but still applied to a number of BP 1988 radiopharmaceuticals. The disadvantages of this medium are the poor resolution compared with other planar thin layer support media and the long development times required for both ascending and descending techniques. In radiopharmacy these are often outweighed by the ease of cutting a developed paper chromatogram into strips or segments for counting or scanning the radioactivity profile.

It is good practice to mark the (starting) line of application and the expected solvent front (finishing line) with a sharp, soft pencil before applying the sample. Paper is manufactured with a 'grain' lying in one direction (the machine direction) and it is recommended that the machine direction be marked on the paper and the chromatogram run in the same direction to ensure reproducibility between runs.

On a multiple sample paper chromatogram the width of the chromatographic lanes should be wider than customary on TLC plates to accommodate the greater lateral diffusion of bands in this technique. Edge effects are also common; band development and band shape are affected by the solvent flow characteristics induced by evaporation at the paper edges. It is prudent to ensure that samples are not applied too close to the edges – a margin of 10 mm is satisfactory – and to spot at intervals of not less than 25 mm across the width of the paper.

Single sample paper chromatograms are perhaps more common in the radiopharmacy, using strips about 20 × 200 mm dimensions. These have the advantage of simple development in a tall jar such as a measuring cylinder with minimum mobile phase volumes. A typical procedure is illustrated in SOP 6.

Chromatography Papers

Whatman No 1 Paper is a good, general purpose medium for PC, but easily tears when wetted with aqueous solvents. It is unsuitable for ascending chromatographic techniques (unless supported in some kind of frame, or wrapped and clipped into a cylinder) because of this property. *Whatman 3MM Paper* is a thicker paper having similar chromatographic characteristics to No. 1. The advantage lies in the increased mechanical strength and the ability to absorb a sample spot with less spreading. The paper is used quite successfully in miniature chromatography systems. *Whatman 31ET* is a more open textured paper which runs faster than No. 1 or 3MM but has a lower intrinsic resolution.

A number of ion exchange papers are also available. They are weak acid or weak basic ion exchangers which can be used to advantage in the separation of differently charged species. Control of mobile phase pH is essential with these materials to ensure the correct degree of ionisation of both the paper-bound exchanger groups and the migrating solute.

9.3.2.2 Thin Layer Chromatography

Thin layer chromatography (TLC) is the most popular planar chromatographic method. The technique is simple and acceptable results are easily obtained. For radiopharmaceutical work TLC is probably the most useful method although development times of several hours can be a disadvantage with radiopharmaceuticals containing short-lived radionuclides.

Thin layer chromatoplates may be prepared 'in-house' using glass plates and spreading equipment, but these do not always give reproducible chromatograms. Commercial TLC materials are preferable for radiopharmaceutical quality control applications. The normal thickness of the layer is 0.25 mm (250 μm). Glass-backed plates are traditional, but are not easily cut or segmented. Plastic- and metal foil-backed plates are more versatile; they can cut with scissors or a sharp scalpel to any required size. Similarly, after development these chromatoplates can be cut into suitable segments for counting and quantitation. Some plates have a tendency to flake or crumble when being cut, leading to loss of radioactivity. This can be overcome by covering the layer with sellotape before cutting.

Many different stationary phases are available for TLC work, but for radiopharmaceutical purposes silica gel is to be preferred in view of the large number of chromatograms reported. Plates incorporating a fluorescent indicator, although useful for locating the solvent front (by virtue of the concentation of uv-absorbing impurities at the solvent front) and location of UV absorbing species, are not normally required in radiopharmacy since the quantitation is made through the radioactivity distribution on the plate.

ITCL Materials

The Gelman Company produce several Instant Thin Layer Chromatography (ITLC) materials. They consist of a glass fibre web impregnated with the modified silica stationary

Table 5
Mini-Chromatography Systems for Tc Radiopharmaceuticals

No.	*Support*	*Mobile phase*	*Useful for*
A Free TcO_4^- *determinations only*			
1	Whatman 3MM	95% acetone	MDP, GH, DTPA, DMSA, HSA, MAA and uS
2	Whatman 3MM	saline	SC, MAA, SbC, PhyT
3	ITLC-SG	85% MeOH	SC, MAA
B Free TcO_4^- *and hydrolysed Tc (remains at origin)*			
4	Whatman 3MM	(a) 95% acetone (b) saline*	DTPA, HIDA
5	ITLS-SG	(a) 95% acetone** (b) saline*	MDP, PyP, PP, EHDP

*secondary solvent runs to 20 mm above the origin. **wet spot – do not dry before development.

KEY:

MDP – Medronate (methylene diphosphonate)
DTPA – diethylenetriamine penta acetic acid
HSA – human serum albumin
uS – HSA microspheres
SbC – antimony sulphide colloid
EHDP – editronate (hydroxyethyl diphosphonate)
GH – glucoheptonate
DMSA – dimercaptosuccinic acid
MAA – macroaggregated albumin
SC – sulphur colloid
PyP – pyrophosphate
HIDA – 2,6-dimethylacetanilidoiminodiacetate.

Table 6
Planar Chromatography of Selected Radiopharmaceuticals

Radiopharmaceutical	*Mobile phase*	*Support medium*	*Complex*	*Rf values* TcO_4^-	*Colloid*	*Reference*
Pertechnetate	acetone	ITLC-SG		1.0	0.0	Robbins, 1984
	0.9% NaCl	ITLC-SG		1.0	0.0	
	acetone	Wh 1		1.0	0.0	
Colloids						
Tc-S (sulphur colloid)	acetone	Wh31ET		1.0	0.0	Robbins, 1984
Tc-SbS (antimony sulphide)	0.9% NaCl	ITLC-SG		1.0	0.0	,,
Lung Imaging Agents						
Tc-MAA (macroaggregates)	acetone	Wh31ET	0.0	1.0		Robbins, 1984
Tc-HAM (microspheres)	acetone	Wh31ET	0.0	1.0		,,
Renal Agents						
Tc-pentetate (DTPA)	acetate	Wh31ET	0.0	1.0	0.0	Robbins, 1984
	water	ITLC-SG	1.0	1.0	0.0	
Tc-ferpentate	acetone	Wh31ET	0.0	1.0	0.0	,,
	water	ITLC-SG	1.0	1.0	0.0	
Tc-Gluceptate	acetone	Wh31ET	0.0	1.0	0.0	,,
	water	ITLC-SG	0.0	1.0	0.0	
Tc-succimer (DMSA)	n-BuOH + 0.3M HCl	ITLC-SA	0.5	1.0	0.0	,,
Tc-ethylene-dicysteine (ECD)	acetone	ITLC-SG	0.0	1.0	0.0	Verbruggen, 1992
	0.5M HAc	ITLC-SG	1.0	1.0	0.0	
Albumin						
Tc-HSA (human albumin)	acetone	Wh31ET	0.0	1.0	0.0	Robbins, 1984
	EtOH + ammonia + water	ITLC-SG	1.0	1.0	0.0	
Bone Agents						
Tc-editronate (EHDP)	acetone	Wh31ET	0.0	1.0	0.0	Robbins, 1984
	water	ITLC-SG	1.0	1.0	0.0	
Tc-medronate (MDP)	acetone	Wh31ET	0.0	1.0	0.0	,,
	water	ITLC-SG	1.0	1.0	0.0	
Tc-oxidronate	acetone	Wh31ET	0.0	1.0	0.0	,,
	water	ITLC-SG	1.0	1.0	0.0	
Tc-pyrophosphate (PyP)	acetone	Wh31ET	0.0	1.0	0.0	,,
	water	ITLC-SG	1.0	1.0	0.0	
Hepatobiliary agents						
Tc-lidofen (HIDA)	20% NaCl	ITLC-SA	0.0	1.0	0.0	Robbins, 1984
	water	ITLC-SG	1.0	1.0	0.0	
Tc-iprofen (PIPIDA)	20% NaCl	ITLC-SA	0.0	1.0	0.0	,,
	water	ITLC-SG	1.0	1.0	0.0	

Table 6 *(cont)*
Planar Chromatography of Selected Radiopharmaceuticals

Radiopharmaceutical	*Mobile phase*	*Support medium*	*Complex*	*Rf values* TcO_4^-	*Colloid*	*Reference*
Tc-diosfenin (DISIDA)	20% NaCl	ITLS-SA	0.0	1.0	0.0	,,
	water	ITLC-SG	1.0	1.0	0.0	
Brain Imaging Agents						
Tc-exametazime (HM-PAO)	butanone	ITLC-SG	0.0	1.0	0.0	Neirinckx, 1987
	0.0% NaCl	ITLC-SG	0.1	1.0	0.0	,,
	$MeCN{:}H_2O$	Wh 1	1.0	1.0	0.0	,,
	butanone	Wh DE 81	1.0	0.0	0.0	Solanki, 1988
	Et_2O	Wh 1	1.0	0.0	0.0	Hung, 1988
Tc-ECD	acetone + 0.5 M NH_4Ac	WhMKC18				Leveille, 1992
Heart Imaging Agents						
Tc-MIBI	EtOH	alumina	0.5–1	0–0.5	0.0	Proulx, 1989
	acetone	ITLC-SG	0.5–1	0.75–1	0.0	
	saline	ITLC-SG	0–0.25	0.75–1	0.0	
	$CHCl_3{:}MeOH$ (9:1)	ITLC-SG	0.5–1	0–0.5	0.0	
	acetone	Wh 1	0.75–1	0.75–1	0.0	
	0.9% NaCl	Wh 1	0–0.5	0.5–1	0.0	
	$CHCl_3{:}MeOH$ (9:1)	Wh 1	0.5–1	0–0.25	0.0	
	butanone	ITLC-SG	0.5	1.0	0.0	Van Wyk, 1991
Tumour Imaging Agents						
Tc(V)-DMSA	BuOH:AcOH: H_2O (3:2:3)	silicagel	0.5	0.7	0.0	Westera, 1985
	butanone	silicagel	0.0	1.0	0.0	

phases, silica gel (ITLC-SG) and silicic acid (ITLC-SA). The ITCL-SG material is very popular among radiopharmacists for routine radiochemical purity determinations. ITLC supports/stationary phases are fast-running variants of conventional TLC systems. The mobile phase migration speed is increased by the fine random mesh construction of the material, but the resolution is poorer than conventional TLC supports and is similar to paper. ITLC chromatographic systems for radiochemical purity determinations of radiopharmaceuticals are listed in Tables 4 to 6. A typical method for ITLC chromatography is illustrated in SOP 7.

9.3.2.3 Sample Application Techniques

Chromatographic separation and quantitation depends in part on the technique, accuracy and reproducibility of the sample application. For optimal resolution the sample spot must be kept small, about 3 mm for standard 200 mm length plates, and proportionally smaller for shorter length plates. The volume applied will depend on the radioactivity of the sample and the purpose of the chromatogram. Detection of small amounts of impurities will require higher applied radioactivity than studies aimed at determining the major radiolabelled components.

The BP 1988 suggests volumes equal to or less than 10 μL should be applied to the line of application, or origin. Volumes between 2 and 5 μL are generally applied in practice, either from a micro-syringe or, more conventiently with radiopharmaceuticals, from disposable capillary micropipettes. These are available in several volumes with an accuracy of about ±2% of the stated volume. This is sufficient since the main purpose of controlling the sample volume is to control the chromatographic conditions, not the amount of sample because percentage purities are computed from the distribution of radioactivity along the chromatogram.

One drawback with capillary pipettes is that they must be loaded by capillary rise while dipping into the sample and this may be operationally difficult with some radiopharmaceuticals. One solution is to withdraw a sample from a vial into a syringe, remove the needle, and insert the capillary into the hub of the syringe for filling. The technique does carry a penalty in terms of increased radiation dose to the fingers and exposure of the sample to the atmosphere.

Many radiopharmacists prefer to apply samples by expelling a single hanging drop from a narrow bore needle attached to a 1 mL syringe, and touching the drop onto the application line of the chromatoplate. There are many advantages to this technique; with practice a single drop of reproducible size can be formed and transferred to the chromatoplate. The size of the drop does not depend too much on the needle size and a 25G (orange) needle is very satisfactory.

Multiple sample applications may be necessary to load the chromatoplate with sufficient radioactivity, but care should be taken in drying the spots between applications. Heating the plate between applications is not advised with $^{99}Tc^{m}$ radiopharmaceuticals since sample decomposition or oxidation may occur during the drying, leading to overestimation of impurities. If spots have to be dried between applications then the use of a gentle current of nitrogen directed at the spot through a Pasteur pipette is a better option than a heat lamp or hot air blower.

9.3.2.4 Radiopharmaceutical Applications

Size of Chromatogram

Radiopharmacists have developed a number of miniature and microchromatographic methods for speed and ease of handling in the radiopharmaceutical quality control laboratory.

Mini-Chromatography: was introduced by Zimmer and Pavel (1977) and described in the UK by Frier and Hesslewood (1980). A practical guide and methods manual based on this technique was produced for the USA Society of Nuclear Medicine by Robbins (1984). Mini-chromatography employs single strips, about 10 × 50 mm, for each chromatogram. The support is usually ITLC—SG although some workers have used paper. The strips are marked in pencil 8 mm (origin) and 46 mm (solvent front) from the base and the sample is applied as a single spot on the 8 mm line. Without drying the spot, the strip is placed in a suitable vial (a liquid scintillation vial, or Universal container is suitable) containing a layer of mobile phase some 1–2 mm deep and allowed to develop to the marked solvent front. A typical procedure is shown in SOP 8 and Table 4 shows some applications of the method.

It can be difficult to observe the progress of the mobile phase on these small chromatograms. Back illumination from a diffused source (e.g. X-ray viewer) is helpful since the wetted strip is translucent and the solvent front can be seen. Some authorities recommend marking the support with a dye marker pen just below the marked solvent front. The dye moves with the solvent/mobile phase enabling the progress to be monitored visually near the end of the development.

The main difficulties with the method are its reproducibility and poor resolution of migratory species. It is most useful when the radiolabelled species either remain at the origin or move with the solvent front. Chromatogram scanning is not easy, but cutting and counting is rapid and simple. Millar has reported the results of a survey into the use of this method by a panel of UK radiopharmacists and concluded that the results from this method improve with experience (Millar, 1989).

Seprachrom System: a proprietary system marketed by the Gelman Company which employs 50 × 100 mm TLC supports mounted in a plastics tank. The chromatoplate is loaded by capillary pipette through small holes punched in the face of the tank which is then gently lowered into the pre-filled solvent reservoir. Development is quite rapid, but visualisation of the rising solvent front can be difficult. Back diffused lighting is useful, but sometimes the upper tank has a large label on its rear face which obscure the progress of the solvent. When development is complete, the tank is removed from the solvent reservoir, the faces separated and the chromatoplate removed for drying and examination. The tanks can be reloaded with ITLC material cut to size from 200 × 200 mm sheets. SOP 9 shows a typical method.

Standard Chromatography: most scientists will have used conventional TLC methods in their training and few words are needed here to describe the technique. In radiopharmaceutical quality control samples are applied and the chromatoplate is developed in a closed tank, often after an equilibration period with the plate suspended in the mobile phase vapour before developing. The BP 1988 specifies standard TLC methods for a number of the radiopharmaceuticals listed in Table 3. Reversed phase TLC plates can be used for a number of radiochemical purity determinations and SOP 10 shows a typical procedure. Some planar chromatographic methods for ^{99m}Tc radiopharmaceuticals are shown in Table 6.

9.3.2.5 Examination and Quantitation of Chromatoplates

In conventional chromatography separated bands or spots on the developed chromatoplate are visualised by spraying with a chromogenic reagent or some other treatment and the band positions and intensities assessed in a semi-quantitative manner. Radiochromatograms can be evaluated in a quantitative manner provided that the detection and measuring systems are properly calibrated.

Autoradiography

Radiochromatograms can be visualised by autoradiography in which a sheet of photographic film is placed on the radiochromatogram, exposed for a suitable period of time, then developed. The method is very good for ^{14}C and ^{3}H-labelled radiochemicals and special film can be obtained for the purpose. Very low radioactivities of these isotopes can be detected with long exposures since the film responds to all the beta particles detected over the exposure and the density of blackening is proportional to the number of particles captured.

Conventional double-sided X-ray film can be used for autoradiography of $^{99}Tc^{m}$ radiopharmaceuticals. A piece of the film is clipped to the chromatogram and left to expose for 30 to 60 minutes in the dark. Over development in X-ray developer usually heightens the contrast of the spots. Although autoradiograms from ^{14}C and ^{3}H sources can be quantitated, this is less convenient with the gamma emitting radionuclides employed in radiopharmaceuticals and the method is used primarily to provide a permanent record of the radiochromatogram. A typical method is shown in SOP 11.

Chromatogram Scanning

Scanning of radiochromatograms with a suitable detector-ratemeter-recorder combination is perhaps the most satisfactory way of examination and quantitation of gamma emitting radiopharmaceuticals.

A simple scanner may be constructed from a slit-collimated NaI(T1) detector coupled to a scaler-ratemeter with the ratemeter ouput signal passed to a chart recorder. If the radiochromatogram is attached to the chart recorder than a full-size tracing of the radioactivity profile may be obtained. A useful addition is a chromatography integrator to measure the area of radioactive peaks and generation of percentage purity reports. The exact details of the system will depend on availability of equipment.

Commercial radiochromatogram scanners are available which work along the lines described above, and others (known as linear analysers) which simultaneously count the activity detected in a fixed number of channels along the length of the chromatogram and present the result as a histogram. Some departments of Nuclear Medicine use their gamma cameras as chromatogram scanners by displaying an image of the chromatoplate and generating an activity profile along the image.

Calibration and Validation

Whichever system is used, it is important to confirm that it is capable of producing reproducible radioactivity profiles from the chromatogram. It is also important to check the detection system for resolution and linearity using the tests described below.

Scanner resolution is difficult to evaluate quantitatively, but a working estimate can be obtained by scanning a dummy chromatogram prepared with spots about 2 mm in diameter placed at decreasing intervals along the line of the scan (say 32, 16, 8, 4, and 2 mm). The 'chromatogram' is scanned scanning under a variety of conditions, and inspection of the radioactivity profile will determine which pair of spots is incompletely resolved. A more elegant solution is to construct a test plate having narrow strips of a long-lived radionuclide (e.g. ^{57}Co) permanently embedded at decreasing intervals and to periodicially scan this plate and check the resolution is satisfactory. Test plates are available commercially for ^{14}C and ^{3}H scanners, but are not yet available for gamma emitters. Constructional details have been described by Carpenter (1986).

The resolution of the scanner will depend on the design of the collimator, the detector-chromatoplate distance, and the window settings on the scaler. The optimum conditions for any system must be found by experiment.

Scanner response linearity must be checked and verified if quantitation is wanted. The band or peak area is the quantity sought, not simply the count rate so that the linearity must be checked under normal scanning conditions.

Stability of band area must be evaluated under the normal operating conditions. The radioactivity peak profile of bands on the chromatogram will depend on their activity and resolution but the area of the band should remain constant and proportional to the radioactivity. The condition can be tested by applying the same radioactivity as different sized spots onto the chromatoplate and scanning under normal operating conditions. A typical set of instructions for these tests is shown in SOP 12.

Measurement of Band Area

Measurement of band area from the radioactivity profile is an important state in quantitating the radiochromatogram. The precision of the final radiochemical purity value will depend on the reliability of these band area measurements.

Chromatographic band areas can be determined by a number of methods. The simplest is triangulation where the area is calculated from the formula

$$\text{Area} = 0.5(h.w)$$

where H is the band height and w the full width at half the maximum height (also known as FWHM – full width at half maximum), both expressed in the same arbitrary units (e.g. mm on the chart). The method is acceptable only where the bands are perfectly symmetric.

In most radiochromatograms the bands are far from symmetric; tailing and distortion are commonly seen. A chart recorder fitted with an integrator is much more useful in determining the areas of these bands. A dedicated chromatography integrator is the best option. These instruments although designed for HPLC and other CC, are easily connected to a ratemeter and act just like a chart recorder with the advantage of producing a report on the percentage radioactivity in each detected band. Peak positions are expressed in time units, but these are easily converted to distances along the chromatogram if the scan speed is accurately known. Their one disadvantage is the tendency to assign peaks to a noisy background; this can be overcome by (a) increasing the time constant of the ratemeter and accepting some distortion in the band shape, or (b) resetting the signal threshold for initiation of peak integration.

An alternative to band area determination is to cut the radiochromatoplate into segments corresponding to the peaks identified from the radioactivity profile and to count the radioactivity in each one as described in the next section.

Chromatogram Counting

If chromatogram scanning is not possible then cutting and counting is the only practical alternative. The chromatoplate can be cut into sections each corresponding to a component, main or impurity, and the segments counted in a suitable counting equipment. If the radioactivity distribution is unknown the chromatoplate can be cut into equal width segments, the radioactivity counted, and the radioactivity profile constructed as a histogram. This method will have to be used where the applied radioactivity is too low for reliable peak discrimination by scanning but has the definite advantage of allowing extended counting times for each segment and improvement of counting statistics.

The counting efficiency will depend on the design and operating characteristics of the detector, but for most NaI(Tl) well detectors an efficiency approaching or exceeding 10% can be expected with $^{99}Tc^{m}$ and radionuclides of similar gamma energy. When counting in a well detector it is important to maintain the same counting geometry for all segments of the chromatogram, large or small pieces. This is achieved by rolling or compressing the material into the bottom of a counting vial before placing in the detector.

The linearity of detection should be verified by counting a series of dilutions (or simulated spots on the chromatogram) covering the range 1 to 200% of the expected radioactivity and plotting the count rate against applied radioactivity (in kBq) as described under chromatogram scanners. A suitable SOP for linearity checking and use of a well crystal counter is shown in SOP 13.

Artifacts in Planar Chromatography

Artifacts and non-reproducible results can arise from a number of sources in radiochromatography. The following checklist is based on Levitt (1978).

1. Reaction with the support, especially by drying the spots.
2. Splashing when spotting.
3. Interaction with dyes used to visualise the solvent front.
4. Grease from fingers.
5. Strips touching wet walls of the developing chamber.
6. Contamination with other radiopharmaceuticals when spotting.
7. Incorrect mobile phase.
8. Correct, but contaminated mobile phase.
9. Insufficient mobile phase to allow full development to the required solvent front.
10. Contaminated forceps and scissors.
11. Poor mixing of mobile phase components.
12. Uneven sample spotting.
13. Sample washed off by using too much mobile phase in the chamber.
14. Selective evaporation of mobile phase component on storage.

9.3.3 Column Chromatography

A number of column methods have been used in radiopharmaceutical quality control. The most useful are gel filtration and HPLC techniques.

9.3.3.1 Gel Filtration of Radiopharmaceuticals

Gel filtration, or size chromatography is a technique in which a sample is applied to a vertical column and eluted under gravity or low pressure with a solvent. Small solute molecules can penetrate the interstices of the 3-dimensional mesh in porous beads of the gel while larger molecules are excluded. Consequently, unlike other forms of chromatography, the smaller solutes are retained longer than larger molecules which elute first from the column. The eluate can be collected as fractions for radioassay, or an on-line detector can be constructed as described in the section on HPLC to give the eluted radioactivity profile. Alternatively, the column may be scanned using a modified radiochromatogram scanner.

The gel filtration method is applied mainly to macromolecules but has several interesting uses in radiopharmacy. The obvious applciation is in the assessment of radiolabelling of proteins, iodinated or In-labelled through a bifunctional chelate. The radiolabelled protin is eluted first, followed by the radiolabelled unbound bifunctional chelate and other small radiolabelled species. The technique is easily adapted as a purification method for radiolabelled macromolecules by using short bed columns in 10 mL polypropylene syringe barrels and collecting the first few fractions eluted. A suitable method is described in SOP 14 on radioiodination of proteins, (see also Chapter 8).

Another application is in the assessment of radiolabelled colloids. These will move down the column to a degree related to their particle size distribution and the radioactivity profile of the scanned column can act as a non-specific indicator of suitability (Persson, 1977).

9.3.3.2 High Performance Liquid Chromatography

Introduction

High performance liquid chromatography (HPLC) is a natural development of conventional column chromatography which uses very small particles of absorbent coated with stationary phase (5-10 μm) tightly packed in small diameter columns (4 × 100–200 mm). The large surface area available for exchange and partitioning within the compact column gives excellent resolution of many substances including radiopharmaceuticals. The pressure drop across the length of an HPLC column can be considerable, and driving pressures of 1000 psi are not unusual, necessitating the use of specially designed pumps and sample injector systems.

HPLC is a highly popular technique in pharmaceutical analysis and development since it allows separation of most, it not all, impurities and degradation products, and permits the development of stability-indicating assays. The method has a place in radiopharmaceutical quality control but is more expensive in first cost and running costs for consumables.

Equipment

The basic equipment for HPLC consists of a reservoir of mobile phase which is pumped through a sample injector device and chromatographic column to a detector and a collection vessel. A wide range of commercial equipment is available and the over-riding consideration with radioactive materials is reliability and ease of decontamination. Chromatography pumps for HPLC are mainly piston actuated pumps and come in a variety of pump actions, some with damping cylinders to smooth the pulses from the piston stroke (essential with high sensitivity UV detectors).

Injection systems vary from the on-column injector module fitted with a rubber septum which is punctured by the needle of the sample injection syringe. More useful with radioactive materials, are sample injector valves in which a sample loop is pre-loaded and the mobile phase flow is switched through the loop during injection. These allow safe filling of the constant volume loop. The normal technique is to inject excess sample through the sample loop into a plastics tube fitted with a needle inserted in a shielded vial. Preliminary injection of an air bubble helps in visualising the progress of the loop filling.

Radiopharmaceutical Applications

Radiopharmaceutical applications of HPLC have been reviewed by several authors (de Groot, 1988; Wieland, 1986) and should be consulted for practical and specific details of a particular application. HPLC methods are now available for a range of routine diagnostic radiopharmaceuticals and some typical analytical systems are shown in Table 7. The method is now used as an identity test for etifen substance in the BP 1988 Addendum 1991, although not for radiochemical purity determination, and an HPLC-SEC method is specified for [^{99m}Tc] labelled Albumin.

A number of problems have been reported with HPLC of Tc radiopharmaceuticals. The analytical method relies on the complete elution of all radioactive species injected or applied to the column. This is not possible when the sample contains colloidal or reduced Tc_2O since this component will become trapped on the column and purity determinations based on the areas of eluted components will overestimate the purity of the sample. Some kind of radioactivity-balance must be sought, and a method employing calibrated pre-column and post-column detection loops is recommended.

A second problem arises with the use of excess Sn(II) salts as reducing agents in Tc kits. Chromatography usually causes some of the Sn(II) to be retained or trapped at the top of the column: this will reduce any TcO_4^- present succeeding samples. A second and subsequently sample will appear to be free of TcO_4^- impurity due to on-column reduction, again giving falsely high radiochemical purity values. The effect can be detected with the dual detector loop system but the loss may be due to colloid, reduction of free pertechnetate, or both. Under these circumstances planar chromatographic methods have the advantage since all radiolabelled species will be separated or detected under proper conditions.

Radiolabelled Proteins

Radiolabelled protein radiopharmaceuticals require different HPLC conditions from small molecule radiotracers. Radio-HPLC can be used to purify labelled proteins from precursor reagents and unbound radiolabel, and similar systems are applied to the radiochemical analysis of these materials.

Several different physico-chemical processes can be used in the separation and purification of proteins. Separation according to molecular size can be achieved through gel permeation chromatography, the HPLC analogue of size-exclusion chromatography with Sephadex materials. Macromolecules are separated by a 'sieving' process according to their size, the smaller molecules being eluted last. A typical example is the chromatography of ^{99}Tc^{m}-labelled human serum albumin by Hosain and Hosain (1982). This method has been adopted by the Pharmacopoeias for Technetium [^{99m}Tc] Albumin Injection using a TSK G 3000 SW column (size-exclusion) with a phosphate buffer mobile phase.

Separation according to overall charge is performed with ion exchange columns and carefully buffered mobile phases, often by gradient elution to modify the pH (and thus retention) during the chromatographic run. Ionic strength is as important as pH in this separation mode, and gradient elution (either by pH or ionic strength) can be employed to hasten elution.

Separation according to the degree of hydrophobic interaction is achieved with a number of reversed-phase columns. Silica C_{18} rp can be used at acidic pH values, although polymer-based columns (prp-18, etc) are to be preferred because of their wider operating pH range (1 to 13). Newer column materials such as TSK 5PW-phenyl and graphitised carbon (Hypercarb) are reported to be useful. Proteins are strongly retained on these column materials and gradient

Table 7
HPLC of Selected Radiopharmaceuticals

Agent	*Column*	*Mobile phase*	*Reference*
TcO_4^-			
	Spherisorb, amino-bonded	Na acetate pH 4.5	Deutsch, 1982
	Waters sepralyte C_{18}	Bu_4N^+ in 40% MeOH	Bonnyman, 1983
Tc-HSA			
	Sperogel TSK 3000	0.1 M phosphate	Vallabhajosula, 1982
Tc-Diphosphonates			
EHDP	TSK G2000PW	0.9% NaCl, 10 mM EHDP, 1 mM Sn(II)	Huigen, 1988
	Aminex A28	0.85 M Na acetate	Huigen, 1988
	Aminex A-27	0.85 M Na acetate	Pinkerton, 1982 de Groot 1986
	C-18 rp	50 mM EHDP + mM NaAc + 3 mM Bu_4OH	Niewland, 1989
MDP	Aminex	0.85 M Na acetate	Tanabe, 1983
	Vydak C_{18} – RP	I mM NaAc, 2 mM Bu_4OH, 3% EtAc, pH 6.0	Hoch, 1986
Tc-HIDAs			
	uBondapak C_{18}	0.025 M phosphate pH 6.0	Nunn, 1983
	Ultrasphere ODS 5 um	0.01 M phosphate pH 6.8 + methanol (1:1)	Fritzberg, 1980
Tc-DADS derivs			
	Ultrasphere ODS 5 um	0.01 M phosphate + MeCN gradient 1:9 to 4:6 in 10 min	Fritzberg, 1981
Tc-bis-aminoethanethiols			
	PRP-1 RP	MeCN:water (85:15)	Kung, 1984
Tc-$DMPE_2Cl_2$			
	C_8-rp	MeOH:water (7:3) + 0.02 M hexanesulphonic acid + 0.003 M Phosphate	Vandenheyden 1983, 1983a
Tc-MAG_3			
	C_{18}-RP	EtOH:0.1 M phosphate pH 6.5 (5:95)	Fritzberg, 1986 and Taylor, 1988
	C_{18}-RP	10% MeOH in 0.05 M phosphate pH 7	Brandau, 1988
	Hypersil ODS 5 um	0.01 M phosphate pH 6:EtOH (95:5) for 10 min, then water:MeOH (90:10)	Millar, 1989
	C_{18}-RP	0.05 M phosphate pH 5.9:methanol (85:15)	Noll, 1992
Tc-DTC			
	uBondapak phenyl	MeOH:water (85:15)	Baldas, 1982
Tc-HM-PAO			
	PRP-1	20 mM phosphate pH 7.4 with 0–25% linear grad of THF in 6 min)	Neirinckx, 1987
Tc-MRP200			
	PRP-1	Phosphate pH 7.4 with 5%–45% THF gradient after 5 mins	Morgan, 1991
Tc-Fab			
	Zorbax SEC	0.2 M phosphate pH 7.2	Kasina, 1991
[^{123}I] iodo-α-methyltyrosine			
	RP-18	MeOH: H_2O: AcOH (40:60:1)	Biersack, 1989
[^{123}I] iodohippurate			
	Hypersil SAS	MeOH:0.1 M AcOH (30:70) pH 4	Millar, 1982

Table 7 *(cont)*
HPLC of Selected Radiopharmaceuticals

Agent	Column	Mobile phase	Reference
[^{131}I] MIBG			
	uBondapak C18	0.2 M ammonium Phosphate pH 7.0:THF (80:20)	Mangner, 1986
[^{123}I] HIPDM			
	uBondapak Phenyl	1% ammonium acetate pH 5.5:MeOH (30:70)	Mangner, 1986
[^{125}] p-iodobenzylsulphonamide			
	Dupont C18	60% MeOH	Singh, 1991
[^{67}Ga] and [^{111}In]-EHPG and -HBED			
	PRP-1	60% MeOH:0.05 M Na citrate pH 8.0 (60:40)	Hunt, 1988
^{111}In-DTPA			
	Alltech C18	5 nM phosphate: 2.5 nM octylamine in MeCN (86:15)	Vera, 1991
[^{68}Ga] and [^{111}In]-LDL			
	TSK GE1 G500-PW	0.15 M NaCl	Moerlin, 1991

elution methods are frequently necessary, decreasing the proportion of organic modifier and neutral salt concentrations to hasten elution.

An ultraviolet absorbance detector in tandem with the radiation detector is essential to ensure that the radioactivity *and* protein are co-eluted. Aromatic amino acids absorb strongly at 280 nm, the monitoring wavelength usually chosen.

Detector Linearity

The problem of assuring detector linearity has been discussed earlier under planar chromatography. Similar considerations apply here; the detection system must be shown to have a linear response to peak area over the range of radioactivities expected. The normal radioactivity injected in the sample will depend on local conditions and customs. In general, a sample volume of 10 to 50 μL is appropriate and the sample is injected through the loop of the injector set in the fill position which is then switched to sweep the slug of sample through to the column. A test of the linearity and dynamic range of the detector system requires a series of dilutions of a non-retained radiopharmaceutical covering the range 1 to 200% of the expected radioactivities. Equal volumes of these solutions are chromatographed by injection through the sample loop, even though the exact volume of the loop is inknown. The practice of partly filling the injector sample loop with smaller volumes delivered from a microsyringe cannot be relied to give reproducible sample volumes.

The plot of peak area against injected radioactivity will soon reveal any paralysis of the detection system by curvature. If the curvature is unacceptable then one solution is to employ a smaller volume detector loop or coil, and some authorities recommend a set of interchangeable detector loops for specific purposes. A suitable systems performance test is described in SOP 15.

Incomplete Sample Recovery

As mentioned under the discussion of Tc radiopharmaceuticals, some of the radioactivity may not be eluted from the column for various causes and it becomes necessary to check for incomplete elution. One method is to use two detector loops or coils, one connected to the column outlet as normal and another identical loop connected between the injector system and the column. All the injected radioactivity then passes through the pre-column detector and is recorded as a single, large peak which can be used as a standard (area) for the peaks eluted from the column. Eluted component radioactivites can then be reported as percentages of the pre-column standard peak and the recovery easily computed.

The practical application of this idea needs to be rigorously tested before use. The pre-chromatography peak will be sharp and intense compared with the eluate peaks and the detector and recorder settings may not be appropriate for both. A smaller pre-column loop can be used and calibrated against the post-column loop by chromatography of a series of dilutions of a non-retained species such as pertechnetate. Accurate calibration and validation of the assay method must be assured when using these techniques.

If the eluted components are trapped or adsorbed in the detector loop then the recovered radioactivity may be greater than 100%. This is usually indicated as a higher than normal baseline. The only solution is to replace the detector loop with one made from material less prone to adsorbing the component in question. Teflon loops are satisfactory for most post-column purposes even though they cannot be permanently bent or shaped into a neat loop. They cannot be used before the column under the high pressures encountered at this end of the system.

9.3.4 Electrophoretic Methods

Electrophoresis is a separation technique which relies on the different migration velocities of charge solute species dissolved in an electrolyte solution under the influence of an electric field gradient. Solute migration will depend on a number of factors including the sign and multiplicity of the charge, and the effective hydrodynamic volume.

The direction of migration will depend on the sign of the charge: cationic species C^+ will travel towards the cathode (– ve electrode) while anionic species A^- travel towards the anode (+ ve electrode). Neutral molecules and insoluble species will not migrate but may be carried a small distance by the flow of electrolyte generated by electroendosmosis.

The degree of separation can be changed to a small extent by altering the electrolyte environment and thus the hydrodynamic radius. The migration of weak acids and bases can be modified by pH changes which alter the degree of ionisation of these species.

Electrolyte Solutions

Conductive electrolyte solutions are essential for electrophoresis to ensure a uniform electric field gradient and an acceptable current flow. In most radiopharmaceutical applications buffered aqueous electrolyte solutions are used.

When dealing with low solublity lipophilic radiopharmaceuticals a mixed hydro-organic electrolyte solution may be employed such as *n*-propanol containing cetyltrimethylammonium bromide (Cetrimide) or other long-chain alkylammonium halide as conductive electrolyte.

Support Media

Although electrophoresis is possible in tubes of aqueous electrolyte, diffusion and convection currents distort any separation that might be achieved and it is customary to use a fairly rigid support medium to reduce these effects. Paper and cellulose acetate strips soaked in the electrolyte solution are commonly used in radiopharmacy and can be scanned or evaluated in the same way as radiochromatograms described in another section. Starch and polyacrylamide gels are used as supports for protein and macromolecular electrophoresis including radiolabelled antibodies and other proteins.

Of the paper supports, Whatman No. 1 is satisfactory for electrophoresis. It needs careful handling when wetted by electrolyte but has sufficient mechanical strength when dried. Cellulose acetate strips are quite strong when wet but need careful handling when dry, being brittle and prone to cockling. Some mechanical strength can be retained in the dry state by using 10% v/v glycerol in the electrolyte solution. The dried strip retains its flexibility and the added glycerol can sometimes improve the resolution by suppressing band spreading by diffusion.

Electrophoresis Equipment

The horizontal technique is satisfactory for most radiopharmaceutical applications and good commercial equipment is available at a reasonable cost. Home-made equipment is unsuitable for this technique in view of the hazards associated with the high voltages necessary for the technique.

The basic equipment consists of a tank having two electrode compartments and a frame or cooled platen for supporting the strips. The strips are placed on the horizontal supports and connected to the electrode compartments by paper wicks pre-soaked in the electrolyte and placed over the ends of the strip and dipping into the electrode compartments. A transparent cover fitted with a safety cut-out is placed over the tank before electrical connection is made to the power supply.

Power supplies come in many shapes and specifications depending on the nature of the electrophoresis experiment. Constant voltage (V), constant current (i), or constant power (V.i) operation modes are available. Each has its advantages and disadvantages. Constant voltage operation (about 10–30 V/cm of strip = about 300 V) is traditional, but overheating of the strip can occur and in extreme cases, charring with citrate buffers!

Radiopharmaceutical Applications

The main application is in the radiochemical purity determination of labelled proteins where separation cannot easily be achieved with chromatographic techniques. The BP 1988 specifies paper electrophoresis for the radiochemical purity of Iodinated [^{125}] Albumin Injection. A sample of at least 0.5 mg albumin (smaller amounts may not behave properly on migration) is electrophoretised on paper (5 × 30 cm) using a barbitone-acetate buffer at 500 V for 1 hour, dried, and the activity profile determined. At least 95% of the radioactivity must be located in the same region as normal human serum albumin. Cellulose acetate electrophoresis is specified for the protein identity test (the stained electrophoretogram shows no significantly different distribution from normal human albumin treated in the same manner) but no radioactivity measurements are specified for this test.

The radiochemical purity of Chromium [^{51}Cr] Edetate Injection is also determined by paper electrophoresis using a barbitone-buffered electrolyte. A 10 μL sample is applied as a 3 mm band at a point 10 cm from the cathode on 120 g m^{-2} paper. Electrophoresis is performed at 30 V cm^{-1} for 30 mins when the desired anionic edetate complex migrates some 5 cm towards the anode. The expected radiochemical impurities are [^{51}Cr] CrO_4^- which migrates faster towards the anode (about 10 cm), and the cationic $^{51}Cr^{3+}$ ion which migrates in the opposite direction, some 7 cm towards the cathode. The separation of principal components from two differently charged impurities is clearly demonstrated by electrophoresis; chromatographic methods are less successful at this separation. A suitable procedure for electrophoresis of radiopharmaceuticals is shown in SOP 16.

9.3.5 High Voltage Capillary Zone Electrophoresis

High voltage capillary zone electrophoresis (HVCZE) has been hailed as an answer to many difficult analytical separations by virtue of its non-chromatographic electrophoretic mobility mode of separating components. The technique employs fine glass capillaries of about 50 μm internal diameter which allow fast and efficient heat dissipation and permit the use of high voltages in the 15–30 kV range for fast and efficient separation of a variety of analytes including peptides and proteins. Commercial equipment uses on-line UV detection and produces separations seemingly indistinguishable from HPLC traces in terms of speed and resolution. Radiopharmaceutical applications are few, but are expected to increase once the problem of on-line radioactivity detection is solved.

9.3.6 Partition Methods

Recently a number of workers have used a modified form of the classical shake flask solvent partition technique used for determination of log P values. The method has the advantage that equilibrium is established between the phases within a few minutes and samples can be withdrawn and the phases assayed for radioactivity.

In a typical experiment a small sample of the radiopharmaceutical is diluted with aqueous buffer and the same volume of immiscible organic solvent (octanol, chloroform, diethyl ether are all popular) is added. The tube is capped and the phases are mixed (often with a whirlmixer), allowed to separate, then samples counted. The results are expressed as percentage of the 'lipophilic' radioactivity in the organic phase calculated from the expression:

$$\%\ \text{lipophilic} = 100 \times \frac{\text{C(organic at equilibrium)}}{\text{C(aqueous at start)}}$$

The method has been used by Tubergen *et al.* (1991) for extraction of lipophilic $^{99}Tc^{m}$-d,1-HMPAO with diethyl ether. Bossuyt and Morgan (1991) used extraction into water-saturated octanol for rapid radiochemical purity determinations of MRP20.

9.4 PARTICLE SIZING

Two major types of diagnostic radiopharmaceuticals consist of particulate suspensions. One group is used for the investigation of perfusion defects and includes preparations such as macroagregated human serum albumin and microspheres. The other group is used for investigation of the reticuloendothelial system and includes preparations such as colloids and phytate formulations.

9.4.1 Particulate Preparations

Safe and reproducible use of these preparations requires control over the number and size of the particles in the product. The preferred range of particle size is 20 to 80 μm with no particles larger than 100 μm and the minimum of particles below 20 μm.

Light microscopy is the best method for determination of particule number and size in these preparations. A sample is placed in a standard haemocytometer chamber and the number of particles estimated by counting particles in the centre and four corner squares: multiplication by the appropriate factor will give the number of particles per cm^3.

Particle sizing is best done from a photograph of the haemocytometer chamber. At least 600 particles should be examined and their sizes estimated from the known magnification of the photograph. Alternatively a Zahlstreifen eyepiece can be used. This has adjustable parallel counting lines and is used by counting about 200 particles along a section of known length (1–2 mm). From this number the length containing 5000 particles is estimated. This length is then scanned, counting only those particles which are over size. The maximum percentage of over size particles can then be calculated from confidence limits based on the Poisson distribution.

9.4.2 Colloidal Preparations

Not all radiopharmaceutical colloids are true colloids, and the mean particle size of colloidal preparations varies widely between different formulations of the same agent, and between different agents. Some sulphur colloids have mean particle sizes of around 0.4–0.6 μm while antimony trisulphide colloids have mean sizes below 0.1 μm. No single technique is suitable for sizing over such a large range.

Filtration through Nuclepore membranes (polycarbonate membranes having closely controlled etched pores) gives useful data for routine quality control. Samples of the preparation are filtered through a number of separate filters of known, different pore sizes and the percentage of radioactivity retained by each filter is calculated. The percentage retention may be plotted against filter pore size to give an 'activity-size' distribution. The method is not suitable for particles smaller than 0.05 μm. A typical method is shown in SOP 17.

Electron microscopy of samples evaporated on carbon grids can be used for accurate sizing of some colloids but cannot be recommended for routine examination. Some colloidal particles (especially sulphur) will evaporate under the conditions of high vacuum and electron bombardment and results are not easily comparable with those from filtration studies.

Light scattering and photon correlation techniques are now used for estimation of colloidal particle size distributions. These methods are quick and return a weight distribution which may not reflect the radoactivity associated with the individual size fractions.

9.5 PARTICULATE CONTAMINATION

All products for administration by injection should be free from gross particulate contamination. Control is exercised by using glassware, vials and reagents which are themselves free from particulate matter.

Visual examination of the product either directly through a leads glass or screen between illuminated cross-polaroid screens provides adequate control of most small volume radiopharmaceuticals. Those which cannot be examined visually (e.g. colloids, macroagregates, microspheres) must be controlled through strict control of glassware, reagents and containers.

9.6 CONTROL OF pH

Glass electrodes and pH meters are universally employed for measurement and checking of solution pH of pharmaceuticals. They are not always suitable for radiopharmaceutical quality control in view of the health and contamination hazards associated with handling unsealed sources.

Narrow range indicator papers are suitable if standard ph buffers are used in conjunction with the sample to give reference colours corresponding to upper and lower pH limits. A drop of each pH standard should be placed on the paper along with a drop of the sample, so providing a permanent visual record of the pH test.

9.7 BIOLOGICAL DISTRIBUTION TESTS

Biological distribution tests are performed in the development of new radiopharmaceuticals and are specified for some ^{99m}Tc-radiopharmaceuticals in the BP as shown in Table 4. In most cases the test is performed on 3 mice or rats and the test is valid if results in 2 of 3 animals are acceptable. A number of particulate radiopharmaceuticals are controlled in respect of abnormal lung (colloid) or liver (lung perfusion agents) uptake in the subjects. Biological distribution tests are not normally performed in the hospital radiopharmacy; their proper place is in the radiopharmacy research laboratory or in the radiopharmaceutical manufacturer's quality control laboratories.

9.8 SUMMARY AND CONCLUSIONS

Quality control of radiopharmaceuticals is a complex and time consuming activity in the hospital radiopharmacy. It should be evisaged as part of an ongoing scheme of quality assurance which embraces all aspects of the work done in the radiopharmacy. Not all the tests can, or should, be performed on each diagnostic agent every time it is dispensed or manufactured. A proper scheme is necessary to ensure that all radiopharmaceuticals are regularly checked, and a combination of radiochemical analysis, environmental control and monitoring, and adequate training of personnel will go a long way towards achieving satisfactory quality assurance.

REFERENCES

Baldas J., Bonnyman J., Pojer P.M. and Williams G.A. (1982). *The influence of reducing agents on the composition of Tc-99m complexes; implications for ^{99}Tc radiopharmaceutical preparation.* Eur. J. Nucl. Med., **7**, 187–189.

Biersack H.J., Coenen H.H., Stocklin G., Reidmann K., Bockisch A., Oehr P., Kashab M. and Rollmann O. (1989). *Imaging of brain tumours with L-3[^{123}I] Iod-a-methyltyrosine and SPECT.* J. Nucl. Med., **30**, 110–112.

Billinghurst M.W., Abrams D.N., Lawson M.S. (1991). *Stabilisation of [^{99m}] HMPAO-I. Ethanolic preparation.* Appl. Radiat. Isot., **42**, 607–612.

Bonnyman J. (1983). *Effect of milking efficiency on ^{99}Tc content of ^{99m}Tc derived from ^{99m}Tc generators.* Int. J. Appl. Radiat. Isot., **34**, 901–906.

Bossuyt S.M., Morgan G.M., *et al.* (1991). *Tc-99m-MRP20: a potential brain perfusion agent:* in vivo *distribution and SPECT studies in normal volunteers.* J. Nucl. Med., **32**, 399–403.

Brandau W., Bubeek B., Eisenhut M. and Taylor D.M. (1988). *Technetium-99m labelled renal function and imaging agents III. Synthesis of ^{99m}Tc-MAG$_3$ and biodistributiuon of by-products.* Appl. Radiat. Isot., **39**, 121–129.

British Institute of Radiology (1979). *Guidelines for the Preparation of Radiopharmaceuticals in Hospitals.* London, BIR.

Carpenter A.P. (1986). *Radioanalytical techniques: ITLC TLC, Mini-columns, and Electrophoresis. In* Analytical and Chromatographic Techniques in Radiopharmaceutical Chemistry, edited by D.M. Wieland, M.C. Tobes and T.J. Magner pp. 39–70. New York: Springer-Verlag.

Deutsch E., Heinemann W.R., Zodda J.P., Gilbert T.W. and Williams C.C. (1982). *Preparation of* no carrier added *technetium-99m complexes: determination of total technetium content of generator eluates.* Int. J. Appl. Radiat. Isot., **33**, 843–848.

Frier M. and Hesslewood S. (eds) (1980). *Quality Assurance of Radiopharmaceuticals – a Guide to Hospital Practice.* Nucl. Med. Commun., special issue.

Fritzberg A.R. and Lewis D. (1980). *HPLC analysis of Tc-99m iminodiacetate hepatobiliary agents and a question of multiple peaks.* J. Nucl. Med., **21**, 1180–1184.

Fritzberg A.R., Klongensmith W.C., Whitney W.P. and Kuni C.C. (1981). *Chemical and Biological Studies of Tc-99m N,N' bis(mercaptoacetoamide)-ethylenediamine; a potential replacement for I-131 hippurate.* J. Nucl. Med., **22**, 258–263.
Fritzberg A.R., Kasina S., Eshima D. and Johnson D.L. (1986). *Synthesis and biological evaluation of technetium- 99m MAG_3 as a hippuran replacement.* J. Nucl. Med. **27**, 111–116.
de Groot G.J., Das H.A. and de Ligny C.L. (1986). *The separation of $^{99m}Tc(Sn)$ EHDP complexes by HPLC and GPC.* Appl. Radiat. Isot. A., **37**, 23–27.
de Groot G.J., Das H.A. and de Ligney C.L. (1988). *A system for high performance liquid chromatography of $^{99}Tc^m$ complexes with on-line radiometric detection and data processing.* Int. J. App. Radiat. Isot., **36**, 349–355.
Hauser W. and Cavallo L. (1977). *Measurement and Quality Assurance of the Amount of Administered Tracer. In* Quality Control in Nuclear Medicine, edited by B.A. Rhodes, pp. 154–163. St. Louis: Mosby.
Hoch D.J. and Pinkerton T.C. (1986). *Reversed phase HPLC of ^{99m}Tc methylene diphosphonate bone imaging kits with quantification of pertechnetate.* Appl. Radiat. Isot., **37**, 593–598.
Hosain P. and Hosain F. (1982). *High performance size exclusion chromatography of human serum albumin labelled with technetium-99m. In* Nuclear Medicine and Biology Advances, Vol 1. Proceedings of the 3rd World Congress in Nuclear Medicine and Biology, edited by C. Raynaud, pp. 238–241. Oxford: Pergamon Press.
Hnatowich D.J. (1986). *HPLC of radiolabelled antibodies. In* Analytical and Chromatographic Techniques in Radiopharmaceutical Chemistry, edited by D.M. Wieland, M.C. Tobes and T.J. Magner, pp. 279–293. New York: Springer-Verlag.
Huigan Y.M., Gelsema W.J. and de Ligny C.L. (1988). *Effect of the composition of the eluent in the chromatography of ^{99m}Tc-disphosphonate complexes.* Appl. Radiat. Isot., **39**, 381–384.
Hung C.Y., Corlija M., Volkert W.A., Holmes R.A. (1988). *A kinetic analysis of Tc-99m d,1-HMPAO decomposition in aqueous media.* J. Nucl. Med., **29**, 1568–1576.
Hunt F.C. (1988). *Reversed phase high performance liquid chromatography of Gallium-67 and Indium-111 chelates of EHPG, HBED and their derivatives.* Appl. Radiat. Isot., **39**, 349–352.
Kasina S., Rao T., *et al.* (1991) *Development and biologic evaluation of a kit for preformed chelate Tc-99m radiolabelling of an antibody Fab fragment using a diamide dimercapto chelating agent.* J. Nucl. Med., **32**, 1445–1451.
Kloster G. and Laufer P. (1984). *Identification of Radiopharmaceuticals by their retention of HPLC; a caveat.* Int. J. Appl. Radiat. Isot., **35**, 545.
Kung H.F., Molnar M., Billings J., Wicks R. and Blau M. (1984). *Synthesis and biodistribution of neutral lipid-soluble Tc-99m complexes that cross the blood-brain barrier.* J. Nucl. Med., **25**, 326–332.
Leveille J., Demarceau G., Waloriteh R.C. (1992). *Intrasubject comparison between technetium-99m ECD and technetium-99m HMPAO in healthy human subjects. –J. Nucl. Med.,* **33**, 480–484.
Levit N. (1980 (ed.). *Radiopharmacy Laboratory Manual for Nuclear Medicine Technologists.* pp. 69–80, Albuquerque, New Mexico: University of New Mexico College of Pharmacy.
Mangner T.J. (1986). *Protein artefacts in the chromatography of radiopharmaceuticals. In* Analytical and Chromatographic Techniques in Radiopharmaceutical Chemistry, edited by D.M. Wieland, M.C. Tobes and T.J. Mangner, pp. 261–278. New York: Springer-Verlag.
Millar A.M. (1982). *HPLC of Iodohippuric acid [^{123}I] Injection.* J. Pharm. Pharmacol., **34**, , 14–17.
Millar A.M. (1989). *Quality Assurance of Radiopharmaceuticals. In* Radiopharmaceuticals and Radiotracers in Pharmacy, edited by A.E. Theobald, 1989. Chichester: Ellis Horwood.
Mock B.H. and Weiner R.E. (1988). *Simplified solid-state labelling of [^{123}I] m-iodobenzylguanidine.* Appl. Radiat. Isot., **39**, 939–942.
Moerlin S.M., Daugherty A., Sobel B.E., Welch M.J. (1991). *Metabolic imaging with Ga-68 and In-111 labelled low density lipoprotein.* J. Nucl. Med., **32**, 300–307.
Morelli J.L., Rapin J.R., LePoncin L., Lageron A., Saccavini J.C. and Bardy A. (1982). *Dimercaptosuccinic acid complexes: their structure, biological behaviour and renal localisation. In* Radionuclides in Nephrology, edited by A.M. Joekes, pp. 25–31. London: Academic Press.
Neirinckx R.D., Canning L.R., Piper I.M., Nowotnik D.P., Pickett R.D., Holmes R.A., Volkert W.A., Foster A.M., Weisner P.S., Marriot J.A. and Chaplin S.B. *Technetium-99m d,1-HM-PAO: A new radiopharmaceutical for SPECT imaging of regional cerebral blood flow.* J. Nucl. Med., **28**, 191–202.
Niewland R.J.A., Das H.A. and de Ligny C.L. (1989). *Improvement of the reproducibility of ion-pair HPLC of $^{99m}Tc(Sn)$ EHDP complexes and the influence of the Sn(III) concentration on the composition of the reaction mixture.* Appl. Radiat. Isot., **40**, 153–157.
Noll B., Johannsen B., May K. and Spies H. (1992). *Preparation of the renal function and imaging agent Tc-99m MAG3 starting from S-unprotected mercaptotriglycine.* Int. J. Appl. Radiat. Isot., **43**, 899–901.
Nunn A.D. (1983). *Structure-distribution relationships of radiopharmaceuticals: Correlation between the reversed-phase capacity factors for Tc-99m phenylcarbamoylmethyl iminodiacetic acids and their renal elimination.* J. Chromatogr., **255**, 91–100.
Nunn A.D. and Fritzberg A.R. (1986). *Components for the Design of a radio-HPLC system. In* Analytical and Chromatographic Techniques in Radiopharmaceutical Chemistry, edited by D.M. Wieland, M.C. Tobes and T.J. Magner, pp. 103–124. New York: Springer-Verlag.
Persson B.R. (1977). *Gel Chromatography Column Scanning. In* Quality Control in Nuclear Medicine, editer B.A. Rhodes, pp. 210–212. St. Louis: Mosby.
Pinkerton T.C., Ferguson D.L., Deutsch E., Heinemann W.R. and Libson K. (1982). In vivo *distributions of some component fractions of $Tc(NaBH_4)$HEDP mixtures separated by anion exchange high performance liquid chromatography.* Int. J. Appl. Radiat. Isot., **33**, 907–915.
Proulx A., Ballinger J.R. and Gulenchyn K.Y. (1989). *Routine determination of ^{99m}Tc-MIBI.* Appl. Radiat. Isot., **40**, 95–97.
Rhodes B.A. (ed.) (1978). *Quality Control in Nuclear Medicine.* St. Louis: Mosby.
Robbins P.J. (1984). *Chromatography of Technetium-99m radiopharmaceuticals – a practical guide.* New York: The Society of Nuclear Medicine Inc.
Solanki K.K., Mather S.J., Janabi M.Al. and Britton K.E. (1988). *A rapid method for the preparation of $^{99}Tc^m$ hexametazime-labelled leucocytes.* Nucl. Med. Commun., **9**, 753–761.
Scrivastva S.C., Meinken G.E., Richards P., Ford L.A. and Benson R. (1982). *HPLC characterisation of clinically used ^{99m}Tc bone agents – relative tissue distribution of fractionated components in mice. In* Nuclear Medicine and Biology Advances. Vol. 1 – Proceedings of the 3rd World Congress in Nuclear Medicine and Biology, edited by C. Raynaud, pp. 1631–1634. Oxford: Pergamon Press.
Tanabe S., Zodda J.P., Deutsch E. and Heinmann W.R. (1983). Effect of pH on the formation of $Tc(NaBH_4)$-MDP radiopharmaceutical analogues. Int. J. Appl. Radiat. Isot., **34**, 1577–1584.

Taylor A.T. and Eshina D. (1988). *Effects of altered physiologic states on clearance and biodistribution of technetium-99m MAG_3, iodine-131 OIH, and iodine-125 iothalmate.* J. Nucl. Med., **29**, 616–622.

Thoneur C.M., Couch M.W., Creer D.M., Thomas K.D., and Williams C.M. (1988). *Biodistribution and radiation dosimetry of radioiodinated SCH 23982: a potential dopamine D-1 receptor imaging agent.* J. Nucl. Med., **29**, 1668–1674.

Tubergeu K., Corlija M., Volkert W.A., Holmes R.A. (1991). *Sensitivity of Tc-99m-d,1-HMPAO to radiolysis in aqueous solution.* J. Nucl. Med., **32**, 111–115.

Vallabhajosula S., Goldsmith S.J., Pollina R. and Lipszyc H. (1982). *Radiochemical analysis of Tc-99m human serum albumin with high pressure liquid chromatography.* J. Nucl. Med., **23**, 326–329.

Vanderheyden J.-L., Libson K., Nosco D.L., Ketring A.R. and Deutsch E. (1983). *Preparation and characterisation of $[^{99m}Tc(DMPE)_3]^+$, a potential myocardial imaging agent.* J. Nucl. Med., **24**, 9.

Vanderheyden J.-L., Lisbon K., Nosco D.L., Ketring A.R. and Deutsch E. (1983a). *Preparation and characterisation of $[^{99m}Tc(DMPE)_2X_2$, X = Cl, Br, DMPE = 1,2 bis (dimethyl phosphinoethanol).* Int. J. Appl. Radiat. Isot., **34**, 1611–1615.

Van Wyk A.J., *et al.* (1991). *Synthesis and ^{99m}Tc labelling of MMI (MIBI) and its ethyl analogue EMI.* Int. J. Asppl. radiat. Isot., **42**, 687–689.

Verbruggen A.M., *et al.* (1992). *Technetium-99m-L,L,ethylene dicysteine; a renal imaging agent I.* J. Nucl. Med., **33**, 551–557.

Vora M.M. (1991). *HPLC analysis of Indium-111 diethylenetriamine-penta-acetic acid radiopharmaceutical.* Int. J. Appl. Radiat. Isot., **42**, 19–24.

Westera G., Gadze A. and Horst W. (1985). *A convenient method for the preparation of $^{99m}Tc(V)$ dimercaptosuccinic acid ($^{99m}Tc(V)$-DMSA).* Int. J. Appl. Radiat. Isot., **36**, 349–355.

Wieland D.M., Tobes M.C. and Manger T.J. (editors) (1986). Analytical and Chromatographic Techniques in Radiopharmaceutical Chemistry. New York: Springer-Verlag.

Zimmer A.M. and Pavel D.G. 1977). *Rapid miniaturised chromatographic quality-control procedures for Tc-99m radiopharmaceuticals.* J. Nucl. Med., **18**, 1230–1233.

Zucchini G.L., Marinelli M., Pozzato R. and Garuti P. (1987). *Comparison of different chromatographic quality control procedures to determine the radiochemical purity of common ^{99m}Tc diagnostic agents.* Appl. Radiat. Isot., **38**, 283–288.

SOP1

CHELSEA RADIOPHARMACY: STANDARD OPERATING PROCEDURE
CALIBRATION OF IONISATION CHAMBER

1 Ionisation chambers used for routine measurement of radioactivities of received and dispensed radiopharmaceuticals need to be checked for calibration accuracy and linearity of response every three months.

2 **Calibration Accuracy**

For this test a standard radioactive source is required. A suitable source is ^{226}Ra having an activity of about 3.7 MBq (100 μCi) obtainable from Amersham International and provided with a calibration certificate traceable to NPL.

a Set the ionisation chamber controls to read ^{226}Ra

b Place the standard source in the measuring volume of the ionisation chamber. Allow the instrument to settle for several minutes before taking a reading. It may be necessary to switch to a 'slow' setting of the readout device to reduce the random fluctuations.

c Take at least three readings of the source activity at about 5 minute intervals and record their average and standard deviation.

d If necessary with an indirect reading instrument, calculate the radioactivity of the standard source.

e Compare the measurements with the stated radioactivity of the standard source.

f Confirm that the measured radioactivity lies within 5% of stated radioactivity. If the measurement lies outside this tolerance the instrument must be taken out of use and services or recalibrated by the manufacturer.

3 **Linearity Checks**

The linearity of response over the dynamic range of the instrument should be confirmed as follows.

a Obtain a sample of the highest Tc-99m activity expected in the Radiopharmacy, usually in the GBq range.

b Taking all radiation safety precautions, measure the radioactivity of this sample. Note the activity and time of measurement.

c Repeat the measurement at intervals of 6 to 12 hours, noting the time and activity at each measurement, until the radioactivity has fallen to a level indistinguishable from background.

d Convert the recorded radioactivities to their logarithms and plot as ordinate against elapsed time since the initial observations.

e Examine the plot visually for linearity. If programs are available, then perform a linear regression on the data and examine the residuals for evidence of non-linearity.

f Carefully note the radioactivity regions which appear nonlinear (usually the high and low ends of the overall range) and record the usable range on the instruction sheet for the instrument.

SOP2

CHELSEA RADIOPHARMACY: STANDARD OPERATING PROCEDURE
Determination of Beta Absorption Curves

Beta absorption curves are specified in the BP as a means of identification of beta emitting radionuclides. The equipment consists of a lead castle fitted with shelves for the source and interposed screens all below a GM detector. Aluminium screens or filters are placed between the source and the GM detector and the decrease in count rate with increasing aluminium thickness is followed until all the particles are absorbed s shown by a fairly constant background count rate. The absorption curve is compared to that of a standard sample measured under identical conditions.

Preparation of the radioactive source is critical; the BP directions for source preparation must be followed.

Method

1 Check the controls and operation of the scaler. Set the high voltage to its specified level.

2 With no source present in the assembly, count the background for 5 minutes.

3 Place the metal shield on SHELF 1 of the castle and leave it in position at all times EXCEPT WHEN TAKING A COUNT.

4 Place the unknown source in a plastics holder and insert in SHELF 4 of the castle. Place an absorber holder on SHELF 3.

5 Take 1 minute counts (or longer as appropriate) with increasing thickness of aluminium absorbers placed in SHELF 3. *At least six screens should be used, of increasing mass per unit area (mg/cm^2) with the thickest screen absorbing all the particles and thus giving a background count.*

6 Correct all counts for background and paralysis using the formula:

$$C_{true} = \frac{C_{obs}}{1 - C_{obs}\,\tau}$$

where C_{obs} is the observed count rate cpm after background subtraction and τ is the paralysis time of the equipment expressed in seconds.

7 Repeat steps 4 to 6 with the standard source of the radionuclide being identified.

8 Plot the logarithm of the true count rate (ordinate) against the superficial density (mg/cm^2) for both sample and standard.

9 Calculate the coefficient of mass attenuation by the following method:

a inspect the plots and identify the portion of the curve that is the most linear.

b identify the lightest screen, m_1 and the heaviest screen, m_z, lying within the linear region of the plots.

c calculate the coefficient from the formula:

$$\mu_m = \frac{2.303}{m_z - m_1}(\log A_1 - \log A_z)$$

where A_1, A_z are the corrected count rates obtained with the lightest and heaviest screens within the liner part of the curve.

10 Compare the mass absorption coefficients of the sample and standard.

11 Accept the sample identity if the difference between the coefficients is less than 10%.

SOP3

CHELSEA RADIOPHARMACY: STANDARD OPERATING PROCEDURE
Molybdenum-99 Breakthrough Test for Tc-99m Eluates

Every eluate obtained from a Mo-99/Tc-99m Generator system should be examined for Mo-99 breakthrough. The rapid method described below depends on the selective transmission of high energy gamma photons from M0-99 impurity through a 7 mm thick lead shield.

The maximum permissible radioactivity due to the parent Mo-99 is 0.1% of the measured Tc-99m radioactivity (or 1kBq of Mo-99 activity for every 1 MBq of Tc-99m activity).

Method

1 Measure the Tc-99m radioactivity of the generator eluate as described in the SOP for the ionisation chamber.

2 Reset the ionisation chamber to measure M0-99 radioactivity by changing the attenuator settings to those appropriate to Mo-99

2 Transfer the eluate vial to the 7mm wall lead shield and replace in the ionisation chamber.

3 Note the reading corresponding to Mo-99 activity and calculate the percentage present.

SOP4

CHELSEA RADIOPHARMACY: STANDARD OPERATING PROCEDURE
SCINTILLATION DETECTOR PERFORMANCE OPTIMISATION

Scintillation detectors must be set to maximum counting efficiency by adjustment of the photomultiplier high voltage and the pulse threshold or window settings. This SOP describes a generic procedure for optimising scintillation counters, either plastics or thallium-activated sodium iodide.

1 Set the threshold to about 20% of its maximum value. If an energy window is available, then set this to 'integral' or a wide value to ensure collection of high numbers of pulses.

2 Place a gamma emitting sample of activity 1-5 kBq near the detector (or in the well of well detector).

3 Slowly increase the HV setting until the scaler begins to count.

4 Set the equipment to record 10 second counts.

5 Starting at a rational value just below the HV determined above, increase the HV in steps of 10 volts and record the 10 second count. Continue as the count rises with voltage and stop when it is obvious that the counter is 'racing'

6 Remove the radioactive source and repeat the previous step to obtain a series of background counts at the same voltages.

7 Plot the S(ample) and B(ackground) count rates against HV to determine the length of the counting plateau and to select an operating voltage within that range.

8 Alternatively, calculate the function S^2/B and plot at each HV setting. The optimum HV corresponds to the peak on this plot.

9 As a further check the detector linearity should be determined with standards of known radioactivity.

SOP5

CHELSEA RADIOPHARMACY: STANDARD OPERATING PROCEDURE
SCINTILLATION DETECTOR LINEARITY CHECKING

The working voltage and energy window of a NaI(Tl) scintillation detector must be adjusted to detect the photopeak of the specified radionuclide ($^{99}Tc^{m}$ in this case) to ensure maximum counting efficiency. The instrument settings should have already been adjusted for optimum counting dfficiency according to SOP: SCINTILLATION DETECTOR PERFORMANCE OPTIMISATION and should not be changed.

Method

1 Prepare a stock solution containing about 1MBq mL^{-1} of ^{99m}Tc radioactivity by dilution from a generator eluate. Note the eluate label details (radioactivity, volume, time of measurement) for use in calculations later on.

2 Prepare a series of calibration standards by diluting 0.2, 0.4, 0.6, 0.8 and 1.0 mL of the stock solution to 100 mL with water. Label the calibration standards.

3 Dispense 1 mL aliquots of each standard into 5 mL plastic counting vials by using a <u>fresh</u> 1 mL disposable syringe for each. Ensure the tubes are securely capped and label them.

4 Take a 10 second background count and then count each calibration standard for 10 seconds. Correct the counts by subtracting the background. Note the time of measurement.

5 Calculate the radioactivity of the standards counted from the expression

$$A(\text{dps}) = \frac{S(\text{MBq mL}^{-1}) \times V(\text{mL}) \times 10^{6} \times f}{100}$$

Where S(MBq mL^{-1}) is the radioactive concentration of the stock solution (from label details), V(mL) is the volume of eluate taken for dilution, and f is the <u>decay factor</u> for ^{99m}Tc obtained from tables for the <u>elapsed time</u> $(t - t_{ref})$ between the reference time and completion of the counting in step 4. The factor 10^6 converts radioactivity in MBq to disintegrations per second.

6 Convert the observed 10 second counts to count rate (in cps) and plot observed count (cps) against the true radioactivity (in dps, step 5). Examine the plot and check that points at the higher radioactivities are linear and do not show a drop in count rate.

7 By drawing the best line through the points or using a graphics/statistics program to generate the best line, calculate the counting efficiency from the slope of the graph. (A slope of 1 indicates 100% efficiency, 0.2 is 20%)

SOP6

CHELSEA RADIOPHARMACY: STANDARD OPERATING PROCEDURE
Paper chromatography of Radiopharmaceuticals

Whatman 3MM paper is recommended for radiochromatography as it is fast running and mechanically strong in the wet condition.

Method

1 Cut a piece of Whatman 3MM paper and mark in sharp, soft pencil as in the diagram:

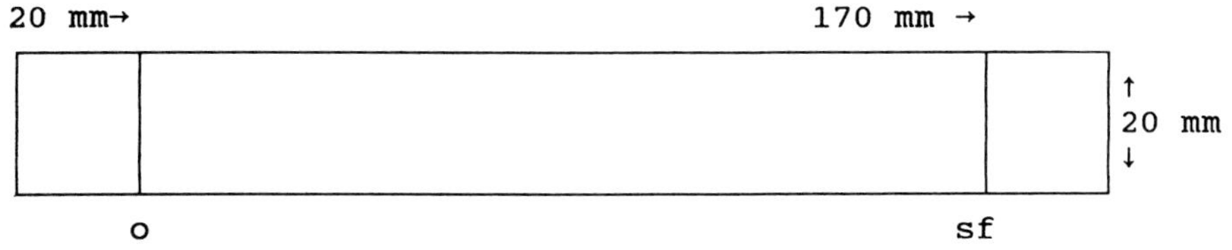

2 Take a tall cylinder (250 x 40 mm diam) and place enough mobile phase to give a 10 mm deep pool at the bottom. Moisten a solvent saturation pad with the mobile phase and slide it down the inside wall of the cylinder until it touches the pool of mobile phase.

3 As an aid to visualising the solvent migration make a mark about 3 mm below the solvent front line with a suitable felt-tip marker.

3 Using either a 5 μL capillary pipette or a drop hanging from the end of a 25G (orange) needle, place a single spot of the radiopharmaceutical at the origin of the ITCL strip.

4 Immediately clip the strip to the hanger and lower gently into the cylinder until the bottom edge is immersed some 2-3 mm in the pool.

5 Place the assembly in front of the cold light and allow development to proceed until the mobile phase reaches the solvent front line.

6 Immediately remove the strip from the cylinder and dry under the infrared lamp or in a stream of warm air.

7 Examine and quantitate the strip by any of the approved methods for the particular radiopharmaceutical.

SOP7

CHELSEA RADIOPHARMACY: STANDARD OPERATING PROCEDURE
ITLC chromatography of Radiopharmaceuticals

The ITLC system consists of a glass microfibre mat impregnated with silica gel or silicic acid. The material is extremely fragile and should be handled with great care. In particular the surfaces should not be touched with the bare fingers as fingerprints are known to cause artefacts in the chromatograms.

Method

1 Cut a piece of ITLC material and mark in sharp, soft pencil as in the diagram:

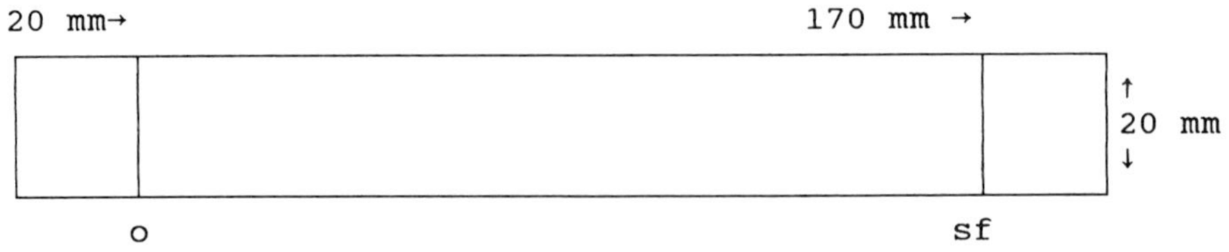

Activate the silica by heating in an oven at 110°C for 10 minutes, then allowing the strip to cool before use.

2 Take a tall cylinder (250 x 40 mm diam) and place enough mobile phase to give a 10 mm deep pool at the bottom. Moisten a solvent saturation pad with the mobile phase and slide it down the inside wall of the cylinder until it touches the pool of mobile phase.

3 As an aid to visualising the solvent migration make a mark about 3 mm below the solvent front line with a suitable felt-tip marker.

3 Using either a 5 μL capillary pipette or a drop hanging from the end of a 25G (orange) needle, place a single spot of the radiopharmaceutical at the origin of the ITCL strip.

4 Immediately clip the strip to the hanger and lower gently into the cylinder until the bottom edge is immersed some 2-3 mm in the pool.

5 Place the assembly in front of the cold light and allow development to proceed until the mobile phase reaches the solvent front line.

6 Immediately remove the strip from the cylinder and dry under the infrared lamp or in a stream of warm air.

7 When dry, protect the ITLC strip by sandwiching between two layers of sellotape.

8 Examine and quantitate the strip by any of the approved methods for the particular radiopharmaceutical.

SOP8

CHELSEA RADIOPHARMACY: STANDARD OPERATING PROCEDURE
Minichromatography for $^{99}Tc^{m}$ Radiopharmaceuticals

Method

1 Prepare strips of Gelman ITLC-SG material or Whatman 3MM paper according to the diagram:

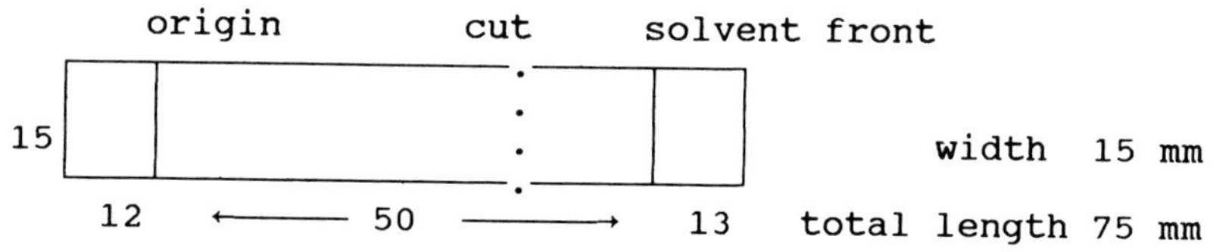

2 Prepare developing tanks by placing about 1 ml of the mobile phase into glass Universal tubes or scintillation vials.

3 Apply 5μL spots of samples to separate strips using calibrated capillary pipettes.

4 Immediately develop the chromatograms until the mobile phase reaches the solvent front line.

5 Remove the strips from the developing tube and dry them under the IR lamp.

6 Divide each strip into upper and lower sections by cutting across the pre-marked line.

7 Roll each section and place in a counting tube.

8 Determine which is the most radioactive section and count this for 50 or 60 seconds, or until at least 10 000 counts have been accumulated, whichever is the longer, C_h

9 Count the less active section for the same time period, C_l

10 Count the background for the same period of time, B

11 Calculate the percentage of radioactivity in each section of the strip from the formula:

$$\% = 100 \times \frac{C_{h \text{ or } l} - B}{C_h + C_l - 2 \times B}$$

SOP9

CHELSEA RADIOPHARMACY: STANDARD OPERATING PROCEDURE
Seprachrom System for Radiochromatography

The Gelman Seprachrom system consists of a moulded polyethylene two-piece chromatoplate developing chamber which fits into a base tank containing the mobile phase. The chromatoplate, either ITLC or paper, is mounted between the faces of the upper chamber after spotting then inserted into the base tank for development.

Method

1 Cut a piece of ITLC material or Whatman 3MM paper 95 x 50 mm and mark with a sharp, soft pencil according to the diagram:

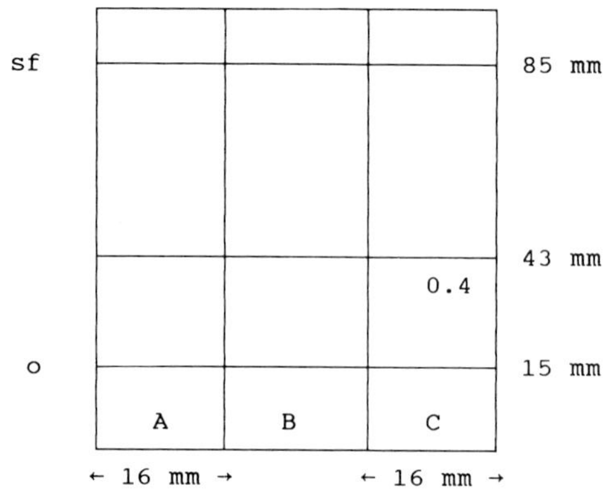

2 Prepare the chamber by pipetting about 4 mL of mobile phase into the lower tank.

3 In the case of Whatman 3MM paper, carefully check that the strip is not curled. If it is, gently remove the curve by running it between the fingers in the opposite curvature several times.

4 Load the chromatoplate by spotting T(est) samples or Standard) at the centre of each channel at the origin.

5 Mount the chromatoplate in the upper chamber by slipping the top of the strip under the retaining bar fitted to the rear face of the upper chamber, then pressing the upper face in position to sandwich the chromatoplate between the faces by the upper retaining bar and the lower gripping row of studs on each face.

6 Check that the chromatoplate is not curved or touching either face of the upper chamber. If it is, then disassemble the upper chamber, remove the plate and de-curl the material before reassembly.

7 Gently place the upper chamber assembly into the top of the solvent tank and allow to equilibrate for about 5 minutes.

8 After equilibration, gently push the upper chamber fully down into the solvent tank without splashing to start development.

9 Place the Seprachrom chamber infront of a cold light as an aid to viewing migration of the mobile phase.

10 When development is complete, remove the upper chamber and separate the two faces. Remove the chromatoplate and dry under an infrared lamp.

11 Examine and quantitate the chromatogram by any of the methods approved for the radiopharmaceutical being evaluated.

SOP10

CHELSEA RADIOPHARMACY: STANDARD OPERATING PROCEDURE
Reversed Phase High Performance TLC for $^{99}Tc^m$ Radiopharmaceuticals

Reverse phase HPTLC is suitable for lipophilic radiopharmaceuticals and those containing lipophilic components or impurities. Careful attention to sample application techniques and development conditions is essential for successful application of this technique. Suitable plates include Merck C18RP

Method

1 Prepare the developing tank containing a solvent saturation pad and place about 5 - 10 mL of the mobile phase in the tank, ensuring the solvent pad is saturated. Replace the lid and allow the system to equilibrate for about 15 mins.

2 Meanwhile mark up the 100 x 100 mm plate with a sharp, soft pencil according to the diagram:

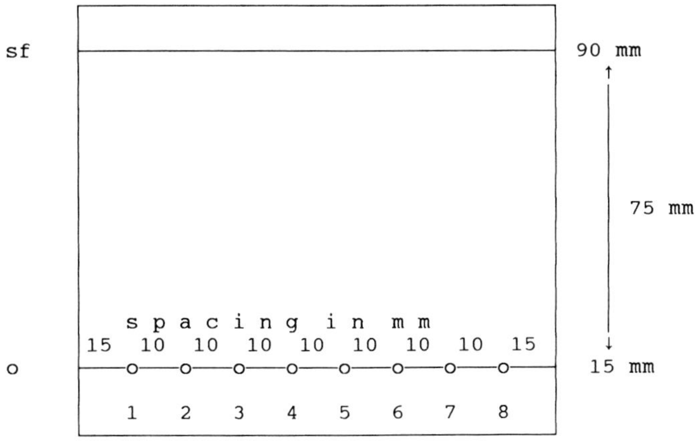

Activate the plate by heating in an oven at 110°C for 10 minutes, then allowing the plate to cool before use.

3 Using a 1 or 2 μL capillary pipette, spot samples onto the plate at marked locations. *Ensure that spot diameter does not exceed 2mm. Use multiple applications if necessary.*

4 Adopt a systematic arrangement of test sample and standard spots. If a single radiopharmaceutical is being examined the following sequence of S(tandard) and T(est) is recommended:

S T T S T S S T

If several radiopharmaceuticals are being examined, reduce the number of S(tandards) accordingly e.g.

S T1 T2 S T3 T1 T3 T2

5 If multiple applications are required dry each spot with a current of nitrogen gas between applications. A suitable gas line can be constructed from a 1 mL disposable syringe barrel cut and fitted into the gas tube and a wide bore (green?) needle fitted to the syringe hub.

6 When the plate is loaded, place it in the developing tank suspended above the mobile phase and leave for about 10 - 15 mins to equilibrate with the lid closed.

7 After equilibration, carefully lower the plate into the mobile phase, close the lid and leave to develop until the mobile phase reaches the pre-marked solvent front line.

9 When development is complete, remove the plate from the tank and dry under the infrared lamp.

10 Examine the chromatoplate by any of the scanning techniques available. Recommended settings for high resolution scanning should be adopted.

SOP11

CHELSEA RADIOPHARMACY: STANDARD OPERATING PROCEDURE
Autoradiography of Chromatograms

Autoradiography of radiochromatograms provides a permanent record of the distribution of radioactivity on the chromatoplate but cannot give reliable information on the distribution of radioactivity between peaks, spots or regions.

1 Develop and dry the chromatogram as usual.

2 Take the chromatoplate and light-proof cassette or envelope into the darkroom.

3 Once in the darkroon switch on the safelight and switch off the normal lighting. Wait a few minutes for the eyes to adjust to the new lighting level.

4 Unwrap a sheet of X-ray film and cut a piece the same size as the chromatoplate. Replace unused film in its envelope. Fix the plate and film together using clips and mark the orientation and identity of both by clipping a distinctive pattern on one edge of the plate-film pair. Place the assembly in the light proof cassette and leave for at least 30 mins or preferably overnight.

5 After exposure of the film re-enter the darkroom and assemble the developing tanks and dishes. Half fill the developing tank with developer, and similarly half fill the stop tank with stop solution and fixer tank with fixer solution.

6 Switch on the safelight and switch off the normal lighting. Wait a few minutes for the eyes to adjust to the new lighting level. Remove the plate-film pair from the lightproof cassette. Separate the two components and gently place the film in the developer.

8 Develop the film for about 5 minutes until the radioactive areas are clearly shown as dark spots. gently rock the tank during development to ensure even mixing and exposure to the developing solution.

9 Stop development by transferring the film to the stop bath and immersing in the stop solution for about 1 minute.

10 Transfer the film from the stop bath to the fixer bath and gently rock the bath until the unexposed ares of the film are dissolved and appear uniformly clear when viewed against the safelight.

11 Transfer the film to the wash tank and wash in running water for at least 10 minutes. Remove the finished film, squeeze off excess water and hang on clips to dry.

SOP12

CHELSEA RADIOPHARMACY: STANDARD OPERATING PROCEDURE
Radiochromatogram Scanner: Operation and Performance Checks

The radiochromatogram scanner consists of a motor and gear-box driven scanner baseplate which carries the chromatoplate beneath a slit-collimated 0.5" diameter NaI(Tl) detector. This is connected to a NE 5 scaler ratemeter from which a 100 mV fsd output is fed to a Spectra-Physics integrator.

Operating Instructions

1 Switch ON all units and allow to stabilise for a few minutes.

2 For normal work set the integrator settings as follows:
chart speed - 4 cm/min
attenuation - 128

3 Place the chromatogram on the bedplate underneath the acetate cover sheet and adjust the detector head to scan the required channel on the chromatogram.

4 Set the ratemeter to a sensitive range, set the bedplate gearbox in neutral and manually scan the chromatogram to locate the main peak. Adjust the sensitivity of the scaler to give a reading greater then 0.5 fsd. Also adjust the response time (time constant) of the scaler to remove most, but not all, of the ratemeter fluctuations.

5 Move the chromatoplate so that a low activity (background) region is under the detector. Set the integrator to evaluate the background by pressing PTEVAL on the control panel and wait until the instrument completes its evaluation.

6 Move the chromatoplate so that the lower edge lies under the detector slit. Change the gearbox setting to a speed of 4.41 cm/min (marked on the case.

7 To scan the chromatogram simultaneously press the SCAN button on the bedplate and the INJ A pad on the integrator. The chromatoplate will move under the detector at a speed of 4.41 cm/min and the integrator will plot the radioactivity profile at a chart speed of 4 cm/min.

8 Significant peaks on the chromatogram will be marked with their 'retention time' during the scan.

9 To stop the scan press the INJ A pad on the integrator and then the STOP button on the scanner. The integrator then prints out a report listing the retention times and peak areas of all detected peaks.

Linearity and Resolution Checks

The radiochromatogram scanning system must be periodically checked for linearity of response and resolving power.

Method

1 Prepare a solution of Sodium Pertechnetate containing between 8 and 12 MBq/ mL of Tc-99m radioactivity.

SOP12 *(cont)*

2 Take a piece of Whatman No 1 chromatography paper of size 2 x 20 cm. Draw a central pencil line down the length of the strip and mark off six sets of cross lines 2cm apart.

3 Using a 20 μL syringe, carefully dispense 1, 2, 5, 10, 15 and 20μL volumes at successive cross lines to simulate spots on a chromatogram. Dry the spots under an infrared lamp.

4 Place the prepared strip on the scanner bedplate and scan the 'chromatogram' under the standard conditions to be used for the Tc-99m chromatograms.

5 Examine the radioactivity profile and the peak report. Calculate the amount of radioactivity in each of the spots and plot this against the measured/reported peak areas (expressed as counts) for each simulated peak.

6 Examine the plot and confirm that it is linear over the range of radioactivity examined. In particular ensure that the difference between the measured count for the 20 μL peak and the best fitting line do not differ by more than 3% of the predicted peak count for that sample.

Resolution Checks

The peak resolving power of the scanning system must be checked periodically to ensure that recorded radioactivity profiles are acceptable and are undistorted. Peak profiles may appear distorted through the selection of long time constants (response times) which produce a trailing distortion to the profile.

Method

1 Prepare a solution of Sodium Pertechnetate containing between 8 and 12 MBq/ mL of Tc-99m radioactivity.

2 Take a piece of Whatman No 1 chromatography paper 20 x 2 cm and draw a central line down the length of the paper strip. mark off six sets of cross lines at spacings of 4, 6, 8, 10, 12, 16, 18, and 20 mm.

3 Using a glass micro syringe dispense 5μL volumes of the pertechnetate solution at each cross line. Ensure that the spot diameter is less than 3 mm by making multiple applications if necessary, then dry the spots under an infra red lamp.

4 Place the prepared strip on the scanner bedplate and accumulate the 'chromatogram' under the standard conditions to be used for the Tc-99m chromatograms.

5 Examine the radioactivity profile for the strip and locate the pair of spots where the baseline is not cleanly separated but the height of the trough above the baseline is about one-tenth of the average adjacent peak heights. The distance between the spots is the approximate resolution of the detection system.

SOP13

CHELSEA RADIOPHARMACY: STANDARD OPERATING PROCEDURE
Radiochromatogram Quantitation

Methods for determining the radioactivities of multiple peaks on chromatograms or electrophoretograms are described in this SOP. General principles only are discussed. The user should obtain exact details form the SOP for a particular radiopharmaceutical

If chromatogram scanning is not possible then cutting and counting is the only practical alternative. The Chromatoplate can be cut into sections each corresponding to a component, main or impurity, and the segments counted in a suitable counting equipment. If the radioactivity distribution is unknown the chromatoplate can be cut into equal width segments, the radioactivity counted, and the radioactivity profile constructed as a histogram. This method will have to be used where the applied radioactivity is too low for reliable peak discrimination by scanning.

The counting efficiency will depend on the design and operating characteristics of the detector, but for most NaI(Tl) well detectors an efficiency approaching or exceeding 50% can be expected with $^{99}Tc^{m}$ and radionuclides of similar gamma energy.

When counting in a well detector it is important to maintain the same counting geometry for all segments of the chromatogram, large or small pieces. This may be achieved by rolling or compressing the material into the bottom of a counting vial before placing in the detector.

The linearity of detection should be verified by counting a series of dilutions (or simulated spots on the chromatogram) covering the range 1 to 200% of the expected radioactivity and plotting the count rate against applied radioactivity (in kBq).

DETECTOR LINEARITY

1 Prepare a solution of pertechnetate at approximately the same radioactive concentration as the radiopharmaceutical being examined. Alternatively the radiopharmaceutical itself may be used as the radioactivity standard in this test.

2 Prepare a series of at least five radioactivity standards by dispensing from a micro syringe 1, 3, 5, 7 and 10 μL volumes of the radioactive solution onto small strips of the chromatographic medium to be used in the main radiochemical purity test.

3 Dry the strips and 'Swiss roll' them into counting tubes ensuring that the final size of the rolled strips is similar in all tubes.

4 Count the strips under the standard conditions specified for counting on the equipment used.

5 Plot the count rate (cps) against the decay-corrected radioactivity of the samples applied in step 2.

6 Examine the plot for linearity and ensure that the plotted point for the highest radioactivity does not differ by more than 3 percent from the value predicted from the best fitting line.

SOP13 *(cont)*

CUT AND COUNT

This method can be used when the migration distances of the various radioactive species are known. The developed strip is cut into two or three pieces corresponding to the regions where the radioactive components are expected to lie.

1 Before running the chromatogram mark off in soft pencil the cutting lines (as well as the conventional origin and solvent front lines).

2 Dry the developed chromatogram as usual. Cut the chromatogram into two or three sections according to the method directions. Roll each section and place in a counting tube. mark the tube with a code indicating its contents.

3 Ensure that the detector-scaler is set to the specified operating conditions for that particular radionuclide and that all pre-counting checks have been performed.

4 Count the background radiation for 50 or 60 seconds and calculate the background cps.

5 Count the rolled sections in their counting tubes for 50 or 60 seconds. Calculate the raw cps for each section.

6 Subtract the background cps from each section count.

7 Calculate the percentage of the total radioactivity in each section from the formula:

$$\% \text{ in section} = 100 \times \frac{\text{corrected cps}}{\text{sum of corrected cps for all sections}}$$

HISTOGRAM METHOD

1 Dry the developed chromatogram as usual. In the case of ITLC chromatograms seal the surface by applying a strip of sellotape to each side.

2 Starting from the bottom of the chromatogram mark off 5 mm segments with a soft pencil or ball point pen. *Number each segment before proceeding.*

3 Cut the segments with scissors or a sharp knife and place each one in a coded sample tube.

4 Ensure that the detector-scaler is set to the specified operating conditions for that particular radionuclide and that all pre-counting checks have been performed.

5 Count the background radiation for 50 or 60 seconds and calculate the background cps.

6 Count the rolled sections in their counting tubes for 50 or 60 seconds. Calculate the raw cps for each section.

7 Subtract the background cps from each section count.

8 Plot a histogram of the corrected cps against strip number and use this to identify the main and impurity peaks in the chromatogram. *It is often helpful to plot a second histogram showing the corrected cps on a log scale as an aid in locating small impurity peaks.*

9 Add together the counts for all segments contributing to the particular peak and calculate the percentage of total radioactivity under each peak from the formula:

$$\% \text{ peak} = 100 \times \frac{\text{sum of segment counts for the peak}}{\text{sum of all segment counts}}$$

SOP14

CHELSEA RADIOPHARMACY: STANDARD OPERATING PROCEDURE
RADIO-IODINATION OF IMMUNOGLOBULINS

Method

1 Dissolve 2 mg of the IODO-GEN reagent in 200μL of chloroform.

2 Pipette 100 μL of the chloroform solution into the screw-cap microtube provided.

3 Gently rotate the microtube so that the chloroform solution coats the maximum surface area possible.

4 Plate the iodogen reagent onto the walls of the tube by the following method: Gently place the microtube on its side and leave to stand for 5 minutes in the fume cupboard. Evaporate the remaining chloroform with a gentle stream of nitrogen for about 5 minutes. The tube is now ready for use.

5 Examine the label details of the sodium [^{125}I] iodide solution provided and calculate the volume needed to dispense about 5 MBq of the ^{125}I radioactivity.

6 Place the iodogen-coated tube upright in a rack and add in rapid succession 200 μL human IgG solution (5 mg mL^{-1}) followed by the calculated volume of sodium [^{125}I] iodide containing 5 MBq of ^{125}I radioactivity. Cap the tube, mix well, and allow to react for 10 - 15 minutes.

7 Transfer the solution from the iodogen reaction tube to a clean microfuge tube. (This serves to stop the reaction).

8 Measure the radiolabelling efficiency by ITLC chromatography using 85% methanol as the mobile phase (the free iodide migrates behind the solvent front and labelled protein remains at the origin). After development dry the strip in front of a heat lamp. The chromatogram should then be cut into 10 mm *numbered* segments and the radioactivity counted with a well crystal.

The next step involves purification of the antibody by gel filtration using a PD-10 column. The column is first equilibrated with 20-30 mL of phosphate buffered saline (PBS), the labelled protein added and eluted with more PBS. The purified protein is eluted first.

9 Remove the stopper from the column and allow the equilibrating buffer to run through and leaving a flat surface to the gel. Gently layer the labelled protein mixture on to the gel and allow to soak into the column.

10 Gently add 12 consecutive 2 mL aliquots of PBS to the top of the column and collect 2 mL fractions in plastic counting tubes.

11 Cap the tubes and measure their radioactivity by counting in a well crystal detector. Plot the count data as a histogram and calculate the radiolabelling efficiency from the proportion of radioactivity present in the two peaks.

SOP15

CHELSEA RADIOPHARMACY: STANDARD OPERATING PROCEDURE
HPLC of Radiopharmaceuticals: Performance Checks

HPLC systems must be checked for compliance with performance specifications before use in radiopharmaceutical quality control. The main specification and tests are detector linearity and column resolution performance.

COLUMN RESOLUTION

1 Set up the HPLC system to the operating conditions specified for the particular radiopharmaceutical. Note especially:

a mobile phase flow rate
b detector sensitivity setting and electronic damping
c integrator attenuation
d peak threshold detection setting.
e integrator chart speed

2 Prepare a solution of Sodium pertechnetate at the same radioactive concentration recommended for the radiopharmaceutical. *The use of the radiopharmaceutical itself is not recommended for this test.*

3 Set the HPLC system to its operating conditions and allow the column to equilibrate for about 15 mins before proceeding.

4 Inject a 20μL sample of the pertechnetate solution onto the column through the injector device and record the chromatogram.

5 Examine the chromatogram and ensure:

a the peak is symmetric with little evidence of tailing
b the apex of the peak lies within the upper half of the chart record and does not go off scale.

6 Determine the column efficiency from the expression:

$$N = \frac{5.54}{L} \left[\frac{V_r}{w_h} \right]^2$$

where V_r is the distance along the baseline between the point of injection and a perpendicular dropped from the maximum of the peak of interest, L is the length of the column in metres, and w_h is the width of the peak of interest at half-height, measured in the same units as V_r.

7 When examining radiopharmaceuticals containing several components ensure that the resolution of the column is at least 1.0 as defined by the formula:

$$R = 2(V_{ra} - V_{rb})/(y_a + y_b)$$

where V_{ra}, V_{rb} are the distances along the baseline between the point of injection and perpendiculars dropped from the maxima of two adjacent peaks, and y_a,y_b are the respective baseline peak widths.

DETECTOR LINEARITY

1 Prepare a series of five dilutions of Sodium Pertechnetate solution which contain 20, 50 100, 150 and 200% of the expected activity of the radiopharmaceutical to be chromatographed.

2 *In random order*, inject 20μL samples of each dilution and record the chromatograms and peak areas.

3 If time permits, repeat the injections in a different random order, recording the chromatograms and peak areas as before.

4 Plot the recorded peak areas against the concentrations (expressed preferably in MBq/mL, although % dilutions are acceptable in some situations).

5 Examine the plot and confirm that it is linear over the range of radioactivity examined. In particular ensure that the difference between the recorded peak area for the highest activity (200%) peak and the best fitting line do not differ by more than 3% with reference to the 100% sample.

SOP16

CHELSEA RADIOPHARMACY: STANDARD OPERATING PROCEDURE
Electrophoresis of Radiopharmaceuticals

Introduction

Although planar chromatography (paper, TLC, ITLC) are the most popular techniques, electrophoretic separations add an extra dimension to the purity/impurity profile of radiopharmaceuticals. Unlike chromatography there is no solvent front for determining R_f values. A suitable alternative is to run a spot of Pertechnetate [$^{99m}Tc\ O_4^-$] under the same conditions as the sample and report sample migrations as the ratio:-

$$R_S = \frac{\text{migration (mm) of sample}}{\text{migration (mm) of } TcO_4^-}$$

Since TcO_4^- is anionic any cationic ^{99m}Tc species will have -ve R_S values under this convention.

Method

1 Set up the Shandon electrophoresis tank and fill both compartments with the chosen electrolyte solution (usually a pH 6.8 phosphate, or 9.2 carbonate-bicarbonate buffer) ensuring that the two chambers are equally filled.

2 For paper electrophoresis take a piece of Whatman 1 paper (10 x 30 cm) and mark an application line at the mid-point with a soft pencil, marking off application points along the line at 2 cm intervals.

3 Dip the paper in the electrolyte solution. gently blot between paper towels, and place in position in the electrophoresis tank. Close the lid and pass current for about 5 mins at a voltage of 10V cm^{-1} to equilibrate the paper.

4 Remove the lid (current cuts off automatically) and spot the radiopharmaceutical on the pre- marked spots from a 1 ml syringe fitted with an orange needle. Replace the lid and run the electrophoretogram for 30 t0 40 minutes.

5 For cellulose acetate (Celagram) electrophoresis, carefully remove the strip from its packing and with a soft pencil gently mark the point for application. Place the marked strip shiny side up on the surface of the buffer electrolyte contained in a shallow dish and allow to float for 2-3 minutes (until the pores are filled with the liquid).

6 Remove the strip with forceps and very gently blot semi-dry between paper towels. Transfer the strip to the electrophoresis tank and place paper wicks over each end dipping into the buffer. Replace the lid and pass current for 5 minutes at about 10V $cm^{-1}$to equilibrate the cellulose.

7 Remove the lid (current cuts off automatically), spot the radiopharmaceutical and proceed as in step (4).

8 When electrophoresis is finished, remove the paper or cellulose strips (CARE - soggy paper tears easily) and hang to dry in front of the heat lamp. The cellulose acetate strips tend to curl at this stage and become very friable. One solution is to coat them with a strip of sellotape before they are completely dry. Another solution is to add about 10% glycerol to the electrolyte buffer used to pre-soak the strips to prevent complete dehydration under the heat lamp.

9 The dried electrophoretograms can be examined and quantitated by any of the methods described under chromatography.

SOP17

CHELSEA RADIOPHARMACY: STANDARD OPERATING PROCEDURE
PARTICLE SIZING OF Tc-99m COLLOIDS BY FILTRATION

1 **Introduction**

The biodistribution of any colloid preparation will depend largely on its particle size distribution. Small particles (about 10 - 100nm) are taken up by circulating RES cells and lymph nodes, while larger particles (about 200 - 800nm) are extracted by the liver and spleen.

1.1 **Nuclepore filtration**

Nucleopore filters are polycarbonate membranes which have been treated to produce submicroscopic pores of accurately known diameter; they may be regarded as "sieves" for submicron particles. Unlike sieves, however, the mass of material retained by a particular mesh cannot be measured. With radiolabeled colloids, the radioactivity retained by a filter can be compared to the activity which passes through, and the percentage activity retained can be calculated. The test can be carried out with a range of nucleopore filters and a cumulative particle size distribution curve constructed.

Small samples of the radiolabelled colloid are filtered through a range of filters (0.03 to 8.0μm) and the percentage activity retained is calculated. The results are plotted as a cumulative frequency (percentage oversize) curve and as a normal distribution.

Method

1. Prepare a series of nucleopore filters by fitting membranes to filter holders. Mark each one with its pore size.

2. Dilute the colloid preparation with isotonic saline to a radioactive concentration of about 500kBq/mL

3. Using a 1mL disposable syringe, carefully inject about 0.1mL of the sample into one of the prepared filter holders.

4. Attach a 2ml luer-lock syringe (preloaded with 2mL of saline) to the filter holder and wash the colloid through the filter into a small plastic vial.

5. Remove the syringe, refill it with air, and force the solution remaining inside the holder through the filter by air pressure.

6. Securely cap both vial and filter and count the activity on a calibrated scintillation detector. Correct all counts for background.

7. If necessary, correct the filtrate counts for any free pertechnetate activity found by chromatography of the colloid sample.

8. Calculate the percentage activity retained by the filter using the formula:

$$\text{percent retained} = 100 \times \frac{F - B}{S + F - 2B}$$

   where F, S = count rate of filter and solution respectively,
   B = background

9. Plot the percentage retained against log(pore size) to obtain a sigmoid curve. Locate the 50% retention point and read off the average particle size of the preparation.

10. Replot the data using log probability paper. Determine the mean particle size and the log standard deviation from the plot.

Chapter 10

Factors Which Affect the Integrity of Radiopharmaceuticals

C. Hojelse, K. Kristensen and C.B. Sampson

10.1 INTRODUCTION

The purity and quality of a radiopharmaceutical has a pronounced effect on the accuracy of diagnosis or therapy. It is imperative, therefore, that the radiopharmaceutical is prepared and administered according to established standards of practice (see Kristensen, 1979).

Most radiopharmaceuticals are prepared according to standards laid down in the official pharmacopoeias or in national registration protocols. For research and clinical trial material where fixed standards may not be available levels of purity may need to be set specifically for that product. It should be emphasised that standards for radiopharmaceuticals should always include details of analytical methods as well as the actual specification (see Chapter 9).

If gamma camera scintigraphy indicates the possibility of a defective product samples from the same batch should be quality tested immediately. If the material is found to be defective the diagnostician must be advised as soon as possible in order to avoid the possibility of mis-diagnosis. If the radiopharmaceutical is found to be acceptable in terms of purity then the possibility of drug interference should be considered (see Chapter 19).

At the Danish National Isotope Pharmacy approximately half of all deliveries from manufacturers were inspected before dispatch to hospitals (Pederson, 1984). It was found that in one particular year aboiut 4% of these materials were found to be defective. Of this figure half were so serious that an immediate report was made to the manufacturer concerned. Less serious defects were generally reported on a half yearly basis.

10.2 GENERAL DEFECTS

As discussed earlier defects in radiopharmaceuticals are usually observed in the patient as an unexpected biodistribution. In the case of therapy the patient may be exposed to unnecessary irradiation of organs (Wells, 1980). Other observed defects include fever or pyrogenic reactions due to microbial or pyrogen contamination (for fuller account see Chapter 23).

If there is a possibility of a defect the parameters to be investigated include:

Radionuclidic purity
Radiochemical purity
Specific activity
Particle size (if appropriate)
pH
Sterlity/apyrogenicity

If the radiopharmaceutical fulfils the specifications listed above handling techniques should then be considered and include:

Injection technique into the patient
Possibility of a faulty syringe
Dispensing/dilution technique
Contamination of radiopharmaceutical with swab antiseptic
Contamination of radiopharmaceutical with components of syringe
Contamination arising from the use of the same syringe to dispense several products
Faulty storage conditions
Poor transport conditions

In the following section a number of examples are given of problems that might arise in daily practice. There are few published clinical examples of radiopharmaceutical defects as it is difficult to establish with certainty a direct cause and effect relationship.

10.2.1 Faulty Injection Technique

The classic example of the effect of faulty injection technique is shown in Figure 1. Withdrawal of un-anticoagulated blood

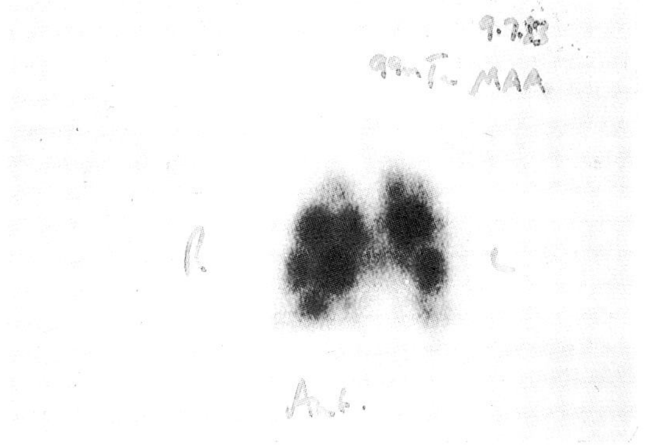

Figure 1.

can form clots in the syringe. The clots become radiolabelled with Tc-99m MAA and on re-injection for hot spots on the lungs as shown (Preston and Greenland, 1970). This technique should therefore be avoided when injections of Tc-99m MAA are given. A similar effect with Tc-99m albumin colloid has also been described (Shile *et al.*, 1986). A potentially harmful efect of poor injection technique is associated with the extravascular injection of injection. The local radiation dose at the site of injection may be significant and could cause radiation 'burn'. This is particularly true for radionuclides such as thallium-201 due to the relatively long half life and the emission of Auger electrons (Castranovo *et al.*, 19887. A case report describing such damage from thallium-201 was reported through the European Scheme for adverse reaction reporting (ENMS, 1988).

10.2.2 Swabbing of Vials During Dispensing Procedures

Another example of the susceptibility of radiopharmaceuticals is the effect of excessive swabbing of the rubber septum of the multidose vial. Thus the pooling of antiseptic on the surface of the septum followed by injection of droplets into the vial was found to produce a colloidal complex in a vial of Tc-99m DMSA (Murray *et al.*, 1986). Only ten microlitres of a 2% solution of centrimide and chlorhexidine were shown to produce this effect. Iodinated antiseptics have been reported to be responsible for the formation of free pertechnetate in technetium labelled radiopharmaceuticals (Fisher *et al.*, 1977). Chlorhexidine may have caused the aggregation of sulphur colloid particles and unacceptable levels in the lung (Sampson, 1985). Early experiences also indicate that ethyl alcohol for swabbing generator vials may impair elution efficiency. It is essential, therefore, that swabbing should be performed only by the system recommended by the manufacturer.

10.2.3 Instability of the Radiopharmaceutical

The radiochemical purity of a radiopharmaceutical can often influence its biodistribution. The most common occurrence is the release of unbound radionuclide from the labelled compound. Examples are iodide in iodinated compounds and free pertechnetate in Tc-99m labelled products. Apart from insufficient labelling or inadequate purification this effect can also be seen as a result of general instability of the product. Radiolytic breakdown of I-131 sodium iodide in the form of gelatin capsules has been reported (Bonneyman and Evers, 1986). More recently it has been reported that the sensitivity of Tc-99m HM-PAO to radiolytic induced decomposition in aqueous solution rapidly reduces the radiochemical purity after reconstitution. High specific activity and high concentration exacerbates this problem (Tubergen *et al.*, 1991). Diminished immunoreactivity of several I-131 radioiodinated murine monoclonal antibodies due to radiolysis is reported to be largely eliminated by freezing at − 70 °C immediately after radiolabelling (Wahl *et al.*, 1990).

Technetium labelled compounds are normally stable for several hours provided they are kept in the original vial and that air is not introduced during dispensing. Introduction of air can lead to oxidation with the release of free pertechnetate. This is observed in the patient as uptake in the salivary glands, thyroid and stomach as shown in Figure 2. When dispensing and dilution is peformed in secondary vials it may be necessary to increase the stability by filling with nitrogen (Sampson and Keegan, 1985). Several reports have described that DTPA is stable only if the vial is unopened; if air is introduced during the removal of doses the radiochemical purity markedly decreases (Millar, 1983; Rattanajuvikoørn,

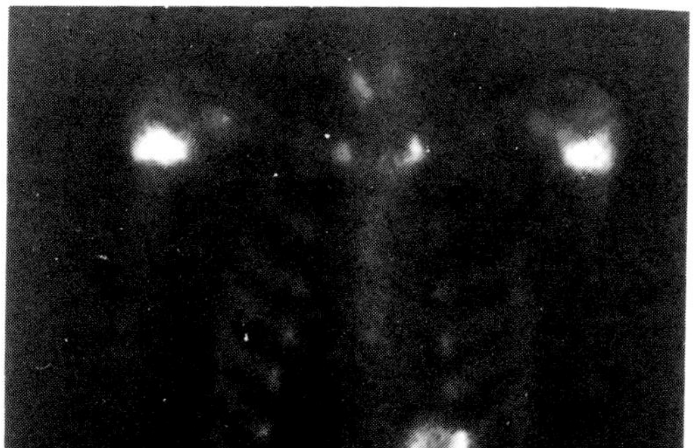

Figure 2. Free pertechnetate in the thyroid, stomach and salivary glands caused by exposure of MDP to air.

1986). Moreover, a number of different brands of DTPA were shown to be markedly unstable if they were diluted or if there was a lengthy delay before injecting the patient (Sampson and Keegan, 1985; Rattanajuvikoørn, 1986). Experimental subdivision and low temperature storage of unlabelled exametazime has been reported to preserve radiolabelling capacity and the ability of Tc-99m exametazime to label leucocytes (Sampson *et al.*, 1991; Hawkins *et al.*, 1991; Piera *et al.*, 1990). One argument against this procedure is that exametazime is recommended by the manufacturer to be used only as a single dose preparation (without preservative) and during handling there might be a risk of microbiological contamination. In addition exametazime is very sensitive to oxidation due to the low content of tin. Also, there is the theoretical risk that during dilution and/or freezing there is a risk of adding oxidative agents (Hewat, 1992). In general, it is recommended that manufacturers' methods be strictly adhered to.

10.2.4 Generators/Kits

Problems occasionally arise as a result of incompatibility between the generator eluate and the actual kit. For example, it has been shown that oxidant in the eluate can markedly affect the stability of Tc-99m DTPA (Sampson and Keegan, 1985).

The amount of Tc-99m available for elution will vary according to the time at which the generator was previously eluted. The specific activity of the eluate will also depend on the status of the generator at the time of elution (Holland *et al.*, 1986). This also applies to the quantity of radiolytic impurity originating from the energy released by the decay of the generator or eluate. The often talked about 'Monday effect' where problems sometimes arise after labelling with eluate from a generator that has not been eluted for several days gives rise to these effects. The problem has been reduced to some extent by the use of generators that are in a dry state between elutions. Other methods include the use of oxidants in the eluate (e.g. sodium nitrate) or copper salts on the column.

The importance of the avoidance of trace metal impurities is well illustrated by a study of the effect of impurities in sodium chloride solutions for the elution of generators (Boyd and Sorby, 1984).

It has been shown that it is essential to prepare Tc-99m exametazime (for cerebral blood flow imaging) using eluate that is not more than two hours old owing to the build up of impurities in older eluates (Amersham, 1989). The addition of small amounts of sodium iodide to generator eluates immediately after elution enables to be used up to at least six hours after elution, with no adverse effect on the radiochemical purity (Baynes *et al.*, 1989).

Another possible impurity in the generator eluate is aluminium ion. The quantity found is usually very low (Vinbeg and Kristensen, 1980) but excess aluminium has been shown to cause flocculation of colloids and their subsequent deposition in the lungs.

There could also be other reasons for the formation of large particles in colloids. Tc-99m tin colloid will form large particles if agitated for a long time or shaken too vigorously (Hilditch *et al.*, 1986). These are not dispersable through a syringe needle as has been observed with some aggregates (Whatley and Steele, 1985).

10.2.5 Heat

The preparation of radiopharmaceuticals from kits is usually a simple one-step procedure. However, a number of products e.g. antimony and sulphur colloids require heat to form the colloid, and it is absolutely essential to adhere to the manufacturer's instructions as regards the heating time. Insufficient heat may lead to poor radiolabelling of the compound or formation of particles of the wrong size (Lovett, 1974).

A number of recently developed materials requiring heat have become available and these include the isonitriles for imaging the myocardium and mercaptoglycine for renal studies. As before, it is essential to heat according to the manufacturer's instructions. During the heating process it may take quite some time for the vial in the lead pot to reach the required temperature. Many institutions recommend the use of special lead pots with holes to allow water circulation round the vial.

10.2.6 Volumes of Reagents Used in Preparation

Experience has shown that the purity of a number of products may depend on the accuracy of volumes of solution used for their preparation. The labelling of monoclonal antibodies requries at present a multi-stage procedure (see Chapter 7). Small volumes of reagents are necessary and accuracy of measurement is essential to obtain a good product. Different brands of injection syringes may have differing dead volumes and inaccuracy can easily occur during preparation. Other examples where accuracy in volume is important include iodination processes (see Chapter 7) and procedures for the radiolabelling of leucocytes where a high labelling efficiency of e.g. exametazime is dependent on a small volume as well as a high concentration of Tc-99m exametazime (Sampson *et al.*, 1991).

The undesirable liver uptake of technetium labelled antibodies directed against non-specific cross-reacting antigen (NCA-95) and carcinoembryonic antigen (CEA) has been reported to be reduced by about one third simply by gentle reconstruction of the lyophilised protein during radiolabelling. Special care was taken to avoid bubble formation or dropping of the tin or pertechnetate solution into the antibody-containing vial. These measures demonstrated that scan quality could be improved and liver dose reduced (Reske and Buell, 1990).

10.2.7 Adsorption/Change in pH

Radiopharmaceuticals are characterised by very small amounts of chemical substances used both in the original kit and in the final product. Also, volumes administered to the patient are usually small. Any reduction in dose volume could therefore result in a marked under-dosage of the patient and poor scan quality.

A frequently reported problem during the administration of radiopharmaceuticals is adhesion to the syringe or to the inside of the container. As much as 50% of the required dose may be lost in this way (author's observation). The degree of adhesion to the glass vials of some colloids has been reported to be dependent on the presence of tin and/or protein in the radiopharmaceutical, agitation time after reconstitution and the length of time the producer remains in the vial. Antimony sulphide colloid is less inclined to adhere compared to other colloids (Elliott *et al.*, 1990). Technetium-99m macroaggregates are known to stick to the glass vial as well as the syringe so special care is needed to shake well before use and to perform regular quality checks to ensure accurate dose volumes are drawn up.

Gallium citrate adheres to most qualities of glassware and siliconising largely reduces this tendency although siliconising may not be effective with highly absorbent glass (Gonda and Swift, 1991). Siliconising of the glass vial of thallium-201 is also necessary to reduce adhesion.

Other adsorption problems occur from carrier free solutions such as iodide and ferric citrate (Smith and Kermaghan, 1969). Such solutions may also be sensitive to changes in pH which can occur by simple dilution of unbuffered solutions. Adjustment of pH and addition of carrier may be needed in these instances (Lovett, 1974). pH changes can also produce colloid formation in Indium-111 chloride solutions and this could affect the labelling of blood cells and antibodies.

10.2.8 Radionuclidic Purity

There are few published reports of radionuclide impurities affecting the visual appearance of a scintigram. However, prolonged use of a I-123 product where the radionuclide is prepared by the (p, 2n) procedure may be such an example. Preparations of this type may contain the impurity I-124 with a half-life of 4.2 days as compared to 13 hours for I-123. The amount of I-124 will therefore increase with time. Only a few percent may affect the quality of the scan due to the high radiation energy emitted. Large differences in the energy of radiation emitted may also be seen with I-126 as an impurity in I-125 labelled preparations. Use of a radioactivity meter for determination of the total activity in I-125 labelled material may therefore lead to gross errors.

10.2.9 Hygiene/Cross-contamination

Dispensing of radiopharmaceuticals must, of course, be performed using aseptic technique. During the radiolabelling of blood products there is always the possibility (although slight) that the blood may be contaminated virally with, for example, Hepatitis B or HIV. Strict asepsis and good hygiene are essential precautions in order to avoid contamination of patients or staff (see Chapter 5). The risk of cross-contamination between blood samples should be decreased by separation of the samples by space or time. To trace a patient's infection to an unsterile product is often difficult because of the difficulty of contacting the patient after the event. This problem has been highlighted by Cooper and Harbert (1973) who showed that a large number of pyrogenic reactions were not accounted for until a special survey was made.

The present standard for sterility: 'a maximum of one contaminated sample per one million' cannot adequately be controlled by testing. It is therefore important to keep the system under regular surveillance (Brown and Baker, 1986). Recently, a case report of an unsterile generator suggested that the contamination was due to inadequate cleaning of the lead container of the eluate vial (Vinberg and Kristensen, 1988). Radiopharmaceuticals are, almost universally, dispensed in multidose vials and do not usually contain bacteriostatic agents. Their use should therefore be limited to a short time and preparation should be routinely stored in a refrigerator.

10.2.10 Interactions of Radiopharmaceuticals with Syringes and Catheters

The administration of radiopharmaceuticals via heparinised catheters occasionally produces defects. For example, when a heparinised catheter is used for *in vivo* red cell labelling with pyrophosphate diminished cardiac activity and increased renal activity has been observed (Hegge *et al.*, 1978). This was thought to be due to the formation of a technetium-heparin complex which localises avidly in the kidneys. Later work (Millar, 1989; Frier, 1992) showed that a complex may be formed between stannous ion and a compound leached from the catheter preventing the stannous ion from entering the cells and performing their reducing role. A few reports

Table 1

Drug Defects Reported in 1988-1991 from Hospitals in Denmark (54), The Netherlands (8), United Kingdom (136), Hungary (11), East Germany (2), Spain (9) and Italy (1)

	Label	*Appearance*	*Total radio-activity*	*Radio-chemical purity*	*Radio-nuclide purity*	*Elution efficiency*	*Particulate contamina-tion*	*Biodistr.*	*Sterility*	*Other*	*Total*
H-3 Tritiated water	1										1
F-18 Flouro-deoxy-glucose		1									1
Cr-51 Sodium Chromate	1										1
Co-58 Cyanocobalamin				1							1
Kr-81 Generator	1										1
Tc-99m Generator	7	3		1	1	52	2	1	2	6	75
Tc-99m											
Albumin			1					5			6
Albumin colloid	1						1	2			4
diethyl-IDA								7			7
diethyl-IODO-IDA		1									1
diisopropyl IDA								1			1
DMSA										3	3
DPD								1			1
DTA				3				1			4
Exametazime				1							1
HMDP	1									1	2
Isonitrile								2			2
MAA		4					2	10		4	20
MAG3								1			1
MDP		1		1			1	6		3	12
microspheres	1	1						3			5
P-bityl-IDA				1							1
Pentate	2	1									3
Phytate		1									1
Pyrophosphate							1				1
RBC-label		1						3			4
Rhenium sulfide colloide	1	1		1							3
Sulphur colloide				1							1
Tin colloide		3						1			4
In-111 Chloride			1			1				2	4
In-111 Oxin										2	2
I-123 MIBG	1										1
I-123 Sodium Iodide	1		1								2
I-125 Hippurate										1	1
I-125 Iothalamate			1								1
I-125 Sodium Iodide	1		1								2
I-131 Lipiodol	1										1
I-131 MIBG	1			1							2
I-131 NaI caps	1	1								1	3
I-131 Sodium Iodide	1									2	3
Xe-133 gas	1		2	1						2	6
Tl-201 Thallous chloride				1				5		3	10
	24	19	7	13	1	53	7	49	2	30	206

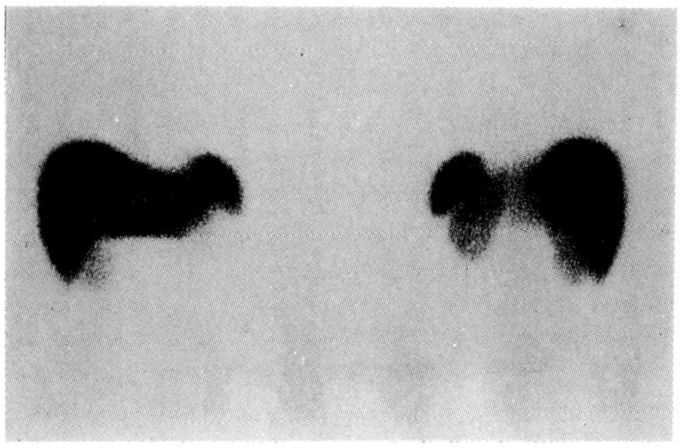

Figure 3. Interaction of Tc-99m tin colloid with the components of a syringe showing the formation of a renally active complex.

have been published of instances where the radiopharmaceutical has reacted in some way with the components of a syringe or needle. It was observed that in one particular brand of sulphur colloid (for liver scintigraphy) 0.25 molar hydrochloric acid had leaked from the kit vial onto the aluminium crimp of a disposable needle. The excess aluminium found its way into the kit vial and the small amount present was sufficient to flocculate the colloidal particles so that they formed macroaggregates which, because of their size, localised in the vasculature of the lung (Adams *et al.*, 1972). The contents of a syringe may occasionally cause problems in scanning and in one published instance the impurity from the rubber plunger of a syringe had reacted with liver scanning material to form a labelled compound which was taken up by the kidneys as shown in Figure 3 (Slater and Anderson, 1983). These problems occurred with one particular brand of syringe – on replacement, the problems disappeared. A similar type of incident occurred with the hepatobiliary agent PIPIDA. On withdrawing the radiopharmaceutical into the syringe an interaction occurred between the components of the syringe and the radiopharmaceutical to form a sticky glue-like substance. Again, the problem disappeared when the particular syringe was replaced with another brand (author's observation).

10.3 REGISTRATION OF DEFECTS

In order to obtain information on defects in radiopharmaceuticals, the European Committee on Radiopharmaceuticals established a reporting system in 1979. The results of those reports are published from time to time, and the latest publication (ENMS 1992) shows that 206 adverse reports were received during the period 1988–1991 (Table 1). It is interesting to obersve that most reports were from the UK and Denmark, both countries of which are particularly active in the collation and dissemination of information on defects.

From Table 1 it can be seen that the majority of defects were associated with generators. It can also be seen that a sizeable number of defects were instances of abnormal biodistribution of which particulates and colloids formed the most prominent part. As regards the Danish experience details are shown in Table 2. Out of a total of 13 reports of abnormal biodistribution approximately half were found to be directly due to a defect in the material. In several instances other causes were thought to be more likely.

Table 2
Reports on Abnormal Biodistribution from Danish Hospitals 1988–1991

		Cases tested for radiochemical purity	
	Number of reports	*Numbers*	*Defect confirmed*
F-18 Fluoro-deoxy-glucose	1	1	1
Tc-99m Generator	1	1	1
Tc-99m			
albumin	3	2	2
EHIDA	2	2	0
DPD	1	1	1
MAA	2	2	0
MDP	2	1	0
1-123 NaI	1	1	0
Total	13	11	5

Since the European Scheme was established all reports have been collated in Denmark. However, from 1993 all reports will be collated in the United Kingdom. All instances of defects should be sent to Dr Stuart Hesslewood, Regional Radiopharmacist, Dudley Road Hospital, Birmingham. New Report Forms are currently being designed and details will be published in due course.

10.4 CONCLUSION

It is essential that rigid controls are applied during manufacture. Developmental work on new radiopharmaceuticals should also include testing of the product under hospital conditions. Such controls should be applied to generators, kit products and materials used in the radiolabelling of blood cells.

Although strict controls can be applied unexpected or unusual sequelae may sometimes occur and these should be monitored regularly by hospital personnel, commercial manufacturers and regulatory authorities. The reporting of defects both locally, nationally, and internationally is vital in order to improve the safety and efficacy of radiopharmaceutical products.

REFERENCES

Adams E.H. *et al.* (1972). *Sulfur colloid flocculation due to acid-leached aluminium.* J. Nucl. Med., **13**, 707–708.
Amersham International plc. (1989). Package insert for Ceretec. UK.
Ballinger J.R. *et al.* (1990). *Radiopharmaceutical factors in the variable quality of Tc-99m HM-PAO images of the brain.* J. Nucl. Med., **31**, 118–122.
Bayne V.L. *et al.*, (1989). *Use of sodium iodide to overcome the eluate age restriction for Ceretec reconstitution.* Nucl. Med. Commun. **10**, 29–33.
Bonneyman J. and van Evers B. (1986). *Radiolytic breakdown of sodium-iodide (I-131) in sodium ipdide (I-131) capsules.* Nucl. Med. Commun. **7**, 839–843.
Boyd R. and Sorby P.J. (1984). *Improved elution efficiency of Tc-99m generators following purification of the eluting saline.* Int. J. Appl. Isotopes, **10**, 993–994.
Castronovo F.P. *et al.* (1988). *The infiltrated radiopharmaceutical injection: dosimetric considerations.* Eur. J. Nucl. Med., **14**, 93–97.
Cooper J.F. and Harbert J.C. (1973). *Bacterial endotoxin as a cause of aseptic meningitis following radionuclide cisternography.* J. Med. Technology, **14**, 387.
Elliott J.S. *et al.* (1990). *Investigation of factors affecting adhesion of Tc-99m labelled colloids to glass vials.* Nucl. Med. Commun., **11**, 375–381.
European Nuclear Medicine Society (1988). *European system for reporting of adverse reactions and drug defects. Third Report 1984–1985.* Eur. J. Nucl. Med., **13**, 4887.
European Association of Nuclear Medicine (1992). *European system for reporting of adverse reactions and drug defects. Ninth Report 1991.* Eur. J. Nucl. Med., **19**, A11–A12.
Fisher S.M. *et al.* (1977). *Unbinding of Tc-99m by iodinated antiseptics.* J. Nucl. Med., **18**, 1139–1140.
Gonda I. and Swift D.L. (1991). *Losses of gallim in common laboratory ware and ways to minimise them.* Eur. J. Nucl. Med. **18**, 511–513.
Hawkins T. *et al.* (1991). The long term stability of reconstituted exametazime: clinical and laboratory evaluation. Nucl. Med. Commun., **12**, 1045–1056.
Hegge F.N. *et al.* (1978). *Cardiac chamber imaging: a comparison of red blood cells labelled with Tc-99m* in vitro *and* in vivo. J. Nucl. Med., **19**, 129–134.
Hewat C.D.R. (1992). *Correspondence.* Nucl. Med. Commun., 121–122.
Hilditch T.E. *et al.* (1986). *Formation of large particles in a Tc-99m tin colloid preparation.* Nucl. Med. Commun., **7**, 845–850.
Holland M.E. *et al.* (1986). *Studies on commercially available Mo-99/Tc-99m generators. Comparison of five analytical procedures for determination of total technetium in generator eluates.* Appl. Rad. Isotopes, **37**, 165–171.
Kristensen K. (1979). *Preparation and control of readiopharmaceuticals in hospitals.* IAEA technical report, No 194. Vienna.
Lovett D,E. (1974). *Radiopharmaceuticals. In* Advances in Pharmaceutical Sciences. Eds. H.S. Bean, A.H. Beckett and A.H. Carless. Academic Press, London.
Millar A.M. *et al.* (1983). *Failure in labelling of red blood cells with Tc-99m: interaction between intravenous cannulae and stannous pyrophosphate.* Eur. J. Nucl. Med. **8**, 502–504.
Millar A.M. *et al.* (1989). *Instability of a commercial Tc-99m DTPA kit; implications for routine quality assurance of Tc-99m radiopharmaceuticals.* Nucl. Med. Commun., **4**, 368–370.
Murray T. *et al.* (1986). *Formation of labelled colloid in Tc-99m DMSA due to the presence of bactericidal fluid.* Nucl. Med. Commun., **7**, 505–510.
Pederson B. (1984). *Drug defects. In* Safety and Efficacy of Radiopharmaceuticals. Eds. K. Kristensen and Norbygaard E. Nijhof, Hague.
Piera C. *et al.* (1990). *Preparation of Tc-99m HM-PAO. Letters to the editor.* J. Nucl. Med., **31**, 127–128.
Preston D.F. and Greenlaw R.H. (1970). *'Hot spots' in lung scans.* J. Nucl. Med., **11**, 422–425.
Rattanajuvikorn K. (1986). *Stability of Tc-99m DTPA.* Unpublished results, Isotope Pharmacy.
Reske S.N. and Buell U. (1990). *Reduced technetium-99m labelled NCA-95/CEA-antibody uptake in liver due to antibody reconstitution.* Eur. J. Nucl. Med. **17**, 38–41.
Sampson C.B. (1985). *Altered biodistribution of radiopharmaceuticals as a result of pharmacological or chemical interaction. In* Radiopharmacy and Radiopharmaceuticals. Ed. A.E. Theobald. Taylor and Francis, London. pp. 189–205.
Sampson C.B. *et al.* (1991). *Tc-99m exametazime labelled leucocytes: effect of volume and concentration of exametazime on labelling efficiency, and clinical protocol for high efficiency multi-dose radiolabelling.* Nucl. Med. Commun. **12**, 719–723.
Sampson C.B. and Keegan J. (1985). *Stability of Tc-99m DTPA injection: effect of delay after preparation, air and oxygen.* Nucl. Med. Commun. **6**, 313–318.
Shile W.J. *et al.* (1988). *Hor spots of the lungs in Tc-99m albumin colloid liver/spleen scintigraphy.* J. Nucl. Med., **16**, 61–63.
Slater D. *et al.* (1983). *Syringe extractables: effect on radio-pharmaceuticals.* Lancet. **ii**, 1431–1432.
Smith H.D. and Kermaghan T. (1969). *Absorption of Fe-59 on glassware.* J. Clin. Path., **22**, 690–695.
Tubergen K. *et al.* (1991). *Sensitivity of technetium-99m HM-PAO to radiolysis in aqueous solutions.* J. Nucl. Med. **32**, 111–115.
Vinberg N. *et al.* (1980). *Fission Mo-99/Tc-99m generators – a study of their performance.* Eur. J. Nucl. Med., **5**, 435–438.
Vinberg N. and Kristensen K. (1989). *Microbiological contamination of Tc-99m eluates.* Nucl. Med. Commun., **9**, 972.
Wahl R.L. *et al.* (1990). *Inhibition of autoradiolysis of radiolabelled monoclonal antibodies by cryopreservation,* J. Nucl. Med., **31**, 84089.
Wells L.D. and Berner D.R. (1980). *Radionuclide Imaging Artefacts.* Yearbook Medical Publishers, London.
Whatley T.L. and Steel G. (1985). *Particle size and surface charge of a tin colloid radiopharmaceutical for liver scinigraphy.* Eur. J. Nucl. Med., **10**, 353–357.

Chapter 11

Documentation, Labelling, Packaging and Transportation

A.M. Millar and K.E. Goldstone

11.1 INTRODUCTION

The subjects covered in this chapter are not the most exciting aspects of radiopharmacy but are, nevertheless, fundamental to good practice. Good documentation and labelling are basic priniples associated with the preparation of all pharmaceuticals. Central radiopharmacies have the added responsibility of packaging the final products and sending them to outlying hospitals in accordance with the regulations which govern the transport of radioactive materials.

Throughout this chapter, the documents illustrated in the various figures are examples of those used in the radiopharmacy, Royal Infirmary of Edinburgh. It is recognised that these will not necessarily meet the needs of many radiopharmacies as the techniques and working practices used in different departments vary considerably. They are presented only to illustrate the information which needs to be documented and to show one way in which this can be achieved.

11.2 DOCUMENTATION

Documentation serves two purposes. Firstly, to describe the procedures involved in the preparation of a radiopharmaceutical and secondly, to record the details of the materials used and that each procedure has been performed in the prescribed manner. A system of recording should be designed to ensure that the history of each radiopharmaceutical can be traced from the details on the label.

11.2.1 Orders

Requests arrive at the radiopharmacy either verbally or in writing depending upon the type of radiopharmaceutical, how soon it is required and the distance to the department where it is to be used. A specimen request form for the supply of radio-pharmaceuticals is shown in Figure 1. However, with the most common radiopharmaceuticals in clinical use today being based on the short half-life Tc-99m it is common practice for radiopharmacies to receive orders by telephone during the afternoon, for Tc-99m radiopharmaceuticals required the following day. Under these circumstances a retrospective written order is desirable. The order can then be retained along with the signed delivery note to record the request, supply and receipt of the radiopharmaceuticals.

In the case of a request for a radiopharmaceutical which is not the subject of a UK Product Licence, a written request is essential and the prescriber should be informed, preferably in writing, that the product is unlicensed. Indeed, the manufacturer may be prepared to supply the radiopharmaceutical only upon receipt of a requesst signed by the prescriber. The situation regarding unlicensed Tc-99m kits is less straightforward since these products are normally supplied in boxes of five vials with each vial being capable of providing up to twenty patient doses. If a Tc-99m radiopharmaceutical prepared from an unlicensed kit is requested for routine use, then a written request for the product to be supplied for administration to the prescriber's patients should be retained in the radiopharmacy as authorisation to purchase and supply the product.

11.2.2 Tc-99m Generator Elution

The first step in the preparation of Tc-99m radiopharmaceuticals is elution of the Tc-99m generator and a specimen worksheet for the procedure is shown in Figure 2. This worksheet contains a description of the elution procedure and the methods used to measure molybdenum-99 (Mo-99) and aluminium breakthrough. Also included is a section in which details of each elution of the generator is recorded, including the results of the Mo-99 and aluminium breakthrough tests.

11.2.3 Tc-99m Radiopharmaceuticals

The preparation of Tc-99m radiopharmaceuticals from commercially available kits represents the major aspect of

Radiopharmaceutical Request / Delivery Note / Receipt

Please submit blue and pink copies

Hospital and Department requesting ______________________

Telephone No. ______________ Extension ______________

Radiopharmaceutical ______________________

Activity ______________________

Volume (if critical) ______________________

Date required ______________________

Time required ______________________

Patient's name (if applicable) ______________________

Delivery point ______________________

Signature ______________________ Date ______________

Send this request to: RADIOPHARMACY
ROYAL INFIRMARY
EDINBURGH
EH3 9YW

Urgent requests can be made by telephone to:
Tel. no. 229 2477 Ext. 2749 or 2600
and must be followed by a written
request marked 'CONFIRMATION'

FOR RADIOPHARMACY USE

Radiopharmaceutical ______________________

Activity supplied ______________________

Time of measurement ______________________

Volume ______________________

Delivery received by ______________________ at ________ hrs

Figure 1. Request/Delivery Note/Receipt for the supply of radiopharmaceuticals.

the work of most, if not all hospital radiopharmacies. The range of Tc-99m radiopharmaceuticals and the number of doses of each Tc-99m radiopharmaceutical requested can vary considerably from day to day. In a typical radiopharmacy, up to ten different Tc-99m radiopharmaceuticals may be prepared during a dispensing session with up to twenty doses of certain ones being required. In conventional pharmaceutical manufacturing practice, each product has its own worksheet on which the preparative procedure is described and relevant recordings are made. Given the diversity of Tc-99m radiopharmaceuticals which can be prepared during a dispensing session, the adoption of such a system for radiopharmacy can prove unwieldy and result in a large volume of paper records being generated. As an alternative, the worksheet in Figure 3 is of a 'free format' design and contains sections in which the radioactive concentrations of the Tc-99m generator elutes are calculated, the radiopharmaceuticals to be dispensed are listed, the dispensed activities are recorded, the names of the personnel who performed the dispensing session are recorded and the signature of the authorised person who released the finished products is recorded. The example of Tc-99m DTPA dispensing included in Figure 3. shows the following details:

(a) the name of the Tc-99m radiopharmaceutical
(b) the departments for which doses of the radiopharmaceutical, are being prepared
(c) the activities to be dispensed
(d) the total activity to be added to the kit
(e) the volume of the reconstituted kit which is required for each dose
(f) the final volume of each dose
(g) the volume of generator elute required for activity d
(h) the total volume to be added to the kit

With the exception of g, which is calculated once the Tc-99m generator has been eluted, all the details can be entered on the worksheet well before the start of the dispensing session. As each dose is prepared, its activity and the time of measurement are recorded in the spaces provided. The batch numbers of the sodium chloride injection and any other raw materials used during the dispensing session are also recorded on this worksheet. The form is printed in duplicate using selfcopying paper. Once all the details of the dispensing session have been entered on the worksheet, one copy is given to the members of staff performing the dispensing and the other copy is used by the member of staff measuring activity and labelling the finished products. The activity of each preparation and the time at which the measurement is made are entered on this second copy which is retained as the record of the dispensing. The worksheet and the worksheets of the Tc-99m generators, provide the complete history of each Tc-99m radiopharmaceutical prepared during the dispensing session. As this style of worksheet contains no details of the procedures used for the preparation of the Tc-99m radiopharmaceuticals, it is important that it is used in conjunction with a procedure manual in which the method for the preparation of each radiopharmaceutical is documented.

11.2.4 Other Radiopharmaceuticals

Radiopharmaceuticals other than Tc-99m radiopharmaceuticals prepared from kits, are probably prepared infrequently enough to justify their own worksheet. In some cases, the procedure will involve nothing more than the dilution of a commercially available radiopharmaceutical to provide injections of a suitable radioactive concentration for clinical use e.g. chromium (Cr-51) EDTA, iodinated I-125 human

ELUTION OF Tc99m GENERATOR (AMERSHAM INTERNATIONAL - MCC 20)

Conditions for elution:	Generator	Specimen label
Aseptic manipulation in Class1 vertical laminar-air-flow workstation in aseptic room	Lot no. ______ Activity ______ GBq Ref. date ______	Tc99m SODIUM PERTECHNETATE 20.0 GBq in 20 ml at 0830 hrs on 01 MAY 85 Lot: A RADIOACTIVE Radiopharmacy - Royal Infirmary of Edinburgh

(Instructions for elution and tests for Mo99 and Al)

Date	Tc99m activity	Volume	Time	Mo99 activity	Mo breakth.	Al breakth.	Lot no. of eluate	Eluted by	Checked by
	GBq	ml	hrs	MBq					

Generator Elution Record

RADIOPHARMACY Royal Infirmary of Edinburgh

Worksheet prepared: May 1985
Amendment no.: 5
Prepared by: AM Millar

Figure 2. Worksheet for the elution of a $^{99}Tc^{m}$ generator.

albumin and sodium iodohippurate (I-131). In other cases, the procedure may involve the preparation of the radiopharmaceutical from raw materials e.g. sodium iodohippurate (I-123) from iodohippuric acid and Na I-123, In-111 monoclonal antibody from monoclonal antibody, cyclic anhydride of DTPA and In-111Cl-3 and Tc-99m leucocytes prepared from autologous blood and Tc-99m hexametazine. The worksheet for a procedure of this type is more in keeping with the conventional pharmaceutical worksheet in that it combines recording of the raw material details, step by step details of the method, recording of the performance of the procedure and any measurements made. An example of this type of worksheet for the preparation of Co-57 bleomycin is shown in Figure 4.

8.2.5 Other Documentation

In addition to activities directly associated with the preparation of radiopharmaceuticals, there are a number of other areas of radiopharmacy practice which need to be documented. The receipt of all raw materials, radionuclide generators, kits and radiopharmaceuticals must be recorded. Techniques used as part of a quality assurance programme should be documented and a record of the results of tests carried out on raw materials, finished products and facilities should be maintained. These might include tests of radionuclidic and radiochemical purity, sterility tests and environmental monitoring. It is often the case that testing such as environmental monitoring and sterility testing are not performed by radiopharmacy staff but are the responsibility of quality assurance staff. Records of these tests might therefore be retained in the quality control department rather than the radiopharmacy. Radioisotope calibrators must be checked periodically and a record of their performance maintained. A record of the radiation dose received by each member of staff must also be kept.

RADIOPHARMACY Royal Infirmary of Edinburgh

Dispensing worksheet

Date ______ Session ___	$^{99}Tc^m$ Eluate A	$^{99}Tc^m$ Eluate ______
Dispensed by ______	35.6 GBq/20 ml @ 0815	____ GBq/__ ml @ ____
Labelled by ______	34.5 GBq/20 ml @ 0830	____ GBq/__ ml @ ____
Released by ______	1725 MBq/ml @ 0830	____ MBq/ml @ ____

a / d / b / f / g	Activities dispensed MBq	Activities dispensed hrs		Activities dispensed MBq	Activities dispensed hrs
$^{99}Tc^m$ DTPA (A: 25)					
W N.MED 500MBq 1.3ml→2.5ml	485	0830			
" (pm) 750 2.0ml→ "	762	"			
R.N.MED 500 1.3ml→ "	509	0840			
C. XRAY 500 "	489	"			
SPARE 800 →2.1ml	820	"			
3050 1.8ml A→8ml					
c / e / i / h					

Figure 3. Radiopharmaceutical dispensing worksheet.

Name of preparation: COBALT (^{57}Co) BLEOMYCIN INJECTION			Date:
Route of admin: Intravenous injection Conditions for prep: Aseptic manipulation in Class 1 vertical laminar-air-flow workstation in aseptic room.	Specimen label: Dept: City Hospital XRay Co57 BLEOMYCIN For Intravenous Injection 50 MBq in 4.0 ml at 1700 hrs on 01 OCT 85 Use before 08 OCT 85 RADIOACTIVE Radiopharmacy – Royal Infirmary of Edinburgh		
Procedure:	**Recording**	**Rec/Prep by**	**Checked by**
1 Record the following: Cobaltous Chloride (Co57) Solution (CIS UK Ltd) — Batch no.; Activity in 1ml Bleomycin (Lundbeck) — Batch no. Sodium Acetate Injection (2 mmol/ml) (L.H.B.) — Batch no. Water for Injections B.P. — Manufacturer; Batch no.	____ ____ MBq ____ ____ ____ ____		____
2 Dissolve the contents of an ampoule containing 15mg bleomycin in 6ml Sodium Chloride Injection B.P. Transfer 1.0ml of this solution to the vial containing the Cobaltous Chloride (Co57) Solution. Incubate the vial at room temperature for 5 minutes.			
3 Inject 0.5ml Sodium Acetate Injection 2mmol/ml) and 9.5ml Water for Injections B.P. into a sterile 10ml vial. Inject 2.0ml of this solution into the Co57/bleomycin solution.			
4 Draw the Co57 bleomycin solution into a 10ml syringe, fit a 200nm sterile filter and fresh needle. Filter the solution into a tared sterile 10ml vial. Withdraw a 0.05ml sample for Qualtiy Assurance into a 1ml syringe fitted with a 25G needle (orange).		____	
5 Reweigh the vial and record the volume of the solution. Measure and record the activity in the vial.	____ ml ____ MBq		
6 Label the vial and its lead pot - see specimen label.		____	____
7 Product released by ______			
Radiopharmaceutical Preparation Sheet RADIOPHARMACY Royal Infirmary of Edinburgh	Worksheet prepared: Oct 1985 Amendment number: 0 Prepared by: A M Millar		

Figure 4. Worksheet for the preparation of ^{57}Co-bleomycin.

11.3 LABELLING

Labelling is a word with two meanings in radiopharmacy and this session deals with the sticky rather than the radioactive variety. A considerable amount of information is required on the label of a radiopharmaceutical, namely:

- name of the radiopharmaceutical
- route of administration
- name and concentration of any added substances
- 'Shake Well', if applicable
- activity
- reference time and date
- volume
- expiry time and/or date
- lot identification
- any special storage conditions
- name of the department in which it is to be used
- name of the radiopharmacy
- 'Radioactive' and the radioactive warning sign.

Figure 5 shows a label for one of the Tc-99m DTPA injections listed on the specimen worksheet shown in Figure 3.

Dept: RIE Nuclear Medicine

Tc99m DTPA
For Intravenous Injection

509 MBq in 2.5 ml
at 0840 hrs on 30 JUN 88
Use before 1700 hrs Lot:A

RADIOACTIVE
Radiopharmacy – Royal Infirmary of Edinburgh

Figure 5. Label for $^{99}Tc^m$-DTPA.

11.3.1 Preparation of Labels

It has been common practice for radiopharmaceuticals prepared in hospitals to be labelled using pre-printed labels on which the day-to-day details such as the activity dispensed and time of measurement are handwritten. The legibility of these details on this type of label is dependent on the legibility of the handwriting, therefore the likelihood of errors in interpretation is greater than with printed labels. As part of the general trend in pharmacy to move away from handwritten labels, computer based label processors have been introduced into radiopharmacy. Millar et al (1984) have described one such system based on a single board computer. The activity of the radiopharmaceutical is read directly from the radioisotope calibrator, the time and date of measurement are read from an internal clock; the name of the radiopharmaceutical, volume, lot number and name of the department for which the radiopharmaceutical has been prepared are entered via a special purpose keyboard; non-standard entries are made through an alpha-numeric keyboard. The label is then printed in duplicate, one label being for the vial and the other for the lead shielding pot. The choice of a printer for use on a label processor is between dot-matrix and daisywheel. Dot-matrix printers are small, fast and cheap but give a low quality print. Some will give a near-letter quality print but only at 12 characters per inch. With the large amount of information required on the label of a radiopharmaceutical and the restricted size of the label, a print density of 15 characters per inch can be advantageous. Only the most expensive of the dot-matrix printer can produce near-letter quality printing at 15 characters per inch. In contrast, daisy-wheel printers are larger, slower and more expensive but provide a high quality print, even at 15 characters per inch.

11.4 PACKAGING AND TRANSPORT

Over half a million packages containing radioactive materials are transported each year in the UK (Advisory Committee on the Safe Transport of Radioactive Materials (ACTRAM) 1987). A considerable proportion of these contain radiopharmaceuticals, including those despatched from central hospital radiopharmacies to outlying hospitals. The packaging and transportation of radioactive materials are required to be in accordance with the criteria laid down by the International Atomic Energy Agency and incorporated into the transport regulations of individual countries. In the UK, transport of radioactive materials in the National Health Service is predominantly by road, with the relevant current regulations being 'The Radioactive Substances (Carriage by road) (Great Britain) Regulations 1974'. However regulations are due for imminent renewal and should be published as The Radioactive Material (Road Transport) (Great Britain) Regulations 1994. Rail is also a possible means of transport and is covered by the List of Dangerous Goods and Conditions of Acceptance by Freight Services & Parcels Services 1990 (BR 22426). At the time of writing transport regulations are in such a state of flux that is especially important to take the advice of your Radiation Protection Adviser prior to transportation of radioactive materials. All aspects of transport of radioactive substances are now subject to mandatory quality assurance programmes; such programmes must be established by each consignor.

11.4.1 Packages

The principle features of a package for the transport of radioactive material are that it must be not less than 10 cm for the smallest external dimension, leakproof with respect to the contents, securely closed, shielded to the required extent and free form external contamination. Although the regulations describe four types of package, only two of these are relevant to the transport of radiopharmaceuticals.

Excepted packages contained such small quantities of radioactive material that they need not comply with most of the packaging and labelling requirements of the regulations subject to certain conditions, for example that the dose rate at the surface of the package does not exceed 5 μSv/h^{-1} For ^{99m}Tc the radionuclide, used most commonly in medicine, the maximum activity that can be contained in an 'excepted package' is 800 MBq; for ^{131}I the figure is 50 MBq. These are therefore of limited value in the transport of radiopharmaceuticals.

Type A packages are those most commonly used for the transport of radiopharmaceuticals. In addition to the features described above, a 'type A package' is expected to withstand normal transport conditions and minor accidents such as penetration by sharp objects and the action of shock and water.

11.4.2 Labelling of Packages

Excepted packages do not require any special labels or markings on the outside but on opening the package a warning of the presence of radioactive material must be visible. Type A packages are classified into three categories depending upon the radiation level at the surface and at one metre, the latter being known as the Transport Index (TI). Before the introduction of SI units for the measurement of radiation dose-rate, the Transport Index was the radiation level in millirem per hour at 1 metre from the external surface of the package. With SI units now being used, the Transport Index is obtained by measuring the radiation level in millisieverts per hour at 1 metre and multiplying the figure obtained by 100, since 1 mSv = 100 mrem. The three categories, which have different identification labels to

Table 1
Categories of Packages and Conditions

Category	Conditions: Transport Index (TI)	Conditions: Maximum radiation level on external surface
I – White	0	not more than 5 μSvh^{-1}
II – Yellow	More than 0 but not more than 1	more than 5 μSvh^{-1} but not more than 500 μSvh^{11}
III – Yellow	More than 1 but not more than 10	more than 500 μSvh^{-1} but not more than 2 mSvh^{-1}

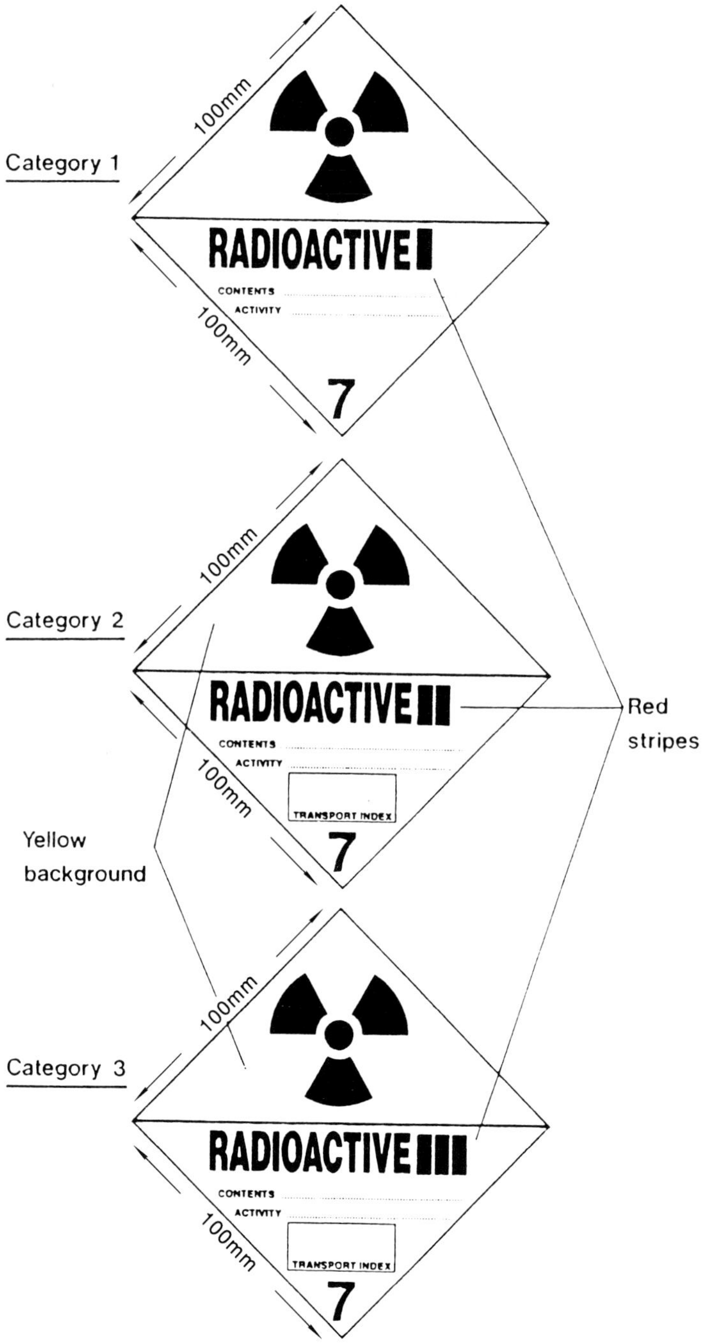

Figure 6. Category I (white), Category II (yellow) and Category III (yellow) hazard labels for packages containing materials.

simplify recognition and to facilitate control by workers when handling packages, are described in Table 1 and an example of each is shown in Figure 6. Each package must bear the appropriate identification label on two opposite sides.

In addition to the labelling requirement, the consignor must make out and sign a certificate for each consignment of radioactive materials and must give the certificate to the carrier, or if the consignor is himself carrying the goods, to the driver of the vehicle. Drivers of vehicles transporting radioactive materials must be appropriately trained. If the goods should be transferred to another vehicle, the same certificate or a copy should be in the hands of the driver before the journey is continued. The certificate should contain the following particulars.

1. Proper shipping name and UN number specified by IAEA.
2. Name and address of the consignor and, if possible, a telephone number at which he can be notified in the event of an accident.
3. The type of package – this will usually be Type A for radiopharmaceuticals.
4. The name of the radionuclide.
5. A description of the physical or chemical form of the materials, i.e. liquid, solid, powder, gas, etc.
6. The activity of the radionuclide in appropriate becquerel units.
7. The category of the package.
8. The transport index (for Categories II and III only).
9. A signed and dated statement in the following terms: 'This is to certify that the above named goods are properly described and are packed and marked in accordance with the applicable regulations of the The Radioactive Material (Road Transport) (Great Britain) Regulations 1994, or of the International Regulations and are in a proper condition for transport'.

A specimen Consignor's Certificate is shown in Figure 7.

11.4.3 Delivery Vehicle

When radioactive materials are being transported by road, warning placards must be displayed on both sides and rear

Consignor's Certificate

For the Carriage of Radioactive Material by Road

Consignor: Radiopharmacy,
Royal Infirmary, Edinburgh, EH3 9YW
Tel. 031 229 2477 Ext. 2749 or 2600

Radioactive Material UN No 2910

Consignee		Date
Category	Type A	Transport Index
Radionuclide	Form	Activity

This is to certify that the above-named goods are properly described and are packed and marked in accordance with the Radioactive Substances (Carriage by Road) (Great Britain) Regulations 1974 and are in a proper condition for transport.

Signature ....

Figure 7. Consignor's certificate for the transport of radioactive materials.

of the vehicle. The placards should show the radioactive warning sign and the word 'RADIOACTIVE,' and the minimum overall dimensions for commercial vehicles should be 250 mm × 250 mm. The 1994 Regulations have a conditional provision for private vehicles allowing the placards to be only 100 mm × 100 mm. These placards are partly to warn the fire services, police and others in the event of an accident. Care should be taken to remove them when no radioactive consignment of an exempt quantity is being carried.

This vehicle is carrying

RADIOACTIVE
MATERIALS

In case of accident get in touch at once with

THE POLICE

and

(Particulars of owner/operator of vehicle)

Figure 8. Hazard warning notice to be carried in the driving cab of a vehicle being used for the transport of radioactive materials.

There must also be a notice in the driving cab giving details of persons to be contacted in the event of an accident. This notice must be fireproof and have durable black lettering embossed or stamped on a white ground. It must be not less than 12 cm × 12 cm and capital letters must not be less than 12 mm high for the word 'RADIOACTIVE' and 5 mm high otherwise. The notice must be securely posted in the cab where it is plainly visible to the driver. The object of this notice is again to warn emergency services in the event of an accident and should be removed when no radioactive material is being carried. The form of this notice is shown in Figure 8. The vehicle must carry a fire extinguisher.

In general, a vehicle is limited to a total Transport Index of 50.

The 1994 Regulations no longer allow the professional user partial exemption.

11.5 SUMMARY OF RECORDS TO BE KEPT IN A RADIOPHARMACY

Activity	**Details to be recorded**
Receipt of materials	Quantity, manufacturer lot no.
Elution of radionuclide generators	Manufacturer, lot no, activity, reference date. Activity and volume eluted. Mo-99 and Al breakthrough.
Preparation of radiopharmaceuticals	Manufacturer and lot no. of materials used. Volumes used. Activities dispensed.
Supply of radiopharmaceuticals	Signed request. Materials supplied. Signature of person taking delivery.
Quality assurance	Calibration of radioisotope calibrators. Physical measurements made on final products (e.g. radiochemical purity). Environment/monitoring. Sterility tests.
Radiation Safety	Radiation dose received by each member of staff.

REFERENCES

Advisory Material for the IAEA Regulations for the Safe Transport of Radioactive Material (1985 Edition) Third Edition (as amended 1990). IAEA Safety Series No. 37. Third Edition, IAEA Vienna (1990).

Code of Practice for the Carriage of Radioactive Materials by Road. (1986). HMSO, London.

Dangerous Goods by Freight Services and by Parcels Services, List of Dangerous Goods and Conditions of Acceptance, BR Publication BR22426, 1977.
Millar A.M., Brydon J., Williamson D. and Forsyth I.F. (1984). *A radiopharmacy label processor.* British Journal of Radiology, **7**, 740–743.
Regulations for the Safe Transport of Radioactive Material 1985 Edition (as amended 1990). IAEA Safety Series No. 6, IAEA Vienna (1990).
The Radioactive Substances (Carriage by Road) (Great Britain) Regulations, SI No. 1735, HMSO London 1974.
The Radioactive Material (Road Transport) (Great Britain) Regulations 1994.

Chapter 12

Microbial and Radiation Monitoring in the Radiopharmacy

S.R. Hesslewood

12.1 INTRODUCTION

Radiopharmacies are used for the preparation of a wide range of products in a variety of dosage forms. The majority of radiopharmaceuticals are administered parentally and hence need to be sterile and prepared in conditions which satisfy both pharmaceutical and radiation safety requirements. There is therefore the need to develop two monitoring protocols:

(a) for particulate and microbial contamination
(b) for radioactive contamination in order to assess levels present and prevent uncontrolled spread.

One of the difficulties that has arisen in radiopharmacies is that official guidance has tended to concentrate on one or other of these aspects, whereas an integrated approach is clearly advantageous in order to develop safe working systems. In certain situations, this may require a compromise where there is a difference in requirements, for example for pharmaceutical reasons, a positive room pressure is advantageous but this is potentially hazardous when handling radiopharmaceuticals since radioactive contamination may be dispersed to the surroundings.

Within the United Kingdom, radiopharmaceuticals are classified as Medicinal Products and as such are subject to controls under the Medicines Act (1968). One aspect of the Act is the control of premises in which Medicinal Products are prepared. The Guide to Good Pharmaceutical Manufacturing Practice (1973), commonly referred to as GMP, gives general guidance on the basic environmental standards required for manufacture of sterile products. More recently, guidance has been provided in The Rules Governing Medicinal Products in the European Community Volume IV Guide to Good Manufacturing Practice for Medicinal Products (EEC GMP). In particular, this reference includes Supplementary Guidelines for the Manufacture of Radiopharmaceuticals.

These documents do not cover radiation monitoring of such facilities although such monitoring is clearly necessary to ensure that contamination does not create hazardous conditions. In the United Kingdom the required for monitoring of areas in which radioactive materials are handled is specified in the Ionising Radiations Regulations (1985). Much practical information is given in the accompanying Approved Code of Practice (1985) and the Guidance Notes for the Protection of Persons against Ionising Radiations arising from Medical and Dental Use (1988). Reference to these publications is essential to ensure that monitoring techniques are suitably selected and employed.

This chapter will discuss potential sources of both particulate and radioactive contamination of radiopharmacies, methods available for their measurement and suggestions for suitable monitoring protocols. However, because of differences in working practices, it is unlikely that a uniform approach can be adopted in all departments and hence it is necessary for each department to adopt testing protocols relevant to their own situation which meet the requirements laid down.

12.2 SOURCES OF PARTICULATE CONTAMINATION IN RADIOPHARMACIES

For parentally administered radiopharmaceuticals, there is the requirement to control the particulate contamination of the environment in which they are prepared, the underlying philosophy being that reducing this level lowers the chance of contamination in the final product. Particulate contamination can also arise from personnel or equipment in the radiopharmacy and can be either microbial or inanimate. The ultimate aim is of course the total avoidance of particulate contamination in the radiopharmaceutical and knowledge of the level and type of contamination arising from the environment, personnel or equipment is advantageous. One type of particulate contamination that is particularly important is microorganisms which could produce an infection if administered to patients. The microorganisms may be bacterial or fungal and may be present as individual particles or in association with other particles such as human hair or skin flakes.

12.2.1 Airborne Contamination

Atmospheric air can contain between 10^7 and 10^{11} particles per cubic metre ranging in size from below 0.5 microns to above 10 microns. The level and nature of contamination will vary considerably according to the district (urban or rural) and prevailing weather conditions. It is likely that inanimate particles such as dust and fibres will be present together with other contamination such as pollen grains and material of human origin e.g. skin microorganisms. Larger particles (5 microns or greater) tend to settle out under gravity, leaving the majority of airborne particles in the smaller size ranges which remain suspended due to air movements. The level of atmospheric contamination can be reduced by the incorporation of filtration systems for air entering safety cabinets and rooms in which radiopharmaceuticals are prepared (see Section 10.3).

12.2.2 Contamination Arising From Personnel

People represent a major source of particulate contamination and it has been estimated that they contribute 80% of particulate contamination generated within a room. On average, a person sitting at rest sheds approximately 10^5 particulate per minute and this can rise by a factor of 4 with movement. These particles will include skin flakes, hairs and liquid droplets from the respiratory traces. Some of these particles will also carry microorganisms. Sampson (1985) quotes a value of 10^4 bacteria-carrying particles per minute being shed by a person during average activity. The number of organisms present is therefore dependent on the number of people present and their degree of activity. Bacteria in air samples are usually Gram-positive cocci of skin origin and associated with skin scales. It is likely that each scale will contain more than one bacterium and different species may be present. Of these organisms, less than 1% are viable pathogens, mainly Staphylococcus aureus (Ayliffe *et al.*, 1982). This organism is present in the anterior nares of approximately 40% of the healthy population and may also be present to a lesser extent in the perineum and axillae which all contain similar glands. It may also be present transitorily on the fingers and face (Casewell and Hill, 1986). Other microorganisms may arise as a result of human activity e.g. Gram-negative bacteria in the air are usually associated with aerosols from contaminated fluids (Aycliffe *et al.*, 1982).

12.2.3 Contamination Arising From Equipment and Materials

Particles can be generated from all types of equipment and materials used in radiopharmacies e.g. paper wrappings of disposable syringes and needles.

Wearing of gloves is essential when working in radiopharmacies to provide an impervious barrier to prevent both particulate contamination of the environment by the operator and radioactive contamination of the operator by the materials being handled. However, certain types of glove contain approximately 5 million particles of talc or starch per square centimetre. This is to facilitate putting them on, but could also contribute to particulate contamination of the environment.

Other potential sources of particulate contamination of radiopharmaceuticals include the vials and closures supplied by commercial manufacturers. The majority of radiopharmaceuticals in current use are either supplied in their final form in rubber capped vials or are prepared within the radiopharmacy by closed techniques using kits supplied by manufacturers. Any particulate contamination occurring during the commercial manufacture of these vials or kits will inevitably be present in the final radiopharmaceutical unless a filtration step is used to remove it.

Autologous blood labelling procedures could also give rise to microbial contamination in the working environment, since if blood is spilled, there is the potential risk of dispersal of any organisms that it may contain.

Other types of particulate contamination in radiopharmaceuticals can be introduced during their preparation. Firstly, the opening of ampoules can lead to small particles of glass or paint flaking off, falling into the contained solution, being drawn into a syringe and introduced into the radiopharmaceutical vial. Secondly, repeated puncture of the closure of the vial with a needle may lead to coring of the rubber and the subsequent shedding of rubber particles into the radiopharmaceutical. This situation is also potentially hazardous, since it may permit leakage of radioactive solution when the vial is subsequently inverted.

12.3 PROCEDURES FOR REDUCING MICROBIAL AND PARTICULATE CONTAMINATION

Reduction of airborne contamination in working areas can be achieved by passing the air through suitable filters. Safety cabinets incorporate High Efficiency Sub-micron Particulate Air (HESPA) filters capable which reduce particulate contamination to below 3000 particles per cubic metre of size 0.5 microns and no particles exceeding 5 microns. This

Table 1
Comparison of Grades of Air Cleanliness

Standard		*Document*			
Maximum number of particles per cubic metre				*British Standard 5295*	
0.5 Micron	*5 Micron*	*EEC GMP*	*GMP*	*1976*	*1989*
3,500	0	A & B	1	1	F
350,000	2,000	C	2	2	J
3,500,000	20,000	D	3	3	K

level corresponds to the requirements of Class A as defined in the EEC GMP. Different documents (GMP and British Standards) have used alternative terminology to describe the same standards and there is therefore potential for confusion. The relationship between these documents is shown in Table 1 which gives the nearest equivalent grades. In situations where room air is filtered, HESPA filters may also be used as terminal filters just before air enters the room, although, in addition, it is normal to use coarser pre-filters capable of removing larger particles and thus prolonging the effective life of HESPA filters. When installing terminal filters, attention must be paid to ensure that they are effectively sealed in position and air is not allowed to bypass the filter. Air is commonly supplied at a positive pressure in these situations, thereby displacing contaminated air as quickly as possible and maintaining low particulate counts in the environment.

Particulate contamination generated from equipment within the radiopharmacy can be reduced by having the minimum amount necessary which should be of suitable design and construction. Steps should also be taken to ensure that equipment and materials are suitably cleaned to remove loose particles from their surface prior to their introduction into radiopharmacies. Wherever possible, equipment should be retained specifically for the radiopharmacy. In addition to minimising the cleaning procedures, this helps to avoid the spread of radioactivity when equipment has inadvertently become contaminated.

Since the majority of particles generated within radiopharmacies arise from personnel, attempts are made to reduce this by adopting suitable protective clothing, which itself must not generate particles and be comfortable to wear. The major items used are:

(a) head coverings e.g. hats or hoods which completely cover the hair;
(b) overalls which completely cover ordinary clothes;
(c) gloves to prevent transfer of contamination from the hands;
(d) overshoes.

GMP (1983) recommends that a non-linting face mask, capable of preventing the shedding of droplets should be worn in aseptic areas. However, direct spread of Staphylococci into the air from the nose or mouth during normal breathing or talking is uncommon. The value of fact masks in all circumstances has therefore been questioned (Ayliffe *et al.*, 1982). Of more importance is the health and personal hygiene of operators and they should report conditions e.g. colds, skin infections that may cause shedding of abnormal types or numbers of organisms.

12.3.1 Radiopharmaceutical Preparation Techniques

One of the most important factors helping to achieve low levels of particulate contamination of radiopharmaceuticals is the widespread use of closed procedures in which the product is prepared by transfers between rubber-closed vials and is not allowed to come into contact with the environment. Experiments have suggested that transfers between such vials are one sixth as liable to microbial contamination as transfers between open bottles (Abra *et al.*, 1980a). Such closed procedures should therefore be adopted wherever possible.

12.4 CONSEQUENCES OF PARTICULATE CONTAMINATION OF RADIOPHARMACEUTICALS

Parentally administered radiopharmaceuticals should ideally be free of all particulate contaminants in order to minimise the risk of untoward reactions in the patient. Injected particles may produce discomfort or anaphylactic reactions.

The British Pharmacopoeia (1988) requires that injectable solutions 'when examined under suitable conditions of visibility are clear and practically free from particles'. The presence of large particles, visible to the naked eye requires that the product be discarded unless the contamination can be removed without affecting the safety, quality and efficacy of the product. However, it is possible that particulate contamination not visible to the naked eye is also present. The British Pharmacopoeia (1988) does not specify limits unless the injection is supplied in containers with a nominal content of 100 ml or more. This does not therefore apply to radiopharmaceuticals which are supplied in much smaller volumes.

Standards of particulate contamination for small volume parenteral products are specified in the United States Pharmacopoeia XXI. Products meet the requirement of the test if they contain not more than 10^4 particles per container equal to or greater than 10 micrometres and/or 1000 particles per container equal to or greater than 25 mircometres in effective spherical diameter. Discussions currently taking place may result in similar specifications in the European Pharmacopoeia although no time scale has been set for their introduction.

Microbial contamination of radiopharmaceuticals for parenteral administration manufactured in hospitals is also possible. Preparing radiopharmaceuticals with sterile ingredients and using closed procedures within suitable safety cabinets greatly reduces the opportunity for contamination. The number of organisms required to initiate an infection in a patient is difficult to define and depends on a variety of factors e.g. the susceptibility of the host, which may be affected by existing desease state or therapy. In addition the virulence of the causative organism is important. Ayliffe *et al.*, (1982) suggest that 10^5 cells of Staphylococcus aureus may not necessarily cause in infection, although in the presence of a foreign body such as a suture, 10^2 organisms may be sufficient. However, appropriate faclities and procedures to minimise the possibility of any microbial contamination must be used.

It is probable that there are no reliable figures indicating the frequency of microbially contaminated radiopharmaceuticals prepared in hospitals. One of the reasons for this is the fact that the value of retrospective sterility testing of technetium radiopharmaceuticals after decay of radioactivity has seriously been questioned (Wind 1985, Brown and Baker 1986). They found that microorganisms may not survive for prolonged periods in many radiopharmaceuticals because of the poor nutritional value and the degree of radiation damage incurred. In particular, both papers showed a decrease in the viability of *Staphylococcus aureus* over a few days in a range of technetium radiopharmaceuticals.

However, since most radiopharmaceuticals are prepared and used in the same working day and the key issue is what is the fate of any microbial contaminants during this period? Abra *et al.* (1980b) assessed the growth of five different microorganisms (including Gram positive and negative bacteria and fungi) in nine technetium kits over a period of eight hours. They inoculated each vial with a relatively small number of microorganisms in an attempt to simulate possible contamination during preparation. They did not find any consistent pattern of growth although *Escherichia coli* appeared to double in numbers in eight hours at 25° C in Macro-aggregated albumin (MAA) and Diethylene triamine pentaacetic acid (DTPA). The fungi, *Aspergillus niger* and *Candida albicans* grew in Human Serum Albumin in the same time period at 25° C. Results with *Staphylococcus aureus* were variable and were difficult to interpret in view of the very low number of organisms inocculated. For safety and convenience, these experiments were performed with kits that had been reconstituted with Sodium Chloride Injection rather than Sodium ($^{99}Tc^{m}$) Pertechnetate and thus the survival of organisms may have been overestimated since the potential deleterious effects of radiation were avoided. Brown and Baker (1986) demonstrated that the presence of radioactivity adversely affected the survival of *Psudeomonas aeruginosa* and *Staphylococcus aureus* in some technetium kits when compared with non-radioactive controls. Abra *et al.* (1980b) calculated that a vial containing 555 MBq of technetium-99m would deliver 10 Gy over a period of 8 hours which would cause a 44% reduction in the numbers of *Pseudomonas aeruginosa* which was the organism most susceptible to radiation damage. However, even with higher activities of technetium-99m, the radiation dose delivered is insufficient to guarantee sterilisation of radiopharmaceuticals by self-irradiation. The British Pharmacopoeia (1988) states that 25 kGy is generally accepted as being an adequate dose of ionising radiations to achieve sterility.

12.5 DETECTION OF MICROBIAL AND PARTICULATE CONTAMINATION IN THE RADIOPHARMACY

Techniques for microbial and particulate monitoring have been reviewed by Sampson (1985). Of the techniques available for microbial monitoring of the environment, settle plates are the easiest to use since they simply require exposure of suitable nutrient agars to the atmosphere at critical sites for a specified period of time. The plates are then incubated and inspected for microbial growth. This technique does not give a reliable quantitative estimate of microorganisms present since the volume of air sampled is not measured and whether or not organisms settle on to the agar is largely a matter of chance. However, by using constant exposures at the same sites, gross variations in microbial contamination can be detected. Settle plates may also be useful in helping to identify the type of microorganisms present in a particular environment.

Accurate quantification requires the use of either a slit sampler or centrifugal air sampler (see Sampson 1985) in which a known volume of air is sampled and any contained microorganisms impinged on to the solid culture medium which are then incubated and examined for growth. The number of viable microorganisms per cubic metre of air can then be calculated. The EEC GMP specifies the basic environmental standards for the manufacture of sterile products. Within unidirectional airflow workstations (Grade A), the maximum permitted number of microorganisms is less than one per cubic metre. In a Grade B environment a maximum of five microorganisms per cubic metre of air is permitted.

The microbial contamination of work surfaces can be assessed by the use of contact plates. This involves placing appropriate solid culture medium on the surface to be examined. Any microorganisms present adhere to the agar, which is then incubated and examined for growth. Sampling sites should be selected such that critical areas are assessed. It is essential when using this technique that scrupulous cleaning of the sites takes place after sampling such that traces of culture medium are not left on the work surface.

Particulate contamination of the environment is most commonly determined using instruments which measure the scattering of a beam of light when particles pass through it (e.g. Royco sampler). The instruments can be calibrated to measure particles of given size ranges and by sampling a known volume of air, it is possible to calculate the number of particles per cubic metre of air (see Sampson, 1985).

The maximum number of particles permitted by the EEC GMP within a unidirectional airflow work station is a maximum of 3000 particles per cubic metre equal to or greater than 0.5 micrometres with no particles exceeding 5 micrometres i.e. Grade A.

Practical experience has shown that it is impossible to maintain Grade A conditions in any working area when personnel are present, no matter how well clad they are in protective clothing or how good is the quality of the incoming filtered air. Most radiopharmaceuticals are prepared using closed procedures which are less prone to particulate contamination (Abra *et al.*, 1980b). This was recognised in 'Guidance Notes for Hospitals on the Premises and Environment for the Preparation of Radiopharmaceuticals' issued in 1982 by the Department of Health and Social Security which states that it may be satisfactory to prepare such radiopharmaceuticals under less demanding conditions provided they are made and used within one working day. The Guidance Notes state that manipulations should be performed in a workstation complying with Class 1 BS 5295 (corresponding to Grade A of the EEC GMP, see Table 1) conditions and that the workstation should be situated in a room with a good standard of hygiene preferably supplied with filtered air. The highest standard of cleanliness suggested for the room environment was Class 3 BS 5295.

The frequency of monitoring is not laid down in any official guidance and it therefore needs to be determined locally and is dependent on the type and number of radiopharmaceuticals prepared and the standard of the facilities in which this takes place. A strategy has been suggested by Frier *et al.*, (1988) and is shown in Table 2. These recommendations were based on current practices in radiopharmacies in the United Kingdom and provide a sound basis for on-going monitoring.

Table 2
Suggested Frequency of Environmental Monitoring in Radiopharmacies

	Test	*Frequency*
(a)	Microbial Contamination	
	Settle Plates	Weekly
	Contact Plates	Monthly
	Air Sampling	Monthly
(b)	Particulate Contamination	
	Air Sampling	6 Monthly

12.6 RADIOACTIVE CONTAMINATION OF RADIOPHARMACIES

Preparation of radiopharmaceuticals involves the use of unsealed sources of radioactivity and as such the possibility of spillage can never be discounted. Such spillage could result in direct contamination of personnel or of work surfaces. Personnel could therefore also become contaminated by contact with spillages on work surfaces. Further hazards also arise if volatile or gaseous materials are being handled, since spillage may result in an increase in the air concentration of radioactivity, which may then be ingested.

Within the United Kingdom, the Ionising Radiations Regulations (1985) require the definition of Controlled Areas where dose rates exceed 7.5 microsieverts per hour or where the air concentration or surface contamination level of a radionuclide exceeds levels stated in the Regulations.

Where a Controlled Area has been defined, entry is restricted to either Classified Workers, as defined in the Regulations, or persons entering under a written system of work, which specifies how staff should carry out procedures. It is also necessary to define the boundaries of the Controlled Area in the local rules of the department and provide warning signs stating 'Controlled Area' and displaying the radioactive trefoil symbol.

Radiopharmacies will need to be defined as Controlled Areas, since the instantaneous dose rate, measured over 1 minute, will exceed the limit of $7.5 \mu Svh^{-1}$ wherever a technetium generator is situated. Stores used for radioactive substances or waste are also likely to be Controlled Areas. The Ionising Radiations Regulations do contain exemptions to this limit, but they will not apply to radiopharmacies in view of the levels of radioactivity handled.

The air concentration and surface contamination levels of commonly ued radiopharmaceuticals at which the definition of a Controlled Area becomes necessary are shown in Table 3.

It is to be hoped that these levels of contamination can be avoided and the largest factors enhancing safety are the skill of staff adhering to suitable working practices and careful design of premises and equipment used. However, accidents can occur and complacency is dangerous.

The Guidance Notes require that monitoring for external radiation and surface contamination should be carried out on a systematic basis.

Table 3
Contamination Levels Requring Designation as Controlled Areas

Radionuclide	*Air concentration*	*Surface contamination*
	$Bq\,m^{-3}$	$Bq\,cm^{-2}$
Ga-67	6×10^4	4×10^4
Tc-99m	6×10^5	4×10^5
In-111	3×10^4	2×10^4
I-125	3×10^2	1×10^2
I-131	2×10^2	1×10^2
Xe-133	6×10^6	Does not apply
Tl-201	9×10^4	7×10^4

12.7 MONITORING OF RADIOACTIVITY LEVELS IN RADIOPHARMACIES

12.7.1 External Dose Rates

Monitoring of the external dose rate in the radiopharmacy can be performed continuously with an appropriate instrument, capable of detecting gamma and beta radiation placed at a suitable position in the department. The advantages of such an arrangement are that an instantaneous reading of the dose rate can be obtained and it is also possible to incorporate an audible alarm, set to sound at a selected dose rate. Potential hazards are thus immediately apparent.

The used of portable instrument (e.g. Geiger Muller detector or Ionisation Chamber) allows measurement of instantaneous dose rates at a variety of sites in the radiopharmacy and store rooms used for radioactive materials. This is particularly useful to demonstrate the adequacy or otherwise of local shielding round radioactive sources. Depending on local circumstances, weekly or monthly measurements at selected sites in the department should be made. In addition monitoring should be performed whenever a change in working practice occurs.

Cumulative measuremetns of external radiation can be made by placing Thermoluminescent dosemeteres or film badges at strategic points in the radiopharmacy. Results from such determinations are not, of course, immediately available.

12.7.2 Surface Contamination

The measurement of surface contamination is necessary for all work surfaces, but especially internal surfaces of safety cabinets and fume cupboards in which radiopharmaceuticals are manipulated. They should be monitored at the end of each working session. Protective clothing worn by personnel, particularly gloves and overshoes also requires monitoring at the end of each working session to minimise the spread of any radioactive contamination. In addition, the equipment used in the radiopharmacy will need to be monitored. Floors should also be monitored as any contamination present may be spread on the feet of personnel to other areas. A weekly assessment has been proposed (Frier *et al.*, 1988).

12.7.3 Techniques for Measurement of Surface Contamination

Surface contamination can be performed either by direct monitoring using a suitable instrument or wipe testing of the surface with subsequent measurement of the removed activity. The UK Guidance Notes (1988) recommend that direct monitoring should be used for preference. A portable monitor is recommended for use in radiopharmacies and should be equipped with a sensitive scintillation detector, capable of measuring low levels of gamma radiation. Such monitors usually have scales which may be calibrated in count rate, rather than dose rate. Thus it is valuable to observe count rates measured by the instrument with known activities of specified radionuclides in order to achieve an approximate calibration.

In some situations, direct monitoring of contamination of work surfaces is not possible (e.g. those adjacent to technetium generators where there is a high external dose rate). In these circumstances, wipe testing can be performed. The technique involves wiping a specified area with a moist swab which removes radioactivity. The swab is then placed in a suitable detector to measure the radioactivity on it. Depending on the detector used, it may be necesary to construct a calibration curve such that the number of Becquerels at a particular radionuclide present can be calculated. The Approved Code of Practice (Paragraph 147) states that it should be assumed that only 10% of radioactivity is removed from the surface, unless other evidence is available. The amount removed may be considerably different and has been shown to be dependent on the radiopharmaceutical, the nature of the worksurface, and the type of swab used for wiping (Scott and Gibson, 1991). Where experiments can safely and conventiently be performed, they may help to determine the actual amount of a range of commonly used radiopharmaceuticals removed by a technique standard in the department. In this way, far more accurate estimations of contamination levels can be achieved.

The Ionising Radiations Regulations do not specify any levels of contamination which are acceptable and at all times the concept of 'as low as reasonably practicable' must be adopted. The Guidance Notes quote derived limits for surface contamination from which the National Radiological Protection Board has proposed levels of contamination that should not be exceeded. For the interior surfaces of work stations, fume cupboards etc., no specific level is mentioned and 'the minimum reasonably achievable' is stated. For other work surfaces in Conrolled Areas, the level should not exceed 300 Bq cm $^{-2}$ for $^{99}Tc^{m}$, ^{125}I, ^{67}Ga and ^{201}Tl. A lower level of 30 Bq cm $^{-2}$ is specified for ^{111}In and ^{131}I. It is therefore necessary that the contamination monitor used is capable of detecting radioactivity at these levels and below.

REFERENCES

Abra R.M., Bell N.D.S. and Horton P.W. (1980a). *An evaluation of some radiopharmaceutical transfer techniques.* Journal of Clinical and Hospital Pharmacy, **5**, 3–9.

Abra R.M., Bell N.D.S. and Horton P.W. (1980b). *The growth of micro-organisms in some parental radiopharmaceuticals.* International Journal of Pharmaceutics, **5**, 187–193.

Ayliffe G.A.J., Collins B.J., Taylor L.J. (1982). *Hospital-acquired Infection.* Bristol. John Wright Sons Ltd.

Approved Code of Practice, The Protection of Persons Against Ionising. Radiations arising from any Work Activity. The Ionising Radiation Regulations (1985). London, HMSO.

Brown S. and Baker M.H. (1986). *The sterility testing of dispensed radiopharmaceuticals.* Nuclear Medicine Communications, **7**, 327–336.

Casewell M.W. and Hill R.L.R. (1986). *The carrier state: methicillin-resistant* Staphylococcus aureus. J. Antimicrob. Chemother. (Suppl A) **18**, 1–12.

Frier M., Hardy J.G., Hesslewood S.R. and Lawrence R. (1988). *Hospital Radiopharmacy: Principles and Practice Report 56.* Institute of Physical Sciences in Medicine, York.

Guidance Notes for the Protection of Persons Against Ionising Radiations Arising from Medical and Dental Use (1988). London, HMSO.

Guide to Good Pharmaceutical Manufacturing Practice (1983). London, HMSO.

Scott L.E. and Gibson C.J. (1991). *Wipe tests to assess $^{99}Tc^{m}$ surface contamination: Effects of surface type, swab type and chemical form.* Nuclear Medicine Communications, **12**, 127–133.

Sampson C.B. (1985). *Environmental Control and Monitoring in the Radiopharmacy. In* Radiopharmacy and Radiopharmaceuticals, edited by A.E. Theobald, p. 145–156. London: Taylor and Francis.

The Ionising Radiations Regulations (1985). London, HMSO.

The Rules Governing Medicinal Products in the European Community. Volume IV. Good Manufacturing Practice for Medicinal Products. Commission of the European Communities, Luxembourg.

Wind K. (1985). *The Sterility Testing of Radiopharmaceuticals. In* Radiopharmacy and Radiopharmacology Yearbook 1, edited by P.H. Cox. p. 25–46. New York: Gordon and Breach Science Publishers.

Chapter 13

Waste Management in the Radiopharmacy

A.T. Elliott

13.1 INTRODUCTION

Within every radiopharmacy, the waste management policy should be an early consideration discussed with the Radiation Protection Adviser. Public apprehension about the disposal of radioactive and clinical waste is at a high level and may be mirrored in the approach of a Local Authority. The overriding aim should be to discharge the minimum possible quantities from the facility, by adopting appropriate production procedures, utilising on-site storage to permit radioactive decay and by including safety features to guard against accidental discharges.

13.2 RADIOACTIVE WASTE MANAGEMENT

Radioactive waste can be defined as radioactive material for which there is no further use; in the present context, this would include stock residues, contaminated materials from laboratory or patient procedures and materials used in connection with contamination incidents. As much use as possible should be made of radioactive decay to reduce the quantities of waste to be disposed of.

In order to facilitate waste management, a policy of strict segregation according to half-life should be employed. Within laboratories, separate cinbins and waste sacks should be provided for Tc-99m, I-131, Xe-133 and long-lived radionuclides. This permits early disposal of waste containing only the short-lived materials, minimising storage space required. Otherwise, bins and sacks with perhaps only one long-lived item will have to be stored for protracted periods before disposal is possible. Care should be taken to establish that shorter-lived radionuclides are not subject to long-lived contaminants, for example that I-123 does not contain I-125, which confounds such an approach.

A rotational storage system should be employed within the store, each item being marked with the radionuclides involved, an estimate of the activity involved and the date of deposit. Given the difficulty of disposal of solid waste, every effort should be made to minimise the amount of waste generated. Particularly for long-lived radionuclides, waste should be disposed of as liquid wherever possible, always taking into account the additional hazard (to staff and facility) of, for example, emptying vials.

13.3 RADIOACTIVE WASTE STORE

This should be designed to comply with the permissible radiation levels about to be introduced (ICRP, 1990), which are more stringent than the current levels by a factor of three. It will be necessary to estimate the maximum quantities of radionuclides likely to be placed into storage and to calculate the resulting radiation dose rates. Dependent upon its situation, the resultant dose rates outside may have to comply with those for members of the public. For a facility handling large quantities of radioactive materials and storing dose residues, this may require the walls to be lined with lead-ply panels containing 2–5 mm thick lead sheet, the joints being covered doors will have to contain shielding also. This thickness will be adequate for all lower energy radionuclides but if therapeutic quantities of I-131 are to be held, additional local shielding may need to be utilised; since the half-value thickness at this energy is 2.8 mm, it would be uneconomic (and impractical) to put the necessary thickness of lead into the walls.

Within the store, racking should be fitted to permit rotation and separation of various types of waste. It is a requirement that the store should be constructed to be readily decontaminated and should be weathertight and rodent-proof. It should be protected by high-security locks.

13.4 DISPOSAL OF RADIOACTIVE WASTE

The disposal of radioactive waste, other than for very small quantities specified in the Radioactive Substances (Hospital

Exemption) Order, must be covered by a certificate of authorisation issued by HM Inspectorate of Pollution. Note that certain types of clinical waste may offer other hazards and fall into the scope of the Control of Pollution (Special Waste) Regulations. Where therapeutic procedures are undertaken, solid patient waste may be generated – contaminated crockery, cutlery, linen etc; since this may contain organic matter and may have to be stored for some time, it constitutes a potential biohazard to the radiopharmacy facility and should not be stored there. Provided that no alpha-emitters are included, the following disposals of waste from a hospital site are permitted without complying with the specific conditions of a certificate of authorisation:

(a) total activity of less than 400 kBq in a minimum volume of 0.1 m^3 or a single item of activity 40 kBq in the same volume;
(b) a total of 25 MBq of carbon-14 and tritium, together with 5 MBq of all other radionuclides, for site incineration. The activity in the residual ash must not exceed 400 kBq per 0.1 m^3;
(c) activity less than 1 GBq of technetium-99m and 500 MBq of other radionuclides in human excreta disposed of via the public sewer per month and less than 50 MBq of other aqueous liquid waste.

Since these limits apply to a site as a whole, it is unlikely that a hospital with a nuclear medicine department will be able to operate under these exemptions. It should be noted that, if a site is covered by a waste disposal authorisation, the exemptions no longer apply and all disposals must be made under the terms of the certificate.

13.4.1 Solid Waste

This usually comprises the greatest volume of waste. For most of this material, the radioactive contaminant will be Tc-99m and, after two weeks in the radioactive waste store, it can be sent out as non-radioactive waste under the terms of (a) above. Prior to disposal, all labels indicating that the contents are radioactive should be removed; in hospitals utilising colour-coded refuse bags, it may be necessary to place the original bag into another of the correct colour for ordinary waste.

The usual route of disposal for higher-activity waste (and all waste posing a biohazard) is via the hospital incinerator. It is important to ensure that any radioactive waste is burned in the middle of the operative period in order to ensure complete combustion. If it is fed in too early, the operating temperature may not have been reached and plastics (vials, gloves etc) may not ignite properly while, if fed in near the end of a run, the material may not have been completely consumed and the ash residue will be overly active.

It will be necessary to demonstrate that the flue lining does not accrete radioactivity and that the residual ash is below the limit for disposal through the local authority as given in (a) and (b) above. These measurements will be required on, probably, an annual basis.

Note that the ash measurements are particularly difficult. Given that low energy gamma and beta emitters may be contained in the waste, it will probably be necessary to employ liquid scintillation counting, limiting the amount of sample which can be measured. Since only a very small sample can be counted, any statistical error in the result can give spurious results for the bulk material.

The alternative to incineration is deep burial, which requires a special arrangement with HM Inspectorate of Pollution and the local authority and is limited to certain council tips. Some authorities require a user representative to be present on each occasion – it is advisable to be present on at least the first occasion to ensure that the burials are in accordance with regulations, in particular the 4 m depth.

13.4.2 Aqueous, Non-Toxic Liquid Waste

Within strict limits agreed by the relevant authority (in the UK, Her Majesty's Inspectorate of Pollution), aqueous liquid radioactive waste is disposed of to the drainage system. The regulations require discharge into a main drain, but fail to define the latter. In practice, it is considered to be one in which there is adequate and reasonably constant flow, i.e. no possibility of stagnant pools of radioactive waste. In some circumstances, it may be necessary to increase the flow artificially by use of a flushing tank connected to the highest point in the drainage system to meet these criteria.

Waste must be poured carefully to avoid splashing adjacent surfaces and the sink rinsed carefully. It is good practice to run water into the sink for a few moments afterwards to clear radioactive liquid from the trap. Where heated sink traps are used, care should be exercised in the disposal of solutions of radioiodine to ensure that no radioactive vapour is produced when the heater is activated.

Where small animal work is carried out, the most convenient method of carcase disposal is via maceration, converting solid waste into a liquid slurry which can be disposed of via the sewerage system. Care must be taken to ensure that the macerator is readily maintained and, during operation, that it does not jam.

A hazard assessment must be carried out by the Radiation Protection Adviser to assure the local authority that there is no danger to sewage workers. This will involve the calculation of the amount of activity which could be ingested by consuming 0.8m^3 of discharge liquid (equivalent to the annual water consumption of reference man) and comparison with the Annual Limit of Intake. The external hazard will be calculated on the basis of immersion in discharge liquid at the hospital outfall.

13.4.3 Non-Aqueous/Toxic Liquid Waste

Liquids immiscible with water or toxic liquids cannot be disposed of through the drainage sytem. An example is liquid scintillator, although there are some available which are biodegradable, non-flammable and of low toxicity which have been developed specifically for discharge into the drainage system; note that even the latter may not be acceptable to the local water authority.

Conventional scintillator in counting vials may be disposed of by incineration, provided that the batch is not too large and that the type of incinerator is suitable – manual loading systems should not be employed because of the risk of flashback (premature ignition). Similar considerations apply to flammable solvents.

If incineration is not possible, the vials should be capped firmly, placed in a heavy-gauge plastic bag and stored in a metal drum. Bulk scintillant should be decanted into a metal drum. Since the quantity of radioactivity will be low, the drums may be stored in a fire-proof solvent store until a preset limit has been reached and then removed by special collection by a firm licensed for such disposals – the Radiation Protection Adviser should be consulted over these arrangements. It is vital to maintain accurate records of the contents of individual drums, since an inventory will be required by the disposal firm.

11.4.4 Gases

The outfall of any gaseous discharge must be at a height of 50% above the highest point of the building. Curiously, the regulations do not mention surrounding buildings. Tests should be carried out to ensure that the discharge is dispersed successfully and does not return to ground level or become entrained in any adjacent air intake to other buildings.

Although it may be considered that a radiopharmacy does not handle radioactive gases, the exhaust from a laminar flow cabinet (LFC) may become contaminated in the event of accident.

In most cases, laminar flow cabinets will operate purely in recirculating mode. Particularly in cases where volatile materials are to be handled, the exhaust should be ducted. Where experimental work is carried out, the LFCs may operate normally in recirculating mode but are fitted with an emergency button which switches them into total exhaust; since the intake air in the latter mode is all drawn from the room, this drops the room pressure below ambient and so prevents the spread of any material from the room.

Dependent upon the quantities and type of radionuclides to be handled, one or two filters may be employed in the outlet duct. The first is a HEPA type and should remove all particulates and aerosols, while the second contains activated charcoal to absorb any gaseous materials. Such filters should be of the 'safe change' type and would be handled only by physics staff if contaminated, when they must be treated as solid waste. If more than one LFC is fitted, the outlet ducts should be kept separate to avoid the possibility of cross-contamination.

13.5 RECORDS

Records must be kept of the radionuclide, activity, chemical form, route of disposal and date of disposal. Note that the requirements for keeping an inventory of radioactive materials do not apply to waste. An annual return is required by the Pollution Inspectorate.

REFERENCES

The Ionising Radiations Regulations 1985 (Statutory Instrument 1333), HMSO, London.

The Radioactive Substances (Hospitals) Exemption Order 1990 (Statutory Instrument 2512), HMSO, London.

Radioactive Substances Act 1960, HMSO, London.

Guidance notes for the protection of persons against ionising radiations from medical and dental use 1988, HMSO, London.

Control of Pollution Act 1974, HMSO London.

The Control of Pollution (Special Waste) Regulations 1980 (Statutory Instrument 1709), HMSO, London.

Chapter 14

Operator Safety in the Handling of Radiopharmaceuticals

S.R. Hesslewood

14.1 INTRODUCTION

In any discussion on operator safety, it is necessary to consider all potential sources of hazard and the nature of the task to be undertaken when designing a safe system of work. Thus systems for preparing and dispensing of radiopharmaceuticals need to take into account the fact that, in addition to being radioactive, the majority of currently used materials are administered parenterally. This means that pharmaceutical implications are important and there will be differences in techniques and facilities to those which may be used for handling radioactive substances not intended for administration to patients. The protocols for dispensing radiopharmaceuticals and design of radiopharmacy laboratories are discussed in Chapters 5 and 4 respectively. It is also necessary to consider any biological hazard to the operator arising from the radiopharmaceutical being handled, for example when labelling blood cells. In particular, great care must be taken to avoid needle-stick injuries when handling blood. Requirements for blood labelling are discussed in Chapters 5 and 6. This chapter will, therefore, concentrate on the radiation hazards to the operator. These can arise from either ingested activity or external radiation. Methods of minimising both sources are necessary to achieve maximum safety. Minimising ingested activity means that there must be a total ban on all hand to mouth operations e.g. eating, drinking, pipetting, applying cosmetics in departments where radiopharmaceuticals are handled. It also requires that all the facilities must effectively remove gaseous or volatilised radioactivity from the working environment.

The principles of radiation protection in radiopharmacy are based on the recommendations of the International Commission on Radiological Protection (ICRP) as laid down in Publication 26 (ICRP 1977). Three basic guidelines are laid down:

(a) No practice shall be adopted unless its introduction produces a positive net benefit;
(b) All exposures shall be kept as low as reasonably achievable (the 'ALARA' principle);
(c) The dose equivalent to individuals shall not exceed recommended limits for the appropriate circumstances.

14.2 REGULATIONS AND CODES OF PRACTICE

The manner in which the ICRP recommendations are applied is determined by individual countries. Within the European Economic Community, a Council Directive (the 'Euratom Directive') laid down basic safety standards for the protection of patients against the dangers of ionising radiations. This has been implemented in the United Kindom by means of The Ionising Radiations Regulations (1985), which are legally enforceable. The regulations are supplemented by an Approved Code of Practice, 'The protection of persons against ionising radiation arising from any work activity' (1985). In addition, the practices within hospital radiopharmacy are also governed by 'Guidance Notes for the Protection of Persons Against Ionising Radiations arising from medical and dental use' (1988). Each of these documents initially appears complex, but a thorough study of them is essential when designing safe systems of work. In view of their comprehensive nature, the majority of discussion in the remainder of the chapter is based on them and while it must be remembered that, whereas they are strictly only applicable within the United Kingdom, most of the features will also have relevance elsewhere. Individual Regulations or sections of the Approved Code of Practice or Guidance Notes are detailed at appropriate points in the text. This chapter should be read in conjunction with Chapter 15.

The current applicable dose limit for employees aged 18 years or over within the United Kingdom are specified in the Ionising Radiations Regulations (Schedule 1). The whole body limit is 50 mSv per annum, while that for individual organs or tissues, other than the lens of the eye, but including any body extremity or over any area of skin is 500 mSv. There are also separate limits for the lens of the eye (150 mSv per annum), the abdomen of a woman of reproductive capacity (13 mSv in any consecutive three month interval) and the abdomen of a pregnant woman (10 mSv during the declared term of the pregnancy).

Working practices adopted must therefore ensure personnel do not exceed these limits. Within the United Kingdom, any person likely to exceed 3/10 of any relevant dose limit must be designated a Classified Worker (Regulation 9). The worker must then have his health reviewed at least once a year by an appointed doctor and be monitored by an Approved Dosimetry Service.

Publication 60 of the ICRP (1990) has recommended more stringent dose limits and it is expected that these will eventually be introduced into new regulations. The timetable for this will be dependent on national authorities. Within the United Kingdom, it is anticipated that new regulations will be made in 1995.

14.3 HANDLING OF RADIOACTIVE MATERIALS IN THE RADIOPHARMACY

Three basic factors affect radiation doses to personnel. They are:

(a) The distance between the worker and the radioactive source. The radiation dose decreases proportionally with the square of the distance – the so called 'inverse square law';
(b) The time spent manipulating the radioactive source;
(c) The amount of shielding used to reduce the dose rate from the radioactive source.

The optimal procedure for handling radiopharmaceuticals may require a compromise of these parameters. For example, if extra shielding means that handling times increase, there may not be a significant reduction in the radiation dose absorbed by the fingers.

14.3.1 Distance Between the Radioactive Source and the Worker

The dose rate from a radioactive source decreases with the square of the distance from the source. Thus doubling the distance will reduce the dose rate four-fold. Working practices should therefore be designed to ensure that the maximum distance, compatible with ease of manipulation, is maintained between personnel and radioactive sources. Since the elution of technetium generators proceeds automatically once the evacuated vial has been placed in position, it is good practice to move away until the process has been completed.

Vials containing radiopharmaceuticals should be removed from shielding with tongs or forceps rather than gloved fingers (Regulation 6, paragraph 5). The devices must permit rapid and safe manipulation and not cause an increase in the handling time or the risk of the vial being dropped or damaged during manipulation.

Whenever handling unshielded syringes is unavoidable, e.g. when being placed in the dose calibrator, they should be handled by the end remote from the needle. It has been calculated the dose rate over a 0.5 ml volume of technetium-99m in a 2 ml syringe is forty times that at the end of the syringe barrel (Henson 1973). Some departments therefore advocate the use of syringes with a capacity greater than the volume to be transferred (e.g. 5 ml for an injection volume less than 2 ml) in order to increase the distance between fingers and the radioactive solution. Further support for this concept is given in the Guidance Notes which recommend that syringes should not normally be filled to more than 50% of their capacity (Paragraph 10.44).

14.3.2 Time Spent Handling Radioactivity

Radiation exposure of personnel can be reduced by minimising the time spent performing manipulations. This requires that all procedures are carefully evaluated to avoid unnecessary exposure and emphasises the need for new members of staff to practise techniques with non-radioactive materials in order to gain familiarity with the apparatus used before commencing to work with radioactivity. A particular situation is that spending undue time extracting the final volume of a radioactive solution from a vial will significantly increase the operator's finger dose which in view of the comparatively small increase in extracted activity may not be justified.

14.3.3 Shielding

Shielding appropriate for the type of radiation encountered should be used whenever practicable. Shielding may be constructed from a variety of materials including lead, tungsten, aluminium or perspex. Lead should be painted or otherwise covered to provide a cleanable surface and to protect operators from accidental ingestion of lead.

14.3.4 Generators

Technetium generators have one of the highest surface dose rates of materials currently used in radiopharmacies and these can exceed 7 mSv h^{-1}, depending on the amount of shielding incorporated by the manufacturer. Increasing the amount of shielding within the generator can present practical problems in that it may become too heavy to be lifted into the radiopharmacy. It s therefore sensible to store and elute the generators behind additional lead shielding within the department. This may be either in the form of a wall of lead bricks or a custom built castle supplied the generator's manufacturer.

Table 1
Half Thickness of Lead for some Radionuclides

Nuclide	*Photon energy (KeV)*	*Half thickness (mm)*
Tc-99m	140	0.26
In-111	172	0.4
	247	1.1
I-123	159	0.37
I-131	364	2.6

14.3.5 Work Stations

Operator protection can be enhanced by the incorporation of local shielding into the structure of the work station in such a way that air flow patterns are not affected. Acrylic lead or lead glass visors offering protection are readily available and can be fitted by the manufacturer. Shielding in the form of lead sheeting can also be fitted beneath the work surface of the work station. Extra shielding in the form of lead bricks or screens inside the work station will inevitably affect air flow patterns and care must, therefore, be taken to ensure that in open-fronted work stations, operator protection is not compromised by permitting escape of air through the front aperture. For this reason, the minimal amount of equipment and materials should be introduced into the work station. The use of totally enclosed work stations (isolators), in which manipulations are performed through glove ports, removes the risk of air escaping towards the operator. The design and use of isolators is discussed in Chapter 5. Drip trays should, however, always be used in order to contain any spillage that may occur during manipulations.

14.3.6 Vials

During preparation and dispensing of radiopharmaceuticals, vials should be kept within appropriate shielding except during activity measurements. Since vials are usually inverted during dispensing, the design of shielding should be such that the vial is still retained under such circumstances without the need of being held with fingers.

For technetium-99m radiopharmaceuticals (gamma energy 140 KeV), a lead shield of 2 – 3 mm is sufficient to reduce dose rates substantially, whilst retaining the ease of handling. Other radiopharmaceuticals (emitting higher energy gamma rays, e.g. those based on iodine-131, principal gamma energy 364 KeV) need thicker shields to achieve significant reduction in dose rate. The thickness of lead required to reduce the transmission of gamma rays of various energies to 50 per cent of its value (the half thickness), is shown in Table 1.

When handling radionuclides that emit only beta minus particles, it is possible to use materials of lower atomic number such as aluminium to reduce the bremsstrahlung produced. Perspex is also useful for this purpose. Pure beta minus emitting radionuclides commonly encountered in radiopharmacies include phosphorus-32 (maximum beta energy 1.7 MeV) and yttrium-90 (maximum beta energy 2.3 MeV). However, it is usual for phosporus-32 and yttrium-90 to be supplied in lead pots which are sufficiently thick to absorb the generated bremsstrahlung. Measured dose rates at 10 cm from unshielded and shielded soiurces of phosphorus-32 and yttrium-90 are shown in Table 6.2. It can be seen that attentuation by 3 mm lead exceeds that produced by 10 mm perspex.

Table 2
Dose Rates at 10 cm from Phosphorus-32 and Yttrium-90

	Dose rate (μSv h^{-1} MBq^{-1})		
Nuclide	*Unshielded*	*10 mm perspex*	*3 mm lead*
P-32	10.1	0.03	0.006
Y-90	39.2	0.07	0.02

14.3.7 Syringes

Many radiopharmaceutical manipulations require the use of syringes and during preparation of technetium-99m radiopharmaceuticals, it is common for several gigabequerels to be transferred between vials. It has been calculated that surface doses of 260 μSv s^{-1} could be experienced over a 0.5 ml volume of 370 MBq of technetium-99m in a 2 ml syringe (Henson, 1973). Inappropriate handling of syringes will therefore mean that the annual limit for fingers, currently 500 mSv, is reached rapidly. Syringe shields may be used to attenuate radiation emanating from the syringe and the Guidance Notes state that syringes used for handling gamma or high energy beat emitters should be shielded (Paragraph 10.44).

Shields are usually made of lead or tungsten and incorporate a lead glass window. Lead has the disadvantage that it is soft and easily deformed and tungsten is therefore often preferred. Lead glass does not have the same attentuation as either lead or tungsten. However, for preparation and dispensing of radiopharmaceuticals, the lead glass window should be sufficiently wide to ensure good visibility of the graduations on the syringe and the volume of solution within. Lead glass is also brittle and care must therefore be taken to prevent damage.

The attenuation factor of tungsten in commercially available syringe shields has been calculated to be between 27 and 178 (Harding *et al.*, 1985). In practice, the dose to the fingers was not reduced by this amount since the syringe is not totally enveloped and it is necessary to remove the syringe from the shield for activity measurements. For manufacturing and dispensing of technetium-99m radiopharmaceuticals, it was found that syringe shields reduced the operator's finger dose by a factor of two. Syringe shields did, however, produce an eight fold reduction in finger doses of personnel injecting radiopharmaceuticals, providing they did not also install the syringe into the shield. In addition to being expensive, syringe shields are generally heavy and bulky, making venepuncture difficult. For these reasons, they are often unpopular with staff giving injections.

In view of the small reduction in finger dose compared with the large attentuation factors of the materials used, Thomson *et al.* (1986) questioned whether a less bulky design of shield with a lower attenuation factor would give similar protective effect when giving injections. They found that a 0.8 mm lead sheet with an attenuation factor of 10 for technetium-99m was suitable. The design of the shield was modified by replacing the lead glass window with a slot, since visibility of syringe graduations is not important, and also by remove a crescent shaped section from the underside of the shield to facilitate venepuncture. Further work by this group has found that a bismuth shield with an attenuation factor of 6 for technetium-99m offered similar protection to that afforded by lead (Thomson *et al.*, 1987). Bismuth has the advantage that it is lighter than other materials used for shielding and is easier to machine. Further evaluation of this material in syringe shields for manufacture and dispensing of radiopharmaceuticals, as opposed to their injection, seems justified.

14.4 PERSONNEL MONITORING

Such monitoring is necessary to ensure radiation doses received by personnel are maintained within relevant dose limits. It also permits monitoring of new techniques to ensure that their introduction does not cause an unacceptable radiation exposure.

A range of dosemeters can be used, but the most common device utilised for personnel monitoring is the film badge

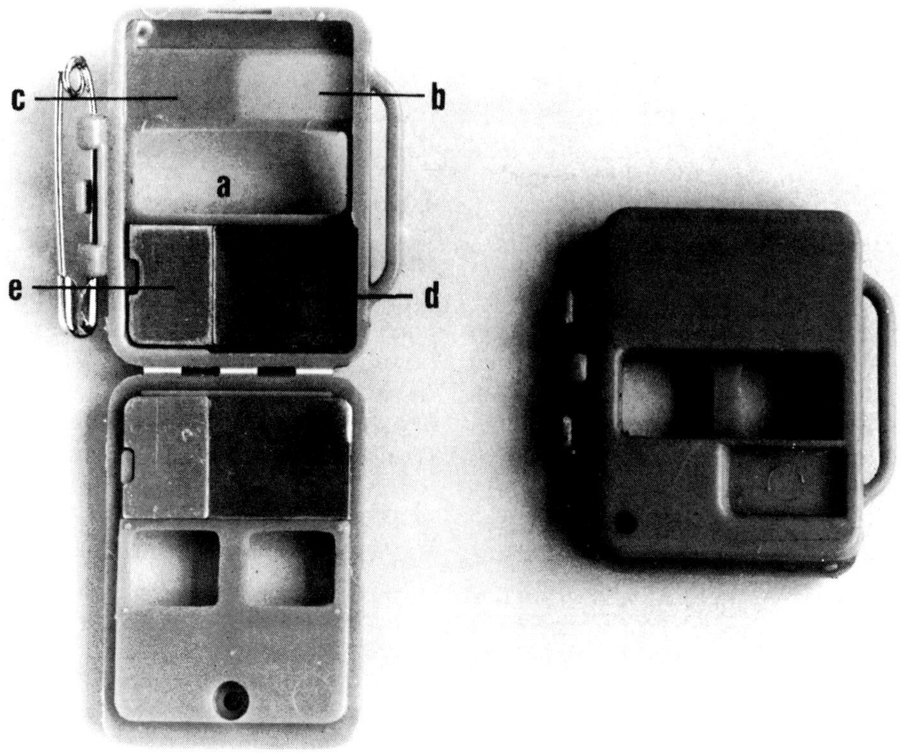

Figure 1

(Figure 1). It consists of a piece of X-ray film inside a paper envelope. The badge is contained within a plastic holder which has five windows of different size and shape. These aid in the identification of the types of radiation falling on the X-ray film. The windows are as follows:

(a) An open window, which allows unobstructed access of all types of radiation to the film badge;
(b) A plastic window, approximately 0.5 mm thick;
(c) A plastic window, approximately 3 mm thick;
(d) A composite window of plastic and light alloy;
(e) A composite window of plastic, tin and lead.

Particulate emissions (e.g. beta particles) and low energy gamma photons will affect the open window the most, while high energy gamma rays (> 500 KeV) will affect all areas of the film equally.

Personnel issued with a film badge must wear it at all time when at work. They must also take care that the film badge is not lost or damaged in such a way that assessment of the absorbed radiation dose is not impaired (e.g. by being exposed to heat or being sent to the laundry). It is also important that the film badge is not exposed to ionising radiation while not being worn (e.g. by being left adjacent to a radioactive source overnight).

The film badge is normally worn on the trunk at either chest or waist height and this is taken as monitoring the dose to the whole body. The monitoring period is normally 1 month but can range between 2 weeks and three months, depending on the likely level of exposure (Guidance Notes, Paragraph 1.18). At the end of the monitoring period, the film badge is processed by an approved dosimetry service. The pattern of irradiation on the film is compared with that observed on samples from the same batch irradiated with calibrated sources of activity and an estimate made of radiation absorbed by personnel.

Other types of dosemeter suitable for monitoring whole body doses include direct reading meters in which a small ionization chamber is incorporated to measure absorbed radiation. The meters are frequently supplied with a clip such that they can conveniently be located in a pocket in protective clothing worn during procedures. The absorbed dose can be read at any desired interval, either from a calibrated scale or digitally. Some models also include audible alarms which can be set to sound at predetermined dose levels. The advantage of this type of meter is that instant monitoring is possible.

Within the United Kingdom, the Guidance notes recommend that more than one dosemeter is used if it is suspected that other parts of the body could exceed 1/10 of the appropriate dose limit (Guidance Notes, Paragraph 1.19).

14.4.1 Monitoring of Doses to Hands and Fingers

During the dispensing of radiopharmaceuticals, it is likely that the hands and fingers will receive the highest radiation dose, since many techniques require the manual transfer of radioactive materials between vials with syringes. Therefore, it is advisable that a separate assessment of the radiation dose absorbed by these tissues is made. This can conveniently be achieved by means of a thermoluminescent dosemeter (TLD). The most frequently used TLD contains activated lithium fluoride crystals. A few milligrams are placed in a small sachet in such a way that they can be conveniently worn on the hand. The TLD should be worn inside non-permeable gloves worn during manipulations. The crystal lattice of the lithium fluoride is able to absorb the incident radiation and retain the excited state of the atoms for several weeks. A monitoring period of one month is again convenient, at the end of which, the absorbed radiation is assessed by an approved dosimetry service. The TLD is placed in a furnace which rapidly heats it to 250 °C. This produces vibrations within the crystal lattice which causes the return of the stored electrons to the ground state. This is accompanied by the emission of the visible photons. The light intensity emitted is measured and is proportional to the radiation dose absorbed. The dose to personnel is calculated by reference to calibration curves.

Two designs are shown in Figure 2. In one type, the sachet is incorporated into a plastic strip which can be made into a ring with adhesive tape and worn round the finger or taped to the palm of the hand. Whereas this type can conveniently be worn round the base of the finger, practical difficulties were encountered at the finger tip, since it was found that the TLD was uncomfortable to wear and tended to slip off during use (Williams *et al.*, 1987). The other design consists of a finger stall with the TLD sachet attached at its tip. The advantages of this design are that it can conveniently be worn beneath gloves and allows accurate measurement of radiation dosage to the finger tip, which has been found to be approximately three times higher than at the base of the finger or on the palm of the hand (Williams *et al.*, 1987).

Measurements have also demonstrated that the radiation dose absorbed by the thumb during manufacture of radiopharmaceuticals can be approximately twice that received by the index finger (Table 3). This is due to the fact that the thumb was used to depress the plunger of the syringe when adding radioactive solutions to vials in these manipulations. This indicates the importance of careful choice of areas to be monitored with TLDs.

Table 3
Comparison of Radiation Doses Absorbed by Index Finger and Thumb

	Dose ($mSv\ mo^{-1}$)		
Operator	*1*	*2*	*3*
Index finger	5.6	4.1	5.7
Thumb	9.9	8.6	9.6

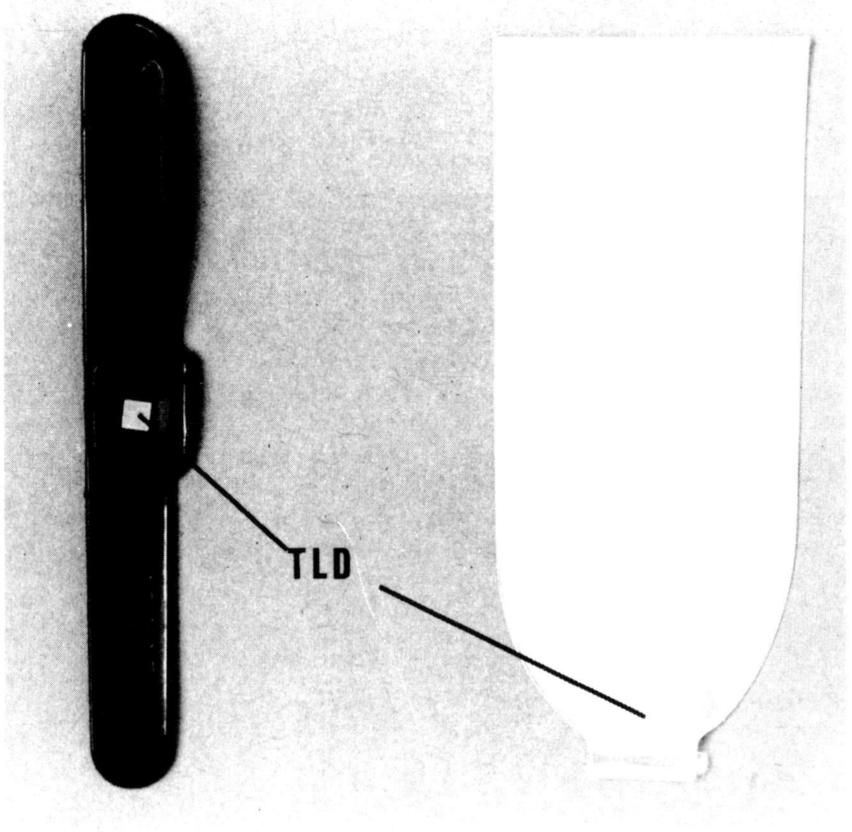

Figure 2

14.5 ACCIDENTS IN THE RADIOPHARMACY

No matter how well a radiopharmacy is designed and how carefully it is operated, the possibility of an accident involving radioactive materials can never be totally ruled out. It is therefore a requirement that contingency arrangements exist to deal with accidents should they occur. Extensive guidance is given in the Guidance Notes (Chapter 16), to which reference should be made when drawing up plans.

In radiopharmacies, the most likely accident is the spillage of a radioactive solution. One of the most important features is therefore containment of the spillage to the greatest extent possible in order to minimise decontamination procedures. For this reason, drip trays should always be used when manipulating radioactive solutions. Each radiopharmacy should be equipped with a decontamination kit containing suitable absorbant materials, protective clothing, decontaminating magnets and monitoring equipment. This kit must be instantly available and be accompanied by instructions for its use such that contingency plans can be brought into use as quickly as possible. The basic items that should be present in the kit are shown in Table 4, but these may need to be supplemented or modificed depending on local circumstances. Greater emphasis must, however, always be placed on prevention of contamination rather than relying on procedures to deal with the results of contamination.

Direct body contamination of personnel can be minimised by the use of appropriate protective clothing which covers vulnerable areas of the body. Obviously, gloves are essential when handling radioactive materials. Overalls should be designed such that they can be overlapped at the wrists by gloves in order to prevent contamination of the forearms. Other protective clothing should be worn as appropriate. In situations where manufacture and dispensing of radiopharmaceuticals occurs within clean rooms, the protective clothing required for pharmaceutical reasons will normally be adequate.

Direct body contamination can also occur by needle stick injuries and if such an incident occurs, monitoring and appropriate decontamination procedures must be carried out. If a needle stick injury occurs whilst handling blood, it is also necessary to consider potential biological hazards (e.g. risk of hepatitis) to which the operator may be exposed.

Table 4
Contents of Radiopharmacy Emergency Box

Protective Clothing	*Personnel Decontamination Items*
Overalls	Plastic sponge
Hats or Hoods	Nail brush
Overshoes	Soft brush
Disposable rubber gloves	Bar of soap
	Bottle of liquid detergent
	Box of tissues
	Box of paper towels
Surface Decontamination Items	*Other Items*
Polythene bucket	Long forceps
Plastic sponge	Roll of "Radioactive" labelled tape
Scrubbing brush	Felt pen for demarcation
Can of aerosol decontaminant or	Contamination monitor
Bottle of liquid decontaminant	
Rolls of adsorbent paper	
Polythene bags for waste disposal	

14.5.1 Decontamination Procedures

Such procedures are required for personnel and also for surfaces and equipment used during manufacture or dispensing procedures since any radioactivity present on them may lead to personnel contamination.

14.5.1.1 Personnel Decontamination Procedures

In situations where it is suspected that personnel contamination has occurred, the body should be monitored to locate the contaminated area. If this is on the protective clothing, the latter should be removed immediately and either disposed of (e.g. gloves) or decontaminated as appropriate. This may require storage of the clothing before it can be sent for laundering (Guidance Notes paragraphs 10.90 and 10.91). Having removed contaminated protective clothing, it is then necessary to monitor the skin and clothes of the operator to determine whether they too have been contaminated.

Any contamination detected on the skin of personnel should be removed as soon as practicable. Hands should be washed with soap or mild detergent and water. The hands should then be monitored and the washing procedure repeated if contamination is still present. For this reason, it is essential to have washing facilities immediately adjacent to those in which radiopharmaceuticals are manipulated. Sinks should be equipped with foot, knee or elbow operated taps (Guidance Notes paragraph 10.15). This prevents transfer of radioactivity from the hands. Vigorous scrubbing that may break the skin must be avoided (Guidance Notes paragraph 10.79). Activity on unbroken skin will usually wash off quite easily but activity at any break in the skin or around the fingernails can be extremely difficult to remove. A soft nailbrush must therefore be provided as part of the decontamination facilities. In the case of cuts, irrigation with tap water should be performed, being careful not the wash further contamination into the wound. When parts of the body other than the hands are contaminated, local washing should be performed in the first instance. Showers can also be taken provided this does not result in contamination being transferred to other parts of the body from which it is difficult to remove e.g. radioactivity being washed into the eyes, particularly as there is a separate, more stringent dose limit for the lens of the eye. It is, however, unlikely that showers will be necessary to deal with contamination arising from hospital manufacturing and dispensing procedures.

Incidents involving personnel contamination must be reported to the Radiation Protector Supervisor who will arrange further treatment or medical advice if thought necessary where decontamination procedures have failed to remove activity (Guidance Notes paragraph 10.80).

14.5.1.2 Decontamination of Surfaces and Equipment

It is important that contaminated surfaces or equipment are identified as soon as possible so that the necessary remedial action can be taken. For surfaces, it is also important that the extent of the contamination is clearly demarcated. This can be achieved by a felt tip pen in the emergency kit.

The majority of work in radiopharmacies involves technetium-99m. In view of its six hour half-life, it may be convenient to cover surfaces from which it is difficult to remove with suitable shielding for a period of 24 hours to allow activity to decay prior to attempting further decontamination procedures. Similarly, it may be convenient to remove contaminated equipment e.g. tongs, shielding vials to a suitable store prior to performing decontamination procedures. In the first instance, decontamination should be performed by washing with detergent and water. Monitoring for residual activity should then be performed and the procedure repeated if necessary. Monitoring of work surfaces adjacent to technetium generators with a scintillation meter is not usually possible because of the high background. In such circumstances, it may be necessary either to remove the generator or to perform wipe testing of the contaminated surface. The Approved Code of Practice suggests that it should be assumed that 10% of the activity is removed by wiping unless otherwise demonstrated (paragraph 147). This, however, is a broad generalisation and may represent a gross underestimation of activity removed and should therefore be treated with caution (Scott and Gibson, 1991). Where it can safely be performed, it may be worthwhile determining experimentally the amount of each type of radiopharmaceutical in use that can be removed by wiping surfaces and equipment.

Where contamination persists, it may be necessary to resort to stronger cleaning agents. Decontamination solutions containing surface active or chelating agents are commercially available in the form of towelettes or sprays which lift the contamination from the surface. However, these must be chosen such that they do not damage the material under treatment. If small pieces of equipment become contaminated with long lived radionuclides, or short lived radioactivity which is difficult to remove, it may be economically preferable to discard them as radioactive waste rather than attempting extensive decontamination procedures.

4.6 CONCLUSIONS

Radiation protection in the radiopharmacy requires the design of safe systems of work that can readily be followed by all personnel working in the department. In practice this means that all procedures must be made as simple as possible and incorporate the three basic criteria of radiation protection: distance, time and shielding. It is also necessary that individuals are well trained and always vigilant when handling radioactive materials to reduce radiation exposure of themselves and other personnel in the department. In view of the fact that the majority of radiopharmaceuticals are administered parenterally, expertise is aseptic manipulations is also required and must not be compromised by radiation protection requirements.

Prevention of radioactive contamination must always be the goal rather than relying on decontamination procedures, although the latter must be available in case of accidents.

REFERENCES

Approved Code of Practice, The Protection of Persons Against Ioinizing Radiation Arising from any Work Activity. The Ionizing Regulations (1985). London, HMSO.

Guidance Notes for the Protection of Persons Against Ioinizing Radiations Arising from Medical and Dental Use (1988). London, HMSO.

Harding L.K., Hesslewood S.R., Ghosh S.K. and Thomson W.H. (1985). *The value of syringe shields in a nuclear medicine department.* Nuclear Communication, **6**, 449 – 454.

ICRP (1977). *Recommendations of the International Commission on Radiological Protection. Publication No. 26.* Annals of the ICRP (3) (Oxford: Pergamon). The Ionizing Radiation Regulations (1985). London, HMSO.

ICRP (1990) *Recommendations of the International Commission on Radiation Protection* (Oxford: Pergamon).

Scott L.E. and Gibson C.J. (1991). *Wipe tests to assess $^{99}Tc^{m}$ surface contamination: Effects of surface type, swab type and chemical form.* Nuclear Medicine Communications, **12**, 127–133.

Thomson W.H., Hesslewood S.R. and Harding L.K. (1986). *How effective are syringe shields?* Nuklearmedizin Supplementum, **22**, 49–51.

Thomson W.H., Mills A.P., Hesslewood S.R., Ghosh S.K., Copeland J. and Harding L.K. (1987). *Twoards a lighter syringe shield.* Nuclear Medicine **26**, 211–212.

Williams E.D., Laird E.E. and Forster E. (1987). *Monitoring radiation dose to the hands in nuclear medicine: Location od dosimeters.* Nuclear Medicine Communications, **7**, 499–503.

Chapter 15

Regulatory Requirements for the Dispensing and Supply of Radiopharmaceuticals

J.R. Gill and J.L. Turner

15.1 INTRODUCTION

Radiopharmaceuticals are amongst the most highly regulated of materials administered to patients because they are controlled both as medicinal products and as radioactive substances.

The Regulations arise from three main sources, the Medicines Act 1968, the Health and Safety at Work etc. Act 1974, and the Radioactive Substances Act 1960, all of which are concerned with public safety.

Regulations made under the Medicines Act control the manufacturer, sale and supply of all medicinal products through a system of licences and exemptions.

Regulations made under the same Act also control the administration to humans of radioactive substances through a system of certification. Regulations made under the Health and Safety at Work etc Act 1974 lay down requirements for the radiation protection of workers and of persons affected by ionising radiations at work. These requirements include provisions for the control of radioactive substances used at work. The Health and Safety at Work etc Act only applies in Great Britain; however similar requirements exist in Northern Ireland.

The Radioactive Substances Act 1960 requires that premises where radioactive substances are held be registered with the Environment Departments and requires authorisation for the accumulation and storage, and for the disposal, or radioactive waste. For further information, reference should be made to 'The Radioactive Substances Act 1960 – a Guide to the Administration of the Act' (HMSO).

These Acts are specific to the United Kingdom but they must be considered within the framework of European Community (EC) legislation. The EC Pharmaceutical Directives oblige member states to operate a system of authorisation for the manufacture and marketing of medicinal products. Euratom Directives oblige member states to take certain measures to protect the health of workers and the general public against the dangers of ionising radiation. These Community obligations may be met in each member state by different combinations of primary legislation, statutory regulation and administrative arrangements but the end result should be a harmonised and effective system of controls throughout the Community so that free movement of goods may result.

Two exemptions affecting radiopharmaceuticals in the United Kingdom were removed during 1991. The so-called 'Crown Immunity' exempting National Health Service (NHS) hospitals from the need to comply with the Medicines Act was removed with effect from 1 April 1991. And the exemption of radiopharmaceuticals from the obligations of the EC Pharmaceutical Directives, along with that of blood products and immunologicals, was removed with effect from 1 January 1992.

The Medicines Act and subordiante legislation arising from it are administered and enforced by the Health Ministers. The Health and Safety at Work etc Act and the regulations made under that Act are enforced either by the Health and Safety Executive (HSE) or by local authorities. The latter are concerned with premises such as shops, offices, hotels, restaurants and the like. Other premises are the concern of HSE. In particular it may be assumed that all work involving radiopharmaceuticals will be covered by HSE.

The different sets of regulations are essentially complementary and should not be seen to conflict in any way. Together they provide for comprehensive protection for all those involved with radiopharmaceuticals, whether worker, patient or member of the general public. It is the responsibility of those handling the products to know how the regulations apply to their particular work and to comply with them.

15.2 THE MEDICINES ACT 1968

15.2.1 General

The Medicines Act provides legislation for consumer protection which regulates the importation, manufacture and sale or supply of medicinal products. Under the Act these activities must either be conducted in accordance with a licence or certificate granted for the purpose or in accordance with the terms of one of the specified exemptions from licensing. To do otherwise is to commit an offence.

The Medicines Act established a Licensing Authority, being one or more of the Health and Agrilculture Ministers of the United Kingdom, and a Medicines Commission to advise the Ministers. The day to day administration of the Act, in so far as it relates to licensing of medicinal products for human use and the granting of administration certificates, is conducted by officials of the Department of Health (DoH) in England and Wales and the corresponding bodies in Northern Ireland and Scotland. The majority of officials concerned with licensing are employed within the Medicines Control Agency (MCA) of the DoH. The Medicines Commission is supported by expert committees established under Section 4 of the Act, including the Committee on Safety of Medicines (CSM) and the Administration of Radioactive Substances Advisory Committee (ARSAC). A further committee, the Committee on Radiation from Radioactive Medicinal Products, was also established under Section 4 but has since been discontinued, its functions having been taken over by the CSM and ARSAC. Two sub-committees of the CSM, for Chemistry, Pharmacy and Standards (CPS) and for Safety, Efficacy and Adverse Reactions (SEAR), give particular advice relating to the CSM to the quality and to the safety and efficacy respectively of products which are, or may be, licensed.

A 'Next Steps' Agency, the MCA is required to be self-supporting financially and thus charges fees for its work, including assessment of licence applications and inspections.

15.2.2 Product Licences

Any person wishing to market a medicinal product, that is to promote its sale or supply in a normal commercial sense (and in particular to advertise it) must hold a Product Licence relating to that product. The criteria which are considered by the Licensing Authority when determining an application for a licence include in particular the safety, efficacy and quality of the product. The cost and comparative efficacy of the product may not be considered. The licence when granted is conditional on compliance with certain standard provisions given in Statutory Instrument 1971:972 as amended and with specific conditions including the indications for which the product may be promoted, its recommended dosage, where it may be manufactured and the specification with which it must conform during its shelf life. Thus a licence closely defines the product and changes may only be introduced with the approval of the Licensing Authority.

If the product contains a chemical substance not previously used in a licensed product the application is always referred for consideration by the CSM and its expert sub-committees. Much more numerous are the abridged applications where the chemical substance has been used before in a licensed product and its safety and efficacy are already established. The main assessment required is of the specific indications to be claimed and of the quality of the product. This assessment is usually made entirely by the professional staff of the MCA, who may seek further information from the applicant before being satisfied that a licence may be granted. Reference is made to the CSM for advice on any novel issue or, as required by law, if it is proposed to refuse the application. There are several levels of appeal against a rejection, up to the Medicines Commission (see 'Guide to the Licensing System' [1988].

The text of labels, package inserts and any data sheet are also assessed. A licensed product must display its product licence number on the label and in literature. Thus the presence of the PL number differentiates licensed products from unlicensed. Licenses are renewable usually at five yearly intervals. There is a general requirement on the licence holder to apply to vary the licence in order to maintain certain technical attributes, such as the analytical methods used for quality control, comparable to the 'state of the art'. Licence holders are required to notify the Licensing Authority of any information which casts doubts on the continued validity of the data submitted to support the quality, safety or efficacy of the product and of any decision to recall products. They must also keep and make available any records of reports of adverse reactions to their products.

The data required to support an application for a Product Licence are determined largely by EC rules and are outlined in Section 15.4.3.

15.2.3 Product Licences of Right

When licensing was introduced in the United Kingdom in 1971 products already on the market were entitled to Product Licences of Right (PLR). These were granted without consideration of safety, efficacy or quality but were subject to review at any time by the then established Committee on Review of Medicines.

The review of all PLRs of products then covered by EC pharmaceutical directives was completed by the end of 1990. The review of radiopharmaceutical products must be completed by 31 December 1992 (see Section 15.4.3).

15.2.4 Clinical Trial Certificates and Clinical Trial Exemption Scheme

A clinical trial is performed primarily to determine what effects a product has in man when there is evidence that these may be beneficial. It is usually organised by a company wishing to obtain data to support a product licence application or variation. In these circumstances the supply of the product must be authorised either by a product licence, a clinical trial certificate (CTC) or under the clinical trial exemption (CTX) scheme. The supplier makes application, referring to data to support the safety and quality of the product and its likely benefit or utility. For novel or complex products applications must be made for a CTC and the full data assessed by the Licensing Authority. In the majority of cases application may be made for consideration under the CTX scheme and only a summary of the data and conclusions need be submitted. The CTX is allowed unless the Licensing Authority raises an objection within a short period (see 'Guide to the Licensing System' [1988]) Certificates and exemptions are subject to certain conditions which the holder must draw to the attention of the practitioner conducting the trial.

15.2.5 Doctors' and Dentists' Exemption Scheme

If a practitioner, rather than a supplier, wishes to initiate a clinical trial using an unlicensed product he may only lawfully be supplied with the product if it is prepared under the supervision of a pharmacist in a registered pharmacy, hospital or health centre or if it is supplied in accordance with the Doctors' and Dentists' Exemption Scheme (DDX). (See 'A Guide to the Provisions Affecting Doctors and Dentists', 1985). To use the DDX scheme the practitioner must notify the Licensing Authority and provide details of the product, the trial and the supplier. In the absence of an objection from the Authority within 21 days the trial may take place. An objection would be raised if the Authority knows of a safety hazard of which the practitioner is unlikely to aware, but this in no way reduces the responsibility of the practitioner concerned.

15.2.6 Exemptions for Supply to Particular Patients ('Specials')

Apart from the arrangements designed to permit the supply of unlicensed products for clinical trials conducted on behalf of suppliers (CTC or CTX) or practitioners (DDX), Section 9 of the Medicines Act allows a doctor either to prepare himself or to obtain an unlicensed product for administration to a particular patient of his or hers. In this situation the Licensing Authority may have made no assessment of the safety, efficacy and quality of the product or may have assessed these matters and found the evidence incomplete or otherwise unsatisfactory. The practitioner prescribes the unlicensed product entirely on his own responsibility.

The supplier of the unlicensed product may only do so in response to a bona fide unsolicited order and the product may not be advertised. The order need not name the patient concerned so the common term 'named patient exemption' is a misnomer; however the supplier should satisfy himself that an 'audit trail' could be established back to the patient if necessary. If the product is made in the United Kingdom this must either be under the supervision of a pharmacist in a registered pharmacy, hospital or health centre (see 15.2.9) or by a manufacturer holding a 'Specials' Manufacturing Licence. (See 'Special Dispensing Services' 1972). If the product is imported this may be to the order of a doctor for adminsitration to a particular patient of his under Section 13 of the Act, or it may be imported in the absence of an order under the terms of the Medicines (Exemptions from Licences) (Importation) Order 1984. In the latter case the importer must notify the Licensing Authority in advance and the quantity which may be imported on each occasion is limited to not more than 25 doses or courses of treatment.

15.2.7 Licences for Manufacture, Wholesale Dealing and Importing

The Medicines Act also requires anyone in the United Kingdom who manufactures, wholesales or imports medicinal products to hold the relevant licence (see Applications for Manufacturer's Ordinary Licences 1990). Before a licence is granted the quality management system of the applicant, including the facilities provided and the procedures to be followed for production, quality control and storage, is assessed by Medicines Inspectors of MCA against the standard provisions for licences as amended. The latest (1992) amendment to these 1971 Regulations has the significant addition of requiring compliance with the principles of Good Manufacturing Practice (GMP) as interpreted in Volume IV of The Rules Governing Medicinal Products in the EC: the Guide to Good Manufacturing Practice. The 1992 reprint of the 'Guide' includes an annex on the manufacture of radiopharmaceuticals.

A Manufacturer's Ordinary Licence (ML) is required if licensed products are to be made. If the unlicensed products mentioned above (section 15.2.6) are to be made, a Manufacturer's ('Specials') Licence must be held. Many manufacturers hold both types of licence. When manufacture occurs overseas the Licensing Authority still requires assurance that production and quality control complies with GMP before granting a Product Licence. For countries within the EC or the Pharmaceutical Inspection Convention (PIC) sufficient assurance can be obtained from the relevant regulatory authority but when manufacture occurs in a third country the UK Inspectors will inspect the manufacturing site.

Wholesale dealing may be considered as the supply of products by one organisation (legal entity) to another organisation for the purpose of further sale or supply. A Wholesale Dealer's Licence (WL) is required to wholesale medicinal products, except that (a) the holder of a ML does not require a WL to supply the products he has made and (b) a registered pharmacy is allowed to wholesale up to 5% by value of the total medicinal products purchased without holding a WL. If products are imported from outside the EC a Wholesale Dealer's (Import) Licence is required. To obtain and maintain a WL the requirements of good pharmaceutical wholesaling practice described in the Guide to Good Pharmaceutical Manufacturing Practice (1983) should be met.

Inspectors are required to inspect sites routinely after licences have been granted in order to ensure that standards are maintained and the provisions in product licences relating to production and quality control are followed.

15.2.8 The 'Qualified Person'

One of the standard provisions of a Manufacturer's Ordinary or a Wholesale Dealer's (Import) Licence is that the licence holder has 'permanently and continuously at his disposal' the services of a 'Qualified Person' as defined in Article 23 or 24 of Directive 75/319/EEC. The Qualified Person is named on the Licence. The duties of the Qualified Person include ensuring that each batch of medicinal product has been manufactured in accordance with GMP and with the details in the Product Licence. In the case of products imported from outside the EC the Qualified Person must ensure that each batch has been fully tested in the importing country and found to comply with its Product Licence. In both cases the Qualified Person must certify the batch record before the batch may be released.

The Licensing Authority has delegated to the three professional bodies, the Institute of Biology, the Royal Pharmaceutical Society and the Royal Society of Chemistry, the tasks of assessing the eligibility of their members to be Qualified Persons and of maintaining a register of these persons. The three bodies have also produced, in consultation with the MCA, a Study Guide and a Code of Conduct for Qualified Persons. The Licensing Authority expects Qualified Persons to adhere to this Code and a disciplinary procedure may be followed if gross breaches occur.

There is no requirement or possibility for a Qualified Person to be named as such on a Manufacturer's ('Specials') Licence because this does not authorise the manufacture of licensed products; neither does working on the manufacture of 'Specials' count as qualifying experience towards becoming a Qualified Person for the same reason.

15.2.9 Production Within the National Health Service

Since the removal of 'Crown Immunity' for the NHS on 1 April 1991, the preparation and supply of medicinal products by Health Authorities has been subject to all the requirements of the Medicines Act. The arrangements are described in a Mdeicines Act Advisory Leaflet (MAL 1992). If a Health Authority wishes to make a market a product in the fullest sense it must obtain a Product and a Manufacturer's Licence to cover this activity. More usually a radiopharmacy will prepare unlicensed products under one of the following arrangements:

either (a) the radiopharmacy holds a Manufacturer's 'Specials' Licence:

or (b) the radiopharmacy operates under the exemption for hospitals or registered pharmacies in Section 10 of the Medicines Act.

To hold a 'Specials' Licence the radiopharmacy must comply with the relevant good manufacturing practices and have the persons responsible for production and quality control named on the licence. As there is no licensed product involved there is no requirement for a 'Qualified Person'. There is also no specific requirement for the direct involvement of a pharmacist, although a source of pharmaceutical expertise is almost certainly required in order to comply with GMP. The operation will of course be inspected routinely by the Medicines Inspectorate.

To operate under a Section 10 exemption the operation must be under the supervision of a pharmacist. No application for exemption is required and the Medicines Inspectorate is not involved. Operation in this way may be more appropriate for relatively small scale of preparation and local distribution.

15.2.10 Administration of Radioactive Substances

Section 60 of the Medicines Act enables the Health Ministers to make regulations requiring practitioners to hold certificates to administer certain classes of products where this administration requires specialised knowledge. Such regulations are the Medicines (Administration of Radioactive Substances) Regulations 1978. A doctor or dentist who wishes to use a radioactive medicinal product in man must hold a certificate, which specifies the products concerned and the purposes for which they may be administered, or he must be acting in accordance with the directions of such a person.

An application for a certificate should include details of the experience and qualifications of the applicant, the products to be administered, the purpose of administration and the equipment, staff and other facilities available for the preparation, storage, dosimetry and administration of the product and for patient monitoring. The Radiation Protection Adviser is required to sign the application confirming that acceptable arrangements exist for dealing with contamination accidents. Certificates usually remain in force for a period of 5 years and towards the end of this period an application for renewal, if required, must be made.

The Administration of Radioactive Substances Advisory Committee (ARSAC) has been appointed to advise Ministers on matters relating to the certification scheme. Under a medical chairman the Committee is comprised of people with wide and recent relevant experience and has included physicists, pharmacists and radiographers in addition to clinicians. The Committee usually meets twice a year and advises both on individual applications and on matters of general principle such as the experience to be expected in a successful applicant or the nature of the support facilities required. Notes for Guidance (1984) plus an updated supplement (1986), agreed by ARSAC, have been issued to assist applicants. (A revision is planned during 1992). In particular when an applicant wishes to use a diagnostic product in a manner listed in the Notes a simple reference to the Notes is sufficient. For unlisted products the application should include full details of the investigation and estimates of dosimetry for the maximum usual activities proposed. If the use is for research, information is expected on the purpose, size and design of the study and on whether the permission of the local Ethical Committee has been sought (Bourdillon *et al.*, 1983). The activity to be administered for therapy is not expected to be stated in an application as this is considered to be a matter entirely for clinical judgement. The Regulations do not cover the use of nuclear powered pacemakers or teletherapy apparatus.

When applications for product licences are being considered by the Licensing Authority the ARSAC recommendations on dosage and use are borne in mind so that any conflict between these and the indications and dosage defined in the licence is avoided.

15.3 THE HEALTH AND SAFETY AT WORK ETC. ACT 1974

15.3.1 Introduction

The Health and Safety at Work etc. Act 1974 (HSW Act) lays down general duties on employers, employed persons, manfucturers and others to ensure the safety both of work people and those affected by work activities. Failure to comply with those duties consitutes an offence in criminal law. The Act applies to all kinds of work with the sole exception of domestic work in the home.

15.3.2 Duties on Employers to Their Employees

An employer must ensure so far as is reasonably practicable the health, safety and welfare at work of all his employees. This duty extends to include safe equipment and systems of work; safety in the use, handling, storage and transport of articles and substances; providing information, instruction, training and supervision; keeping places of work safe including the means of access and egress; and providing a safe and adequate working environment.

Employers, unless they employ fewer than five employees, have to draw up a written statement of their safety policy which includes the arrangements for carrying out that policy. They must consult the trades union safety representatives and must set up safety committees if the safety representatives so wish.

15.3.3 Duties on Employers and Self Employed to Non-Employees

Employers and the self employed have a duty to conduct their work in such a way as to ensure so far as is reasonably practicable that persons not in their employment are not exposed to risk to their health and safety. The self employed have a similar duty to protect themselves.

15.3.4 Duties on Those in Control of Premises

Where people use premises as a place of work or a place to use equipment or substances provided there, the person in control of the premises has a duty to ensure so far as it reasonably practicable that the premises are safe, including the means of access and egress and that the equipment or the substances provided are safe and without risks to health.

15.3.5 Duties on Manufacturers etc.

Section 6 of the HSW Act, which was substantially modified by the Consumer Protection Act 1987, places duties on designers, manufacturers, importers and suppliers of articles for use at work. The duties cover safety in the design and construction of such articles, the testing and examination of them and the provision of adequate information to the user to ensure safety. It requires designers and manufacturers to carry out research into the safety of articles and places duties on those who erect or install articles for use at work to ensure, so far as it is reasonably practicable, that nothing about the way they are erected or installed makes them unsafe or a risk to health.

The Section also places similar duties on the manufacturers, importers and suppliers of substances with a view to ensuring so far as is reasonably practicable that substances will be safe and without risks to health to those at work who use, handle, process store or transport them.

15.3.6 Duties on Employees at Work

The Act places duties on employees to take reasonable care for the health and safety of themselves and of others affected by what they do at work. They are required to cooperate with their employers to enable the latter to discharge their own statutory duties.

15.3.7 The Health and Safety Commission and the Health and Safety Executive

The HSW Act established two bodies – The Health and Safety Commission (HSC) and the Health and Safety Executive (HSE).

The general functions of HSC, which consists of a full time chairman and nine part-time members, include the promotion of health, safety and welfare of persons at work and the protection of others against risks arising from work activities. Its duties extend to carrying out research and providing training, information and advice on health and safety matters. It is also responsible for drawing up proposals for regulations and for approving codes of practice.

The HSE is a body consisting of three persons appointed by the HSC. It is responsible for enforcing the general duties of the HSW Act and of a range of health and safety legislation referred to as the 'relevant statutory provisions'. These include acts and regulations made before the HSW Act was passed and also the regulations which have been made subsequently using the powers of the HSW Act. There are a number of inspectorates employed by the HSE. These are the Factory Inspectorate, the Agricultural Inspectorate, the Mines and Quarries Inspectorate, the Nuclear Installations Inspectorate and the Explosives Inspectorate. Inspectors appointed under the HSW act have wide ranging powers to enable them to enforce the relevant statutory provisions in the premises which they inspect. These powers include powers of entry, powers to carry out investigations including taking samples, measurements, photographs, etc. and powers to issue notices for requiring dangerous activities to be stopped (prohibition notices) or requiring contraventions of the law to be remedied within a specified period of time (improvement notices). In England and Wales, inspectors are empowered to prosecute in a magistrate's court for offences under the relevant statutory provisions.

15.3.8 Local Authorities

Besides the HSE, local authorities are charged with enforcing the relevant statutory provisions in certain types of premises. These are mainly premises such as offices, shops, hotels and restaurants, and places of entertainment. Local authorities appoint their own inspectors, who have similar powers to those of the HSE.

15.3.9 The Ionising Radiations Regulations 1985

There are three main reasons for introducing the Ionising Radiations Regulations 1985 (IRR 1985)

(a) *The HSW Act*

Prior to the HSW Act, there was a wide range of piecemeal legislation for health and safety. There were requirements which applied in factories; different requirements applied in offices and shops, in mines and quarries, etc; and a large number of work places had no health and safety legislation in force at all. It was an express purpose of the HSW Act for all this pre-existing legislation to be progressively replaced by a system of regulations and approved codes of practice. This system would be designed to maintain or improve standards of health, safety and welfare at work.

In the case of protection against ionising radiations there were regulations which applied in factories, and voluntary codes of practice in hospitals, research establishments, etc. These codes of practice had no statutory force and there were therefore no penalties for failing to follow the advice they contained. All these regulations and codes were therefore replaced by a comprehensive set of regulations applying to all work activities in which there was a hazard from exposure to ionising radiations and radioactive substances.

(b) *Euratom Directives*

As a consequence of joining the European Communities the UK became subject to European legislation, including directives made under the terms of the treaties. The Euratom treaty requires the laying down by directive of the basic safety standards for the protection of workers and the general public against risks arising from ionising radiations. Members states are obliged to put such directives into effect, although the means whereby they are put into effect is up to individual states to decide.

The latest Euratom directive is that of 1980 as amended by an amending directive in 1984. Most of the provisions in the directive cover the protection of workers and those affected by work activities. In Great Britain these provisions are put into effect by the IRR 1985.

(c) *International Commission on Radiological Protection*

All the regulations and voluntary codes of practice for protection against ionising radiations (see para 15.3.9 (a) above) were based on the recommendations of the International Commission on Radiological Protection (ICRP). In 1977 ICRP published new recommendations which replaced those issued previously. As a consequence the provisions which applied in the UK were out of date in that they did not reflect the ICRP's latest recommendations. Consequently, even without the constraints of the HSW Act and of the Euratom directive,'there would have been pressure to replace the regulations and codes with new provisions based on the 1977 ICRP recommendations.

15.3.10 Regulations and Guidance

In 1985 therefore the IRR 1985 were made by the Secretary of State for Employment, having been proposed by the HSC. They were laid before parliament on the 4th September 1985 and came fully into operation on the 1st January 1986. At the same time, the HSC approved a code of practice entitled 'The Protection of Persons Against Ionising Radiation Arising from any Work Activity'(1985). The purpose of the code of practice is to give practical guidance on ways of complying with the IRR 1985.

An 'approved' code of practice has a special significance in law when it comes to criminal proceedings. Failure to comply with the code is not in itself an offence. However such a failure can be used as evidence that the relevant regulation has been contravened. It would be necessary for the defence to show that the regulation had been complied with in a different way.

In addition to the regulations and approved code of practice, there a number of guidance documents available which are designed to help those engaged in work with ionising radiation to carry out that work in accordance with good radiation protection practice. The guidance documents do not have any legal force but they are generally consistent with regulatory requirements. Following the guidance will normally ensure that the legal requirements are observed. In the fields of radiopharmacy and nuclear medicine, as with other medical applications of ionising radiations, the relevant guidance is given in 'Guidance Notes for the Protection of Persons Against Ionising Radiation Arising from Medical and Dental Use' (1988).

What follows is a description of some of the requirements of the IRR 1985 which are particularly relevant to radiopharmacy work and nuclear medicine. It is not however intended as a comprehensive guide and anyone who has a need to comply with the regulations should consult the regulations themselves and the guidance mentioned above, or they should seek the advice of a radiation protection adviser.

15.3.11 Arrangement of Regulations

The reglations are arranged in groups or 'parts'. Within each part is a number of regulations which have a common purpose. There are in all 41 regulations arranged in nine parts. Finally there are 10 schedules of information relevant to specific regulations.

15.3.12 Part I – Interpretation and General

Regulation 2 contains definitions of certain terms which have a particular meaning in the regulations. In reading the regulations it is necessary to be aware of these definitions, and the other paragraphs of regulation 2. This is because the intention of particular regulations can otherwise be misunderstood. Perhaps the most important is the term 'work with ionising radiation'. This defines the processes to which the regulations are relevant. These include any work involving radioactive substances or the operation or use of radiation generators. Similarly, 'radioactive substance' and 'radiation generator' are defined in regulation 2.

Regulation 4 places an obligation on employers to cooperate with one another in situations where the work done by one employer affects the employees of another. This can happen for example if a maintenance contractor comes into the department to do work on the drains used for the disposal of radioactive waste. The contractor must be informed of the possible hazards from contamination and advised of any necessary precautions.

Work with ionising radiation is required to be notified to the HSE under regulation 5. The details that have to be notified are listed in schedule 4, and HSE has power to ask for further information – listed in schedule 5 – if it so decides. There are exceptions to the notification requirement and these are listed in schedule 3. Among these exceptions is where the only work with ionising radiation is caring for persons to whom a radioactive medicinal product has been administered. This means that if a hospital receives patients who have been treated with a radioactive substance at another centre, that hospital does not have to notify HSE under this regulation.

15.3.13 Part II – Dose Limitation

The ICRP recommendations (see section 15.3.9) are based on three main principles, often referred to as justification, optimisation and dose limits. The justification principle, that is, no practice involving exposure of persons to ionising radiation should be adopted unless there is a positive net benefit, is not explicitly included in the regulations. Rather the regulations are intended to control the risks from ionising radiation arising from a work activity. They do not bear on the decision whether or not the work activity should be permitted to take place. However, it is argued in the preface to the approved code of practice that the optimisation principle can be taken to the extent of questioning the justification of a practice involving exposure to ionising radiation.

The optimisation principle (all exposures should be kept as low as reasonably achievable, economic and social factors being taken into account) is reflected in regulation 6 (restriction of exposure). This regulation places an obligation on employers (and the self employed) who undertake work with ionising radiation to take all necessary steps to restrict, so far as is reasonably practicable, the exposure of employees and others. The regulation goes on to prohibit the handling of sealed sources directly by hand, and this applies also so far as is reasonably practicable to unsealed sources and to articles containing radioactive substances. Finally there is a prohibition on eating, drinking, smoking etc. in working areas where there is likely to be contamination.

Guidance on the necessary steps to take to restrict exposure in accordance with this regulation is given in the approved code of practice. General guidance is given in part 1 of the approved code, paras 8–27. Part 2 of the approved code is devoted entirely to giving guidance on ways to comply with this regulation as it applies to particular processes. In the second part there is a section on radioactive substances used in or on the body. The purpose of the section is to provide guidance on the radiation protection of any person who comes near to a patient undergoing diagnostic procedures or radiotherapy with radioactive substances.

15.3.14 Part III – Regulation of Work with Ionising Radiation

Regulation 8 requires the designation of controlled and supervised areas in the work place. Controlled areas are areas where doses are likely to exceed 3/10 of the dose limits for adult employees. Supervised areas are the remaining areas where doses are likely to exceed 1/10 of those limits.

Controlled areas have to be physically demarcated and access must be controlled. Entry to controlled areas is confined to classified persons and to those who enter a written system of work designed to keep the dose received below 3/10 of the dose limit. Furthermore, where a written system of work is operated there must be monitoring to demonstrate that it is being effective.

In order to decide on the need for an area to be designated in this way, reference should be made to schedule 6 of the regulations. This sets out criteria for designation of controlled areas on the basis of radiation dose rates, levels of airborne or surface contamination, quantities of radioactive substances present and so on. There is guidance on the design and equipment requirements for areas in which radioactive substances are used in the Guidance Notes for the protection of persons against Ionising Radiations arising from Medical and Dental Use, Chapter 10.

Persons who are likely to receive doses greater than 3/10 of the dose limits must be designated classified persons under regulation 9. Only adults who are certified by an appointed doctor or employment medical adviser as being fit may be classified persons.

Employers are normally required by regulation 10 to appoint a suitably qualified and experienced person to be a radiation protection adviser (RPA). They must make written local rules, and must ensure that the work with ionising radiation is supervised by a radiation protection supervisor (RPS) whom they must appoint. The RPA may be appointed from outside the department, but the RPS must be one of the employees. Regulation 12 requires that information, instruction and training should be provided for employees, trainees and others. This includes information to women employees about the possible hazards from ionising radiation during pregnancy.

15.3.15 Part IV – Dosimetry and medical Surveillance

The provisions of this part of the regulations are mainly concerned with classified persons. They include the requirement to measure all significant doses of ionising radiation received and to keep dose records. These requirements for dosimetry are contained in regulation 13, which makes it obligatory to use an approved dosimetry service, approved that is by HSE.

All classified persons must be under adequate medical surveillance by an employment medical adviser or appointed doctor. 'Adequate' medical surveillance is elucidated in the approved code of practice. It includes a pre-employment medical examination and periodic reviews of health. The doctor must certify in a health record that the person is fit (or otherwise) to be engaged as a classified person. However, regulation 16 provides a right of appeal for the person who is aggrieved by the decision of the employment medical adviser or appointed doctor.

15.3.16 Part V – Arrangements for the Control of Radioactive Substances

This part includes four regulations aimed at the safe keeping of radioactive substances, together with a further two on the provision and maintenance of washing and changing facilities and on personal protective equipment. Whenever reasonably practicable, radioactive substances should be used in the form of a sealed source built in such a way as to prevent leakage. Tests for leakage have to be carried out at periodic intervals.

Regulation 19 requires steps to be taken to account for and keep records of all radioactive substances. Regulation 20 is about storage arrangements and regulation 21 is concerned with transport and moving of radioactive substances. Both requirements refer to the provision of suitable receptacles.

Adequate washing and changing facilities must be provided for persons entering and leaving controlled areas where there is a risk of contamination. The approved code of practice (paras 133–136 of part 1) gives advice on what facilities are considered to be adequate.

15.3.17 Part VI – Monitoring

Since the only way to detect the presence of radiation or of contamination is by the use of some kind of monitoring instrument, it is most important that a suitable programme of monitoring be drawn up. Part VI of the regulations consists of a single regulation on the monitoring of levels of radiation and of contamination. The requirement is for adequate monitoring for each controlled area or supervised area, the objective being to ascertain the efficacy of the precautions being used. The results of this monitoring must be recorded. It is important that persons who are required to carry out this monitoring are trained to be able to do it properly and to understand the significance of the results obtained.

Regulation 24 goes on to consider the equipment used for monitoring. This is subject to a regime of examination and testing by a qualified person appointed by the employer.

15.3.18 Part VII – Assessment and Notifications

This part is concerned with what could go wrong during work with ionising radiation: identifying what hazards can arise out of accidents and incidents and being prepared for them. This applies to any work with ionising radiation at whatever level. However in the case of users of large amounts of radioactivity, a special hazard assessment is required with a report which is sent to HSE. If the assessment of hazard shows that an accident could lead to overexposure, then the employer must draw up contingency plans to cope with the accident should it occur.

Regulation 28 requires a formal investigation to be carried out if any employee receives a dose exceeding 3/10 of the dose limit in a year. The purpose of the investigation is to determine whether all necessary steps have been taken to restrict exposure as required by regulation 6. In the event of actual or suspected exposure beyond the dose limits there are further investigation requirements, and requirements to notify HSE and others of the occurrence. Regulation 31 contains further notification requirements in the event of releases, spills or losses or radioactive substances.

15.3.19 Part VIII – Safety of Articles and Equipment

Section 6 of the Health and Safety at Work etc. Act 1974, as modified by the Consumer Protection Act 1987, places duties on manufacturers and others concerning the safety of articles for use at work. This duty is extended by regulation 32 to include a duty to ensure that such articles are designed and constructed so as to restrict exposure to ionising radiation. The regulation also provides for new installations to be subject to a critical examination by an RPA to ensure that the safety features and warning devices operate correctly and that there is sufficient protection from ionising radiation.

Regulation 33 is concerned with equipment used for medical exposure. Any equipment used in connection with medical exposure must be designed to restrict the exposure of the person undergoing the exposure to the extent that this is compatible with the purpose of the exposure. Any incident whereby a malfunction or defect in radiation equipment leads to the person undergoing the medical exposure receiving a dose much greater than intended must be notified to HSE.

Regulation 34 prohibits the misues of or interference with sources of ionising radiation.

15.3.20 Part XI – Miscellaneous and General

The final part of the regulations brings together various provisions such as exemption certificates, extensions of the scope of the regulations outside Great Britain, transitional provisions, and modifications for the Ministry of Defence.

15.3.21 New ICRP Recommendations

The recommendations of the ICRP have recently been revised and were published as the 1990 Recommendations of the International Commission on Radiological Protection. There are a number of important changes in these latest recommendations, including the use of new dose quantities for measurement, reduced dose limits, and the introduction of dose constraints below the dose limits. At the present time the EC is engaged in revising the basic safety standards directive (see 15.3.9(b)) in the light of these new ICRP recommendations. A new Euratom directive will lead in due course to the revision of IRR 1985.

Meanwhile, to take account of the higher risk estimates for exposure to ionising radiations which are explained in the ICRP publication, in 1991 the HSC approved additional guidance on the restriction of exposure to ionising radiations.

This fourth part of the Approved Code of Practice on the Ionising Radiations Regulations 1985 has two main thrusts:

(a) Employers should review the decisions which were made previously about the restriction of exposure, and perhaps take steps to further restrict that exposure.
(b) Employers should conduct a special investigation whenever an employee reaches a recorded cumulative total of 75 mSv or more within any five years after 1 January 1988. The investigation would be centred round that employee and would be aimed at reaching an acceptable strategy for the future exposure of that employee to ionising radiations.

15.4 THE EUROPEAN COMMUNITY

15.4.1 General

The United Kingdom is required as a member of the EC to adapt its national legislation to comply with the Community obligations arising from the EC Directives. If there is a conflict between national legislation and a Directive, or in the absence of a national law, the Directive will prevail. Radioactive medicinal products are subject to obligations arising from Euratom Directives and Pharmaceutical Directives; UK laws and administrative arrangements have been introduced or adapted in order to comply with these.

15.4.2 Euratom Directives

Directive 80/836/Euratom, as amended by 84/467, requires member states to have a system of prior authorisation with respect to radioactive substances. Article 5a of the Directive requires prior authorisation to administer a radioactive substance for the purpose of diagnosis, treatment or research. In the United Kingdom this requirement is met by the Medicines (Administration of Radioactive Substances) Regulations (see section 15.2.10). Article 5c requires prior authorisation for the importation for commercial purposes and the preparation of medicinal products containing radioactive substances. This requirement is met in the United Kingdom by the licensing of manufacturers and importers under the Medicines Act.

Mention has already been made of Euratom directives in section 15.3.9 (b) as a reason for the introduction of the Ionising Radiations Regulations 1985.

15.4.3 Pharmaceutical Directives

The first Pharmaceutical Directive 65/65/EEC, as amended, requires a marketing authorisation (A Product Licence in the UK) to be held for medicinal products marketed within the Community. Certain classes of products, including radiopharmaceuticals, were exempted until recently from the scope of this Directive by Article 34 of Directive 75/319/EEC so there was no Community requirement, as opposed to a UK requirement, for a radiopharmaceutical to have a marketing authorisation. This exemption was removed by the Extension Directive 89/343/EEC, for new products with effect from the end of 1991 and for all existing products not later than the end of 1992. (An exception to this general exemption was that any product of biotechnology, which includes some radiopharmaceuticals, was already required by Directive 87/22/EEC to have a marketing authorisation after assessment under the centralised procedure referred to below).

The requirement for a marketing authorisation applies to generators, kits, precursor radiopharmaceuticals and industrially prepared radiopharmaceuticals. Products prepared in a hospital from these authorised generators, kits or precursor radiopharmaceuticals do not themselves need a marketing authorisation provided they are made in accordance with the manufacturer's instructions at the time of use by a person authorised to use them.

The data required to support an application for a marketing authorisation was agreed by the EC Committee for Proprietary Medicinal Products (CPMP) and is specified in technical Directive 91/507/EEC. This updates and largely replaces Directive 75/318/EEC, mostly with effect from 1 January 1992. Guidance on how to apply for a marketing authorisation is given in Volume II of the Rules Governing Medicinal Products in the European Community: Notice to Applicants and in the amendments applicable to radiopharmaceuticals adopted in October 1991. Guidance on the data required to support an application is given in Volume III of the Rules and its Addendum 1991; additional guidance has been agreed by the CPMP for radiopharmaceuticals (published in Pharmacology and Toxicology, *68*, 228–232, 1991) and for radiopharmaceuticals based on monoclonal antibodies (published in Pharmacology and Toxicology, *69*, 212–222, 1991). The text of all the pharmaceutical Directives is given in Volume I of the Rules.

In order to facilitate the application of the new requirements to many existing radiopharmaceuticals a harmonised procedure has been agreed between the regulatory authorities and industry for the submission of quality-related data and Summaries of Product Characteristics to all involved member states.

Manufacturers within the EC are required by Directive 75/319/EEC as amended by 89/341/EEC to comply with Good Manufacturing Practice. Directive 91/356/EEC states the principles and guidelines of GMP and in addition requires importers in the EC to ensure that their manufacturers in third countries also comply with standards of GMP at least equivalent to those in the EC. Volume IV of the Rules: The Guide to Good Manufacturing Practice gives detailed guidance and includes an annex of additional guidance for the manufacture of radiopharmacteuticals. The official status of the Guide is as interpretation of the GMP Directive and within the UK it replaces the DHSS 'Orange Guide'.

15.5 THE PREPARATION AND SUPPLY OF RADIOPHARMACEUTICALS IN THE NATIONAL HEALTH SERVICE

15.5.1 General

Because of training, background and professional contacts the radiopharmacist is the ideal person in the health service to be involved in the purchase and distribution of radiopharmaceuticals, their preparation from purchased kits or their production when necessary from primary starting materials and their quality control. He or she should ensure compliance with the requirements of the Health and Safety at Work etc Act 1974, the Ionising Radiations Regulations 1985 and the Medicines Act 1968 which are relevant to the local work area and that the principles of the codes of practice and guidelines are followed. In so far as is possible the detail of any guidance should also be adhered to unless it can be argued that an alternative gives at least equally satisfactory results. When the preparation is done in an establishment with a Manufacturer's Licence seperate persons must be designated as responsible for 'Production' and 'Quality Control'. When the licence is not for 'Specials' (unusual within the NHS – see section 15.2.9) a designated 'Qualified Person' must also contribute to the batch release procedure.

As has been shown, the statutory requirements and the accompanying guidance relating to radiopharmaceuticals come from several sources, cover many situations and may be enforced by a variety of officials each concerned primarily with his or her own duties. The responsibility for determining what is relevant and what needs to be done in any particular work situation rest with the staff and management of the unit.

When in doubt, and in particular in view of the changes under the Medicines Act at the time of writing, advice should be sought from the relevant regulatory body.

15.5.2 Preparation

The unit in which radiopharmaceuticals are prepared, whether licensed or exempted under the Medicines Act, must also be listed on the certificate held by the practitioner who is responsible for administering the products. General guidance on the appropriate standards of premises, procedures and control relevant to the quality of the product are given in Volume IV of the Rules: the Guide to Good Manufacturing Practice (1992) and the Guidance Notes for Hospitals (1982), although it should be noted that the latter were written before contained workstations or isolators became generally available for use in radiopharmacies and use of these may modify the requirements. The latest advice may be obtained from the Medicines Inspectorate.

Guidance on radiation protection requirements including the use of contained workstations will be found in the Guidance Notes for the protection of persons against Ionising Radiations arising from Medical and Dental Use (1988).

15.5.3 Supply

When obtaining supplies of radiopharmaceuticals the person placing the order should be aware of whether or not the product is licensed. When an unlicensed product is required the supplier will need evidence with or in advance of the order that the product has been ordered by a practitioner for administration to a particular patient. Such orders may not be solicited, for example, by a commercial supplier, and the products may not be advertised.

If an unlicensed product is supplied by the radiopharmacy the fact that it is unlicensed should be brought to the attention of the person responsible for its administration. It would seem prudent to ensure that this person is aware of the significance of using unlicensed products and whether or not there is an alternative licensed product. No particular importance should be attached to a manufacturer's claim that an application has been made for a product licence. The MCA is not at liberty to divulge details of applications under assessment, or whether an application has been or is likely to be refused. As the requriement for radiopharmaceuticals to hold marketing authorisations (product licences) is extended throughout the EC by the end of 1992 the availability of unlicensed products in the UK is likely to decline.

When medicinal products are supplied form one Health Authority or Trust to another by way of wholesale dealing, a Wholesale Dealer's Licence may be requried (see section 15.2.7), depending on the seale and route of supply. A distinction may be made between supply to another body as stock or for administration; at the time of writing the arrangements have not been finalised.

15.5.4 Administration

The person administering a radioactive medicinal product to man must either hold a certificate issued by the Health Ministers in respect of the product, or be acting in accordance with the directions of a certificate holder. The radiopharmacy forms one of the support facilities which are described in the application for the certificate so any significant changes in the radiopharmacy should be drawn to the attention of the certificate holder and the DoH, in particular when application is made to renew the certificate.

15.5.5 Adverse Reactions and Defective Products

Those involved in the supply and administration of products should ensure that the Medicines Control Agency is made aware of any adverse patient reaction to a product (the 'Yellow Card' scheme) and of any suspected possible defect in the quality of a product (the Defect Reporting Scheme). The holder of a Manufacturer's or Product Licence under the Medicines Act is obliged to report such adverse ractions and product defects.

15.6 SUMMARY

The requirements of the Medicines Act 1968, the Health and Safety at Work etc Act 1974 and the Radioactive Substances Act 1960 impact the dispensing and supply of radiopharmaceuticals in many and various ways. The simple objective is to ensure that the patient only receives a safe, effective and consistent product and the workers and general public are not put at risk from ionising radiation.

The Medicines Act allow prescribers flexibility to use unlicensed products under certain circumstances, but it must be understood that these do not have the assurance of quality, safety and efficacy given to licensed products by the assessment and intervention of DoH staff and independent expert advisors, the arrangements for their manufacture and quality control when these are overseas or are manufactured under the exemption in Section 10 of the Medicines Act will not normally be audited by Medicines Inspectors, and there is not the statutory requirement to keep the MCA informed about doubts over their quality, safety or efficacy.

From 1 January 1992 the manufacture and supply of radiopharmaceuticals throughout the European Community has been subject to the Pharmaceutical Directives, as it has been for many years to the Euratom Directives. This change should have little effect in the United Kingdom on products which already have full product licences, but it will affect those with product licences or right and possibly the availability of previously unlicensed products from other member states.

The ending of 'Crown Immunity' for NHS units in 1991 necessitated other arrangements to comply with the Medicines Act and the Pharmaceutical and Euratom Directives.

REFERENCES

Medicines Act 1968. London, HMSO.
Health and Safety at Work etc Act 1974. London, HMSO.
The Medicines (Standard Provisions for Licences and Certificates) Regulations 1971. (SI 1971:972).
The Radioactive Substances Act 1960. London, HMSO.
Radioactive Substances Act 1960 – A Guide to the Administration of the Act; HMSO.
Guidance Notes on Applications for Product Licences (MAL 2) 1989. London, HMSO.
Guide to the Licensing System (MAL 1) 1988. London, DHSS.
A Guide to the Provisions Affecting Doctors and Dentists (MAL 30) 1985. London: DH.
Special Dispensing Services (MAL) 1972. London: DHSS.
The Medicines (Exemptions from Licences (Importation)) Order 1984. SI 1984:673.
Applications for Manufacturer's Ordinary Licences (MAL 5) 1990. London: DH.
Guide to Good Pharmaceutical Manufacturing Practice, 3rd edn. 1983. London, HMSO.
Health Services Circular (Interim Series) HSC (IS) 128, 1975. London: HMSO.
The Application of the Medicines Act to Health Authorities (MAL x): to be published during 1992 by DH, London.
Guidance Notes for Hospitals on the Premises and Environment for the Preparation of Radiopharmaceuticals 1982, (unpublished). London, DHSS.
The Medicines (Administration of Radioactive Substances) Regulations SI 1978/1006. London, HMSO.
Notes for Guidance on the Administration of Radioactive Substances to Persons for Purposes of Diagnosis, Treatment or Research. HN (84)5 1984. And Supplement. London, DHSS.
Bourdillon P.J., Godfrey B.E. and O'Brien R. (1983). *The Administration of Radioactive Substances* Radiological Protection Bulletin 53.
The Ionising Radiations Regulations 1985 – Statutory Instrument 1985 No. 1333. London: HMSO.
Health and Safety Commission (1985). *Approved Code of Practice – the protection of persons against ionising radiation arising from any work activity.* London, HMSO.
Health and Safety Commission (1991). *Approved code of Practice, Part 4 – 'Dose limitation – restriction of exposure; additional guidance on regulation 6 of the Ionising Radiations Regulations 1985'.*
Guidance notes for the protection of persons against ionising radiations arising from medical and dental use 1988. London, HMSO.
The Rules Governing Medicinal Products in the EC, the Commission for Official Publication of the European Communities, Luxembourg: – Vol I, The Rules Governing Medicinal Products for Human Use in the EC, 1991. – Vol II, Notice to Applicants, 1991. – Volume III, Guidelines to Quality, Safety or Efficacy of Medicinal Products, 1991. – Volume IV, Guide to Good Manufacturing Practice for Medicinal Products, 1992.

FURTHER READING

The control of Medicines in the United Kingdom of Great Britain and Northern Ireland (MAL 99) 1981. London, DHSS. (Under revision 1992).
The International Commission on Radiological Protection (1987). *Protection of the patient in nuclear medicine, ICRP publication 52 (Annals of the ICRP volume 17 No 4).* Pergamon Press.
International Commission on Radiological Protection (in press): *Radiation dose to patients from radiopharmaceuticals* (ICRP publication 53).
Guidelines for the Planning and Operation of a Radiopharmaceutical Service at a National and Local Level – proceeding of a WHO workshop for administrators in the field of radiopharmaceuticals, Copenhagen April 1987. Geneva 1988: WHO.

Chapter 16

Official and Non-Official Radiopharmaceuticals and Their Properties

P.J. Maltby

16.1 INTRODUCTION

Radiopharmaceuticals have been in use throughout the nuclear medicine community for approximately fifty years. In the early days of radiopharmacy (1950s–1960s) radiopharmaceuticals were generally prepared 'in-house' and were not regarded as true medicines. They were as often as not prepared on the open bench and proper quality testing was not officially encouraged. With the tragic events of the thalidomide disaster many nations took it upon themselves to introduce legislation for the proper preparation and testing of radioactive diagnostic and therapeutic agents and it was not until the Medicines Act of 1968 that proper standards of safety, quality and efficacy were laid down. With the advent of the portable generator system in the early 1960s fresh impetus was given to the development of chemical moieties which could be easily radiolabelled, and since those early years many routinely used radiopharmaceuticals have become the subject of official monographs.

This review will summarise the most commonly used official and non-official radiopharmaceuticals. It should be emphasised that although a product may be the subject of an official monograph it may not necessarily be available. As with all manufactured items market forces dictate their availability and official products may, from time to time, become unavailable. This may be particularly relevant in a clinical context as withdrawal of a product which has been in use for many years may lead to difficulty in selecting a suitable replacement.

On the subject of Produce Licences it should be emphasised that whether a radiopharmaceutical is official or not, the onus is on the pharmacist to check that the material is the subject of a Product Licence in the country of use. Also, the product must be used only for the clinical indication for which it is licensed. If it is not so licensed the burden of responsibility for any adverse effect falls on the pharmacist and/or clinician (see Chapter 14).

16.2 OFFICIAL RADIOPHARMACEUTICALS

Most of the routinely used official radiopharmaceuticals are listed below. Because of the difficulty of listing products from different pharmacopoeias in alphabetic sequence, products are shown in order of increasing mass number (in accordance with the method used by ARSAC). The list does not represent a complete description of all official radiopharmaceuticals but reflects those products which, in the opinion of the author, are likely to remain clinically useful in the forseeable future.

Sodium Phosphate [^{32}P] Injection B.P. E.P. U.S.P.

A sterile colourless solution of sodium and disodium orthophosphates containing phosphorous-32. It may contain sodium chloride and a buffer. Its specific activity is not less than 11.1 MBq per mg of orthophosphate ion.

pH:	5.0 to 8.0.
Storage:	Room temperature.
Clinical use:	Treatment of haemoproliferative disease.
Usual injected activity:	185 MBq.

Sodium Chromate [^{51}Cr] Injection B.P. E.P. U.S.P.

A sterile colourless solution of sodium chromate (^{51}Cr) made isotonic with sodium chloride. It has a specific activity of not less than 370 MBq per mg of chromate ion at expiry.

pH:	6.0 to 8.5.
Storage:	Room temperature.
Clinical use:	Red blood cell labelling agent.
Usual injected activity:	1–4 MBq.

Chromium [^{51}Cr] Edetate Injection [^{51}Cr-EDTA) B.P. E.P.

A sterile violet coloured solution containing chromium-51 in the form of a complex of Cr(III) with an excess amount of E.D.T.A. It may contain sodium chloride and a suitable antimicrobial preservative. It contains a variable amount of chromium (Cr) not exceeding 1 mg per ml, with a specific activity of 37–74 MBq per mg Cr at calibration.

pH:	3.5 to 6.5.
Storage:	Room temperature.
Clinical use:	Determination of glomerular filtration rate.
Usual injected activity:	4 MBq.

Cyanocobalamin [^{57}Co] and [^{58}Co] Solution B.P. E.P. U.S.P.

A colourless to slightly pink solution of cyanocobalamin labelled with cobalt-57 or cobalt-58 respectively and intended for oral administration. It may contain a stabiliser and antimicrobial preservatives. The specific activity is not less than 0.02 MBq per microgram of cyanocobalamin.

pH:	4.0 to 6.0.
Storage:	2°–8°C protected from light.
Clinical use:	Gastro-intestinal absorption tests.
Usual injected activity:	18.5 kBq.

N.B. These solutions may be incorporated into capsule formulations for oral administration.

Ferrous and Ferric [^{59}Fe] Citrate Injection B.P. U.S.P.

A sterile colourless solution containing iron-59 in the iron (II) or (III) state respectively, complexed with citrate ions, and includes sodium chloride. The specific activity is not less than 185 MBq or 37 MBq per mg. Fe respectively at calibration.

pH:	5.0 to 8.0.
Storage:	Room temperature.
Clinical use:	Measurement of iron absorption and utilization.
Usual injected activity:	0.4 MBq.

Gallium [^{67}Ga] Citrate Injection B.P. E.P. U.S.P.

A sterile, colourless, essentially carrier-free solution of gallium-67 citrate. It may contain sodium chloride and a suitable antimicrobial preservative.

pH:	4.5 to 8.0.
Storage:	Room temperature.
Clinical use:	Diagnosis of inflammation and infection; tumour visualization.
Usual injected activity:	111 MBq.

L-Selenomethionine [^{75}Se] Injection B.P. E.P. U.S.P.

A sterile, colourless solution of selenium-75 L-Selenomethionine (the analogue of methionine in which the S atom is replaced by an Se atom). It may contain sodium chloride, carrier methionine, suitable antioxidants and preservatives.

pH:	3.5 to 8.0.
Storage:	2°–10°C protected from light.
Clinical use:	Pancreas visualization.
Usual injected activity:	9.25 MBq.

Krypton [^{81m}Kr] gas U.S.P.

A gas suitable for inhalation obtained from a generator containing rubidium-81 adsorbed on an immobilised suitable column support. It is eluted by passage of humidified air or oxygen through the column.

Storage:	The generator is stored at room temperature.
Clinical use:	Lung ventilation studies.
Usual administered activity:	200 MBq/min for 3 mins.

Sodium Pertechnetate [^{99m}Tc] Injection B.P. E.P. U.S.P.

A sterile colourless solution containing sodium pertechnetate-99m made isotonic with sodium chloride. Technetium-99m is formed by the radioactive decay of molybdenum-99m, which may be produced either by neutron bombardment of stable molybdenum, or by uranium fission. Hence there are monographs for the injection produced by each method. The injection may be prepared by manipulation of a sterile preparation of molybdenum-99, under aseptic conditions.

pH:	4.0 to 8.0.
Storage:	Room temperature.
Clinical use:	For diagnostic imaging either by direct injection or after chelation to a range of organ specific pharmaceuticals.
Usual injected activity:	10 to 1000 MBq.

Technetium [^{99m}Tc] Albumin Injection B.P. E.P. U.S.P.

A sterile colourless to pale yellow solution containing human albumin labelled with technetium-99m. It may contain reducing agents, buffers and antimicrobial preservatives. The reducing agent, if tin, should not be present in a concentration exceeding 1 mg Sn per ml.

pH:	2.0 to 6.5.
Storage:	2°–8°C.
Clinical use:	Blood pool visualization.
Usual injected activity:	200 to 750 MBq.

Technetium [^{99m}Tc] Macrosalb Injection (Albumin Aggregated; MAA) B.P. E.P. U.S.P.

A sterile white suspension of albumin in the form of irregular aggregates of human albumin produced by heat denaturation: The particles are labelled with technetium-99m. It may contain reducing agents, antimicrobial agents, buffers and denatured human albumin. The reducing agent, if tin, should not be present in a concentration exceeding 3 mg Sn per ml.

Particle size:	The particle size of the suspension should be between 10 and 100 micrometers with no particle greater than 150 micrometers.
pH:	3.8 to 8.0.
Storage:	2°–8°C. Shake well before use.
Clinical use:	Lung perfusion studies.
Usual injected activity:	100 MBq.

Technetium [^{99m}Tc] Microspheres Injection B.P. E.P.

A sterile white, yellow or artificially coloured suspension of albumin in the form of spherical insoluble particles of human albumin produced by heat denaturation: The particles are labelled with technetium-99m. It may contain reducing agents, buffers and wetting agents. The reducing agent, if tin, should not be present in a concentration exceeding 3 mg Sn per ml. The radioactivity is not less than 185 MBq of ^{99m}Tc per 10^6 particles at the time of injection.

Particle size:	The particle size of the suspension should be between 10 and 50 micrometers.
pH:	4.0 to 9.0.
Storage:	2°–8°C.
Clinical use:	Long perfusion studies and isotope venography.
Usual injected activity:	100 MBq to 400 MBq.

Technetium [^{99m}Tc] Tin Pyrophosphate, and Pyrophosphate Injection B.P. E.P. U.S.P.

A sterile colourless solution of stannous pyrophosphate or sodium pyrophosphate respectively; labelled with technetium-99m. The former contains sodium pyrophosphate decahydrate varying in concentration from 1 to 50 mg per ml., with a tin content not greater than 3 mg Sn per ml. The latter may contain other reducing agents, antimicrobial agents, buffers and stabilizers.

pH:	4.0 to 7.5.
Storage:	2°–8°C.
Clinical use:	Myocardial and bone imaging agent.
Usual injected activity:	500 MBq.

Technetium [^{99m}Tc] Disofenin Injection (D.I.S.I.D.A.) U.S.P.

A sterile colourless solution of disofenin labelled with technetium-99m. It contains a suitable reducing agent.

pH:	5.8 to 6.6.
Storage:	Room temperature.
Clinical use:	Hepatobiliary imaging agent.
Usual injected activity:	100 MBq.

Technetium [^{99m}Tc] Etifenin Injection (E.H.I.D.A.) B.P. E.P.

A sterile colourless solution of etifenin labelled with technetium-99m, utilising stannous chloride as the reducing agent. The tin content should not exceed 0.2 mg Sn per ml.

pH:	4.0 to 6.0.
Storage:	Room temperature.
Clinical use:	Hepatobiliary imaging agent.
Usual injected activity:	100 MBq.

Technetium [^{99m}Tc] Medronate Injection (M.D.P.) B.P. E.P. U.S.P.

A sterile colourless solution of sodium medronate and a stannous salt labelled with technetium-99m. It may contain antimicrobial agents, antioxidants and buffers. The tin content should not exceed 3 mg Sn per ml.

pH:	3.5 to 7.8.
Storage:	Room temperature.
Clinical use:	Bone imaging agent.
Usual injected activity:	400 to 740 MBq.

Technetium [^{99m}Tc] Oxidronate Injection (H.D.P.) U.S.P.

A sterile colourless solution of sodium oxidronate labelled with technetium-99m. It contains a suitable reducing agent, and may contain buffers and preservatives.

pH:	2.5 to 7.0.
Storage:	Room temperature.
Clinical use:	Bone imaging agent.
Usual injected activity:	400 to 740 MBq.

Technetium [^{99m}Tc] Pentetate Injection (D.T.P.A.) B.P. E.P. U.S.P.

A sterile colourless or slightly yellow solution of sodium pentetate or calcium trisodium penetate complexed with technetium-99m. It contains a stannous salt as the reducing agent and may also contain antimicrobial preservatives, antioxidants and buffers. The tin content should not exceed 1 mg Sn per ml.

pH:	3.8 to 7.5.
Storage:	2°–25°C.
Clinical use:	Brain and renal imaging agent.
Usual injected activity:	100 to 800 MBq.

Technetium [^{99m}Tc] Gluceptate Injection (Glucoheptonate; G.H.A.) U.S.P.

A sterile colourless solution of sodium gluceptate labelled with technetium-99m. It may contain antimicrobial preservatives, antioxidants and buffers. The tin content should not exceed 1 mg Sn per ml.

pH:	3.8 to 7.5.
Storage:	2°–25°C.
Clinical use:	Brain and renal imaging agent.
Usual injected activity:	100 to 800 MBq.

Technetium [^{99m}Tc] Succimer Injection (D.M.S.A.) B.P. E.P. U.S.P.

A sterile colourless solution of succimer labelled with technetium-99m. It may contain stabilisers and antioxidants. The reducing agent, if tin, should be present in a concentration not exceeding 1 mg Sn per ml.

pH:	2.0 to 3.5.
Storage:	15°–30°C. Protected from light.
Clinical use:	Renal imaging agent.
Usual injected activity:	80 MBq.

Technetium [^{99m}Tc] Sulphur Colloid Injection B.P. E.P. U.S.P.

A sterile colloidal dispersion of sulphur, the micelles of which are labelled with technetium-99m. It is clear to opalescent and colourless to pale yellow. The colloid may be stabilised with a protecting substance. It may contain chelating agents and buffers. The particle size range of the dispersed colloid is 100 nanometers to 3 micrometers.

pH:	4.0 to 7.5.
Storage:	Room temperature.
Clinical use:	Liver imaging agent.
Usual injected activity:	100 MBq.

Technetium [^{99m}Tc] Antimony Sulphide Colloid Injection B.P. E.P.

A sterile colloidal dispersion of antimony sulphide, the micelles of which are labelled with technetium-99m. It is a clear orange liquid. The colloid is stabilised with pividone. It may contain a buffer. The antimony concentration should not exceed 0.2 mg Sb per ml. The particle size range of the dispersed colloid is from 3 to 50 nanometers.

pH:	4.0 to 7.0.
Storage:	Room temperature.
Clinical use:	Lymphoscintigraphic agent.
Usual injected activity:	40 MBq.

Technetium [^{99m}Tc] Rhenium Sulphide Colloid Injection E.P.

A sterile colloidal dispersion of rhenium sulphide, the micelles of which are labelled with technetium-99m. It is a light to dark brown liquid. The colloid is stabilised with gelatin. It may contain a buffer. The rhenium concentration should not exceed 0.2 mg Re per ml. The particle size range of the dispersed colloid is from 4 to 12 nanometers.

pH:	5.0 to 8.0.
Storage:	Room temperature.
Clinical use:	Lymphoscintigraphic agent.
Usual injected activity:	40 MBq.

Technetium [^{99m}Tc] Tin Colloid Injection B.P. E.P.

A sterile clear or opalescent colourless dispersion of colloidal tin labelled with technetium-99m. The colloid may be stabilised with a protecting substance. It contains fluoride ions and may contain buffers. The tin concentration should not exceed 1 mg Sn per ml. The particle size range of the colloid is from 50 to 600 nanometers.

pH:	4.0 to 7.0.
Storage:	Room temperature.
Clinical use:	Liver imaging agent.
Usual injected activity:	80 MBq.

Indium [^{111}In] Pentetate Injection (D.T.P.A.) B.P. E.P. U.S.P.

A sterile colourless solution of Indium-111 in the form of ^{111}In-diethylenetriaminepentaacetate. It may contain calcium, sodium chloride and buffers. Its radioactive concentration is 24 MBq to 74 MBq per ml.

pH:	7.0 to 8.0.
Storage:	Room temperature.
Clinical use:	Cisternography, ventriculography and C.S.F. studies.
Usual injected activity:	20 MBq–40 MBq.

Indium [^{111}In] Oxine Injection U.S.P.

A sterile colourless solution of Indium-111 complexed with 8-hydroxyquinoline. It may contain sodium chloride, a suitable non-ionic surfactant and a buffer.

pH:	6.5 to 7.5.
Storage:	Room temperature.
Clinical use:	An ingredient in blood cell labelling.
Usual injected activity:	3.7 MBq–20 MBq.

Sodium Iodide [^{123}I] Solution/Injection E.P. U.S.P.

A sterile colourless solution suitable for either oral administration or for intravenous use if sterilised. It contains Iodine-123 in the form of sodium iodide and may contain a preservative and stabiliser (buffer). The specific activity is not less than 185 GBq per mg I at calibration.

pH:	7.0 to 11.0.
Storage:	Room temperature.
Clinical use:	Throid visualization and function tests.
Usual injected activity:	20 MBq.

N.B. Sodium Iodide [^{123}I Capsules may also be used.

Sodium Iodohippurate [^{123}I] Injection B.P. E.P.

A sterile colourless solution containing sodium *o*-iodohippurate iodinated with Iodine-123. It may contain a suitable buffer and preservative. The specific activity is 0.74 GBq to 7.4 GBq per g of sodium *o*-iodohippurate at calibration.

pH:	3.5 to 8.5.
Storage:	8°–11° C protected from light.
Clinical use:	Functional renal imaging.
Usual injected activity:	20 MBq.

Iodinated [^{125}I] Albumin Injection B.P. E.P. U.S.P.

A sterile colourless to faintly yellow solution of iodine-125 attached to normal human albumin. It contains sodium chloride and a suitable antimicrobial preservative. The protein content is not less than 1%.

pH:	6.5 to 8.5.
Storage:	2°–8°C.
Clinical use:	Plasma volume studies.
Usual injected activity:	185 kBq.

Sodium Iodide [^{125}I] Solution E.P. U.S.P.

A sterile colourless solution suitable for oral or intravenous administration. It contains iodine-125 in the form of sodium iodide. The solution may contain a reducing agent and a buffer.

pH:	7.5 to 9.0.
Storage:	Room temperature.
Clinical use:	Thyroid uptake measurement.
Usual injected activity:	0.4 MBq.

N.B. Sodium Iodide [^{125}I] Capsules may also be used.

Sodium Iodide [^{131}I] Solution B.P. E.P. U.S.P.

A sterile colourless solution suitable for oral or intravenous administration. It contains iodine-131 in the form of sodium iodide. The solution may contain a suitable reducing agent, buffers and preservatives. The specific activity should not be less than 185 GBq per mg Iodine at calibration.

pH:	7.0 to 10.0.
Storage:	Room temperature.
Clinical use:	Diagnosis and treatment of thyroid disease.
Usual injected activity:	0.2 Mbq to 4 MBq diagnosis 200 MBq to 600 MBq therapy 3.7 GBq to 9.25 GBq ablation.

N.B. Sodium Iodide [^{131}I] Capsules may also be used.

Sodium Iodohippurate [^{131}I] Injection B.P. E.P. U.S.P.

A sterile colourless solution containing *o*-iodohippurate sodium labelled with iodine-131. It may contain a suitable buffer and antimicrobial preservative. The specific activity is 0.74 GBq to 7.4 GBq per g of sodium *o*-iodohippurate.

pH:	6.0 to 8.5.
Storage:	8°–15°C protected from light.
Clinical use:	Renal function measurements.
Usual injected activity:	2 MBq.

Xenon [^{133}Xe] Gas U.S.P.

A gas supplied at standard pressure at room temperature, containing 74 to 148 MBq ^{133}Xe per ml of gas. It is suitable for inhalation, and may be diluted with air or oxygen.

Storage:	Normal room temperature and pressure.
Clinical use:	Lung ventilation studies.
Usual administered activity:	185 MBq.

Xenon [^{133}Xe] Injection B.P. E.P. U.S.P.

A sterile colourless solution of Xenon-133 in sodium chloride injection. The radioactive concentration is 3.7 MBq to 55 MBq per ml.

pH:	4.5 to 8.0.
Storage:	2°–10°C. The container must exclude air.
Clinical use:	Regional blood flow measurements.
Usual injected activity:	370 MBq.

Colloidal Gold [^{198}Au] Injection B.P. E.P.

A sterile red colloidal suspension of metallic gold stabilised with gelatin and containing various reducing agents. It has a specific activity of not less than 37–740 MBq per mg Au at calibration. The particle size range is 5 to 20 nanaometers (nm) if used for therapeutical purposes.

pH:	4.0 to 8.0.
Storage:	Room temperature.
Clinical use:	Treatment of malignant ascites.
Usual injected activity:	Up to 7400 MBq.

Thallous [^{201}Tl] Injection B.P. E.P. U.S.P.

A sterile colourless solution containing thallium-201 in the form of thallous (1) chloride. It may contain sodium chloride, stabilizers and a suitable antimicrobial preservative. Its specific activity is not less than 3.7 GBq per mg Tl.

pH:	4.5 to 7.5.
Storage:	Room temperature.
Clinical use:	Myocardial visualization.
Usual injected activity:	74 MBq.

16.3 NON-OFFICIAL RADIOPHARMACEUTICALS

Chromium [^{51}Cr] Chloride Injection

A sterile colourless solution of chromic (III) chloride labelled with chromium-51. It contains sodium chloride. The specific activity is 3.7 to 13 GBg per mg Cr at calibration.

pH:	2.0 to 4.0.
Storage:	Room temperature.
Clinical use:	G.I. tract protein loss determination.
Usual injected activity:	4 MBq.

L-methyl [^{75}Se] Selenomethylnorcholesteno Injection

A sterile straw coloured solution of 6-methylselenomethyl-norcholestenol labelled with selenium-75. It contains antioxidants, solubilizing agents and sodium chloride. The specific activity is 74 to 704 MBq per mg Se at calibration.

pH:	2.5 to 3.5.
Storage:	Room temperature.
Clinical use:	Adrenal cortex imaging agent.
Usual injected activity:	7.4 MBq.

Tauro-23 [^{75}Se] Selena-25 Homocholic Acid (SeHCAT)

An analogue of taurocholic acid containing selenium-75 supplied as a solid dosage form (capsules). It is absorbed on disodium hydrogen phosphate dihydrate. The specific acticity is between 0.37 and 3.7 MBq per mg tauro-selenahomocholic acid.

Storage:	Room temperature.
Clinical use:	Bile acid pool loss measurement.
Usual administered activity:	37 to 370 MBq.

Strontium [^{89}Sr] Chloride Injection

A sterile colourless solution of strontium chloride labelled with strontium-89. It contains strontium chloride in a concentration of 10.9 to 22.6 mg per ml. The specific activity is 2.96 to 6.17 MBq per mg Sr at calibration.

pH:	4.0 to 7.0.
Storage:	Room temperature.
Clinical use:	Palliative agent in the treatment of secondary bone metastases.
Usual injected activity:	150 MBq.

Yttrium [^{90}Y] Silicate Injection

A sterile opalescent dispersion of yttrium silicate labelled with yttrium-90. It contains sodium silicate. The specific activity is between 259 MBq and 1295 MBq per mg Yt at calibration. The particle size is 100 nanometers.

pH:	10.0 to 11.5.
Storage:	Room temperature.
Clinical use:	Radiaton synovectomy agent.
Usual injected activity:	185 MBq.

Technetium [^{99m}Tc] Albumin Colloid Injection.

A sterile opalescent colourless dispersion of colloidal human albumin labelled with technetium-99m. It contains a stannous salt as the reducing agent. It may contain chelating agents, buffers non-denatural human albumin and dispersion agents. The particle size range of the colloid is 100 nanometers to 5 micrometers.

pH:	7.5 to 8.5.
Storage:	2°–8°C.
Clinical use:	Liver imaging agent.
Usual injected activity:	80 MBq.

Technetium [^{99m}Tc] Albumin Colloid (Nanosized) Injection

A sterile clear to opalescent dispersion of colloidal human albumin labelled with technetium-99m. It contains a stannous salt as the reducing agent. The particle size of the colloid is less than 80 nanometers.

pH:	4.5 to 8.0.
Storage:	Room temperature.
Clinical use:	Bone marrow imaging and lymphoscintigraphic agent.
Usual injected activity:	40 to 400 MBq.

Technetium [^{99m}Tc] Teboroxime Injection

A sterile clear to slightly opalescent solution of teboroxime labelled with technetium-99m. It contains a stannous salt as the reducing agent. It may contain chelating agents, buffers and stabilizers.

pH:	3.3 to 4.1.
Storage:	Room temperature.
Clinical use:	Myocardial perfusion imaging agent.
Usual injected activity:	550 to 1850 MBq.

Technetium [^{99m}Tc] Exametazime Injection (H.M.P.A.O.)

A sterile colourless solution of exametazime labelled with technetium-99m. It contains a stannous salt as the reducing agent. It may contain sodium chloride.

pH:	9.0 to 9.8.
Storage:	Room temperature.
Clinical use:	Cerebral blood flow imaging agent and white blood cells labelling agent.
Usual injected activity:	200 to 750 MBq.

Technetium [^{99m}Tc] Mebrofenin Injection (Trimethyl-bromo-HIDA)

A sterile colourless solution of mebrofenin labelled with technetium-99m. It contains a stannous salt as the reducing agent. It may contain antimicrobial preservatives.

pH:	4.0 to 6.0.
Storage:	Room temperature.
Clinical use:	Hepatobility imaging agent.
Usual injected activity:	80 MBq.

Technetium [^{99m}Tc] Tiatide Injection (Mercapto-acetyltrigylcine).

A sterile colourless to slightly opalescent solution of tiatide labelled with technetium-99m. It contains a stannous salt as the reducing agent. It may contain a trans-chelating agent.

pH:	5.0 to 6.0.
Storage:	Room temperature.
Clinical use:	Renal imaging agent.
Usual injected activity:	100 MBq.

Technetium [^{99m}Tc] Sestamibi Injection (M.I.B.I.)

A sterile colourless solution of hexakismethoxyisobutyl-isonitrile labelled with technetium-99m. It contains a stannous salt as the reducing agent. It may contain buffers and stabilizers.

pH:	5.3 to 5.9.
Storage:	Room temperature.
Clinical use:	Myocardial perfusion imaging agent.
Usual injected activity:	400 to 800 MBq.

Indium [^{111}In] Chloride Injection

A sterile colourless solution of indium (III) chloride labelled with indium-111. It contains hydrochloric acid. The specific activity is greater tha 185 GBq per microgram In at reference.

pH:	1.5
Storage:	Room temperature.
Clinical use:	An ingredient for labelling injectable preparations of proteins and blood cells which are subsequently used for imaging.
Usual injected activity:	10 to 150 MBq.

Indium [^{111}In] MAb. B72.3 – GYR D.T.P.A. Injection

A sterile colourless to pale opalescent solution of a conjugate of monoclonal antibody MAb B72.3 labelled with indium-111. It contains various buffers and sodium chloride.

pH:	4.0 to 6.0.
Storage:	Room temperature.
Clinical use:	Diagnostic agent for detection of malignant disease.
Usual injected activity:	111 to 148 MBq.

Indium [^{113m}In] Indium Chloride Injection

A sterile colourless solution of indium (III) chloride as indium-113m. This radionuclide is formed by the radioactive decay of tin-113. The injection may be prepared by the manipulation of a sterile preparation of tin-113 under aseptic conditions. It contains hydrochloric acid and may contain an antimicrobial preservative.

pH:	1.3 to 1.5.
Storage:	Room temperature.
Clinical use:	Diagnostic imaging, either by direct injection or after manipulation to prepare a range of organ specific radiopharmaceuticals.
Usual injected activity:	20 to 370 MBq.

Meta [^{123}I] Iodobenzylguanidine Injection

A sterile colourless solution of metaiodobenzylguanidine labelled with iodine-123. It may contain antimicrobial preservatives and buffers. The specific activity should not be less than 250 GBq per mmo1 MIBG at calibration.

pH:	5.5 to 6.5.
Storage:	2° to 8°C.
Clinical use:	Adrenal medulla imaging agent.
Usual injected activity:	185 MBq.

N.B. This compound may also be labelled with ^{131}I and used both for diagnosis and therapy.

16.4 CONCLUSION

The radiopharmaceuticals described above are those products which have been used for many years for a wide spectrum of disease. Also described are a number of comparatively new products which have been developed specifically for one particular disease.

It should be emphasised that in a brief summary of currently used radiopharmaceuticals it is difficult to include all new and clinical trial products (see Chapter 23). As with therapeutic drugs new radiopharmaceuticals may emerge for a brief period, enjoy a short time of popularity and then disappear owing to lack of clinical interest. However, it is important that the formulation and development of new materials is encouraged as the introduction of new diagnostic methods in nuclear medicine is a vital factor in the advancement of the speciality.

FURTHER READING

British Pharmacopoeia (1988). London, HMSO.
European Pharmacopoeia (1980). 2nd edition.
Santaruffine France, Maisonneuve.
United States Pharmacopeia and The National Formulary (1990). USP XXII rev.
NF XVII rev. Rockville MD, USP Convention.
Martindale: The Extra Pharmacopoeia (1989). 29th edition.
London: The Pharmaceutical Press.

Chapter 17

Mechanisms of Localisation of Radiopharmaceuticals

M. Frier

Queens Medical Centre, Nottingham

17.1 INTRODUCTION

In his respected treatise, Albert (1965) defined selective toxicity as being the injury of one kind of living matter without harming some other kind with which the first is in intimate contact. The injury could be reversible or permanent. The same principles defined by Albert for the activity of selectively toxic agents underlie the biodistribution of the agents used in nuclear medicine. Here the prime requirement is selective uptake or exclusion of a radioactive agent by an organ or lesion. Injury of that organ or lesion is required during therapeutic applications but is to be avoided if possible during diagnostic procedures. The degree of reversibility or permanence of the uptake depends on the study being performed, but in any event, the physical decay of the radionuclide introduces reversibility to the radioactivity associated with the organ or lesion.

Radiopharmaceutical agents exhibit a huge range of physical and chemical properties. Mechanisms of biodistribution may depend on the physical form, as in the uptake of particulate material by phagocytosis, or may be brought about by the similarity of the radiopharmaceutical agent to a substrate or metabolite, as in the uptake of iodine isotopes by the thyroid gland. Some radiopharmaceuticals are distributed by well-understood mechanisms while the actions of others are poorly defined. Significant advances in the understanding of the biodistribution of radiopharmaceuticals labelled with technetium-99m have been made recently with the elucidation of the likely structures of some technetium complexes. The earlier empirical approach adopted towards radiopharmaceutical development tended to assign the same behaviour to the labelled compound as to the substrate, which may be true for larger molecules. However, for smaller complexes, the radionuclide label such as techntium-99m can form an integral part of the molecular structure and produce a molecules with very different characteristics.

An important factor to bear in mind is that the observed biodistribution of a radiopharmaceutical cannot be explained in terms of a single mechanism but rather as the result of interaction between many different mechanisms involving initial dilution, passive or active transmembrane transport, protein binding, possible metabolic incorporation and elimination and excretion. The molecule may also undergo degradation and it must be borne in mind that the observed distribution is that of the radiolabel and not necessarily that of the intact molecule.

17.2 MODES OF LOCALISATION

17.2.1 Capillary Trapping

Intravenous injection of a particulate suspension results in the trapping of the particles in the pulmonary capillary bed if the particle size exceeds that of the precapillary diamter. Pulmonary precapillaries are only about 8 μm in length and 10–15 μm in diameter. The numbers and diameters of vessels in the pulmonary circulation have been determined from a resin cast of a human lung and by interpolation by Harding (1973) who calculated that one milligram of human albumin in the form of spheres 60–90 μm in diameter would block a maximum of 0.31% of available pulmonary vessels in a normal subject.

The same trapping mechanism applies to particles injected intraarterially but here the capillaries blocked would be the first encountered distal to the injection site e.g. the coronary circulation.

17.2.2 Aerosol Deposition

Liquid and solid aerosols have been in use in nuclear medicine for a number of years for the study of lung function. The main applications of the systems are for ventilation studies in which the aerosol suspension is used as an alternative to radioactive gas, and for clearance studies in which a proportion of the aerosol is required to deposit within the lungs such that the efficiency of the subsequent mucociliary clearance of the deposited activity can be observed.

Many solid aerosol generators are based on the spinning disc system described by Few (1970) for the production of polystyrene particles. Solution aerosols can be produced in several ways including jet nebulisation, ultrasound, condensation methods, the use of propellants, spinning discs or by the passage of solution through a vibrating orifice. The most conventient and widely-used system is the jet nebuliser. The extent of lung penetration and deposition within the airways depends on the size range of the droplets inhaled. It is well established that particles larger than 5 μm in diameter are filtered out in the nasal cavity or are deposited in the mouth and pharynx. Droplets smaller than 0.1 μm in diameter remain suspended and are exhaled without deposition. The ideal diameter for maximum penetration of the small airways together with deposition within the lungs is about 0.5 μm.

In the system described by Royston (1984) a jet nebuliser is used to produce a liquid droplet aerosol. Such nebulisers produce an aerosol suspension with a wide range of droplet sizes, and to overcome this problem, the output from the nebuliser is passed through a column packed with glass beads of varying sizes. Larger droplets impact on the beads and coalesce, resulting in an aerosol comprising droplets of a very narrow size range. Clinical results obtained with the system are comparable to those obtained with krypton-81m gas.

An aerosol system for the production of solid particle dispersions of very small dimensions (0.005 μm diameter) has been described by Burch (1984, 1986). Technetium-99m on a structured ultrafine dispersion of carbon penetrates to the alveoli and adheres to the alveolar walls. More recent studies (Strong, 1990) suggest a somewhat larger particle size, perhaps with an activity mean diameter of 140 nm. The solid matrix may in fact consist of sodium chloride which vapourises at temperatures below those used in the production of the aerosol dispersion.

17.2.3 Gaseous Radiopharmaceuticals

The gases used in nuclear medicine studies, principally istopes of xenon (xenon-133, xenon-127) and krypton-81 m are chemically inert and, at the concentrations used, physiologically inert although xenon is known to have an anaesthetic effect at very high concentrations. The gases pass into the pulmonary venous circulation from the lungs and can exchange freely between the blood and tissues, concentrating in body fat. Xenon entering circulation is released through the lungs by the mechanism of alveolar capillary diffusion. Most of the xenon entering circulation is released in this way after a single pass through the peripheral circulation.

Ion Exchange

As with the phenomena of dilution, and diffusion across permeability barriers, ion exchange plays a part in determining the biodistribution of many radiopharmaceutical agents. Simple electrolytes such as strontium salts, fluoride and phosphate are probably extracted from circulation, initially by a process of ion exchange. In areas of active bone growth or repair, there is an increased turnover of calcium and hydroxyl ions and an exchange can take place involving the substitution of strontium for calcium and fluoride for hydroxyl. Following initial uptake by ion exchange, subsequent fate may involve metabolic incorporation or elimination. Weber (1968) suggested that the deposition of bone tracer radionuclides was generally thought to be the result of rapid ion exchange in or on the hydroxyapatite crystal surfaces, and slow incorporation of ions within the crystal structure by slow, intracrystalline ion exchange.

The phosphate and phosphonate complexes of technetium-99m used for bone scanning are probably not taken up by ion exchange mechanisms, but by adsorption on to the surface of hdyroxyapatite crystals. It has been shown in crystallographic studies that there is a relationship between the coordination parameters of calcium in hydroxyapatite and the spatial arrangement of oxygen donor atoms in the ligands.

17.2.5 Transport Mechanisms

Many radiopharmaceuticals achieve their initial biodistribution by simple dilution in a body compartment such as plasma, following which a simple diffusion process along a concentration gradient takes place allowing the substance to cross a permeability barrier. The use of technetium-99m pertechnetate as a brain scanning agent depends on the fact that pertechnetate is excluded from brain tissue by a permeability barrier. When that barrier is damaged in some way, either through trauma, the presence of a tumour or metastatic lesion, or as the result of a cerebrovascular accident, the permeability barrier is damaged and pertechnetate is free to enter.

Pulmonary vascular permeability increases in patients with clinically defined adult respiratory distress syndrome. The phenomenon is characterised by an increased rate of movement of plasma from the blood into the lung, and may be directly monitored by comparing the activity of radiolabelled plasma proteins relative to a vascular tracer. Basran and Hardy (1988) have performed these studies with indium-113m labelled transferrin as the protein and technetium-99m labelled erythrocytes as the vascular tracer.

Other than simple diffusion along concentration gradients, there are many ways in which substances may cross a permeability barrier. The substance may or may not be associated with a carrier. In the process of facilitated diffusion, factors such as lipophilicity favour passive transport through a lipid membranc. Active transport may be involved in which energy is consumed during the transport process and in which the substance may or may not be coupled. Substances to which the membrane is not normally permeable may enter cells by the process of pinocytosis (see below).

Passive transport of lipophilic agents through the cell membrane is the likely mechanism involved in the brain uptake of technetium-99m hexapropyleneamineoxime. An intracellular change in the form of the complex to one which is less lipophilic probably accounts for the fact that little redistribution of activity is seen in the human brain up to 4.5 hours after injection (Ell, 1985).

Weak bases with suitable pH values such as the radioiodinated amine N-isopropyl-p-iodoamphetamine act as pH dependent tracers. These materials are neutral and lipophilic at blood pH (7.4) and can freely penetrate the cell. Intracellular pH, particularly in actively metabolising tissues such as heart and brain, can be significantly lower, and under these conditions, compounds ionise, becoming less lipophilic and are therefore trapped within the cell. Johanssen (1987) has suggested a similar mechanism for the uptake of gallium in which the uncharged gallium hydroxide can penetrate the cell. Under the lower pH conditions found within the cell, the material ionises and becomes bound.

Carrier-mediated processes, involving active transport are involved in the uptake of iodine isotopes and pertechnetate by thyroid, in the excretion of iodinated hippuric acid by the kidneys involving the hippurate transport system, and in the uptake of hepatobiliary agents. Here, radioiodinated dyes such as rose bengal, or technetium-99m labelled agents such as the iminodiacetic acid derivatives, are transported by the anion transport system of the liver.

Active transport mechanisms have also been invoked in the uptake of radiopharmaceutical agents by the myocardium. It has been suggested that thallium-201 thallous ions are taken up by the active transport system for potassium. Although thallium is a group IIIA element as opposed to a group I, its ionic radius is similar to that of potassium. There are differences in behaviour, however, the most marked being the prolonged cellular retention of thallous ions (Strauss 1975). Rinck (1980) has suggested that uptake occurs by the mechanism of facilitated diffusion.

The cationic technetium-99m complexes introduced for myocardial imaging, the hexakis (alkylisonitrile) derivatives (Jones 1982, Gerundini 1986), may also be taken up by some kind of active cation transport system. However, studies have shown (Sands, 1986), that the uptake of the t-butyl compound by myocytes is not affected by preincubation with ouabain, or by the presence of potassium chloride, suggesting that the sodium/potassium/ATPase system is not involved. The observed biodistribution cannot be explained merely in terms of the high lipophilicty of these compounds, and further investigations are needed to understand fully the mechanisms involved.

17.2.6 Phagocytosis and Pinocytosis

Uptake of radiopharmaceuticals by phagocytosis has been exploited for many years in the technique of liver scanning. Particles of colloidal dimensions are engulfed by phagocytic cells such as the Kuppfer cells of the liver or the macrophages of the spleen and bone marrow. Phagocytosis is a multistage process in which particulate material requires to be transported such that it comes into contact with the surface of the phagocytic cell. The particle is then recognised by the cell in some way, following which it becomes attached to the cell surface and is finally engulfed by the cell. The process of recognition is brought about by receptors on the cell surface which respond to material coated with immunoglobulin G (the Fc receptors), material coated with complement (the C3 receptors) and to a foreign surface. The receptors function independently and respond to different molecules. particles may or may not be opsonised.

Particles in the range 25 A to 10 μm can be recognised and phagocytosed. Factors affecting the process, such as particle size, particle number and surface charge have been reviewed by Kuperus (1979) and by Frier (1981). Radiopharmaceuticals which depend for their biodistribution on the phenomenon of phagocytosis include the colloids used for liver scanning such as technetium-99m tin and sulphur colloids, and the microcolloids used for bone marrow imaging such as technetium-99m antimony sulphide and albumin colloids. Methods have been devised for the labelling of phagocytic blood cells in whole blood using technetium-99m tin colloid to be used for the detection of abscesses (Schroth 1981, Pullman 1988).

Pinocytosis is the mechanism whereby macromolecules and dissolved substances affect entry into a cell when the cell membrane is not normally permeable to those substances. It is brought about when microvilli on the cell wall engulf small, fluid-filled vacuoles containing the substance in solution. It has been suggested that increased pinocytosis may contribute towards the increased localisation of radiotracers in tumours (Schall 1971, Winchell 1976) and Anghileri (1984) has cited pinocytosis as being a potentially useful phenomenon for the selective introduction of specific solutes into tumour cells.

17.2.7 Metabolic Incorporation and Metabolic Analogues

Iodine-131 is probably the longest established and best characterised radiopharmaceutical in existence. It still retains a major role in therapy for treatment of benign lesions such as hyperthyroidism, and in malignant thyroid disease such as the irradiation of remnants of thyroid following surgical resection. The high radiation dose associated with iodine-131 makes it less suitable for diagnostic application and its use has largely been superceded by iodine-123. Radioactive iodine follows identical metabolic pathways to those of the natural non-radioactive substrate.

A major problem in the development of radioactive tracers is the lack of suitable isotopes of the natural elements present in metabolites, i.e. carbon, nitrogen, oxygen and sulphur. The positron-emitting nuclides carbon-11, nitrogen-13 and oxygen-15 have been used as for example in the form of carbon-11 glucose for the study of glucose metabolism. There are major limitations to the use of these radionuclides in terms of the lack of suitable cyclotron production facilities, the short half lives of the radionuclides themselves (e.g. carbon-11 20.4 minutes) and the need for suitable cameras for detection of the emissions resulting from positron decay. Thus much of the work on metabolically active materials has involved the incorporation of foreign labels such as fluorine-11, selenium-75 or isotopes of iodine into naturally occurring molecules or the production of labelled foreign molecules which themselves are metabolic analogues.

Selenomethionine was developed as a selenium-75 labelled analogue of the amino acid methionine. Its use in pancreas scanning is based on the fact that digestive enzymes produced by the pancreas are secreted with each meal, and to keep up with this turnover, the pancreas must synthesise new protein at a very rapid rate (Blau 1961, Blau 1962). Selenium-75 can be detected in proteins within an hour of intravenous injection.

Scanning of the adrenal cortex may be performed using steroid derivatives labelled with selenium-75 (Reschini 1984, Hawkins 1980) or isotopes of iodine. 6B-iodomethyl-19-norcholest-5(10)-en-3B-ol and 6B-methylselenomethyl-19-norcholest-5(10)-en-3B-ol are acumulated in the adrenal cortex as precursers of cholesterol synthesis. The adrenal medulla may be imaged with the radioiodinated guanidine derivative meta-iodobenzylguanidine (Wieland, 1980; Sisson, 1981). The compound is specifically trapped by the cells of the adrenal medulla because of the similarity in molecular structure to norepinephrine.

Other compounds which owe their action, at least in part, to the similarity in structure to norepinephrine and serotonin are the iodinated amines N-isopropyl-p-iodoamphetamine and N,N,N′-trimethyl-N′-(2-hydroxy-3-methyl-5-iodobenzyl)-1,3-propanediamine used for the detection of regional perfusion disturbances in the brain. It has been proposed (Winchell 1980) that localisation in the brain is due to the presence of high capacity, non-specific amine-binding sites and selective inhibition of the uptake of serotonin and norepinephrine in synaptosomes by these agents can be demonstrated.

The myocardium can utilise fatty acids as an energy source in conditions of reduced oxygen availability. Non-isotopically-labelled substances such as terminally-iodinated long chain fatty acids or phenyl substituted fatty acids are recognised and utilised by the myocardium under the same conditions, and provide a means of imaging regional myocardial metabolism.

17.2.8 Passage Through the Blood/Brain Barrier

Capillaries supplying the brain are specialised into a structure called the blood/brain barrier. In most other tissues there is free communication between the blood plasma and the interstitial fluid for the interchange of all small molecules and ions. In the brain the barrier impedes the movement of water-soluble substances e.g. glucose, although fat-soluble substances exchange readily between blood and cerebral tissues. There are a number of mechanisms responsible for the effective operation of the blood/brain barrier.

Endothelial cells of the cerebral vessels are special in that the intercellular junctions are modified to form tight junctions – one close to the capillary lumen and one at the basement aspect of the endothelial cells (see Figure 1a, b and c). Also there is a lack of contractility in the brain capillaries due to the lack of actomyosin, which ensures that the tight junctions are not pulled open. Thus molecules capable of entering cerebral tissue must be small enough to enter via the tight junctions or be lipophilic. It is this latter mechanism which allows the lipophilic complex exametazime to enter the brain. Free diffusion out is prevented by a molecular conformational change leading to the formation of a less lipophilic species.

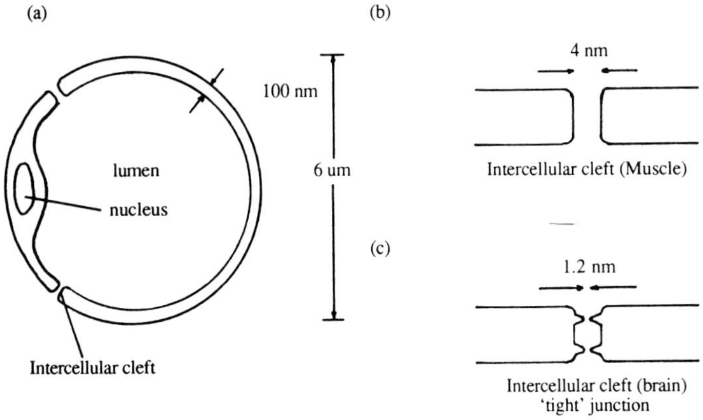

Figure 1 Capillary structure showing wide intercellular clefts of muscle capillaries and narrow intercellular clefts (tight junction) of brain capillaries.

17.2.9 Receptors

Paul Ehrlich invoked the concept of receptors during his experimental studies on chemotherapeutic agents in the early part of this century. Receptors can be thought of as macromolecules with which a drug or radiotracer interacts to produce a characteristic biological effect (Goldstein, 1974; Gerald, 1974). Many types of receptor can be defined, and potentially a more complete understanding of receptors could result in the production of highly specific radiotracers. Receptors which have been investigated include those for polypeptide hormones, acetylcholine, glucocorticoids, the beta-adrenoceptors and the muscarinic-cholinergic receptors.

Specific interactions of radiolabelled derivatives with receptor proteins have been used extensively in biochemistry and physiology in determining the fate of soluble and membrane-bound receptors. The radiolabels used in many of these studies are carbon-14 and tritium, and are therefore not directly relevant to nuclear medicine studies. Currently however, there is interest in developing radiopharmaceuticals which will specifically target groups of receptors, giving the potential for the quantitative estimation of receptors in diseased conditions, or the monitoring of efficacy of drug therapy.

Studies have been published on the alpha-1 adenoceptor ligand 2-[B-(4-hydroxyphenyl)ethylaminomethyl]tetralone, an antihypertensive drug acting by means of peripheral and central alpha adrenoceptor antagonists. The iodinated derivative has higher *in vitro* affinities for the alpha-1 adrenoceptor than does the parent compound and animal studies with iodine-125 and iodine-123 labels have shown the potential of the compound as a diagnostic radiopharmaceutical in SPECT studies of the brain (Couch, 1988).

The presence of receptor sites for the neuropeptide somatostatin can be demonstrated using small radiolabelled peptides (Bakker 1991a, b). Comparison of the structures of somatostation and the small peptide octreotide shows the presence of a similar sequence of amino acids, presumed to be the bioactive site.

Somatostatin

Ala-Gly-Cys-Lys-Asn-Phe-*Phe-Trp-Lys-Thr*-Phe-Thr-Ser-Cys

Octreotide D-Phe-Cys-*Phe-D-Trp-Lys-Thr*-Cys-Thr(ol)

Use of radiolabelled forms of this material makes possible the imaging of tumours with somatostatin receptors, such as carcinoids, pancreatic endocrine tumours, neuroblastomas and paragangliomas (see also Chapter 25).

In the simplest case where the radiopharmaceutical in neither metabolised nor bound to serum proteins, the target to blood ratio is a function of the ratio between the concentration of receptors and the dissociation constant of the radioligand for the receptors. The possibility of determining this ratio *in vitro* opens up the potential for screening compounds for suitability as *in vivo* imaging agents. On this basis, Gibson (1979) has suggested that the muscarinic antagonists are potentially useful myocardial imaging agents.

17.2.10 Autologous Products

Products which are isolated from the body of a subject, radiolabelled and subsequently readministered to the same subject are known as autologous products. Probably the best known and most widely used autologous products are radiolabelled blood cells which have a well established role in diagnostic nuclear medicine. (For a fuller discussion see Chapters 6 and 7).

In the earliest stages of development of blood cell labelling techniques, erythrocytes were separated and labelled with chromium-51 for simple dilution volume measurements of red cell mass. More recently, white cell separation and labelling has been developed, and imaging for infective and inflammatory lesions using granulocytes labelled with indium-111 is now routinely performed. Lymphocytes and granulocytes have also been isolated and labelled. In most instances, white cell labelling is performed using lipophilic complexes of indium-111 such as oxine or tropolone. It is generally considered that the ligand transports the indium-111 through the cell membrane by passive diffusion. Once inside the cell, the complex dissociates and the indium is transferred to some other intracellular component which holds it firmly within the cell. Oxine has been observed to elute from labelled leucocytes (Thakur, 1977) and from labelled platelets (Mathias, 1979).

The mechanism of action of the radiolabelled cells depends on maintenance of the blood cells under study in a condition which allows them to behave in a way identical to that of the unlabelled cell population. An exception to this is the use of deliberately damaged erythrocytes for imaging of the spleen. Here, cells are damaged by heating for 15 minutes at 50 °C to produce spherocytic forms which, on reinjection, are sequestered by the spleen in the same way that old or damaged cells are normally removed.

Cells can suffer incidental as opposed to deliberate damage during the separation and labelling procedures used. For example, centrifugation at high relative centrifugal forces or rapid withdrawal of cell suspensions through narrow gauge needles can bring about mechanical damage. Chemical damage can be caused by a change in pH of the suspending medium used, by chemical toxicity of the agents used in the labelling procedure such as oxine, and by absorbed radiation arising from the radiolabels themselves. It has been calculated that in a population of 10^8 granulocytes labelled with 37 MBq indium-111, the dose to each cell would be 180 Gy (Goodwin 1978). Methods of handling cells and methods of minimising the associated cell damage have been reviewed by Danpure (1984).

17.2.11 Immunological Mechanisms

The use of antibodies as a means of targeting diagnostic and therapeutic radiopharmaceuticals is currently being extensively investigated. The concept of targetting in this way is simple, but in practice is difficult to achieve. Monoclonal antibodies, derived from cultured hybridoma cells, have the capacity to recognise and interact with single antigens, and potentially can identify and target specific groups of cells such as blood cells and tumours. A major problem in applying the technique to imaging and therapy of tumour cells is that the antigens expressed do not necessarily differ qualitatively from those expressed by cells of unaffected tissues. Differences may therefore be only of a quantitative nature, and significant levels of activity may be taken up by tissues other than those of the target. (For a fuller discussion see Chapter 8).

Table 1.
Mechanisms of Localisation of Radiotracers.

Substrate nonspecific

1. Diffusion
   a. Technetium-99m pertechnetate for brain imaging
   b. Xenon-133 and krypton-81m for lung ventilation
2. Isotope dilution
   a. Iodine-125 human albumin for plasma volume
   b. Chromium-51 erythrocytes for red cell mass
3. Capillary blockade and cell sequestration
   a. Technetium-99m macroaggregated albumin for regional lung perfusion studies
   b. Technetium-99m heat-damaged erythrocytes for splenic sequestration
4. Phagocytosis
   a. Technetium-99m tin colloid for liver scanning

Substrate specific

1. Metabolic pathway (isotopic substitution)
   a. Carbon-11 glucose for regional brain studies
   b. Iodine-123 iodide for thyroid studies
2. Metabolic pathway (non-isotopic substitution)
   a. Iodine-123 iodoheptadecanoid acid
3. Metabolic trapping
   a. Technetium-99m pertechnetate for thyroid studies
   b. Fluorine-18 2-deoxy-2-fluoro-D-glucose for regional brain studies
4. Enzyme substrate
   a. Selenium-75 substituted norcholestenol for adrenal scanning
   b. Selenomethionine for pancreas scanning
5. Receptor binding
   a. Alpha-1 adrenoceptor antagonists
   b. Octreotide for somatostatin receptor-positive tumours
6. Antibodies
   a. Anti CEA antibodies for tumour imaging
   b. Antithrombocyte antibodies for thrombus detection
   c. Antimyosin antibodies for myocardial studies

17.3 SUMMARY AND CONCLUSION

Suggested mechanisms by which radiopharmaceuticals accumulate are summarised in Table 1.

The mechanisms may be passive or active and may be substrate non-specific (not participating in a specific chemical reaction) or substrate specific (participate in a chemical reaction or interact with a specific ligand). Understanding the mechanisms of biodistribution of radiopharmaceutical agents requires not only a thorough knowledge of the pharmacokinetic and metabolic processes involved but also an understanding of the structure and fate of the radiopharmaceutical agents themselves. This is particularly the case when considering agents labelled with the radionuclide technetium-99m. It is only recently that the chemical structures of technetium labelled complexes are beginning to be understood and this in turn has led to the development of several potentially useful diagnostic agents.

REFERENCES

Albert A. (1965). *Selective Toxicity*, 3rd edn., Wellwyn Garden City: The Broadwater Press Ltd.

Anghileri L.J., (1984). *Non-specific tumour-seeking radiopharmaceuticals – report and future aspects.* Nuklearmedizin, **23**, 9–14.

Bakker W.H., Albert R., Bruns C., Breeman W.A.P., Hofland L.J., Marbach P., Pless J., Pralet J., Stolz B., Koper J.W., Lamberts S.W.J., Visser T.J. and Krenning E.P. (1991). *(In-111-DTPA-d-Phe)-octreotide, a potential radiopharmaceutical for imaging somatostatin receptor-positive tumours: synthesis, radiolabelling and* in vitro *validation.* Life Sciences, **49**, 1593–1601.

Bakker W.H., Krenning E.P. Reubi J.C., Breeman W.A.P., Setyono-Han B., de Jong M., Kooij P.P.M., Bruns C., van Hagan P.M., Marbach P., Visser T.J., Pless J. and Lamberts S.W.J. (1991). In vivo *application of (In-111-DTPA-d-Phe)-octreotide for detection of somatostatin receptor-positive tumors in rats.* Life Sciences **49**, 1593–1601.

Basran G.S. and Hardy J.G. (1988). *Monitoring pulmonary vascular permeability using radiolabelled transferrin.* J.Thorac.Imag., **3**, 28–35.

Blau M. and Manske R.F. (1961). *The pancreas specificity of Se-75 Selenomethionine.* J. Nucl. Med. **2**, 102–105.

Blau M. and Bender M.A. (1962). *Se-75 Selenomethionine for visualisation of the pancreas by isotope.* Radiology, **78**, 974.

Burch W.M., Tetley I.J. and Gras J.L. (1984). *Technetium-99m 'Pseudogas' for diagnostic studies in the lung.* Clin. Phys. Physiol. Meas. **5**, 79–85.

Burch W.M., Sullivan P.J. and McClaren C.J. (1986). *Technegas – a new ventilation agent for lung scanning.* Nucl. Med. Commun. **7**, 865–871.

Couch M.W., Greer D.M., Thonoor C.M. and Williams C.M. (1988). *In-vivo* binding in rat brain and radiopharmaceutical preparation of radioiodinated HEAT, and alpha-1 adrenoceptor ligand. J. Nucl. Med., **27**, 356–362.

Danpure H.J. (1985). *Cell labelling with 111In-complexes. In* Radiopharmacy and Radiopharmaceuticals, edited by A.E. Theobald, pp. 51–85. London: Taylor and Francis.

Ell P.J., Hocknell J.M.L., Jarrit P.H., Cullum I., Lui D., Campos-Costa D. *et al.* (1985). *A Tc-99m labelled radiotracer for the investigation of cerebral vascular disease.* Nucl. Med. Commun., **6**, 437–441.

Few J.D., Short M.D. and Thompson M.L. (1970). *Preparation of Tc-99m-labelled particles for aerosol studies.* Radiochem. Radioanal. Letters., **5**, 275–277.

Frier M. (1981) *Phagocytosis. In* Progress in Radiopharmacology vol. II, edited by P.H. Cox, PP. 249–259. Elsevier: Biomedical Press.

Gerald M.C. (1974). Pharmacology: an introduction to drugs. Engelwood Cliffs, N.J.: Prentice-Hall.

Gerundini P., Savi A., Gilardi M.C., Margonato A., Vicedomini G., Zecca L. *et al.* (1986). J. Nucl. Med. **27**, 409–416.

Gibson R.E., Eckelman W.C., Rzeszotarski W.J., Jiang V., Maziatis A., Paik C. *et al.* (1979). *In* Principles of Radiopharmacology, vol II, edited by L.G. Colombetti, pp. 17–39. Boca Raton, Florida: CRC Press.

Goldstein A., Aronow L. and Kalman S.M. (1974). *Molecular mechanisms of drug addiction. In* Principles of drug action, New York: John Wiley and Sons.

Goodwin D.A., Busberg J.T., Doherty P.W., Lipton M.J., Conley F.K., Diamanti C.I. *et al.* (1978). *Indium-labelled autologous platelets for localisation of vascular thrombi in humans.* J. Nucl. Med. **19**, 626–634.

Harding L.K., Horsfield K., Singhal S.S. and Cumming G. (1973). *The proportion of lung vessels blocked by albumin microspheres.* J. Nucl. Med., **14**, 579–581.

Hawkins A.L., Britten K.E. and Shapiro B. (1980). *Selenium-75 selenomethyl cholesterol; a new agent for quantitative functional scintigraphy of the adrenals; Physicals aspects.* Brit. J. Radiol., **53**, 883–889.

Johannsen B. (1987). *Principles, problems and trends in radiopharmacology. In* Principle of Radiopharmacology, edited by H. Deckart and P.H. Cox, pp. 166–182. Jena: Gustav Fischer Verl.

Jones A.G., Abrams M.J. and Davison D.A. (1982). J. Nucl. Med. All. Sci., **26**, 149.

Kuperus J.H. (1979). *The role of phagocytosis and pinocytosis in the localisation of radiotracers. In* Principles of Radiopharmacology, vol. III, edited by L.G. Colombetti, pp. 267–276. Boca Raton, Florida: CRC Press.

Mathias C.J. and Welch M.J. (1979). *Labelling mechanism and localisation of indium-111 in human platelets.* J. Nucl. Med. **20**, 659.

Pullman W.E., Sullivan P.J., Barratt P.J., Lising J., Booth J.A. and Doe W.F. (1988). *Assessment of inflammatory bowel disease activity by technetium-99m phagocyte scanning.* Gastroenterology **95**, 989–996.

Reschini E. and Peracci M., (1984). *Uptake of Se-75 Selenocholesterol by adrenal cortical carcinoma and its metastases.* Eur. J. Nucl. Med. **9**, 291–293.

Rinck P.A. and Beckmann H.O. (1980). *Myocardial uptake of thallous ions by facilitated diffusion.* Naturwissenschaften, **67**, 567–568.

Royston D., Minty B.D., Houston A., Jones J.G. and McCleod M. (1984). *A simple separator to generate half micron particles for lung imaging.* Brit. J. Radiol., **57**, 223–228.

Sands H., Delano M.L. and Gallaher B.M. (1986). *Uptake of hexakis(t-butylisonitrile) technetium I and hexakis-(isopropylisonitrile) technetium I by neonatal rat myocytes and human erythrocytes.* J. Nucl. Med. **27**, 404–408.

Schall G.L. and Quinn J.L. (1971). *Diagnosis of central nervous system disease. Brain Scanning. In* Nuclear Medicine, edited by W.D. Blahd. New York: McGraw-Hill.

Schroth H.J., Oberhausen E. and Berberich R. (1981). *Cell labelling with colloidal substances in whole blood.* Eur. J. Nucl. Med. **6**, 469–472.

Sisson J.C., Frager M.S., Valk T.W., Gross M.D., Swanson D.P., Wieland D.M. *et al.* (1981). *Scintigraphic localisation of phaeochromocytoma.* N. Eng. J. Med., **305**, 12–17.

Strauss H.W., Harrison K., Langan J.K., Lebowitz E. and Pitt B., (1975). *Thallium-201 for myocardial imaging; relation of thallium-201 to regional circulation.* Circulation, **51**, 641–646.

Strong J.C. and Agnew J.E. (1989). *The particle size distribution of technegas and its influence on regional lung deposition.* Nucl. Med. Commun., **10**, 425–430.

Thakur M.L., Lavender P., Arnot R.N., Silvester D.J. and Segal A.W. (1977). *Indium-labelled autologous leucocytes in man.* J. Nucl. Med., **18**, 1014–1021.

Weber D.A., Greenberg E.J., Dimich A., Kenny P.J., Rothschild E.O., Myers W.P.L. *et al.* (1968). *Kinetics of radionuclides used for bone studies.* J. Nucl. Med., **10**, 8–17.

Wieland M., Wu J.L., Brown L.E., Mangner T.J., Swanson D.P. and Beierwaltes W.H. (1980). *Radiolabelled adrenergic neuron-blocking agents: Adrenomedullary imaging with iodine-131 iodobenzylguanidine.* J. Nucl. Med., **21**, 349–353.

Winchell H.S. (1976). *Mechanism for localisation of radiotracers in neoplasms.* Semin. Nucl. Med., **6**, 371–378.

Winchell H.S., Horst W.D., Braun L., Oldendorf W.H., Hattner R. and Parker H. (1980). *N-isopropyl-[123I] p-iodamphetamine: Single-pass brain uptake and washout; binding to brain synaptosomes; and localisaton in dog and monkey brain.* J. Nucl. Med., **21**, 947–952.

FURTHER READING

Principles of Radiopharmacology (1979). Vols I, II and III, edited by L.G. Colombetti. Boca Raton, Florida: CRC Press.

Progress in Radiopharmacology (1981). Vol. II, edited by P.H. Cox. Elsevier: Biomedical Press.

Radiopharmacy and Radiopharmaceuticals (1985). Edited by A.E. Theobald. London: Taylor and Francis.

Principles of Radiopharmacology. (1987). Edited by H. Deckart and P.H. Cox, Jena: Gustav Fischer Verlag.

Technetium in chemistry and nuclear medicine (1987). Edited by M. Nicolini, G. Bandoli and U. Mazzi. New York: Raven Press.

Chapter 18

Pharmacology, Pharmacokinetics and Metabolism of Radiopharmaceuticals

M. Frier

18.1 INTRODUCTION

Radiopharmaceuticals in general do not exert any pharmacological effects on the organism, either because they are pharmacologically inert or because they are administered at dose levels too low to exert any measurable influence. There are exceptions to this. For example radioiodinated *meta* – iodobenzylguanidine, a noradrenaline analogue, can exert adrenergic side effects including tachycardia and transient hypertomia especially if injected rapidly. Esentially, radiopharmacology can be regarded as the study of the biological distribution of radioactive medicinal products, and as such incorporates radiopharmacokinetics, transport mechanisms, interaction with binding sites, and metabolic fate. The present chapter investigates the radiopharmacology of a number of radiopharmaceuticals, principally those compounds containing technetium-99m.

The kinetics and biodistribution of the radiolabel has been extensively studied, but less well understood are the fates of the radiopharmaceuticals. These may differ as the result of disassociation or metabolic changes in *vivo.* An early example of this phenomenon was reported by Rosenthall (1976) who demonstrated differences in uptake between normal and rachitic rats of phosphate complexes when labelled with technetium-99m but not of the same complexes when labelled with phosphorus-32.

An understanding of the fate of radiotracers is essential to the design of agents for use in nuclear medicine. Indeed some agents depend on known in-vivo changes for their effect. For example, exametazime undergoes alterations in molecular conformation which result in changes in lipophilicity and an increased retention in brain tissue.

Biodistribution at the whole body level, or at the organ level are relatively easy to observe and to quantify. Biodistribution at the cellular or even the subcellular levels are less easy to determine, but can generate important information, particularly with respect to radiation dosimetry. (This Chapter should be read in conjunction with Chapter 3).

18.2 MYOCARDIAL AGENTS

Many disparate agents have been used to study myocardial perfusion. As early as 1962, Carr reported the use of rubidium-86 for this purpose, exploiting the similarity in behaviour to that of natural potassium. Rubidium can sub stitute for potassium in the NA/K/ATPase system. Nitrogen-13 in the form of ammonia has also been used (Harper, 1972). Non-ionic ammonia diffuses into the myocardial cells where ionisation takes place, and the ionic species are trapped by the glutamate/glutamine reaction.

The most significant advance in studies of the myocardium was made by Kawana in 1970, by his suggestion to use thallium-199 as a potassium analogue for imaging. The 201 isotope was introduced later by Leibowitz (1973). Although belonging to group III, thallium is thought to be transported in to the myocardium by the Na/K/ATPase system, although the mechanism of facilitated diffusion has been suggested. Its efflux, however, is slower than that of potassium. Within 30 minutes of injection, 3–4% of the injected dose accumulates in the myocardium. Redistribution occurs within the following 12 to 18 hours, during which time the heart remains clearly visible.

The search for cationic technetium-99m complexes which could be used instead of thallium led to the development of the *hexakis* – isonitrile technetium complexes, firstly the butyl derivative (t-BI) and secondly the methoxyisobutyl compound (MIBI). t-BI showed high uptake in lung, liver and skeletal muscle, followed by redistribution, whereas MIBI has reduced extramyocardial uptake with minimal redistribution. Although these are cationic compounds, their kinetics and mechanisms of uptake differ considerably from those of thallium. Experiments with isolated myocytes (Sands, 1986) showed that uptake was not affected by ouabain, indicating no involvement of the Na/K/ATPase system. The lipophilicity of this class of compound certainly contributes to the uptake, but does not totally explain it. MIBI does show an affinity for a cytosolic protein of molecular weight 10^4 Daltons to which it binds with a dissociation constant of 0.77×10^{-5} (Mousa 1987), and this may serve to explain the slow clearance from the myocardium, activity remaining comparatively stable for some hours at between 2 and 3% of the administered dose.

A myocardial agent with very different kinetics belongs to the BATO group complexes. This compound is neutral, hightly lipophilic and shows a rapid uptake into the myocardium amounting to 7 or 8% of the administered dose within the first five minutes of injection. This clears very rapidly, however, to a residual activity of 2–3% at one hour post injection. Some change takes place following injection, either in the structure of the complex, or through binding to plasma components, which renders the complex less extractable with time.

18.3 SKELETAL AGENTS

Technetium-99m diphosphonates are the current agents of choice for the performance of bone scans. They show rapid bone uptake, low background uptake in non-skeletal areas and clearance of non-bound activity by urinary excretion. Better than 50% of the injected dose is taken up by bone, with less than 2% remaining in circulation at four hours post injection. Uptake in bone is thought to result from the interaction of the diphosphonates with the surface of the hydroxyapatite crystal, and there is crystallographic evidence to suggest a relationship between the spatial arrangements of the O-donor atoms on osteophilic ligands and the coordination parameters of calcium in hydroxyapatite (Johanssen, 1987). Bidentate, bidentate binding is postulated for methylene diphosphonate and bidentate, tridentate binding for ethylhydroxy diphosphonate (EHDP), because of the presence of the hydroxy group. *In vivo* demonstration of the site of uptake of bone-imaging agents has been investigated autoradiographically. Tilden (1973) examined biopsy specimens obtained from patients after administration of Tc-99m polyphosphate and demonstrated a linear pattern of radioactivity deposition at the junction of bone of different maturities. In thin sections of cancellous bone, the line of radioactivity lies at the interface of the osteoid next to the marrow cavity and the mineralised bone. It is interesting to note that this author makes reference to the potential use of microautoradiography in precise dosimetry calculations at the cellular level. Van Langevelde (1977) found that in rats injected with Tc-99m EHDP, technetium-induced grains were only found in the bone shaft and not in the bone marrow, periosteum or in the layer of osteoblasts immediately against the bone shaft. This, coupled with competitive inhibition studies using non-radioactive EHDP led to the conclusion that hydroxyapatite is the primary binding site. The P-C-P link of diphosphonates is very stable, and is not vulnerable to attack by phosphatase enzymes, whereas the P-O-P link found in polyphosphates and pyrophosphates is readily broken.

18.4 RENAL AGENTS

Radiopharmaceuticals for study of the kidney fall essentially into two groups – those for the demonstration of renal morphology and those for the demonstration of renal function. Of the former group, technetium-99m dimercaptosuccinic acid, (DMSA) is the most commonly used. It depends for its function on specific uptake by and long retention within the parenchymal tissue of the kidney. DMSA was introduced into nuclear medicine practice by Lin (1974). Following intravenous injection to normal subjects, the concentration in kidneys progressively increases from about 25% in one hour to about 40% in six hours (McAfee 1982). Less than 10% of the injected activity is excreted in the urine within the first hour. Early studies by Moretti and his coworkers (1982) indicated that the complex is retained within the cells of the apical part of the proximal convoluted tubules and pars recta, and in the upper part of the loop of Henle. Binding takes place with protein receptors containing sulphydryl groups. Radiopharmaceuticals for the demonstration of renal function can be further divided into agents for the measurement of glomerular filtration rate and those for the determination of effective renal plasma flow. Stable, water soluble chelates of low molecular weight are generally rapidly excreted by glomerular filtration providing that they do not bind significantly to plasma proteins. Chromium-51 EDTA has a long established use for this purpose. Early development work by Eckelman (1970) led to the introduction of Tc-99m diethylenetriaminepentaacetic acid (DTPA) which is excreted exclusively through glomerular filtration. Less than 10% of the activity becomes bound to plasma proteins, leading to a slight underestimation of the glomerular filtration rate.

Radioiodinated o-iodohippuric acid ('Hippuran') has long been the accepted radiopharmaceutical for the determination of effective renal plasma flow. Hippuric acid (benzoyl glycine) is a normal constituent of human urine, being excreted at the rate of approximately 0.7 g per day. It is formed in liver by the combination of benzoic acid and glycine and the ingestion of benzoic acid is followed by the quantitative excretion of hippuric acid by the mechanism of tubular secretion. Several agents labelled with technetium-99m have been developed to replace iodinated hippuran including such materials as N,N'-bis (mercaptoacetyl)-2,3-diaminopropanoate (CO_2 – DADS) (Fritzberg, 1982). The most interesting material is technetium-99m mercaptoacetyl triglycine (MAG-3) developed by Fritzberg in 1986. Comparative kinetics of MAG-3 and hippuran have been evaluated by Pavia (1991) who calculated rate constants, clearance, volume of distribution and protein binding. He concluded that the mean value of renal excretion constant was equal for the two agents. Clearance values were highly correlated (ratio 0.57). Volumes of distribution differed, being 4.1 litres for MAG-3 and 7.0 litres for hippuran. Between 60 and 70% of the tracers are excreted at one hour. Protein binding was found to be variable both between and within subjects, more variable fopr MAG-3 and higher for hippuran. Some authors quote a protein binding value of 60–70% for hippuran but the bond is weak and easily broken.

18.5 PARTICULATE AGENTS

Large particles, ie those with diameters in excess of 10-20 μm cannot pass through the smallest capillaries and are therefore filtered out of circulation on arrival at these vessels. Intravenous injection results in the particles becoming trapped in the arterioles and capillaries of the pulmonary circulation. Arterial injection results in trapping within the capillaries of the perfused organ eg. injection into the hepatic artery leads to entrapment in the liver. The period of residence of the entrapped particles will vary depending on the nature of the particle. Most radiopharmaceuticals of this type ie. microspheres and macroaggragates, are prepared from human albumin, which undergoes metabolic degradation and phagocytosis. Metabolic degradation of microspheres occurs more slowly than that of macroaggregates. When used for lung scanning, macroaggregated human albumin has an effective intrapulmonary half life of between one and two hours (Furth 1965). Radioactivity is released from the degraded particle. Technetium-99m may be observed in the form of pertechnetate in the thyroid gland, and radioactivity may also be eliminated via the kidneys.

Smaller particles (usually less than 1 μm in diameter) are extracted from circulation by the reticuloendothelial system following intravenous injection. The distribution of the reticuloendothelial system within the body is shown in Figure 1.

It has been reported that particles within the size range 0.0025 – 14 μm (Benaccereff, 1975, Griffin, 1974, 1975a) can all undergo engulfment by macrophages. Particles must first leave the vascular compartment. Bundgaard (1983) has described the three types of capillary structure to be found in various organs (see Figure 2), and particles are able to leave the circulation via the sinusoidal type. The fate of these particles will depend on their size and on the material from which they are prepared.

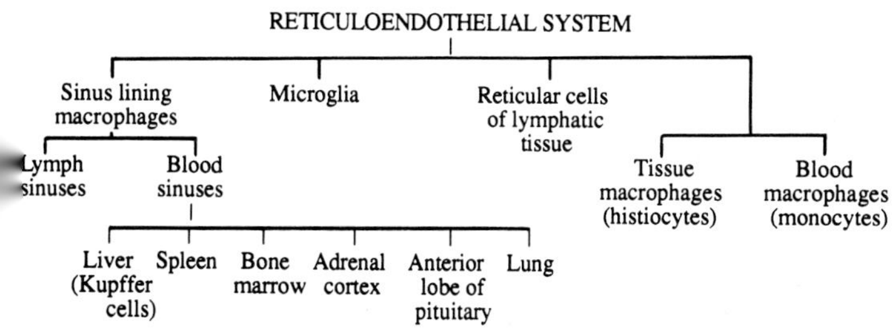

Figure 1 The reticuloendothelial system (after Saba 1970).

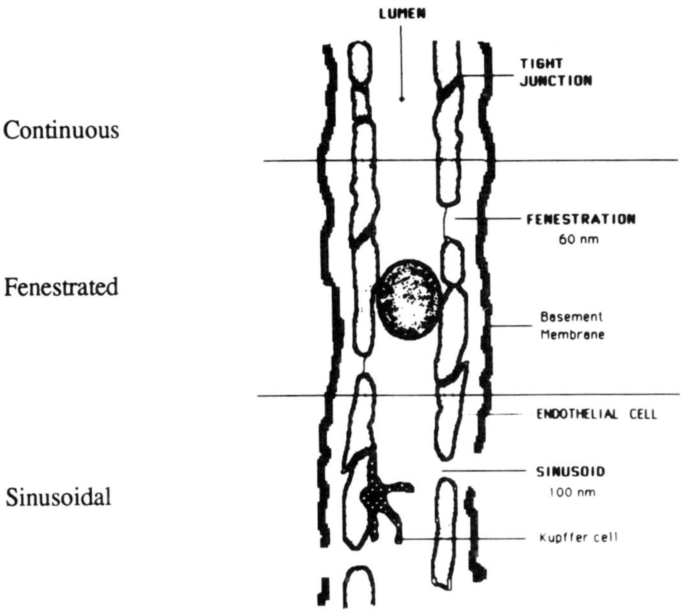

Figure 2 Capillary types of the vascular system (after Bundgaard, 1983).

Particles in the upper size range of this group tend to clear from circulation more rapidly and predominantly go to liver. The smaller size range, eg 10 nm or less, clear more slowly and a larger proportion will be found in spleen and bone marrow. Illum (1987) has demonstrated the influence of surface characteristics on biodistribution by coating particles with poloxamer 407. Uncoated polystyrene particles, 60 nm in diameter are predominantly taken up by the liver. Coated particles go predominatly to bone marrow.

The mechanismn of clearance is that of phagocytosis which is a property posessed by cells of the reticuloendothelial system. Circulating particles may become opsonised – ie undergo reaction with one or a number of plasma components including complement components C3, C4 B and C5, and some alpha and beta globulins. The particles, whether opsonised or not, are then recognised by receptors on the phagocytic cell surface. These receptors have been described by Griffin (1975b) as Fc (being responsive to the Fc portion of immunoglobulin) and C3 (being responsive to the Fc portion of aggregated or antigen-complexed IgG). Other receptors respond to the presence of an unopsonised foreign surface. In response to receptor stimulation, the process of phagocytosis is initiated in which the particles become attached to the cell surface and subsequently become engulfed by the cell. The rate of clearance is determined by the rate of regeneration of the absorbing sites, which involves the ingestion of the occupied site followed by regeneration of the plasma membrane. Inert particles may remain in the cell for long periods. Degradeable particles, eg albumin, will be broken down and the components released. Particle injected interstitially for the performance of lymphoscintigraphy, undergo a similar fate in terms of opsonisation and engulfment by the phagoctyic cells of the lymph nodes. The kinetics of clearance have been extensively studied by Bergquvist (1983) who examined eight different agents. He suggested that the fate of interstitially injected material is strongly dependent on particle size. Small diameter particles (those with diameters less than a few nanometres) will mostly be exchanged through blood capillaries. Larger particles with diameters up to a few tens of nanometres will be absorbed into the lymph capillaries by passage through junctions between the endothelial cells and/or transport in vesicles through the cells by pinocytosis. Large particles with diameters of hundreds of nanometres will spend a long time trapped in the interstitial spaces. Bergquvist (1982) has also examined the radiation dosimetry associated with the administration of colloids for lymphoscintigraphy.

18.6 BRAIN BLOOD FLOW AGENTS

For non-ionic substances without a specific transport mechanism, penetration rate from the blood to the brain is directly related to lipid solubility. Numerous substances are sufficiently soluble to cross the blood/brain barrier including oxygen, carbon dioxide, xenon and the barbiturates. Numerous factors affect the retention of the substance within the brain including degradation, binding within the brain tissue, and metabolism to a polar configuration. Radiolabelled amines, including N-isopropyl-p-iodoamphetamine, can cross the blood/brain barrier because of free diffusion of the unionised lipophilic form. Retention in the brain could be caused by a number of mechanisms. The pH gradient hypothesis proposed by Kung (1980) suggests ionisation within the brain due to the pH shift from 7.4 in the circulation to 7.0. The ionised form would therefore become trapped and unable to diffuse out. Loberg (1980) has calculated that this pH shift is insufficient to account for the observed brain: blood ratios of 37:1 at two hours post injection, predicting a value of no more than 5 or 6:1. Possible alternative mechanisms are demethylation via the n-methyltransferase enzyme, and oxidation via monoamine oxidase, or the presence of high capacity, non-specific binding sites for amines, as proposed by Winchell (1980).

T_c-99m hexamethypropyleneamineoxine (HMPAO) is a lipophilic complex of technetium-99m which has found wide application as a marker for the regional blood flow of the brain. The mechanism of cellular retention is not clearly understood. It has been proposed (Neirinckx, 1987) that it is related to the glutathione content of the cell. El-Shirbing (1989) demonstrated in experimental animals that uptake in brain, lung, kidney, and spleen was not related to glutathione content of these organs, but that glutathione depletion appeared to cause increased liver activity. Costa(1989) has shown in experimental animals that HMPAO can be found attached mainly to cell organelles. There is also a higher concentration of HMPAO in neuronal nuclei than in glial nuclei for all regions of the brain studied. The conclusion from these results is that the higher binding to cytosolic proteins, and preferential neuronal nuclei attachment might indicate more complex mechanisms than simple diffusion for the uptake and retention of this tracer.

18.7 HEPATOBILIARY AGENTS

Structure/activity relationships of technetium-99m radiopharmaceuticals have been reviewed by Muenze (1987). The combination of properties which lead a radiopharmaceutical to be distributed and excreted in its characteristic way can be summarised as follows:

Property	Affects:
Molecular size Molecular charge	Distribution space eg plasma or extracellular fluid
Protein binding	Biokinetics
Lipophilicity	Excretion pattern

Lipophilic molecules tend to be excreted via the hepatobiliary route, and if they possess structural similarities to endogenous bilirubin, may be actively excreted via the anion clearance mechanism.

Rose bengal, labelled with isotopes of iodine, has been used for many years for hepatobiliary studies. It is excreted unchanged via the bile. Bromsulphonphthalein is also excreted by this route but coupled to cysteine and glutathione (Tubis, 1961, Goris, 1973). Many technetium-99m hepatobiliary agents are based on the substituted acetanilide iminodiacetates (the IDAs). These compounds were originally developed during the search for myocardial imaging agents based on Lidocaine (Loberg, 1976, 1978). The free ligand when labelled with carbon-14 is excreted predominantly in the urine. The addition of technetium-99m leads to the formation of two or more compounds but only one undergoes rapid biliary excretion (Fritzberg, 1980). Costello (1983) has suggested that this in the form of a bis-dianionic ligand complex of technetium III. Most observations suggest that the IDAs are transported and excreted in the bile without modification, although some authors have suggesteds conjugation with bile salts (Cox 1981) or with glutathione (Richards, 1981).

Substitution in the benzene ring increases molecular weight and lipophilicity. Higher molecular weight compounds such as butyl IDA undergo less competitive inhibition in the presence of elevated serum bilirubin levels, and consequently lower compensatory renal excretion. Uptake of dimethyl IDA (HIDA) can be reduced by a factor of 3 by an increase in the serum bilirubin levels from 4 to 12 mg%, whereas the uptake of the p-isopropylphenyl derivative (PIPIDA) is reduced by only 30% in the same circumstances.

18.8 CONCLUSION

Knowledge of the fate of parenterally-administered radiopharmaceuticals is of vital importance in the understanding and interpretation of the results obtained during nuclear medicine investigations. What must be constantly born in mind is that nuclear medicine is the study of the functional state of the organ or lesion. Of equal importance is the accurate knowledge of radiation doses received by the patient during nuclear medicine studies. Calculation of radiation dosimetry at both the macro and micro levels can only be performed if the biological fate of the radionuclide is thoroughly understood. This requires knowledge, no only of the normal fate but also of the influences of the disease condition. Intracellular incorporation of radiopharmaceuticals causes additional risks when the radionuclides concerned decay with the emission of Auger electrons. The potential exists for significant genetic damage to occur, as for example in the radiolabelling of lymphocytes with indium-111.

It is not always the case that the fates of the radionuclide and the radiopharmaceutical are identical. While this is important in terms of radiation dosimetry, it is of more significance in the interpretation of results. Monoclonal antibodies labelled with indium-111 or iodine-131 can show apparently different behaviour which is, in part at least, related to the metabolic fate of the iodinated molecule and the subsequent loss of the iodine label.

Knowledge of the pharmacokinetics and metabolic fate of radiopharmaceuticals is essential, not only for the correct interpretation of nuclear medicine investigations, but may permit additional information to be extracted, thus increasing the effectiveness of this already valuable diagnostic technique.

REFERENCES

Benacereff B., Biozzi G., Halpern B.N. and Stiffel C. (1975). *Physiology of phagocytosis of particles by the RES. In* Physiopathology of the reticuloendothelial system. Halpern, B.N., Benecereff B. and Delafresnaye J.F. eds: Blackwell Scientific, Oxford.

Bergquvist L., Strand S-E., Persson B.R.R., Hafstrom L. and Jonsson P-E. (1982). *Dosimetry in lymphoscintigraphy of Tc-99m antimony sulphide colloid.* J. Nucl. Med., **23**, 698–705.

Bergquvist L., Strand S-E., Persson B.R.R. (1983). *Particle sizing and biokinetics of interstitial lymphoscintigraphic agents.* Semin. Nucl. Med., **XIII**, 9–19.

Carr E.A., Beerwaltes W.H., Wegst A.V. and Bartlett J.D. (1962). *Myocardial imaging with rubidium-86.* J. Nucl. Med., **3**, 76–82.

Costa D.C., Lui D., Sinha A.K., Jarritt P.H. and Ell P.J. (1989). *Intracellular localisation of $^{99}Tc^{m}$-d,l-HMPAO and ^{201}Tl-DDC in rat brain.* Nucl. Med. Commun. **10**, 459–466.

Bundgaard, M. (1983). *Vesicular transport on capillary endothelium. Does it occur?* Fed. Proc.; Fed. Am. Soc. Exp. Biol. **42**, 2425–2430.

Costello C.E., Brodack J.W., Jones A.G., Davison A., Johnson D.L., Kasina S. and Fritzberg A.R. (1983). *The investigation of radiopharmaceutical components by fast atom bombardment mass spectrometry: The identification of Tc-HIDA and the epimers of Tc – CO_2 DADS.* J. Nucl. Med., **24**, 353–355.

Cox P.H. (1981). *The radiopharmacological behaviour of IDA derivatives in normal experimental animals, in* Cholescintigraphy., pp 38–42 Cox, PH. ed: Martinus Nijhoff. Dordrecht.

Eckelman W.C., and Richards P. (1970). *Instant Tc-99m DTPA.* J. Nucl. Med., **11**, 761–762.

El-Shirbing A.M., Sadek S., Owunwanne A., Yacoub T., Suresh L. and Abdel-Dayem H.M. (1989). *Is Tc-99m hexamethylpropeneamineoxine uptake in the tissues related to gluthathione cellular content?* Nucl. Med. Commun. **12**, 905–911.

Fritzberg A.R., Kuni C.C., Klingensmith W. C. III., Stevens J. and Whitney W.P. (1982). *Synthesis and biological evaluation of Tc-99m N,N'-Bis(mercaptoacetyl)-2,3-diaminopropanoate. A potential replacement for ($_{131}$I)-o-iodohippurate.* J. Nucl. Med. **23**, 592–598.

Fritzberg A.R., Lewis D. (1980). *HPLC analysis of Tc-99m imidodiacetic acid hepatobiliary agents and a question of multiple peaks: concise communication,* J. Nucl. Med. **21**, 1180–1184.

Fritzberg A.R., Kasiner S., Eshima D. and Johnson D.L. (1986). *Synthesis and biological evaluation of technetium-99m MAG-3 as a hippuran replacement.* J. Nucl. Med., **27**, 111–116.

Furth E.D., Okinaka A.J., Focht E.F. and Becker D.V. (1965). *The distribution, metabolic fate and radiation dosimetry of ^{131}I labelled macroaggregated albumin.* J. Nucl. Med.,, **6**, 506–509.

Goris M.L. (1973). *^{123}I-iodobromsulphonphthalein as a liver and biliary scanning agent.* J. Nucl. Med. **14**, 820–825.

Griffin F.M. Jr. and Silverstein S.G. (1974). *Segmental response of the macrophage plasma membrane to a phagocytic stimulus.* J. Exp. Med. **139**, 323–330.

Griffin F.M. Jr., Griffin J.A., Leider J.E. and Silverstein S.C. (1975a). *Studies on the mechanism of phagocytosis I. Requirements for circumferential attachment of particle bound ligands to specific receptors on the macrophage system.* J. Exp. Med. **142**, 1263–1282.

Griffin F.M. Jr., Bianco C. and Silverstein S.C. (1975b). *Characterisation of the macrophage receptor for complement and demonstration of its functional independence from the receptor for the Fc portion of immunoglobulin G.* J. Exp. Med. **141**, 1269–1278.

Harper P.V., Lathrop K.A., Krizek H., Lembares M., Stark V. and Hoffer P.B. (1972). *Clinical feasibility of myocardial imaging with $^{13}NH_3$.* J. Nucl. Med., **13**, 278–280.

Illum L. and Davis S.S. (1987). *Targeting of colloidal particals to the bone marrow.* Life sciences **40**, 1553–1560.

Johanssen B. (1987). *Principals, problems and trends in radiopharmacology, in* Principals of Radiopharmacology pp 166–182. Deckart H. and Cox P.H. eds: Martinus Nijhoff. Dordrecht.

Kawana M., Krizek H., Porter J., Lathrop K. A., Charleston D. and Harper P.V. (1970). *Use of Tl-199 as a potassium analogue in scanning.* J. Nucl. Med. **11**, (Abstr), 333.

Kung H.F. and Blau M. *Regional intracellular pH shift: a proposed new mechanism for radiopharmaceutical uptake in brain and other tissues.* J. Nucl. Med. **21**, 147–152.

Leibowitz F., Greene M.W., Bradley-Moore P., Atkins H., Ansari A., Richards P. and Belgrave E. (1973). *Thallium-201 for medicinal use.* J. Nucl. Med. **14** (Abstr), 421.

Lin T.H., Khentigan A., Winchell H.S. (1974). *A Tc-99m chelate substitute for organomercurial renal agents.* J. Nucl. Med. **15**, 35–35.

Loberg M.D., Cooper M., Harvey H., Callery P. and Faith W. (1976). *Development of new radiopharmaceuticals based on N-substituted imidodiacetic acid.* J. Nucl. Med., **17**, 633–638.

Loberg M.D. and Fields A.T. (1978). *Chemical structure of technetium-99m labelled N-(2,6 dimethylphenylcarbamoyl-methyl)imidodiacetic acid (Tc-HIDA).* Int. J. Appl. Radiat. Isot., **29**, 167–173.

Loberg M.D. (1980). *Radiotracers for cerebral functional imaging – a new class,* J. Nucl. Med., **21**, 183–186.

McAfee J.C., (1982). *A review of radiopharmaceuticals in nephrorology. In* Radionuclides in nephrology pp. 3–8. Joekes A.M., Constable A.R., Brown N.J.C. and Tauxe, W.N. eds: Academic Press, New York.

Moretti J.L., Rapin J.R., Saccavini J.C., Lageron A., Le Poncin M. and Bardy A. (1982). *2,3-dimercaptosuccinic acid chelates: their structure and biological behaviour. In* Nuclear Medcicine and Biology Vol II, pp. 1651–1655. Raynaud, C. ed: Pergamon Press.

Mousa S.A., Williams S.J. and Sands H. (1897). *Characterisation of in-vivo chemistry of cations in the heart.* J. Nucl. Med. **28**, 1351–1357.

Muenze R. (1987). *Technetium-99m radiopharmaceuticals: Structure-activity relationships. In* Principles of Radiopharmacology pp. 100–116. Deckart H. and Cox P.H. eds: Martinus Nijhoff. Dordrecht.

Neirinckx R.D., Harrison R.C., Faster J.F., (1987). *A model for the in-vivo behaviour of Tc-99m d,l-HM-PAO in man.* J. Nucl. Med., **28**, 559.

Pavia J., Ros D., Piera C., Pavia A., Bassa P., Giralt E. and Setoain J. (1991). *Comparative study of the kinetics of the renal tracers Tc-99m-MAG-3 and I-131 hippuran.* Nucl. Med Commun., **12**, 529–537.

Richards A.G. and Brighouse R. (1981). *Nicotinic acid: a cause of failed HIDA scanning* J. Nucl. Med. **22**, 746–747.

Rosenthall L. and Kaye M. (1976). *Observations on the mechanism of Tc-99m labelled phosphate complex in metabolic bone disease.* Semin. Nucl. Med. **6**, 59–67.

Saba T.M. (1970). *Physiology and physiopathology of the reticuloendothelial system.* Arch. Int Med., **126**, 1031–1052.

Sands H., Delano M.L., Gallagher B.M. (1986). *Uptake of hexakis-(t-butylisonitrile) technetium (I) and hexakis-(isopropylisonitrile) technetium(I) by neonatal rat myocytes and human erythrocytes.* J. Nucl. Med. **27**, 404–408.

Tilden R.L., Jackson J., Enneking W.F., DeLand F.H. and McVey J.T. (1973). *^{99m}Tc-Polyphosphate: Histological localisation in human femurs by autoradiography.* J. Nucl. Med. **14**, 576–578.

Tubis M., Nordyke R.A., Posnick E. and Blahd W.H. (1961). *The preparation and use of I^{131} labelled sulfobromophthalein in liver function testing.* J. Nucl. Med., **2**, 282–288.

Van Langevelde A., Driessen O.M.J., Pauwels E.K.J. and Thesingh C.W. (1977). *Aspects of ^{99m}Technetium binding from an ethane-1-hydroxy-1,1-diphosphonate-^{99m}Tc complex to bone.* Eur. J. Nucl. Med. **2**, 47–51.

Winchell H.S., Horst W.D., Braun L., Oldendorf W.H., Hattner R. and Parker H. (1980). *N-isopropyl-[^{123}I] p-iodoamphetamine: Single pass brain uptake and washout; binding to brain synaptosomes; and localisation in dog and monkey brain.* J. Nucl. Med., **21**, 947–952.

Chapter 19

Effect of Patient Medication and Other Factors on the Biodistribution of Radiopharmaceuticals

C.B. Sampson and P.H. Cox

19.1 INTRODUCTION

Nuclear medicine scintigraphy has now been practised throughout the nuclear medicine community for more than forty years. In recent years many reports have been received of unusual or unexplainable changes in the disposition of the tracer which could not be explained by the patient's histopathology. There are many extraneous factors which can influence biodistribution and it is therefore important to identify these and to distinguish the changes which they produce from those induced by disease. On some occasions it was the drug being taken by the patient, on others it was the radiation therapy or surgical procedure that could alter the behaviour of the tracer. Other factors were method of preparation or even the diet regime of the patient. However, most of the adverse reports were those in which there was some interaction between the patient's medication and the circulating radiopharmaceutical. Several authors have reviewed drug induced changes and catalogued them in various ways (Hladik 1982; Deckart 1986; Cox 1985, 1988; Sampson 1985, 1989, 1990). In this chapter the more important drug-radiopharmaceutical interactions will be described and examples taken from general practice. The text will include a tabular summary of the most widely reported interactions. Also to be described will be other factors which can effect biodistribution such as radiation therapy and diet.

19.2 CLASSIFICATION OF DRUG/RADIOPHARMACEUTICAL INTERACTIONS

Many reported instances of drug interference are somewhat anecdotal and difficulties arise as to a direct cause and effect relationship. Other difficulties arise because of almost complete absence of *in-vitro* testing of the drug with the radiopharmaceutical. Also, it is difficult to determine the precise mode of action as little work has been performed on drug interference at a molecular level. Nevertheless, certain classes of drugs have become associated with characteristic changes in the tracer behaviour and this review will concentrate mainly on these effects.

An increasingly large number of drugs e.g. diuretics, antispasmodics and cardiac agents, are being used to enhance nuclear medicine studies. Because, however, the changes in tracer behaviour are those that might be expected they are outside the remit of this review.

Drug/radiopharmaceutical effects may be classified by organ of interest, radiopharmaceutical used, the patient's drug, or the type of deviation. For convenience and simplicity abnormal effects will be categorised under the headings of unusual handling of the radiopharmaceutical by organ, *in-vivo* physico-chemical interaction, drug-induced disease, and drugs which interfere with blood cell labelling.

19.2.1 Unusual Handling of Radiopharmaceutical as a Result of Pharmacological Effect

By far the largest number of reports of drug/radiopharmaceutical incompatibilities are those in which the functional status of the organ is altered as a result of pharmacological action by the patient's medication. For example, narcotic analgesics such as methadone, pethidine and morphine may cause spasm of the biliary tract due to contraction of the sphincter of Oddi (Pope & Bratke 1981). As a consequence, prolonged transit times of hepatobiliary imaging agents from the liver to the duodenum may occur. Enzyme inducers such as phenobarbitone, may enhance biliary excretion of similar imaging agents, and cholinergic drugs such as bethanechol and cholecystokinim, may also induce gall bladder emptying (Feezer 1982). Other drugs which may affect hepatobiliary imaging include a number of anaesthetics. Halothane has been shown to cause a marked decrease in hepatic blood flow and therefore a reduced uptake of colloid into the liver (Lentle & Scott 1979). Another report has shown that total parenteral nutrition (TPN) can influence uptake of tracer into the gall bladder since during TPN the gall bladder is relatively inactive, resulting in bile stasis and reduced uptake into the gall bladder. Prolonged usage of nicotinic acid and its derivatives can cause liver dysfunction (Winter & Boger 1973) and a case report has been published of complete absence of the imaging agent technetium-99m HIDA in a patient on nicotinic acid therapy (Richards & Brighouse 1981).

Cytotoxic drugs such as cyclophosphamide, vincristine, bleomycin and cis-platin are reported to affect the pharmacokinetic response of radiopharmaceuticals, particularly the tumour-seeking radiopharmaceutical gallium-67 citrate. This material localises in some neoplasms as well as other sites such as the liver and regions of infection or inflammation. In patients on cyclophosphamide and vincristine, it has been observed that there is very high uptake of tracer in the blood pool and little or no uptake in the tumour or liver (Lentle & Scott 1979). The exact mechanism of interaction in unclear. A shift of the liver imaging agent technetium-99m sulphur colloid from the liver to the extra-hepatic reticulo-endothelial system is patients being treated with nitrosoureas has also been reported (Lutrin *et al.* 1978). Similar effects, although less frequent, also occur with antimetabolites such as cytosine arabinoside and methotrexate. Intense renal uptake of the blood pool imaging agent technetium-99m pyrophosphate (PYP) has been reported in children on vincristine, adriamycin and cyclophosphamide therapy (Lutrin *et al.* 1978). This effect was observed only in patients who had been treated for one week with chemotherapy. It has been suggested that the altered pattern of behaviour could be due to a reduction in the glomerular filtration rate or an alteration in renal tubular function. Cytotoxic therapy may have other effects in paediatric nuclear medicine and Figure 1 demonstrates a decrease in skeletal uptake of MDP in a child on a multi-cytotoxic regime. After cessation of therapy the skeletal uptake increases markedly.

A recent case report (Mavers *et al.* 1988) described significant abnormal distribution of gallium-67 citrate in a child with chloroquine poisoning. There was a marked increased in gallium uptake in the heart and kidneys. The exact pathophysiologic mechanism for this has not been elucidated. The pattern of gallium uptake, however, correlated well with the known biodistribution of chloroquine. Another deviation from the normal scintigraphic appearance of gallium occurred in an eight year old patient with juvenile rheumatoid arthritis undergoing gold therapy. The study demonstrated no hepatic uptake of the tracer but showed elevated skeletal and renal activity (Moult & Bekerman 1989). It was thought that the unusual biodistribution was due to inhibition of lysosomal enzymes by gold and/or accumulation of gold in lysosomes.

An increasingly large number of drugs are known to alter hormonal status. The effects associated with these changes may produce marked alterations in the expected biodistribution of radiopharmaceuticals. Stilboestrol, digitalis, gonadotrophins, phenothiazines, cimetidine and oral

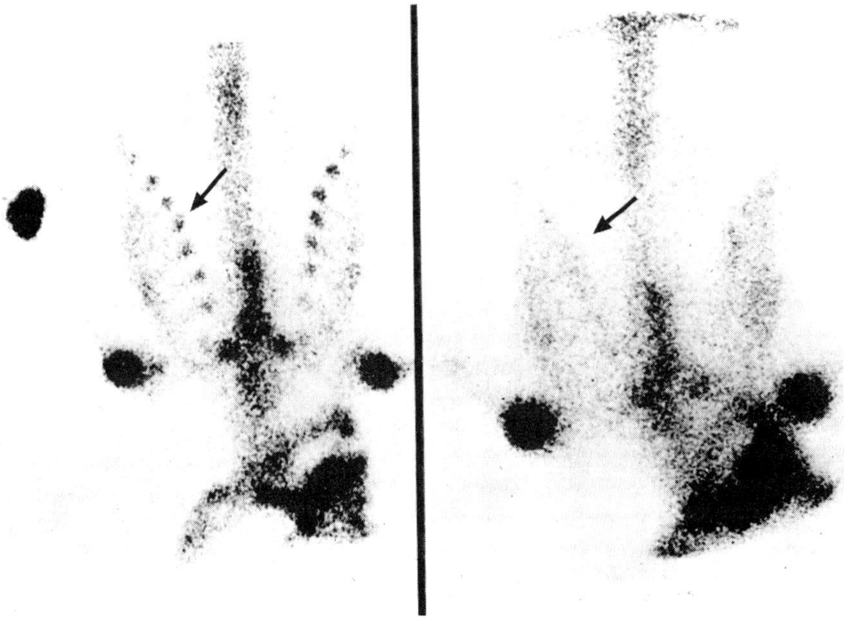

Figure 1 Skeletal scintigram of a child before (right) and after (left) cytotoxic therapy. Note the general suppression of uptake but especially in the areas of active ossification in the ribs (see arrows).

contraceptives increase the production of oestrogens (Lentle & Scott 1979) and may induce gynaecomastia. It has been found that there is increased localisation of gallium-67 citrate (Ajmani & Pincher 1978) and technetium-99m PYP (Ramnsingh *et al.* 1977) in gynaecomastic breasts. Increased levels of oestrogen may be associated with high levels of prolactin and uptake of gallium has been reported in conditions associated with hyperprolactinaemia as shown in Figure 2 (Stephanas & Maisey 1976).

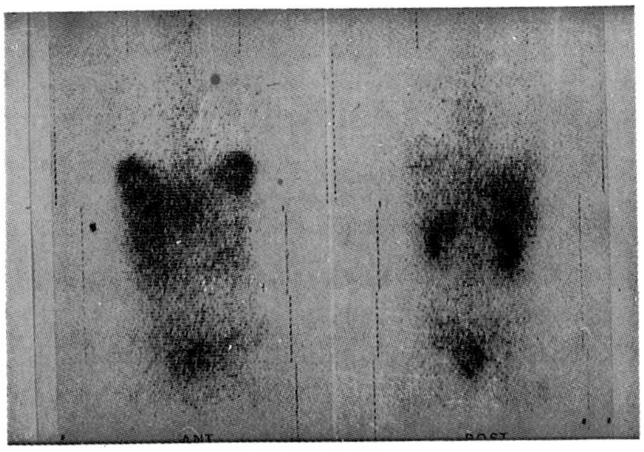

Figure 2 Bilateral uptake of Gallium-67 citrate in a patient with drug-induced hyperprolactinaemia (reproduced with permission).

Although the mechanism of uptake of gallium in drug induced gynaecomastic and prolactin sensitised breasts is not clear, a number of workers have suggested possible mechanism. Hoffer (1960) attributes the uptake in the breast to high concentrations of lactoferrin found in human colostrum and milk, whereas Hayes (1977) attributes it to an increase in lysosomal enzymes which occur during gestation or lactation.

Table 1
Medications Resulting in Hyperprolactinaemia (Adapted from Desai *et al.* 1986)

Pharmacological Class	*Example*
Dopamine Receptor Antagonists	Phenothiazines
	Chlopromazine
	Fluphenazine
	Trifluoroperazine
	Perphenazine
	Thioridazine
	Haloperidol
	Metoclopramide
	Prochlorperazine
Catecholamine Synthesis Inhibitor	Methyldopa
Dopamine Depleting Agent	Reserpine
Calcium Channel Blocker	Verapamil
Opiates	Morphine
	Medorphin
	Methadone

Ramsingh suggests that uptake of gallium is due to the increased enzyme activity of phosphatases. A summary of medications which affect prolactin levels is given in Table 1.

One of the most important groups of drugs that affect the diagnostic accuracy of nuclear medicine tests are those which affect the uptake of radiopharmaceuticals into the thyroid. Thyroid scanning agents in current use include sodium pertechnetate, I-131 sodium iodide and I-123 sodium iodide. Any drug which interferes with the uptake of iodine or blocks its release from the thyroid can interfere with the uptake of tracer and therefore lead to mis-diagnosis. Several drugs, some of which are used daily by diabetics, epileptics and allergy sufferers, have a propensity for affecting thyroid scanning. Other drugs include iodine-containing contrast media, antithyroid medications and thyroid supplements. Table 2 summarises many of the drugs and contrast media which have been reported to affect thyroid scanning (adapted from Grayson 1960).

Table 2
Drugs and Chemicals That Interfere with I-131 Thyroid Uptake (Adapted from Grayson 1960).

Drugs	*Contrast Media*
Lugol's Iodine	Hypaque
Iodides	Dionosil
Anti-tussives	Diodrast
Iodine ointment	
Vitamin preparations	
Anti-thyroid drugs	
Perchlorate	
Sulphonamides	
Steroids	
Phenylbutazone	
Mepbrobamate	
Antihistamines	

Competing anions such as the perchlorate and pertechnetate ions act as competitive inhibitors of the iodine transport mechanism causing decreased uptake of I-131 sodium iodide. Inorganic iodine-containing medications such as Lugol's Iodine and vitamin and mineral supplements are thought to release iodine, thereby decreasing the specific activity of iodide in the body pool resulting in decreased uptake of radioiodine into the thryroid gland (Sternthal *et al.* 1980). Similar mechanisms have been proposed for iodine-containing anti-tussive medicines. Sea foods containing high levels of iodine, e.g. haddock, cod and halibut, may also reduce I-131 uptake in the thyroid. Antithyroid drugs such as propylthiouracil inhibit the metabolic synthesis of thyroid hormones resulting in decreased transport and decreased uptake of I-131 (Steinback & Donoghue 1979). Phenylbutazone is thought to decrease the output of thyroid stimulating hormone (TSH) inducing a secondary depression of thyroid activity (Grayson 1960). A number of workers (Maxon *et al.* 1983) have suggested that low iodide diets could be potentially useful in increasing the radiation dose to the thyroid per megabequeral of administered I-131 radioactivity in ablative therapy.

A few drugs have been reported to cause problems in the interpretation of adrenal scintigrams. For example, oral contraceptives increase the adrenal uptake of the adrenal cortex imaging agent I-131 iodomethylnorcholestenol by producing an elevated plasma renin activity which results in adrenocortical stimulation, increased cortisol secretion and hyperplasia (Gross *et al.* 1981). An increasingly large number of reports have been published on the effects of drugs on the adrenal medulla imaging agent metaiodobenzylguanidine (MIBG). MIBG labelled I-131 has been shown to have a pronounced uptake in the canine and primate adrenal glands and in phaeochromocytoma (tumours of the adrenal medulla). This tracer also localises in the heart and salivary glands. MIBG is an iodinated alkylguanidine which has similarities in structure to noradrenaline and the hypotensive drug gaunethidine. Reserpine is widely known to block the uptake of noradrenaline into storage vesicles, and in some animals to deplete noradrenaline stores from their adrenal glands. Animal sltudies have shown that in dogs previously injected with reserpine there was a decrease in activity of I-131 MIBG in the adrenal glands of 87% (Wieland *et al.* 1981). The effects of tricyclic antidepressants on catecholamine uptake into adrenergic storage vesicles is, again, well known, and in patients taking these drugs I-131 MIBG uptake may be seriously impaired. Thus in patients on imipramine hydrochloride a striking absence of tracer in the heart and salivary glands was observed which reversed on withdrawal of the drug (Nakajo *et al.* 1982).

Drugs which alter acid/base ratios can have important sequelae in nuclear medicine and it has been shown that ammonium chloride and sodium bicarbonate may decrease renal uptake and increase hepatic biodistribution of the renal imaging agent technetium-99m dimercaptosuccinic acid (DMSA) (Yee *et al.* 1981).

One of the most well documented drug/ratio-pharmaceutical interactions is that concerning the suppression of uptake of gallium-67 citrate in cerebral tumours in patients taking cortisone preparations (Waxman *et al.* 1977). It is thought that this occurs as a result of a decrease in extracellular sodium and water content leading to a decrease in oedema. The tracer is often associated with the oedematous fluid so an apparent decrease in the size of tumour is observed on the scintigram. The effect may be so pronounced as to completely suppress uptake into the tumour with possible consequences of complete mis-diagnosis. Cortisone may also affect the sensitivity of detection of bone trauma in technetium-99m MDP bone scintigraphy. Animal studies have shown that sensitivity for detecting fractures in rabbits on high doses of hydrocortisone was 48% compared to 85% for control animals (Alazraki *et al.* 1987). Figure 3 shows a skeletal scintigram of a patient with metastatic disease before and after steroid therapy.

19.2.2 *In-vivo* Physicochemical Interaction Between Radiopharmaceutical and Patient's Medication

Although most drug/radiopharmaceutical incompatibilities are associated with a pharmacological change in the organ of interest, a number of well defined effects occur as a result of a genuine physicochemical interaction between the drug circulating in the blood and the administered radiopharmaceutical. Little is known at a molecular level about the mode of action of such interactions. It is thought that the formation of local complexes could prevent the radiopharmaceutical from its normal distribution pattern. For example, a number of reports have been published on the effect of intramuscular iron dextran on the biodistribution of technetium-99m MDP. Instead of localising throughout the skeleton, a diffuse concentration of activity is usually observed at the site of injection, i.e. the gluteal region of the buttock (Mazzole *et al.* 1976). It is thought that local complexing occurs between reduced technetium and ferric hydroxide as the latter is released from the iron dextran complex.

Aluminium is now increasingly being reported to interact with radiopharmaceuticals. Aluminium ion in patients on aluminium containing drugs such as antacids, could cause flocculation of colloidal particles of sulphur (for liver scanning) so that the particles get trapped in the microvasculature of the lungs (Bobbinet *et al.* 1974). Moreover, elevated plasma levels of albumin may result in an altered biodistribution of the stomach imaging agent sodium pertechnetate. Thus it has been observed that there is a delay in excretion of pertechnetate from the stomach until plasma levels have fallen to normal (Wang *et al.* 1978). In a recent report there was a pronounced alteration in the behaviour of the tumour seeking radiopharmaceutical gallium-67 citrate in a patient with aluminium toxicity and on therapy with desferrioxamine. The patient was also undergoing haemodialysis to clear the aluminium. Whole body images obtained forty-eight hours after injection of the radiopharmaceutical showed diffuse activity and poor tissue localisation and complete absence of normal uptake (Brown *et al.* 1990). Desferrioxamine, a chelating agent used primarily to treat iron overload, is also used to treat aluminium toxicity. Desferrioxamine rapidly forms a complex with aluminium that is readily dialysable (Mulliner *et al.* 1986). However, it also binds gallium forming a complex much stronger than that of gallium with transferrin (the protein to which gallium usually binds), (Weiner *et al.* 1979). Thus in the above patient, desferrioxamine given prior to gallium would have bound some aluminium and would have been removed during dialysis. Excess

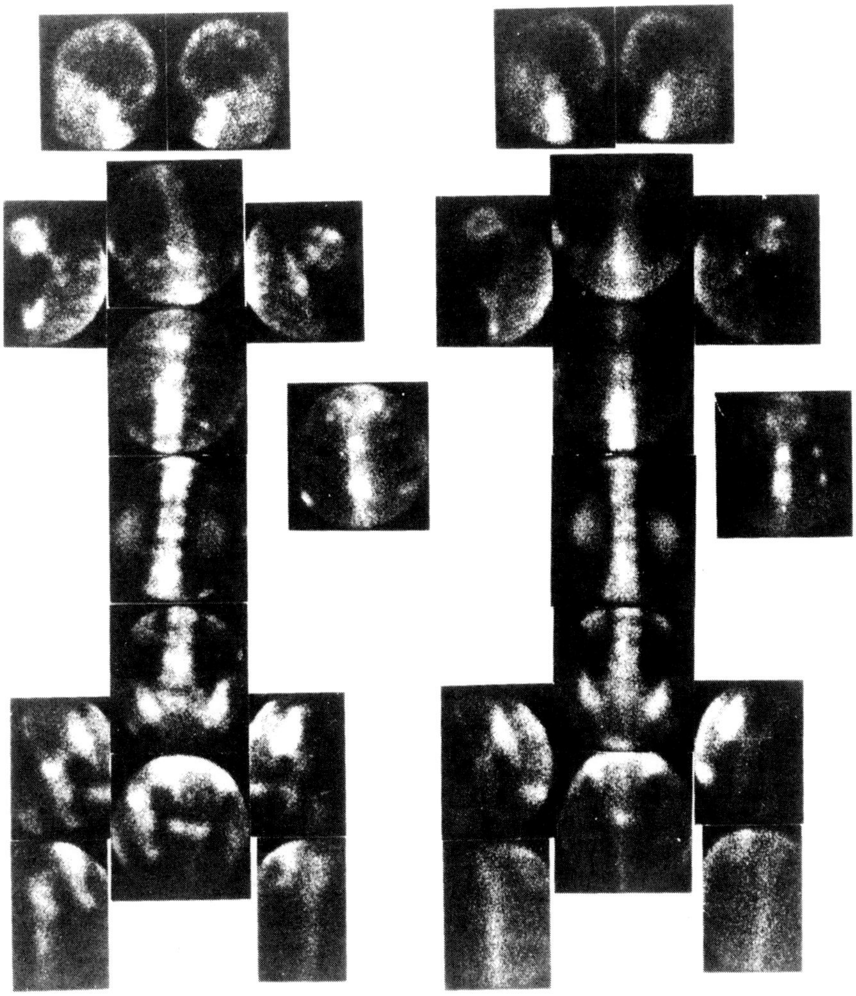

Figure 3. Skeletal scintigram of a patient with metastatic disease before (left) and after (right) steroid therapy. Note the suppression of radioactivity in the metastases although new ones are visible in the ribs.

aluminium could then have interfered with gallium-transferrin binding and subsequent cellular uptake thus altering the normal distribution of gallium. Another aluminium-related case report was that of a patient who was being evaluated for myocardial infarction using technetium-99m pyrophosphate (Eisenberg *et al.* 1989). The patient was taking 4.8 grammes daily of Maalox suspension (containing aluminium hydroxide) for peptic ulcer. Instead of localising in the myocardium, almost all the radioactivity was found to be in the liver and spleen, possibly owing to the formation of colloidal complex of pyrophosphate with aluminium.

The most recent reports of drug interference are those associated with the calcium channel antagonist nifedipine. There have been a number of instances of failure to label red blood cells with technetium in patients taking this compound and also a case report of greatly reduced uptake of MDP in a patient on nifedipine therapy (Figure 4). Blake *et al.* (1988) have also reported that nifedipine may enhance the retention of I-131 MIBG in the localisation of phaeochromocytoma by as much as twofold.

19.2.3 Drug-induced Disease Affecting the Transport of Radiopharmaceutical

It is well known that many drugs in everyday use may cause or aggravate disease, and that the iatrogenic (drug induced) disease itself may then produce an unexpected biological distribution of a tracer. If the clinician is unaware of the presence of the drug-associated disease, it is possible that errors will be made in making an accurate assessment of the patient's primary condition.

On of the largest groups of drugs that can cause iatrogenic diseases, are those which are toxic to the liver. These include paracetamol, aspirin, some cytotoxic agents and tetracylcine. These may, in large doses, cause necrosis of liver cells and

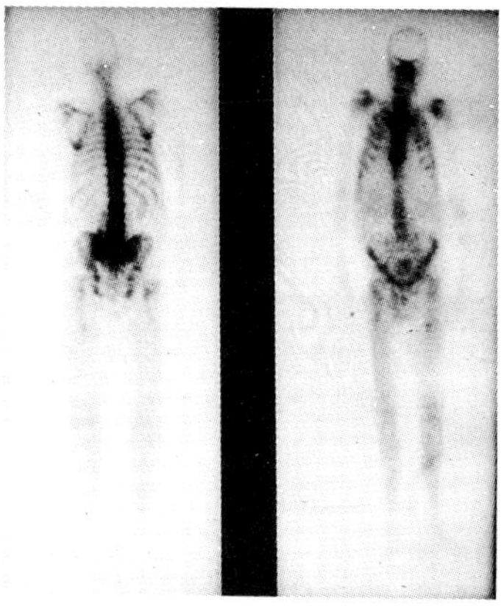

Figure 4. Reduced skeletal uptake of MDP in a patient on nifedipine therapy. Note the increased uptake of tracer in the musculature of the extremities.

a consequent reduction in radioactivity in those regions. The long term use of the contraceptive pill has been associated with the formation of hepatic tumours and these appear as large filling defects on a scintigram (Klatskin 1977). TPN therapy has been reported to cause hepaticdysfunction (Hladik *et al.* 1987) including fatty liver disease, and erythromycin hepatotoxicity has been reported to have resulted in a false positive diagnosis in a patient during scanning with the hepatobiliary imaging agent technetium-99m DISIDA (Swayne & Colc 1986). Hepatobiliary tracers accumulate normally in the gall bladder and from there pass directly into the duodenum. They depend on the presence of bile and bile flow for their effect. It was thought that erythromycin had interfered with bile production, resulting in altered biliary flow dynamics. Because of absence of tracer in the gall bladder it was wrongly thought that the patient was suffering from cholecystitis. A later case report (Flynn & Treves 1987) described the diffuse accumulation of technetium-99m MDP in the liver of a patient with methotrexate induced hepatotoxicity. The authors postulated that inhibition of protein synthesis by methotrexate caused a disruption of the cell membrane high affinity of MDP for calcium lead to diffuse uptake of trac er throughout the liver.

Many drugs are capable of causing acute renal failure, which can cause an abnormal uptake of tracer of a decrease in glomerular filtration rate. Of particular importance are the aminoglycoside antibiotics, penicillins and sulphonamides (Blathenad *et al.* 1978). Other drug induced renal abnormalities include delayed uptake of gallium-67 citrate in patients taking phenylbutazone or frusemide (Linds *et al.* 1983). It was thought that abnormalities occurred as a result of drug-induced interstitial nephritis. Cyclosporin can cause nephrotoxic effects which may become apparent in the post-operative stage as acute renal failure and later as a gradual decrease in GFR. Diuretics such as frusemide can improve renal function so that misleadingly good renograms and flow curves are obtained using the renal imaging agents I-131 Hippuran and technetium-99m DTPA (Clomius *et al.* 1979).

A few drugs are associated with causing lung disease, the most common of which is bleomycin. Toxicity of this drug is well documented and manifests itself as pulmonary interstitial fibrosis. Abnormally high levels of gallium-67 citrate are observed in the lungs of these patients, presumably because of leucocyte infiltration (Crystal *et al.* 1976). Other drugs which produce similar lung uptake abnormalities include amiodarone, busulphan and nitrofurantoin (Hladik *et al.* 1987). Another report suggests that ex-heroin users may have granulomatous lung desease and a resultant abnormal uptake of tracer (Napp 1986).

A number of drugs are cardiotoxic when administered in large doses, e.g. doxorubicin hydrochloride. These agents may impair left ventricular function resulting in changes in the cardiac biodistribution of heart-seeking radiopharmaceuticals such as technetium-99m pyrophosphate. A later report described a marked increase in gallium activity in a doxorubicin-damaged myocardium (Chacke *et al.* 1977). After surgical intervention and cessation of therapy the uptake reverted to normal. Adriamycin is well known to be cardiotoxic in large doses. This is often seen in nuclear medicine investigations as myocardial uptake of technetium diphosphonate complexes in the myocardium. This is probably due to induced changes in cell membrane permeability, possibly related to raised intracellular calcium levels. Contrary to what might therefore be expected, Adriamycin toxicity results in decreased thallium accumulation in the myocardium. Chemotherapy also causes an abnormal uptake of In-111-labelled antimyosin in myocardial muscle (Figure 5).

19.2.4 Drugs which Interfere with the Radiolabelling of Blood Cells

During the past five years there has been a great upsurge throughout the nuclear medicine community in the use of radiolabelled blood cells. In many centres it is now possible to separate and label erythrocytes, neutrophils, platelets, and in a few laboratories, lymphocytes. The main clinical uses for labelled red cells lie in the provision of functional information about left ventricular contraction (MUGA study). In this technique the patient's own red cells are labelled with stannous pyrophosphate or medronate and sodium pertechnetate and the patient imaged under a gamma camera whilst the material is being injected. Sophisticated computer technology enables the contraction and relaxation cycles of the heart to be monitored. In leucocyte scintigraphy the patient's leucocytes are removed by sedimentation and centrifugation, the appropriate radionuclide is added and the cells re-injected. The technique is widely used for the

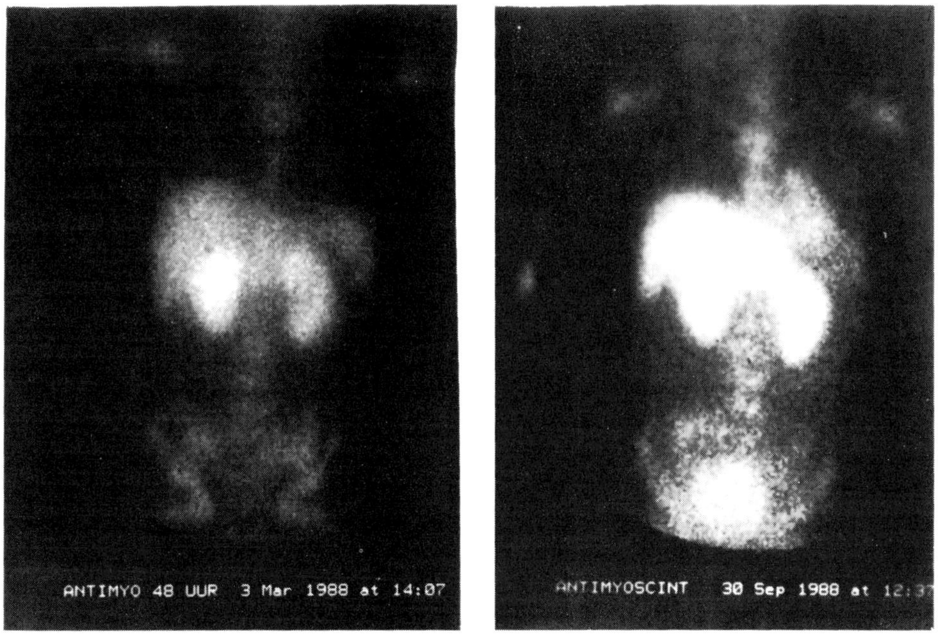

Figure 5. In-111 labelled antimyosin scintigram of a patient before (left) and after (right) steroid therapy. Note the suppression of radioactivity in the metastases although new ones are visible in the ribs.

investigation of loci of inflammation and infection in for example, stomach abscess, inflammatory bowel disease and vasculitis.

During cell labelling procedures many factors need to be taken into account to achieve an optimal labelling efficiency (i.e. proportion of radionuclide actually attached to the cells). These include temperature, number of cells, activity required, and volume of the cell suspension. In addition to these criteria it has recently been established that drugs circulating in the patient's plasma can influence the level of tagging.

Zimmer *et al.* (1981) investigated the effect of five widely used drugs on in-vitro labelling of red blood cells and found that hydralazine and methyldopa significantly decreased the labelling efficiency possibly through oxidation of the stannous ion present in the kit of ingredients. Similar findings in an animal model were reported with prazosin and digoxin (Lee *et al.* 1983). It was thought that the adverse effect with digoxin was associated with the fact that digoxin affects RBC membrane transport by inhibition of the NaK-ATPase dependent pump.

It is well known that the concentration of stannous ion may have a marked effect on the in-vitro labelling efficiency of technetium-99m labelled red cells and it has been shown that optimum yields are achieved with concentrations in the range of 0.03-0.15 ug stannous ion per ml of blood (Zanelli 1982). Any deviation from that range is likely to cause a decreased tagging efficiency of up to 20%. The same worker also showed that propranolol, verapamil, chlorthiazide and frusemide all had quite significant effects on the labelling efficiency.

An interesting observation was made in 1983 (Tatum *et al.*) that patients who had previously received iodinated contrast media produced a sub-optimal red cell tagging efficiency. It was found that the mean labelling efficiency in those patients was 30% as opposed to 90% in patients who had not received the contrast media. It was thought that the poor labelling efficiency could be due to an alteration in the redox potential of the stannous ion and therefore affect its role as a reducer of techneticuml Little is known about the effect of different anticoagulant agents on the labelling efficiency of technetium-labelled red cells, but it has been shown that the choice of either heparin or acid-citrate-dextrose may produce a significant difference (Porter *et al.* 1983). In a series of 23 patients the labelling efficiency using acid-citrate-dextrose was 93.5% +/− 3.8 compared to 87.2% +/− 4 with heparin. Moreover, image quality was improved in that less renal and bladder activity was observed.

In white cell labelling therapy with antibotics, corticosteroids and hyper-alimentation may result in a reduction in chemotaxis of leucocytes and this could effect the results of a diagnosis (Hladik *et al.* 1987). In a recent study in a particular region of the UK a survey showed that there were 15 reports of unusually low labelling efficiencies of indium tropolonate labelled cells (Sampson & Brown 1992). Seven of these patients were found to be on corticosteroids. Although it is not clear whether there is a direct cause and

Table 3
Summary of the Most Frequently Reported Drug Interferences

Drug	*Test*	*Radiopharmaceutical*	*Deviation*
Aluminium	Hepatic	Sulphur colloid	Flocculation of colloid, deposition in lung.
Aluminium	RBC labelling	Tc-99m PYP	Poor labelling efficiency. Free pertechnetate thyroid, stomach, salivary glands.
Aluminium	Renal	Tc-99m DPTA	Abnormal GFR result.
Analgesics	Abdominal	Tc-99m pertechnetate	Delay in gastric emptying, unusual pertechnetate transit time.
Antihistamines	Thyroid	I-131 Sodium iodide	Abnormal uptake.
Amiodarone	Tumour/abscess	Ga-67 citrate	Abnormal uptake in breast.
Ammon. Chlor.	Renal	Tc-99m DMSA	Reduced uptake.
Atropine	Abdominal	Tc-99m pertechnetate	Delay in gastric emptying. Free pertechnetate in thyroid, stomach, salivary glands.
Bethanochol	Hepatobiliary	Tc-99m HIDA and others	Enhanced biliary excretion.
Bisulphan	Tumour/abscess	Ga-67 citrate	Abnormal uptake in breast.
Bleomycin	Tumour/abscess	GBa-67 citrate	Abnormal uptake in lungs.
Cisplatinum	Renal	Tc-99m DMSA/DIPA	Abnormal uptake in kidney.
Cisplatinum	Tumour/abscess	Ga-67 citrate	Abnormal uptake in blood pool, kidneys, skeleton.
Cholecystokinin	Hepatobiliary	Tc-99m HIDA	Enhanced biliary excretion.
Chlorpromazine	Tumour/abscess	Ga-67 citrate	Abnormal uptake in breast.
Colchicine	Schilling Test	Co-57/Co-58	Abnormal result for malabsorption.
Contraceptives	Adrenal	I-131 methylnorcholesterol	Increased uptake in adrenals.
Contraceptives	Hepatic	Tc-99m Sulphur colloid	Filling defect due to drug-induced tumour.
Contraceptives	Schilling test	Co-57/Co-58	Abnormal result for malabsorption.
Cortisone	Tumour/abscess	Ga-67 citrate/Tc-99m	Decrease in apparent tumour size.
Cortisone	Bone	Tc-99m MDP	Decrease in uptake in bone trauma.
Cortisone	Abscess	In-111 WBC	Reduced chlurotaxis of labelled leucocytes
Cyclophosphamide	Tumour/abscess	Ga-67 citrate	Abnormal uptake in blood pool, kidneys, skeleton
Dextrose	Bone	Tc-99m MDP	Reduced skeletal uptake.
Digoxin	Cardiac	Tc-99m RBC	Poor labelling efficiency. Free pertechnetate present.
Doxorubicin	Cardiac	Tc-99m RBC	Abnormal cardiac distribution.
Enterovioform	Thyroid	I-131 Sodium iodide	Abnormal thyroid uptake.
Erythromycin	Hepatobiliary	Tc-99m DISIDA	Increased uptake in liver.
Fluphenazine	Tumour/abscess	Ga-67 citrate	Increased uptake in breast.
Frusemide	Tumour/abscess	Ga-67 citrate	Reduced uptake.
Frusemide	Renal	Tc-99m DTPA/DMSA	Enhanced renal function, misleading diagnosis.
Gentamicin	Renal	Cr-51 EDTA	Decreased GFR.
Haloperidol	Tumour/abscess	Ga-67 citrate	Increased uptake in breast.
Halothane	Hepatic	Liver colloids	Reduced uptake in liver.
Hydralazine	Cardiac	Tc-99m RBC	Poor labelling efficiency. Free pertechnetate present.
Iodides	Thyroid	I-131 Sodium iodide	Abnormal thyroid uptake.
Isoproterenol	Abdominal	Tc-99m pertechnetate	Delayed gastric emptying. Redistribution of pertechnetate.

Isoproterenol	Abdominal	Tc-99m pertechnetate	Delayed gastric emptying. Redistribution of pertechnetate.
Iron salts	Bone	Tc-99m MDP/EHDP	Pronounced abnormal uptake. Diffuse accumulation of tracer at site of injection. High blood pool, renal activity.
Lugol's solution	Thyroid	I-131 Sodium iodide	Abnormal thyroid uptake.
Mepbrobamate	Thyroid	I-131 Sodium iodide	Abnormal thyroid uptake.
Metaclopramide	Tumour/abscess	Ga-67 citrate	Increased uptake in breast.
Methyldopa	Tumour/abscess	Ga-67 citrate	Increased uptake in breast.
Methyldopa	Cardiac/GI bleed	Tc-99m RBC	Poor labelling efficiency. Free pertechnetate in thyroid, salivary glands, stomach.
Morphine	Hepatobiliary	Tc-99m HIDA	Abnormal transit time into duodenum.
Methadone	Hepatobiliary	Tc-99m HIDA	Abnormal transit time into dueodenum.
Methotrexate	Hepatic	Tc-99m Sulphur colloid	Filling defects in liver due to hepatotoxicity.
Methotrexate	Brain	Tc-99m pertechnetate	Increased uptake in ventricles.
Laxatives	Abdominal	Tc-99m pertechnetate	Alteration in pertechnetate pharmacokinetics.
Nifedipine	Cardiac/GI bleed	Tc-99m RBC	Poor labelling efficiency. Free pertechnetate in thyroid, salivary glands, stomach.
Nifedipine	Bone	Tc-99m MDP	Reduced skeletal uptake.
Nifedipine	Phaeochromocytoma	I-131 MIBG	Increased uptake in phaeochromocytoma.
Neomycin	Schilling test	Co-57/Co-58	Abnormal result for malabsorption of vitamin B12
Nitrofurantoin	Tumour/abscess	Ga-67 citrate	Increased uptake in breast.
Nicotinic acid	Hepatobiliary	Tc-99m HIDA	Abnormal or absence of tracer in gall bladder.
Phenylbyutazone	Thyroid	I-131 Sodium iodide	Abnormal uptake in thyroid.

effect relationship there might well be such a link. In the same survey it was reported that there were nine cases of failure to label red cells. Of these, two patients were on nifedipine therapy and two were on iron therapy.

A summary of the most frequently reported instances of drug interference is shown in Table 3.

AUTHORS' NOTE: Part of this text has been reproduced (with permission) from the following paper: Sampson C.B. (1993). Adverse effects and drug interactions with radiopharmaceuticals. In 'Drug Safety', ed. Jinks P; Adis International, Auckland, Hong Kong Sydney, Philadelphia (in press).

19.3 EFFECTS OF RADIATION THERAPY AND OTHER EXTRANEOUS FACTORS

Treatments not associated with the administration of drugs have been observed to influence the biodistribution of radiopharmaceuticals. Radiotherapy is well documented in this respect and depending upon the dose level the affects may be transient or permanent in nature. In the early phase of treatment soft tissue uptake of technetium diphosphonate complexes may be observed on skeletal scintigrams within the radiation field (figure 6). This appears to be associated with an inflammatory response to the radiation and with the passage of time returns to normal. Mineral bone within a radiation field shows a permanently reduced uptake of diphosphonates as a long term effect (Figure 7). This phenomenon appears to reflect reduced blood flow caused by fibrosis.

Renograms reflect altered kidney function in irradiated kidneys with a delayed T maximum and excretory phase. This effect may be transient or permanent depending upon the radiation dose. When assessing this effect it should be remembered that only part of the organ may be affected it lies on the edge of a radiation field. Organs outside the boundaries of a radiation field may still exhibit functional disturbances due to the effect of scatter radiation.

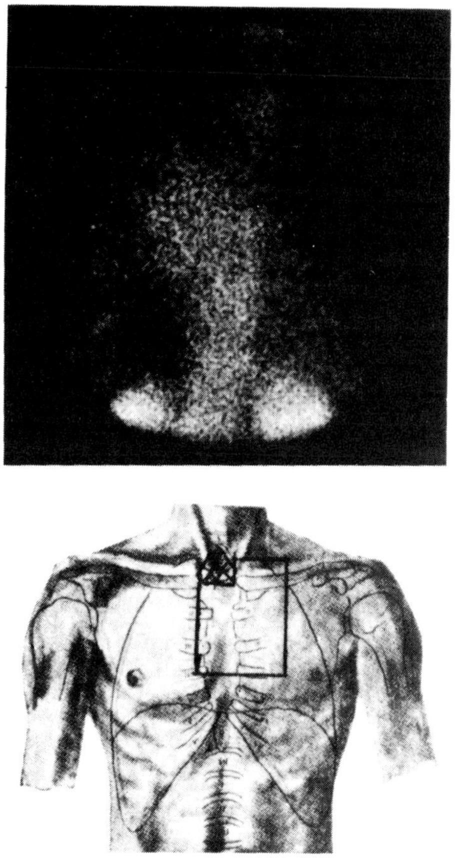

Figure 6. Soft tissue uptake of technetium MDP in muscle associated with the radiation field in the early stages of radiotherapy treatment.

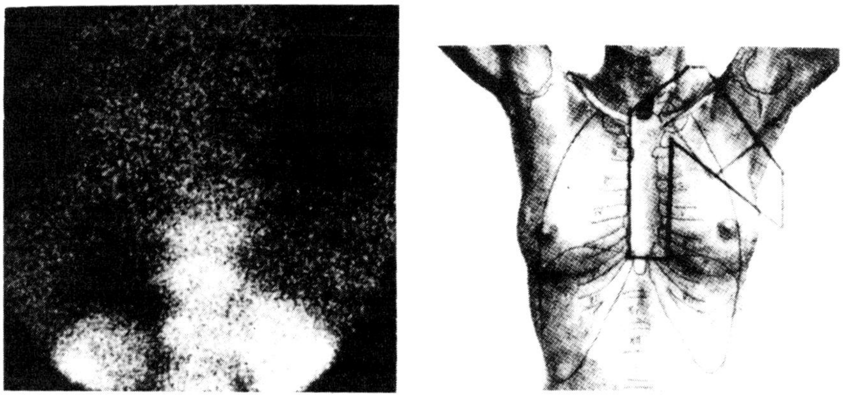

Figure 7. Reduced uptake of MDP associated with radiotherapy field.

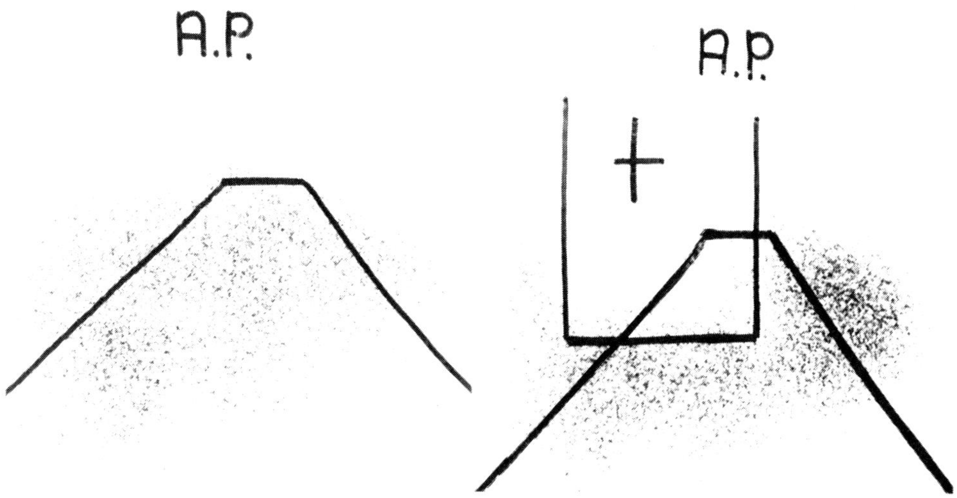

Figure 8. Colloid liver scintigram before (left) and after (right) radiotherapy showing reduced uptake associated with the radiotherapy field.

Analogous to the renogram sodium pertechnetate uptake in salivary glands and excretion in saliva may be depressed and delayed reflecting functional damage to these glands. Radiotherapy has also been reported to cause increased bone uptake and enhanced urinary excretion of gallium-67 citrate.

Few tissues are unaffected by radiation. Phagocytosis in the Kupffer cells of the liver, bone marrow and lymph nodes are readily depressed and is reflected as reduced uptake of radiocolloid (Figure 8).

Whilst on the subject of colloids, recent surgical intervention has been reported as a cause of enhanced spleen uptake. Renal dialysis patients may also show abnormal biodistribution patterns. In the case of gallium reduced liver and enhanced bone uptake have been reported. Also, technetium phosphate complexes have been reported to accumulate preferentially in the gastric mucosa of these patients.

In patients who have recently been exposed to high voltage electric shock accumulation of technetium complexes have been observed in the soft tissue associated with the line of traject of the electrical discharge.

As an extraneous factor effecting biodistribution, the social use of drugs should not be ignored. Chronic alcohol abuse is reflected by increased hepatic retention of xenon-133 whilst radiocolloid uptake is reduced. Acute alcoholic poisoning on the other hand is known to cause rhabdomyolysis in skeletal muscle which can be seen as massive uptake of technetium diphosphonate complexes in the affected muscles. Enhanced thallium-201 uptake can also be associated with this condition. For a fuller account of drug-induced disease as a cause of abnormal biodistribution see Section 19.2.3. Even small doses of alcohol may produce affects and deviations from the expected biodistribution pattern have been observed in I-123 studies to determine fatty acid metabolism in the heart. Tobacco smoking has been observed to reduce both the alveolar and mucociliary clearance of technetium aerosols.

Recent surgery commonly results in the accumulation of radiopharmaceuticals in scars and tissues around the operation site probably reflecting local oedema. Figure 9 shows an example of technetium-MDP uptake at the site of recent thoracic surgery.

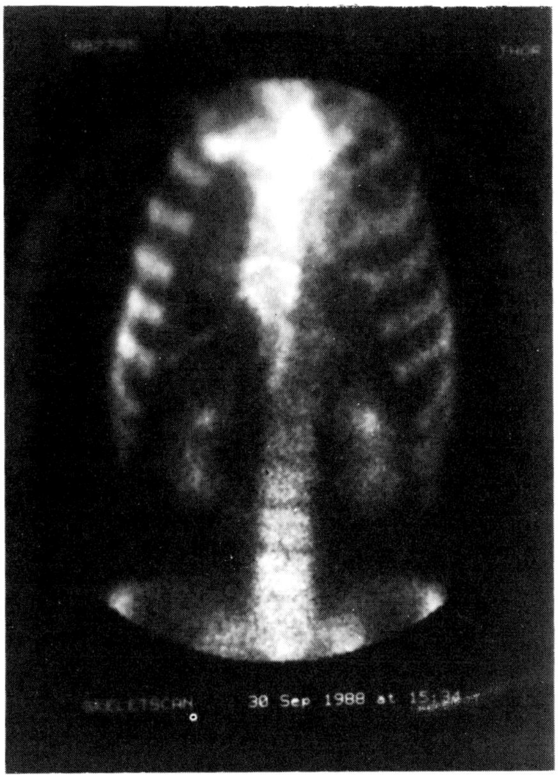

Figure 9. Technetium MDP uptake in the scar tissue at a recent operation site.

19.4 DIET

The nutritional status of a patient can exert a considerable influence upon biodistribution characteristics of many radiopharmaceuticals. The degree of hydration influences the rate of renal excretion and should be particularly taken into account when conducting renal studies with hippuran, DTPA or MAG3 complexes. The ingestion of caffeine, theophylline or theobromine containing beverages can also influence renal excretion because of their diuretic activity. Similarly, the fasting state influences the rate of absorption and the intestinal transport of orally administered compounds. Hepatobiliary function studies with technetium IDA derivatives are particularly sensitive in this respect. If the subject has not been fasting for at least four hours prior to the commencement of the study there is a high probability that the gall bladder will not be visualised. Regional variations in the normal values obtained for bile acid absorption measurements using Se-75 HCAT have also been attributed to variations in diet.

Excessive intake of Vitamin A has been shown to reduce Kupffer cell uptake of technetium colloids in the liver as does iron overload. The latter also causes enhanced renal uptake of gallium-67 citrate. Nicotinic acid and alcohol both influence the uptake of IDA derivatives in the liver and gall bladder.

Iodine-containing foods are well known to affect thyroidal uptake of iodinated compounds and a fuller account has been give in Section 19.2.1.

19.5 REGISTRATION OF INSTANCES OF ABNORMAL BIODISTRIBUTION

It is abundantly clear that many factors, alone and in combination, can affect the biodistribution of radiopharmaceuticals. There would appear to be a clear role for the radiopharmacist to record and document them. The desirability for a centralised registration centre is also clearly evident and has the added advantage that it is then possible to reliably establish the degree of incidence of changes in biodistribution. At the present time the national reporting schemes which exist are voluntary and therefore many incidents go unreported. The British Nuclear Medicine Society, the American Society of Nuclear Medicine and the European Committee on Radiopharmaceuticals all operate adverse reaction reporting schemes which all serve to identify instances of unusual biodistribution. All three publish regular reports of their findings. The European Committee on Radiopharmaceuticals Reporting Scheme also includes the reporting of technical faults and defects associated with generators, ready for use injections and labelling kits. The reporting network is multinational and therefore offers the potential for the early detection of adverse reactions, biodistribution problems and quality defects. From 1993 the British reporting scheme will be combined with that of the European scheme and all instances of adverse biodistribution will be collated in the UK by Dr Stuart Hesslewood (for address, see Frontispiece).

A study of the annual reports, however, clearly shows a reporting bias in favour of certain countries whilst other, apparently have no adverse effects to report which is unlikely. Until there is a high degree of self motivation or until some form of compulsion is introduced, the existing schemes, although of value, will remain relatively ineffective.

REFERENCES

Ajmani S.K., Pincher F.J. (1978). *Gallium-67 citrate in gynaecomastia.* Journal of Nuclear Medicine. **19**, 560–561.

Alazraki N., Scott S., *et al.* (1987). *Effect of glucocorticoids on sensitivity of Tc-99m phosphonate bone imaging for detecting bone trauma.* Journal of Nuclear Medicine, **28**, 606 (abstract).

Blake G.M. *et al.* (1988). *Modification of I-131 MIBG kinetics in malignant phaeochromocytoma.* Nucl. Med. Commun., **9**, 75 (Abstract).

Blathen D., Bullock W., Nuttall C. *et al.* (1978). *A study of renal biopsies of light electron and immunofluoresence microscopy.* Clinical Nephrology, **9**, 103–106.

Bobbinet E.B., Severin M., Zurbriggen M.T. (1974). *Lung uptake of Tc-99m sulphur colloid in patients exhibiting presence of aluminium in plasma.* Journal of Nuclear Medicine, **15**, 1220–1222.

Brown S.J., Slizofski W.J., Dadpavan S. (1990). *Altered biodistribution of Gallium-67 in a patient with aluminium toxicity treated with desferrioxamine.* Journal of Nuclear Medicine, **31**, 115–117.

Chacke A.K., Gordon D.M. *et al.* (1977). *Myocardial imaging with Tc-99m pyrophosphate in patients on adriamycin treatment for neoplasia.* Journal of Nuclear Medicine, **20**, 1029–1037.

Clomius M.H., Dreskoran K., Zeit G. *et al.* (1979). *Renal graft evaluation with pertechnetate and I-131 Hippuran. A comparative clinical study.* Journal of Nuclear Medicine, **20**, 1029–1037.

Cox P.H., Woldring M.G. and Limoris G. (1985). *Progress in Radiopharmacology 1985.* Martinus Nijhof, Dordrevht. pp 224–239.

Cox P.H. (1988). *Radiopharmacy and Radiopharmacology Yearbook 3.* Gordon and Breach Science Publishers, London, New York. pp 17–40.

Crystal G., Fulmer J.D., Roberts W.C. *et al.* (1976). *Idiopathic pulmonary fibrosis; clinical, histologic, radiographic and biochemical aspects.* Annals of Internal Medicine, **85**, 760–788.

Deckart H. and Cox P.H. (1986). *Principals of Radiopharmacology.* Verlag, Netherlands. pp 224–239.

Desai A.G., Interzo C., Bark C. *et al.* (1986). *Drug induced gallium uptake in the breasts.* Clinical Nuclear Medicine. **12**, 703–704.

Eisenberg B., Owens D. *et al.* (1989). *PYP Maalox localisation in liver and spleen.* Clinical Nuclear Medicine, **14**, 636.

Feezer E.A. (1982). *Hepatobiliary imaging; general considerations. The View Box, July issue,* Department of Nuclear Medicine, Wesley Medical Centre, Kansas USA.

Flynn B.M.M., Treves S.T. (1987). *Diffuse hepatic uptake of technetium-99m methylene diphosphonate in a patient receiving high dose methotrexate.* Journal of Nuclear Medicine, **28**, 532–534.

Grayson R.R. (1960). *Factors which influence the radioactive iodine thyroidal uptake test.* American Journal of Medicine **27**, 397–415.

Gross M.D., Valk T.K. *et al.* (1981). *The role of pharmacologic manipulation in adrenal cortical scintigraphy.* Seminars in Nuclear Medicine, **11**, 128–148.

Hayes R.L. (1977). *The tissue distribution of gallium radionuclides.* Journal of Nuclear Medicine **18**, 740–742.

Hegge F.N., Hamilton G.W., Larson S.M. (1978). *Cardiac chamber imaging: a comparison of red blood cells labelled with Tc-99m in-vitro and in-vivo.* Journal of Nuclear Medicine **19**, 129–134.

Hladik W.B., Ponto J.A. *et al.* (1987). *Iatrogenic alterations in the biodistribution of radiotracers as a result of drug therapy. In 'Essentials of Nuclear Medicine Science',* editor W.B. Hladik, Williams and Wilkins, New York. pp189–219.

Hladik W.B. *et al.* (1982). *Drug induced changes in the biodistribution of radiopharmaceuticals.* Semi. Nucl. Med. XIII. 184–218.

Hoffer P. (1960). *Gallium mechanisms.* Journal of Nuclear Medicine. **21**, 282–285.

Klatskin G. (1977). *Hepatic tumours in possible relationship to oral contraceptives.* Gastroenterology **73**, 386–388.

Lee H.B., Wexler J.P. (1983). *Pharmacologic alterations in Tc-99m binding by red blood cells: concise communication.* Journal of Nuclear Medicine, **24**, 894–987.

Lentle B.C., Scott J.R. (1979). *Iatrogenic alterations in radionuclide biodistribution.* Seminars in Nuclear Medicine. **9**, 131–134.

Linds D.S., Saunders J.A., Patel S. (1983). *Delayed renal localisation of Gallium-67: concise communication.* Journal of Nuclear Medicine **24**, 894–897.

Lutrin C.L., McDougall S. *et al.* (1978). *Intense concentration of Tc-99m pyrophosphate in the kidneys of children treated with chemotherapeutic drugs for malignant disease.* Radiology, **128**,165–167.

Mavers P.L., Sty J.R., Wells G. (1988). *Gallium-67 citrate imaging: chloroquine overdosage.* Clinical Nuclear Medicine **17**.

Maxon M.R., Thomas S.R., Bockringen M. *et al.* (1983). *Low iodine diet in I-131 ablation thyroid remnants.* Clinical Nuclear Medicine, **8**, 123–124.

Mazzole A.C., Barker M.M., Belliveal R.E. (1976). *Accumulation of Tc-99m diphosphonate at sites of intramuscular iron therapy.* Journal of Nuclear Medicine and Technology, **4**, 133–135.

Moult R.G., Bekerman C. (1989). *Altered biodistribution of Ga-67 by intramuscular gold salts.* Clinical Nuclear Medicine, **14**, 831–833.

Mulliner D.S., Merz G. *et al.* (1986). *Clearance of aluminium by haemodialysis: effect of desferrioxamine.* Kidney International, Supplement, **29**, S100–S103.

Nakajo N., Shapiro B. *et al.* (1982). *Mechanism of I-131 iodobenzylguanidine accumulation in the salivary glands.* Clinical research, **30**, 721A.

Napp I. (1986). *Pulmonary vascular disease in ex-heroin users.* Clinical Nuclear Medicine. 266–269.

Pope R., Bratke J. (1981). *Two Tec-99m HIDA cases with delayed emptying into the deodenum.* The Monthly Scan. College of Pharmacy, New Mexico. Monthly Newletter, May/June.

Porter W.C., Dees S.M. *et al.* (1983). *Effect of heparin and acid-citrate-dextrose on labelling efficiency of Tc-99m labelled RBCs.* Journal of Nuclear Medicine, **24**, 383–385.

Ramsingh P.S., Pujara G., Iogic J.M. (1977). *Tc-99m pyrophosphate uptake in drug induced gynaecomastia.* Clinical Nuclear medicine, **2**, 206.

Richards A.G., Brighouse R. (1981). *Nicotinic acid: a cause of failed HIDA scanning.* Journal of Nuclear Medicine, **22**, 746–747.

Sampson C.B., Brown A.M. (1992). *Patient medication as a possible cause of unexpected biodistribution of radiopharmaceutical: a regional survey 1981–1991 and a simple algorithm to predict drug/radiopharmaceutical interaction.* Nuclear Medicine Communications **4**, 229 (abstract).

Sampson C.B. (1985). *Altered biodistribution of radiopharmaceuticals as a result of pharmacological or chemical interaction. In 'Radiopharmaceuticals and radiopharmacy practice',* ed Theobald A.E., Taylor and Francis, London.

Sampson C.B. and Hesslewood S.R. (1989). *Adverse reactions to and drug incompatibilities with radiopharmaceuticals. In 'Radiopharmaceuticals, Using Radioactive Compounds in Pharmaceutics and Medicine',* ed Theobald A.E., Ellis, Horwood, Colchester.

Sampson C.B. (1990). *Drugs and chemicals which affect the purity, biodistribution and pharmacokinetics of radiopharmaceuticals.* J. Biopharm. Sci. **1**, 381–400.

Steinbeck J.J., Donoghue G.D. (1979). *Simultaneous treatment of toxic goitre with I-131 and anti-thyroid drugs in a propsective study.* Journal of Nuclear Medicine, **20**, 624–630.

Stephanas A.V., Maisey M.N. (1976). *Hyperprolactinaemia as a cause of Gallium-67 uptake in the breasts. British Journal of Radiology* **49**, 379–380.

Sternthal E., Lipwith G., Starling B. (1980). *Suppression of thyroid radioiodine uptake by various doses of stable iodine.* New England Journal of medicine, **303**, 1083–1088.

Swayne L.L., Kolc J. (1986). *Erythromycin hepatotoxicity: a rare case of a false positive technetium DISIDA study.* Clinical Nuclear Medicine, **11**, 10–12.

Tatum J.L., Burke T.S. *et al. Decreased red cell tagging in patients who had received iodinated contrast media.* Clinical Nuclear Medicine 585.

Wang T.S.T., Fawaz R.A., Esser P.D. *et al.* (1978). *Altered biodistribution of Tc-99m pertechnetate in iatrogenic hyperaluminaemia.* Journal of Nuclear Medicine, **19**, 381–383.

Waxman A.S., Beldon J.R. *et al.* (1977). *Steroid induced suppression of gallium uptake tumours of the central nervous system.* Journal of Nuclear Medicine, **18**, 617 (Abstract).

Weiner M.E., Thakur M. et al. (1979). *Relative stability of In-111 and Ga-67 desferrioxamine and human transferrin complexes. In* 'Radio-pharmaceuticals II. Proceeding of the 2nd International Symposium on Radiopharmaceuticals, Seattle, USA', editor V Sodd.

Wieland D.M., Browne E. *et al.* (1981). *Imaging the primate adrenal medulla with I-123 and I-131 metaiodobenzylguanidine.* Journal of Nuclear Medicine **22**, 358–364.

Winter S.L., Boger J.L. (1973). *Hepatotoxicity from large doses of nicotinamide.* New England Journal of Medicine, **289**, 1180–1182.

Yee C.A., Lee M.B., Blaufox M.D. (1981). *Tc-99m DMSA renal uptake influence of biochemistry and physiological factors.* Journal of Nuclear Medicine, **22**, 1054–1058.

Zanelli G.D. (1982). *Effect of certain drugs used in the treatment of cardiovascular disease on the in-vitro labelling of red blood cells with Tc-99m.* Nuclear Medicine Communications, **3**, 155–161.

Zimmer A.M., Spies, Majewski W. (1981). *Effects of drugs on in-vivo RBC labelling: a proposed mechanism of inhibition.* Proceedings of Second International Symposium of Radiopharmacy, Chicago.

Chapter 20

Use of Drugs to Enhance Nuclear Medicine Studies

S.C.E. Leung and S.R. Hesslewood

20.1 INTRODUCTION

It is well known that patients' medications can interfere with nuclear medicine studies. However, some effects of drug interference can be used to enhance or extend the diagnostic capability of a nuclear medicine examination. For example, though narcotic analgesics have been shown to interfere with hepatobiliary studies by simulating bile duct obstruction, they can be employed to improve diagnosis in conditions that delay or prevent gallbladder visualization (See explanation under hepatobiliary studies). In recent years, there has been increasing interest in the use of this technique known as pharmacological intervention which may be defined as the coadministration of a non-radioactive drug to enhance the diagnostic utility of a nuclear medicine test (Thrall and Swanson, 1989). A specific drug may be administered before, during, or after the administration of radiopharmaceuticals for a given study. The essential purpose of an intervention is to alter organ function and gain diagnostic information by noting the change in the biodistribution, extent of uptake or excretion of the radiotracer. As nuclear medicine procedures are non-invasive, we are sure that the change in response is brought about by the intervention rather than the procedure itself. In the development of each pharmacological intervention, the dosage regimens have been established to reliably achieve the desired or critical change in organ function. For example, the dose of dipyridamole used in cardiac studies must be large enough to produce sufficient change in the coronary blood flow but without unacceptable side-effects. In addition, protocols must be reproducible to allow comparison between patients. Prescriptions for patients scheduled for these studies are often received by hospital pharmacists who are unfamiliar with their intended uses. This chapter aims to discuss the rationale behind the interventions for various organ imaging studies and to summarise information related to the use of such drugs in a tabular form (Table 1) for easy reference. For a more detailed discussion of various imaging protocols using these drugs, the reader is referred to the source material cited at the end of this chapter.

20.2 CARDIAC STUDIES

Nuclear medicine studies of the heart can be divided into two categories: direct imaging of the myocardium to assess regional coronary blood flow, and blood pool imaging to determine ventricular function. The induction of stress may be used to increase the diagnostic sensitivity of these studies as cardiac dysfunction may not manifest itself under basal conditions but may be induced under conditions of stress. When stress increases oxygen and therefore flow demands, vasodilatation will occur in normal coronary arteries, leading to a corresponding increase in coronary blood flow and increased localization of the tracer. Since stenosed vessels are already dilated as a result of the autoregulatory response, stress has relatively little effect on coronary blood flow or tracer deposition. In addition, the local imbalances in the myocardial oxygen supply-demand ratio created by stress, in areas supplied by stenosed coronary arteries, provokes myocardial wall motion abnormalities (Rabinovitch, 1985) which can be detected by blood pool imaging.

However, many patients cannot perform adequate exercise because of anxiety, poor motivation, peripheral vascular disease, musculoskeletal or neurological disorders. Drugs can be used as an alternative to exercise-induced myocardial stress in both myocardial perfusion imaging and blood pool imaging. The advantage of a drug-induced, compared to exercise-induced, increase in coronary flow is that it is reproducible and can be standardized. The disadvantage is that, unlike exercise, it does not provide additional clinically useful information such as the exercise capacity and functional status of a patient. Dipyridamole, adenosine and dobutamine have been used as an alternative, dipyridamole and adenosine are less likely to provoke ischaemia than exercise and are useful in studying patients on beta-blocker therapy which may blunt the response to exercise-induced stress (Botvinck and Dae, 1991).

Dipyridamole is the most frequently used coronary vasodilator in myocardial perfusion imaging (Figure 1), and is associated with the most clinical experience. The exact mechanism of dipyridamole action is not fully established

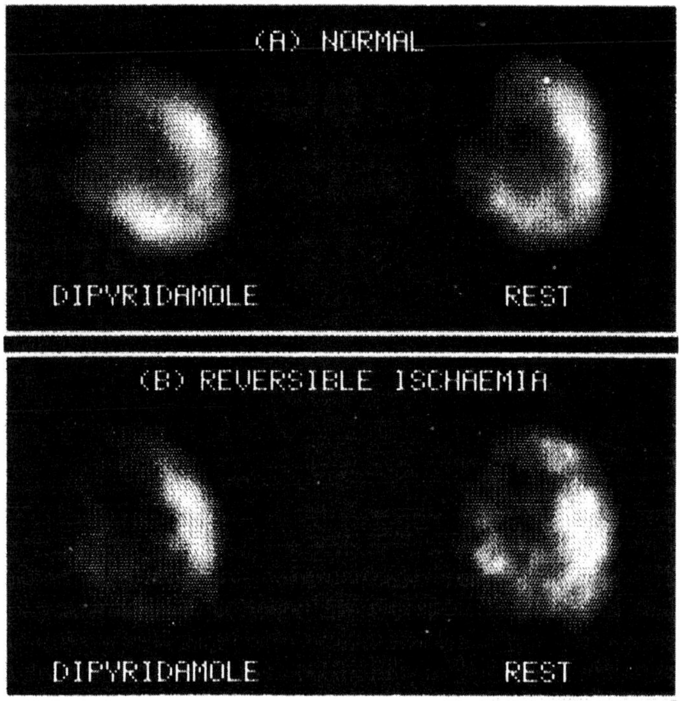

Figure 1. Thallium-201 myocardial scans using dipyridamole to induce stress. In (B) perfusion deficits during the stress test reperfuses to some degree during rest.

(Zeller and Blend, 1987). It prevents the inactivation of intrinsic adenosine by inhibiting the enzyme adenosine deaminase. In addition, dipyridamole may act to inhibit the uptake of adenosine into myocardial, endothelial and blood cells. The resultant increase in myocardial tissue adenosine produces coronary vasodilation predominantly in the small resistance vessels. Adenosine, an endogenous nucleoside, is thought to be a mediator of metabolically induced coronary vasodilatation. It has been proposed that adenosine blocks entry of calcium into vascular smooth muscle cells and therefore causes vasodilatation (Botvinck and Dae, 1991). The administration of dipyridamole or exogenous adenosine causes greater coronary blood flow in the normal arteries and a lesser increase in the stenotic arteries because of diminished flow reserve. As a result, relative differences in tracer uptake between areas of the myocardium that are supplied by stenosed and normal coronary arteries are enhanced by the drugs. Dipyridamole may be administered orally or intravenously (Taillefer *et al.,* 1986). The onset of action is sooner and more predictable with the intravenous form. Absorption via the oral route is erratic and gastro-intestinal intolerance such as nausea is frequent (Beller, 1991). If severe ischaemic symptoms and/or orthostatic hypotension occur during infusion of dipyridamole, they may be treated with intravenous aminophylline (see Table 1). The antagonistic effect of aminophylline is related to its direct action on the small muscle of the coronary vessels (Alfonso, 1970).

Adenosine may be administered by a stepwise infusion method. Its ultra-short half-life of less than 2–10 seconds (Verani, 1991a and b) may increase the safety of pharmacological intervention in high risk patients because of the ability to adjust the dose during infusion. However, as adenosine can decrease atrioventricular conduction, patients with sick sinus syndrome and those with second- or third-degree atrioventricular block should not receive adenosine infusion. Although the side effects of adenosine are more frequent than those of dipyridamole (DePuey and Rozanski, 1991), they disappear rapidly once the infusion is discontinued. Dobatamine is fundamentally a beta-1 agonist with very weak alpha and beta-2 properties. In patients with depressed cardiac function dobutamine causes a significant increase in cardiac output and stroke volume with little or no increase in heart rate or peripheral resistance. Coronary blood flow and myocardial oxygen consumption are usually increased due to increased myocardial contractility (Swanson *et al.,* 1985) It has been used in association with perfusion imaging (Pennell *et al.,* 1991 & Gordon *et al.,* 1987). However, it is more frequently employed in blood pool imaging (Palac *et al.,* 1983) as it has been shown to be superior to dipyridamole in inducing myocardial wall motion abnormality (Lee *et al.,* 1992). The greater risk of cardiac arrhythmias associated with catecholmine stress has limited the use of dobutamine (Rabinovitch, 1985).

20.3 RENAL STUDIES

One of the aims in renal studies is differentiating between dilated, non-obstructed urinary tracts from those with significant mechanical obstruction. The determination is important, since renal atrophy can occur if mechanical obstruction is not surgically corrected, whereas muscular atony causing dilatation can be treated with drugs. The prolonged retention of radioactivity seen in non-obstructed, dilated systems is due to a 'reservoir effect'. Increasing the urine flow rate with diuretic administration results in a prompt washout of the activity from the dilated structure. In contrast, a mechanically obstructed system will demonstrate progressive accumulation of activity which does not respond to diuretic administration (Figure 2). A partial response may indicate partial obstruction or renal dysfunction with an inability to respond to the diuretic. Frusemide is the diuretic of choice because its peak effect is far greater than that observed with other agents (Thrall, 1985). The timing of the frusemide injection may be varied. It may be given 15 minutes before or after the radiotracer injection (Fine *et al.,* 1991). Since the peak effect of intravenous frusemide occurs at 15–20 minutes after injection, a protocol with frusemide given 15 minutes before the radiotracer reduces imaging time. However, the response to frusemide is determined by measuring the change in activity

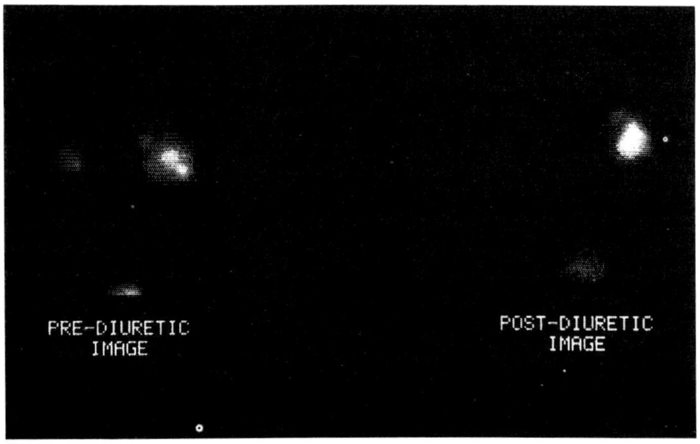

Figure 2. Technetium-99m DTPA renal scan on patient with obstructed right kidney which did not respond to frusemide administration. Clearance of activity is shown in the left kidney.

with time. Measuring the rate of rise of activity before frusemide administration helps to determine whether the rate of fall in activity after administration is appropriate. A moderately poorly functioning kidney would have a moderately impaired rate of rise and a moderately impaired but appropriate rate of fall in response to frusemide in the absence of obstruction. It is, therefore, necessary to evaluate the frusemide response not only as to whether it is good or poor but whether it is appropriate or not (Britton *et al.*, 1991).

Renal studies may also be performed to determine the glomerular filtration rate (GFR) using radiopharmaceuticals excreted by glomerular filtration. Captopril has been shown to reduce the GFR in patients with renal vascular abnormality and is thus used to improve the diagnosis of renal vascular hypertension and detection of renal vascular disease (Majd *et al.*, 1986; Dondi *et al.*, 1989; Dondi *et al.*, 1991). Renal artery stenosis is the most common cause of secondary hypertension, and is potentially remediable by surgery or angioplasty. Captopril, an angiotensin-converting enzyme inhibitor, inhibits the conversion of angiotensin I to angiotensin II. When renal blood flow falls, angiotensin II constricts efferent arterioles to maintain high filtration pressure in the glomerular vessels. In the absence of angiotensin II, the constriction is lost leading to a drop in GFR when perfusion pressure falls, as in the case of renal artery stenosis. Diagnosis is made by comparing a baseline renal study with a captopril enhanced study (Figure 3).

20.4 HEPATOBILIARY STUDIES

The evaluation of hepatobiliary function is accomplished by technetium-99m labelled compounds of iminodiacetic acid (IDA), which are cleared from the circulation by the hepatic cells and secreted into bile by carrier mechanisms in the same way as bilirubin. After intravenous injection, radioactivity appears in the liver promptly followed by movement into the gallbladder and then into the intestine. Various conditions such as the presence of extremely viscous bile in chronic cholecystitis, prolonged fasting or total parenteral nutrition can delay the movement of these radiopharmaceuticals through the hepatobiliary system resulting in delayed gallbladder visualization (Thrall and Swanson, 1989). To promote earlier visualization of the gallbladder and reduce the imaging time required for diagnosis, drugs may be used to evacuate the gallbladder and optimize subsequent filling with rdiotracers. The primary determinant of gallbladder emptying is circulating cholecystokinin (CCK) which is released from the duodenal mucosa in response to the presence of fat and lipolytic products, and to a lesser degree to amino acids and small peptides. In the United Kingdom, CCK prepared from the duodenal mucosa of pigs is available from Ferring Pharmaceuticals Ltd. on a named patient basis. Figure 4 shows the gallbladder contracting after the administration of CCK. Two synthetic and more potent preparations containing the active chemical group of CCK (the terminal heptapeptide) are also available commercially in the United States. Ceruletide is a synthetic decapeptide (Krishnamurthy *et al.*, 1983) and sincalide, a synthetic octapeptide of CCK. Sincalide is five times more potent than CCK, cheaper and more frequently used in the United States (Sanson *et al.*, 1985). These cholecystokinetic agents have essentially replaced the use of a fatty meal to induce gallbladder contractions and emptying of the gallbladder as the response to drugs is quicker and more predictable (Freemann *et al.*, 1981). They act by nerve stimulation and a direct action on gastrointestinal tract smooth muscle. Morever, the agents can be used to assess the effectiveness of gallbladder contraction or ejection fraction (Freeman *et al.*, 1981; Fink-Bennett, 1991; Fink-Bennett *et al.*, 1991).

Morphine has also been used to shorten hepatobiliary studies and to reduce the incidence of gallbladder non-visualization (Fink-Bennett, 1991; Choy *et al.*, 1984; Vasquez *et al.*, 1988; Fink-Bennett *et al.*, 1991). Morphine causes constriction of the sphincter of Oddi with a resultant increase in the pressure in the common bile duct, leading to increased flow of bile and radiotracer into the gallbladder if the cystic duct is patent (Murphy *et al.*, 1980). The imaging time required to determine cystic duct patency is decreased. This intervention is beneficial in the assessment of acute cholecystitis in the presence of chronic cholecystitis or other conditions that usually delay or prevent gallbladder visualization. On the other hand, it is well documented that narcotic analgesics interfere with hepatobiliary studies. This is because no release of radiopharmaceutical into the intestine occurs resuoing in prolonged radiopharmaceutical appearance in the gallbladder or common bile duct, which

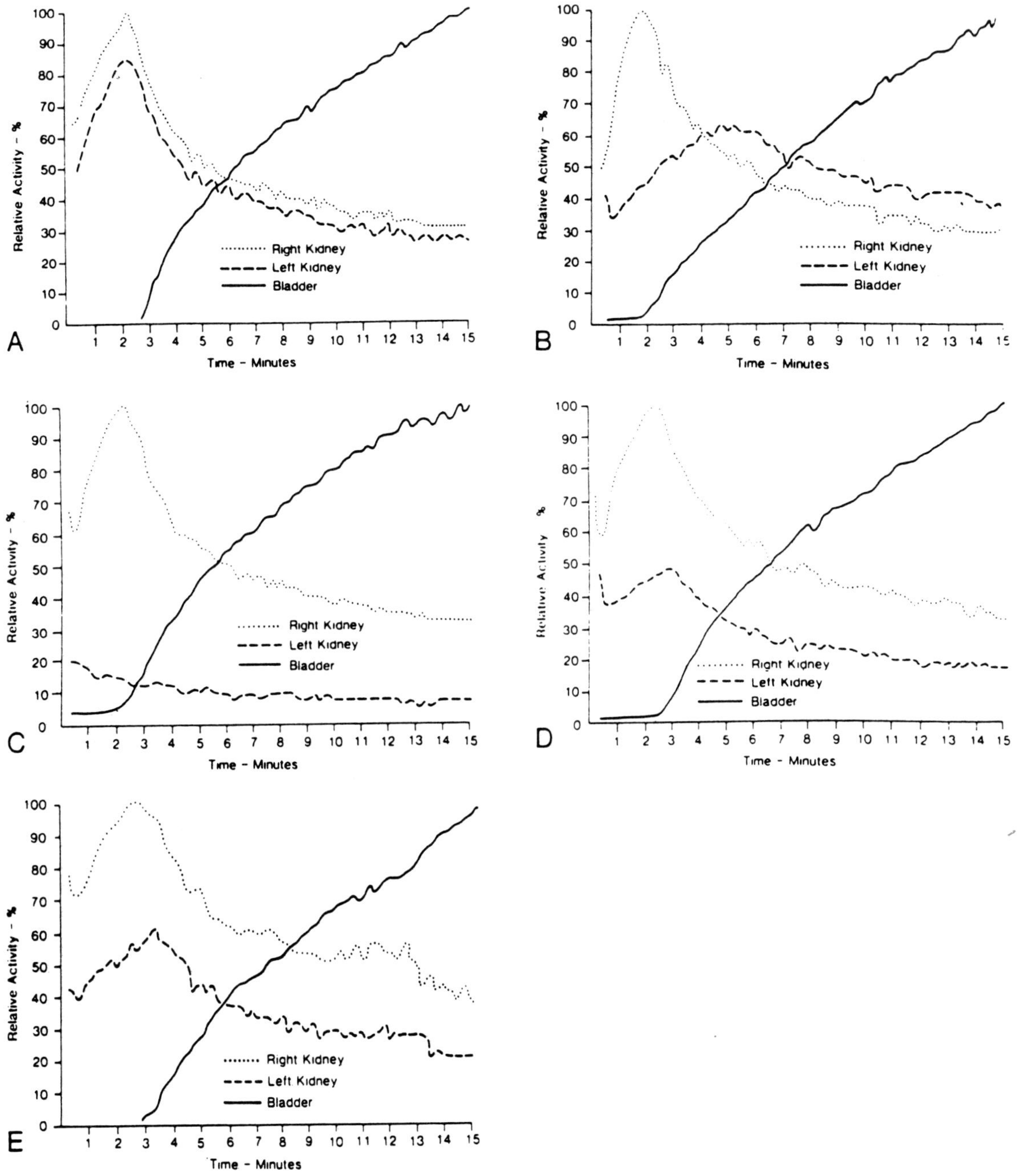

Figure 3. Effect of captopril on excretion of technetium-99m DTPA in a canine model of renal artery stenosis. A shows the curves obtained with left renal artery stenosis. B shows the effect of captopril, producing a decrease in glomerular filtration rate in the affected kidney (reproduced, with permission, from Nally *et al.*, 1986).

simulates the appearance of bile duct obstruction (Chilton & Brown, 1990).

Phenobarbitone is another drug used in conjunction with hepatobiliary imaging. In infants with jaundice, hepatobiliary imaging is comprised by poor hepatic uptake and slow biliary excretion. Administration of phenobarbitone enhances and accelerates biliary excretion of the radiotracer and thereby increases the accuracy of differentiating extrahepatic biliary atresia from neonatal hepatitis. Differentiation is important because appropriate therapy depends on it. Decreased morbidity and mortality are obtainable when biliary atresia is diagnosed and surgically corrected within

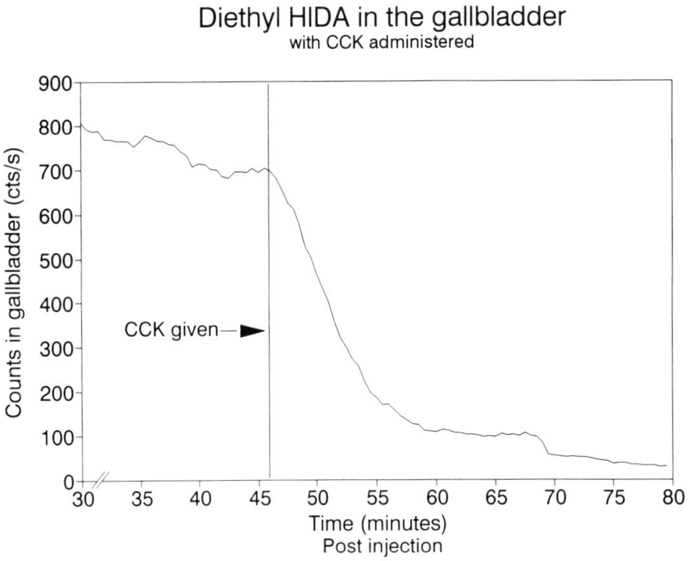

(A)

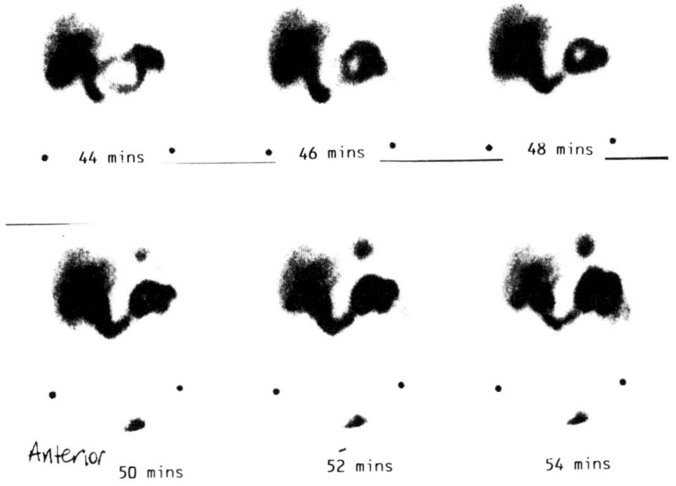

(B)

Figure 4. Effects of CCK on gallbladder function. (A) shows graphically the counts in the gallbladder before and after administration of CCK, and (B) shows the accumulation of activity in the stomach following expulsion of bile from the gallbladder by CCK.

the first two months of life (Fink-Bennett, 1991, Majd *et al.,* 1981). The choleretic effect of phenobarbitone is thought to be independent of its enzyme induction effect, and to be due to its effect upon the whole hepatic transport system for organic anions such as IDA radiolabelled compounds (Majd *et al.,* 1981). By enhancing the uptake of these compounds, the compromised liver is better visualized and its function more readily assessed.

20.5 GASTROINTESTINAL STUDIES

Meckel's diverticulum is an outpouching of the distal ileum and occurs in approximately 2% of the general population. Meckel's diverticulum may contain small bowel mucosa, pancreatic mucosa, or gastric mucosa. More than 90% of patients with lower gastrointestinal tract bleeding caused by Meckel's diverticulum have ileal ulcerations secondary to local acid and pepsin secretions by ectopic gastric mucosa within the diverticulum (Froelich, 1985). The bleeding site can be imaged by the ability of the ectopic gastric mucosa to trap and secrete Tc-99m-pertechnetate. The detectability of the lesion can be enhanced by either reducing the movement of the radiotracer from the abnormal site or by increasing its uptake at the site.

Glucagon reduces gastrointestinal peristalsis, thereby inhibits Tc-99m-pertechnetate secreted by the abnormal site from moving distally and enhances the localization of activity (Froelich and Juni, 1984; Datz *et al.,* 1991). On the other hand, pentagastrin increases gastric mucosal blood flow, stimulates gastric acid secretion and increases the intensity of tracer uptake (Datz *et al.,* 1991; Treves *et al.,* 1978). However, pentagastrin also increases intestinal motility, leading to rapid tracer accumulation in the small intestine and, thus, the possibility of false-positive scans. For this reason, glucagon has been used in combination with pentagastrin (Datz *et al.,* 1991). In addition, cimetidine (Datz *et al.,* 1991; Diamond *et al.,* 1991; Yeker *et al.,* 1984) or ranitidine (Datz *et al.,* 1991) administration has been found to improve pertechnetate imaging of Meckel's diverticulum by decreasing the acidity of the gastric contents. It has been proposed that increased intragastric acidity may enhance the transfer of Tc-99m-pertechnetate from mucosal cells to lumen by promoting stable complex formation in the lumen, and preventing diffusion back into mucosa (Froelich, 1985). Hence, in the presence of cimetidine or ranitidine, the intraluminal release of pertechnetate is inhibited, leading to an accumulation of tracer by mucosal cells.

Tc-99m-pertechnetate is also taken up by the salivary gland due to its chemical similarity to other negatively charged ions contained in the saliva. After an intravenous injection of T_c-99m-pertechnetate, a salivary scan can be performed to provide physiological information about the ability of the salivary glands to take up the radiotracer, and the drainage of saliva. The salivary glands may be stimulated to drain via their ducts into the mouth by asking ther patient to suck a slice of lemon, chew an ascorbic acid 500mg tablet or by placing one or two drops of citric acid on the tongue (Croft and Williams, 1991; Schall *et al.,* 1981). In a normal subject, the salivary glands accumulate the pertechnetate which drains following the secretory stimulus (Figure 5). Duct blockage is demonstrated by the retention of pertechnetate proximal to the obstruction. In xerostomia (dry mouth), there is no uptake into the glands and no discharge into the mouth.

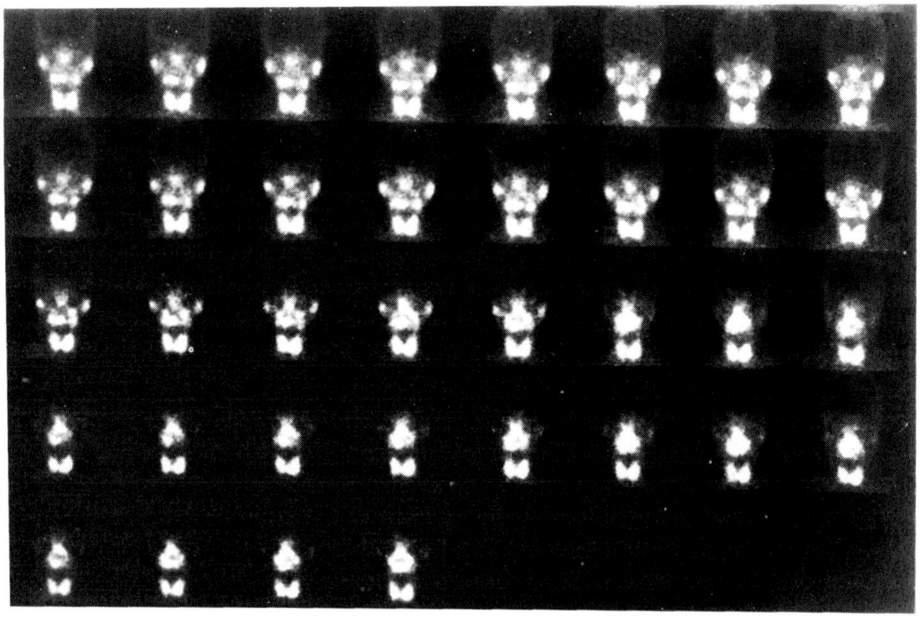

Figure 5. Salivary gland uptake of pertechnetate (read from left to right and from top to bottom). Following oral administration of citric acid, activity in the salivary glands decrease wheras the thyroid activity remains constant.

20.6 ADRENAL STUDIES

Adrenal studies can be divided into adrenal cortical imaging and adrenal medullary imaging.

Radiolabelled cholesterol derivatives are used for imaging the adrenal cortex. The adrenal cortex is divided into three histological zones: the outermost zone, the zona glomerulosa, which is primarily responsible for the synthesis and release of aldosterone; the zona fasciculata which synthesizes and releases cortisol, and the innermost zone, the zona reticularis, which synthesizes and releases androgen and oestrogen hormones. To facilitate scintigraphic evaluation of the zona glomerulosa in hyperaldosteronism or the zona reticularis in hyperandrogenism, dexamethasone is administered to inhibit the release of adrenocorticotrophic hormone (ACTH) from the pituitary and thus suppresses the activity of the zona fasciculata (Gross, 1979). By suppressing the ACTH-dependent component of radiocholesterol uptake which normally accounts for 50% of the adrenal uptake (Khafagi *et al.*, 1991), visualization of the adrenals is delayed. The timing of normal adrenal gland visualization after radiocholesterol administration is dependent on the duration of dexamethasone suppression (DS). Shorter DS regimens using higher doses of dexamethsone have resulted in earlier visualization of normal adrenal activity (Gross *et al.*, 1979). Thus, the interval between tracer injection and normal adrenal visualization has been defined for the 4 mg DS regimen (see table) as ≥ 5 days (Gross *et al.*, 1979). Visualization of adrenal glands earlier than 5 days indicates adenoma or hyperplasia whereas the pattern of activity defines the abnormality. Bilateral visualization indicates bilateral hyperactivity or hyperplasia and unilateral visualization indicates tumour involvement or adenoma (Gross *et al.*, 1979). The distinction between adenoma and hyperplasia in the evaluation of primary aldosteronism and adrenal hyperandrogenism is important, since the treatment is surgical in the former and medical in the latter (Khafagi *et al.*, 1991). However, hyperplasia can produce such marked asymmetry of quantitative uptake as to suggest unilateral disease (Gross *et al.*, 1985). It is therefore useful to quantify the uptake in early unilateral or bilateral visualization as to separate adenoma from hyperplasia. By measuring the level of uptake, adrenal hyperfunction can be separated from normal function as the normal adrenal uptake on DS should not exceed 0.2% of the administered dose (Gross *et al.*, 1985). It is also important to avoid all medications which may affect the adrenal uptake and thus the timing of the normal adrenal gland breakthrough. Spironolactone, diuretics and oral contraceptives have been shown to increase the uptake by the zona glomerulosa by increasing the plasma renin activity (Khafagi *et al.*, 1991).

I-123-metaiodobenzylguanidine (MIBG) and I-131-MIBG have been used for adrenal medullary imaging in the detection of phaeochromocytoma and neuroblastoma. These neuroendocrine tumours may also be treated with therapeutic doses of I-131-MIBG. The therapeutic dose is determined in part by tumour concentration, retention and elimination kinetics. Nifedipine has been shown to increase the tumour retention of MIBG in some patients by changing the tumour kinetics. It may, therefore, be used to improve the clinical effectiveness of therapy by enhancing the radiation dose delivered to tumours without altering the uptake in normal tissue. However, the effect may depend on the plasma nifedipine level achieved and further studies are required (Blake *et al.,* 1988).

Laxatives may also be used to enhance adrenal studies. The excretion of radiolabelled cholesterol derivatives and MIBG by the liver and their subsequent appearance in the colon can interfere with the diagnosis because of excessive tissue activity in the regions of the adrenals (Khafagi *et al.,* 1991, Gross *et al.,* 1985). The interfering colonic activity can be substantially reduced by treating patients from the time of tracer injection through the imaging interval with laxatives. Bisacodyl is ideal here because it acts on the colon only, and does not disturb the enterohepatic recirculation of the radiolabelled cholesterol (Blake *et al.,* 1988).

The in vivo degradation of radioiodinated compounds results in the release of free radioiodine. To block thyroidal uptake of this released radioiodine and radioiodine that may be present as a radiochemical impurity in the injection, patients should be treated with a blocking agent such as potassium iodide. The administration of potassium iodide encourages excretion of unbound radioiodide and thus also decreases background activity (Swanson, 1990; Petry and Shapiro, 1990). Potassium iodide tablets are no longer commercially available but may be given as Aqueous Iodine Oral solution B.P. (Lugol's iodine). Potassium iodate tablets, being more palatable, is an alterantive. Patients who are allergic to iodide may be given anions such as percholorate which acts as a competitive inhibitor of the thyroid gland's anion transport mechanism or triiodothyronine (Khafagi *et al.,* 1991). These blocking techniques are not without side-effects. The hazard of inducing hyperthyroidism in geriatric patients or patients with coronary artery disease, when administering iodide or triiodothyronine must be considered (Ellis *et al.,* 1977, ARSAC, 1992). Blood dyscrasia has also been reported following the use of potassium perchlorate (Ellis *et al.,* 1977, ARSAC, 1992). However, the mortality risk of the blocking procedure is small compared with the estimated risks following these levels of thyroid irradiation (ARSAC, 1992). Treatment should be continued until the estimated level of radioiodine remaining in the body is reduced to an acceptable level. The duration depends on the radionuclide and the dose of radioactivity administered (Khafagi, 1991, ARSAC, 1992). It may be as short as one day when using I-123-MIBG for diagnostic purposes (ARSAC, 1992) or as long as one month when using therapeutic doses of I-131-MIBG (Sisson *et al.,* 1984). In other studies using radioiodinated compounds such as o-iodohippurate, which are stable in the body and not metabolished, blocking is not required.

20.7 BRAIN STUDIES

Tc-99m-pertechnetate is used for conventional brain imaging but of decreasing importance. It does not cross the intact blood-brain barrier (BBB) but accumulates in areas where the BBB has been damaged such as brain tumours and intracerebral haemorrhages. However, the accumulation of pertechnetate in the normal choroid plexus in brain scan causes difficulty in image interpretation. Perchlorate administered as the potassium salt orally or as the sodium salt intravenously may be used to block the uptake of pertechnetate in the choroid plexus (Ellis *et al.,* Hirsch, 1971; Chilton and Thrall 1990). The perchlorate and iodide anions closely resemble that of pertechnetate in having a similar charge and ionic radius (Chilton and Thrall 1990). Hence, pertechnetate uptake by the thyroid is also blocked. Nevertheless, it is now considered unnecessary to administer blocking agents to reduce radiation dose to the thyroid gland when using Tc-99m radiopharmacuticals as the contribution of the thyroid gland to the total radiation dose for this radioisotope is relatively minor (ARSAC, 1992). When Tc-99m-pentetate or Tc-99m-gluceptate are employed for conventional brain imaging, neither normally localizes in the choroid plexus or thyroid gland, therefore patient pretreatment with a blocking agent is not required (Chilton and Thrall, 1990).

Radiopharmaceuticals which cross the intact BBB can be used to assess regional cerebral blood flow (rCBF) in the evaluation of cerebral vascular disease. The normal rCBF at rest need not indicate an adequate vascular supply since vasodilation acts as a compensatory mechanism for proximal stenosis and/or occlusion. However, such areas have a decreased vascular flow reserve which can be assessed by measuring the rCBF at rest and after a vasodilatory stimulus produced by acetazolamide. The mechanism of action responsible for cerebral vasodilatation by acetazolamide is not fully understood, but possible mechanisms include inhibition of the enzyme carbonic anhydrase in red blood cells, brain parenchyma or cerebral vasculature. The direct effect of acetazolamide, independent of carbonic anhydrase inhibition, on the smooth muscle of the cerebral vasculature is another possible mechanism (Yudd *et al.,* 1991).

20.8 THYROID STUDIES

Interventional studies of the thyroid gland were the first to be established in nuclear medicine practice but these are seldomly used in current practice. Substantial uptake of radioiodide in autonomous thyroid tissue can be demonstrated following suppression of normal thyroid tissue with triiodothyronine (T_3) or thyroxine (T_4) (Hurley *et al.,* 1981). Triiodothyronine is preferred as it is more rapid acting and of briefer duration (Swanson *et al.*, 1985). This suppression test is useful in the evaluation of functioning nodules to determine whether they are autonomous.

A second interventional study is the thyroid stimulating hormone (TSH) stimulation test (Swanson, 1990) which is only used occasionally in current practice to differentiate between primary and secondary hypothyroidism. In secondary hypothyroidism, there is a defect in TSH production by the pituitary gland, and the thyroid gland responds to exogenous TSH. On the other hand, in primary hypothyroidism the defect is at the thyroid level, and the gland does not respond to either endogenous or exogenous TSH. TSH stimulation may also be used to enhance tracer localization in follow-up scanning for metastatic disease after thyroid surgery for cancer (Thrall and Swanson, 1989). There is some risk in administering thyroid-stimulating hormone which is of bovine origin because antigen-antibody reactions can occur, especially with repeated studies (Krishnamurthy, 1978).

A third interventional technique in thyroid studies, the perchlorate discharge test, involves the measurement of radioiodine uptake before and after the administration of potassium perchlorate. In patients with organification defects, the perchlorate releases inorganic iodide already taken up by the thyroid gland (Wyngaarden *et al.*, 1952). (Organification is the process whereby inorganic iodide is oxidized and attached to tyrosyl residues which then couple to form the thyroid hormones, thyroxine and triiodothyronine.) The test is usually considered to provide an abnormal result if more than about 10% of the radioiodine uptake in the gland is discharged after perchlorate administration. This indicates a defect in the synthesis of thyroid hormone as a cause of thyroid dysfunction.

20.9 CONCLUSION

In recent years, the diagnostic capability of nuclear medicine testing has been extended not only through the development of new equipment, computers and radiopharmaceuticals but also through the development of new interventional manoeuvers. The change in information obtained from the interventional study offers clues to differentiating various disease conditions. These changes can be brought about by physiological interventions, e.g., exercise in radionuclide ventriculography, and pharmacological interventions. Literally dozens of interventional techniques have been described in the literature (Thrall and Swanson, 1989). This article intends to summarize the more widely used pharmacological interventions which represent an important aspect of current clinical nuclear medicine practice.

REFERENCES

Administration of Radioactive Substances Advisory Committee (ARSAC). Notes for guidance on the administration of radioactive substances to persons for purposes of diagnosis, treatment or research, 1992. Dept. of Health, London.

Alfonso S. (1970). *Inhibition of coronary vasodilating action of dipyridamole and adenosine by aminophylline in the dog.* Circ. Res, **26**, 743–52.

Beller G.A. (1991). *Pharmacologic stress imaging.* JAMA, **26**, 743–52.

Blake G.M. *et al.* (1988). *Modification by nifedipine of I-131-meta-iodobenzylguanidine kinetics in malignant phaeochromocytoma.* Eur. J. Nucl. Med., **14**, 345–8.

Botvinick E.H., and Dae M.W. (1991). *Dipyridamole Perfusion Scintigraphy.* Semin. Nucl. Med., **21**, 242–65.

Britton K.E. *et al.* (1991). *Renal radionuclide studies. In:* Maisey M.N., Britton K.E., Gilday D.L. (eds): Clinical Nuclear Medicine 2nd ed. pp. 91–130. London, Chapman & Hall Medical.

Chilton H.M. and Brown M.L. (1990). *Radiopharmaceuticals for abdominal and gastrointestinal imaging: reticuloendothelial, hepatobiliary and intestinal. In:* Swanson D.P., Chilton H.M., Thrall J.H. (eds): Pharmaceuticals in medical imaging. pp. 462–500. New York, Macmillan.

Chilton H.M. and Thrall J.H. (1990). *Radiopharmaceuticals for central nervous system imaging: Blood-brain barrier, function, receptor-binding, cerebral spinal fluid kinetics. In:* Swanson D.P., Chilton H.M., Thrall J.H. (eds): Pharmaceuticals in medical imaging. pp. 305–42. New York, Macmillan.

Choy D. *et al.* (1984). *Cholescintigraphy in acute cholecystitis: Use of intramuscular morphine.* Radiology, **15**, 1203–7.

Croft D.N. and Williams J.G. (1991). *The gastrointestinal Tract. In:* Maisey M.N., Britton K.E., Gilday D.L. (eds): Clinical Nuclear Medicine 2nd ed. pp. 292–314. London, Chapman & Hall Medical.

Datz F.L. *et al.* (1991). *Physiological and pharmacological interventions in radionuclide imaging of the tubular gastrointestinal tract.* Semin. Nucl. Med., **21**, 140–52.

DePuey E.G. and Rozanski A. (1991). *Pharmacological and other non-exercise alternatives to exercise testing to evaluate myocardial perfusion and left ventricular function with radionuclids.* Semin. Nucl. Med., **21**, 92–101.

Diamond R.H. *et al.* (1991). *The role of cimetidine-enhanced technetium-99m-pertechnetate imaging for visualizing Meckel's Diverticulum.* J. Nucl. Med., **32**, 1422–4.

Dondi M. *et al.* (1989). *Evaluation of hypertensive patients by means of captopril enhanced renal scintigraphy with Technetium-99m DTPA.* J. Nucl. Med., **30**, 615–21.

Dondi M. *et al.* (1991). *Use of Technetium-99m-MAG3 for renal Scintigraphy after angiotensin-converting enzyme inhibition.* J. Nucl. Med., **32**, 424–8.

Ellis R.E. *et al.* (1977). *The use of thyroid blocking agents. A report of a working party of the M. R. C. Isotope Advisory Panel.* Br. J. Radiol., **50**, 203–4.

Fine E.J. (1991). *Interventions in Renal Scintirenography.* Semin Nucl. Med., **21**, 116–27.

Fink-Bennett D. (1991). *Augmented Cholescintigraphy: Its role in detecting acute and chronic disorders of the hepatobiliary tree.* Semin Nucl. Med., **21**, 128–139.

Fink-Bennett D. *et al.* (1991). *Cholecystokinin cholescintigraphy: detection of abnormal gallbladder motor function in patients with chronic acalculour gallbladder disease.* J. Nucl. Med., **32**, 1695–9.

Fink-Bennett D. *et al.* (1991). *Morphine-augmented cholescintigraphy: Its efficacy in detecting acute cholecystitis.* J. Nucl. Med., **32**, 1231–3.

Freeman L.M. *et al.* (1981). *Role of cholecystokinetic agents in Tc-99m-Ida cholescintigraphy.* Semin. Nucl. Med., **11**, 186–193.

Froelich J.W. (1985). *Gasrointestinal studies. In* Thrall J.H., Swanson D.P. (eds): Diagnostic interventions in nuclear medicine. pp. 195–225. Chicago, Year Book Medical.

Froelich J.W. and Juni J. (1984). *Glucagon in the scintigraphic diagnosis of small-bowel haemorrhage by Tc-99m labelled red blood cells.* Radiology, **151**, 239–42.

Gordon L. *et al.* (1987). *Nine thallium stress testing in the detection of sclerotic coronary artery disease.* Investigative Radiology, **22**, 43. (abstract)

Gross M.D. *et al.* (1979). *The normal dexamethasone suppression and adrenal scintiscan.* J. Nucl. Med., **20**, 1131–5.

Gross M.D. *et al.* (1985). *Limited significance of asymmetric adrenal visualization on dexamethasone-suppression scintigraphy.* J. Nucl. Med., **26**, 43–8.

Gross M.D. and Shapiro M.B. (1985). *Pharmacologic manipulation to enhance diagnostic imaging in adrenal gland scintigraphy. In:* Thrall J.H., Swanson D.P. (eds): Diagnostic interventions in nuclear medicine. pp. 76–117. Chicago, Year Book Medical.

Harvey R.F. and Oliver J.M. (1980). *Cholecystokinins and the gallbladder.* Gastroenterology, **78**, 1117–9.

Hirsch J.I. *et al.* (1971). *The role of potassium perchlorate in technetium-99m brain scanning.* Drug Intell. & Clin. Pharm., **5**, 252–7.

Hurley J.R. and Becker D.V. (1981). *Thyroid suppression and stimulation testing: the place of scanning in the evaluation of nodular thyroid disease.* Semin Nucl. Med., **11**, 149–160.

Khafagi F.A. *et al.* (1991). *The adrenal gland. In:* Maisey M.N., Britton K.E., Gilday D.L. (eds): Clinical Nuclear Medicine 2nd ed. pp. 271–91. London, Chapman & Hall Medical.

Krishnamurthy G.T. (1978). *Human reactions to bovine TSH.* J. Nucl. Med., **19**, 284–9.

Krishnamurthy G.T. *et al.* (1983). *Optimization of ceruletide intravenous dose for gallbladder emptying.* J. Nucl. Med., **24**, P38-9.

Lee H.S. *et al.* (1992). *Gated radionuclide ventriculography-comparison of exercise, persantin and dobutamine stress.* Nucl. Med. Commun., **4**, 216. (abstract)

Majd M. *et al.* (1981). *Effect of phenobarbital on Tc-99m IDA scintigraphy in the evaluation of neonatal jaundice.* Semin. Nucl. Med., **11**, 194–204.

Majd M. *et al.* (1986). *Captopril enhanced renal scintigraphy for detection of renal artery stenosis and uptake.* J. Nucl. Med., **27**, 962. (abstract)

Murphy P. *et al.* (1980). *Narcotic anaesthetic drugs. Their effect on biliary dynamics.* Arch. Surg., **115**, 710–1.

Nally J.V., Clarke H.S. Jr., Grecos G.P. *et al.* (1986). *Effect of captopril on ^{99m}Tc diethylene triaminepentacetic acid renograms in two-kidney, one clip hypertension.* Hypertension, **8**, 685–693.

Palac R. *et al.* (1983). *Exercise versus dobutamine infusion during radionuclide ventriculography in patients with coronary disease.* J. Am. Coll. Cardiol., **1**, 642. (abstract)

Pennell D.J. *et al.* (1991). *Dobutamine thallium myocardial perfusion tomography.* Eur. J. Nucl. Med., **18**, 527. (abstract)

Petry N.A. and Shapiro B. (1990). *Adrenomedullary Imaging. In:* Swanson D.P., Chilton H.M., Thrall J.H. (eds): Pharmaceuticals in medical imaging. pp. 368–86. New York, Macmillan.

Rabinovitch M.A. (1985). *Pharmacologic interventions in nuclear cardiology. In:* Thrall J.H., Swanson D.P. (eds.) Diagnostic interventions in nuclear medicine. pp. 31–5. Chicago Book Medical.

Ramsden D.D. *et al.* (1967). *Radioiodine uptakes in the thyroid studies of the blocking and subsequent recovery of the gland following the administration of stable iodine.* Health Physics, **13**, 633–46.

Schall G.L. *et al.*, (1981). *Radionuclide salivary imaging usefulness in a private otolaryngology practice. Arch Otolaryngol,* **107**, 40–44.

Shapiro B. *et al.* (1983). *Value of bowel preparation in adreno-cortical scintigraphy with NP-59.* J. Nucl. Med., **24**, 732–4.

Sisson J.C. *et al.* (1984). *Radiopharmaceutical Treatment of Malignant Phaeochromocytoma.* J. Nucl. Med., **25**, 197–206.

Swanson D.P. (1990). *Adrenocortical Imaging In:* Swanson D.P., Chilton H.M., Thrall J.H. (eds): Pharmaceuticals in medical imaging. pp. 360–8. New York, Macmillan.

Swanson D.P. *et al.* (1985). *Formulary: Pharmacologic interventions in nuclear medicine. In:* Thrall J.H., Swanson D.P. (eds): Diagnostic interventions in nuclear medicine. pp. 247–67. Chicago, Year Book Medical.

Taillefer R. *et al.* (1986). *Thallium-201 myocardial imaging during pharmacologic coronary vasodilatation: comparison of oral and intravenous administration of dipyridamole.* J. Am. Coll. Cardiol., **8**, 76–83.

Thrall J.H. and Swanson D.P. (1989). *Diagnostic interventions in nuclear medicine.* Curr Probl Diag. Radiol., **18**, 1–37.

Treves S. *et al.* (1978). *Pentagastrin stimulation of technetium-99m uptake by ectopic gastric mucosa in a Meckel's diverticulum Radiology,* **128**, 711–2.

Vasquez T.E. *et al.* (1988). *Intravenous administration of morphine sulphate in hepatobiliary imaging for acute cholecystitis: a review of clinical efficacy.* Nucl. Med. Commun., **9**, 217–22.

Verani M.S. (1991a). *Adenosine thallium-201 myocardial perfusion scintigraphy.* Am. Heart. J. **122**, 269–278.

Verani M.S. (1991b). *Pharmacological Stress with adenosine for myocardial perfusion imaging.* Semin. Nucl. Med., **21**, 266–72.

Wyngaarden J.B. *et al.* (1952). *The effect of certain anions upon the accumulation and retention of iodide by the thyroid gland.* Endocrinology, **50**, 537–549.

Yeker D. *et al.* (1984). *Radionuclide imaging of Meckel's diverticulum: cimetidine versus pentagastrin plus glucagon.* Eur. J. Nucl. Med., **9**, 316–9.

Yudd A.P. *et al.* (1991). *Interventions and functional brain imaging.* Semin. Nucl. Med., **21**, 153–8.

Zeller F.P. and Blend M.J. (1987). *The use of intravenous dipyridamole in thallium 201 myocardial perfusion imaging.* Pharmacotherapy, **7**, 178–184.

Table 1
Drugs used in Nuclear Medicine Interventional Studies

Drug & Study	*Dose & Administration*	*Pharmacokinetics*	*Comments*
Acetazolamide Brain studies[51]	IV: 500mg-1g	Rapid onset Peak 25 min. Half-life 90 min.	No additional increase in rCBF has been noted when increasing the dosage from 1 to 2g. Caution in patients with acute strokes (may cause deterioration in the clinical status of the patient).
Aqueous Iodine Oral Solution B.P. (Lugol's iodine) Adrenal studies using radioiodinated compounds[39]	0.1–0.2ml three times a day starting 2 days before radiotracer injection.**		Each ml contains 50mg of free iodine and 130mg of free and combined iodine. Dilute with water or milk before administration to avoid gastrointestinal irritation.
Adenosine Cardiac studies[3,8,9]	IV: start at 50 micrograms/kg /min. increasing to a maximum of 140 micrograms/kg/min., maintained for 4 min. Radiotracer administered after 1 min at maximum dose. or 140 micrograms/kg/min. for 6 min. with radiotracer administered at 3 min.	Peak 2 min. Half-life <2–10 sec.	Caffeine-containing foods, beverages or medications, theophylline-containing preparations and dipyridamole should be withheld for 24 hours before testing. Contraindicated in patients taking oral dipyridamole because of potentiation of hypotension.
Captopril Renal studies[16,20,21]	Oral: 25mg–50mg one hour before radiotracer injection.	Onset within 15 min. Peak 70 min. Half-life 2–3 hr.	Previous medications of captopril should be discontinued for 2 days, lisinopril or enalapril for 1 week, no diuretics for 1 week. Caution: First dose effect (Hypotension) of captopril.
Ceruletide (formerly known as caerulein) Hepatobiliary studies[22,24]	IM:300 nanogram/kg IV;5 nanogram/kg over 3 min.*	Peak IM:5–45 min. IV:19 min.	Never give as a bolus which may cause spasm of the neck of the gallbladder & prevent contracting in a normal gallbladder The incidence of side effects is considerably lower when given IM.
Cholecystokinin (CCK)[23,24,25] Hepatobiliary studies	IV:0.5-1 Ivy dog units/kg, dilute in 20ml normal saline over 5min.* Children: 0.25 Ivy dog units/kg	Onset 1–3 min. Peak 5–15 min. Duration more than 2 hours	Stored at −20°C. Avoid rapid injections-see note for Ceruletide. CCK is standardized in biologic terms either for its gallbladder contracting potency (Ivy Dog units) or its ability to stimulate pancreatic enzyme secretion (Crick Harper Raper units). One CHR unit is about 1.2 times as potent in its effect on the gallbladder as one Ivy dog unit.[55]

Cimetidine Gastrointestinal studies[34,36,37]	Oral: 300mg qds for 24–48 hr. before study; children: 20mg/kg/day IV:300mg in 100ml glucose 5% over 20 min. and imaging begun 1 hr. later.	Oral: Onset 0.5–1hr. Peak 1–2hr. Duration 4–6 hr. IV: Half-life 2 hr.	Rapid injections have been associated with cardiac arrhythmias.
Dexamethasone Adrenal studies[1,11,38–41]	Oral:4mg/day in divided doses for 7 days prior to administration of radiocholesterol and continue until imaging is completed.	Onset immediate Peak 1–2 hr. Duration 2–3 days following cessation of administration	Take with food to avoid G.I. side effects. Patient compliance is required to avoid false positive results. Spironolactone should be stopped for 3–4 weeks and diuretics, at least 2 weeks, before study.
Dipyridamole Cardiac[3–7]	Oral: 300–400mg crushed and administered in a slurry with 30ml water, radiotracer administered after 45 min. IV: 0.14mg/kg/minute, dilute in sodium chloride 0.9% or glucose 5%, infused over 4 min. with patient supine. Radiotracer administered 3–4 min. after end of infusion.	Oral: Peak 45 min. IV: Peak 7–8 min. Duration 30–60 min.	IV aminophylline may be administered to reverse side-effects; 75–100mg given slowly, give up to 250mg if symptoms persist. Nitroglycerin may be used in addition to reverse ischaemia. Concurrent administration of a vasodilator may cause a severe hypotensive effect. Caffeine containing beverages or medications and theophylline containing preparations should be withheld for 24 hours before testing. Not necessary to discontinue oral dipyridamole.
Dobutamine Cardiac studies[11–14]	IV:5 micrograms/kg/min. increasing at increments of 5 micrograms/kg /min every 5–8 min. to a maximum of 20 micrograms/kg/min or until symptoms develop (angina, significant arrhythmia and/or marked hypotension.)	Onset 1–2 min. Peak within 10 min. Half life 2 min.	Discontinue use of beta-blockers and other sympatholytic therapy for at least 48 hours before study.
Frusemide Renal studies[16–18]	IV: 0.3–0.5mg/kg over 1–2 min. 15–20 min. before or after radiotracer injection. Infants and children: 1 mg/kg up to 20 mg	Onset 5 min. Peak 15–30 min. Duration up to 2 hr.	Renal dysfunction can cause an absence of response in cases without significant obstruction. Renal maturation is not complete in infants less than 1 year of age and the effect of the diureti is less predictable.
Glucagon Fastrointestinal studies[11,33,34]	IV:0.25–2 units	Onset 1 min. Peak 2–4 min. Duration 9–17 min. for 0.5 unit dose; 22–25 min. for 2 unit dose.	May be used in combination with pentagastrin. The dueodenum is the most sensitive organ in regard to inhibition of motility with the stomach being the least sensitive.

Table 1 *(cont)*
Drugs used in Nuclear Medicine Interventional Studies

Drug & Study	*Dose & Administration*	*Pharmacokinetics*	*Comments*
Lugol's iodine	See Aqueous Iodine Oral solution B.P.		
Morphine Hepatobiliary studies[25–29]	IV: 40 micrograms/kg diluted in 10ml sodium chloride 0.9% over 3 min., if no gallbladder filling is noted over 40–60 min. following radiotracer administration.	Onset within 5 min. Duration 20–50 min.	
Pentagastrin Gastrointestinal studies[11,34,35]	SC: 6 micrograms/kg 15min. prior to injection of pertechnetate.	Onset within 10 min. Peak 20–30 min. Duration 60–80 min.	May be used in combination with glucagon. High doses of pentagastrin may inhibit gastric acid secretions and negate the desired interventional effects. Pentagastrin should not be combined with cimetidine since the later antagonizes pentagastrin's stimulation of pertechnetate uptake. Since pentagastrin increases acid secretion, it has the potential of causing re-bleeding.
Perchlorate Brain studies[46,49,50]	Oral: as potassium perchlorate Adult: 200mg–400mg Children: 0–2 yrs. 50mg 2–12 yrs. 100mg Give 0.5–1 hr. before radiotracer injection. IV: as sodium perchlorate, 50 mg –100mg at the time of radiotracer injection.	Accumulates in the choroid polexus 30–60 min. after oral administration and the 'blockade' is effective for about 6 hrs. 75% of the oral dose eliminated in 24 hrs.	Iodide uptake by the thyroid is also blocked but at the sub-therapeutic dose and with its relatively short duration of action, it is not contraindicated in hypothyroid patients.
Adrenal studies using radioiodinated Compounds[39,47]	Oral: 200mg every 8 hrs 2 days before radiotracer injection or 400mg initially, then 200mg every 6 hrs starting 0.5–1 hr. before radiotracer injection.**		
Thyroid studies[54]	Oral: 1 g for perchlorate dischare test.		
Phenobarbitone Hepatobiliary studies[24,31]	Oral: 5mg/kg/day in 2 divided doses for 5 consecutive days prior to the test.	Half-life 1.6–2.9 days in children	

Potassium iodate Adrenal studies using radioiodinated compounds[47,56]	Oral: 85–170mg daily starting 2 hours before radiotracer injection.** If first dose >140mg, starting time may be reduced to half an hour before radiotracer injection.		Available as 85mg tablets. 85mg of potassium iodate is equivalent to 60mg of potassium iodate. Potassium iodate has a longer shelf-life. then potassium iodide.
Potassium iodide	Solution: see Aqueous Iodine Oral solution B.P. Tablets: see potassium iodate.		
Ranitidine Gastrointestinal studies[34]	IV: 1mg/kg with a maximum of 50mg, dilute in sodium chloride 0.9%, infused over 20 min.	Half-life 2 hr.	Rapid injections have been associated with cardiac arrhythmias.
Sincalide Hepatobiliary studies[11,23,24]	IV: 20 nanograms/kg over 3 min.*	Onset within 30 sec. Peak 5–15 min. Duration 15–20 min., gallbladder returning to basal size within an hour.	if no gallbladder contraction is observed within 15 minutes, the dose may be repeated at 40ng/kg. Avoid rapid injections–see note for Ceruletide.
Triiodothyronine Thyroid studies[11,52]	Oral: 75–100 micrograms in divided doses daily for 7–10 days.	Onset 1–2 days Half-life 1.5 days	
Adrenal studies using radioiodinated compounds[39]	Oral: 20 micrograms every 8 hours starting 2 days before radiotracer injection.**		
Thyroid stimulating hormone Thyroid studies[11,52,53]	SC or IM: 5–10 units in sodium chloride 0.9% for 1–3 days before study.		Caution: immunogenic because of its bovine origin.

*To evacuate the gallbladder and optimize subsequent filling with radiotracer: give 30 min. before radiotracer injection.
To study contractile function of visualizing gallbladders: give 60 min. after radiotracer injection, or when gallbladder maximally filled.
**Duration of treatment depends on the radionuclide and dose of radioactivity administered.[39,47]

Chapter 21

Diagnostic Applications of Radiopharmaceuticals

L. Smith

21.1 INTRODUCTION

Nuclear medicine studies, using radiopharmaceuticals, have a well established role in the investigation of a wide variety of clinical conditions. Such studies often provide unique functional information about the physiology and pathophysiology of the organ system under investigation and fall into two main categories, imaging and non-imaging.

In imaging studies, gamma camera pictures of a given area are obtained during or after administration of a radiopharmaceutical; these images are usually displayed on X-ray film. The gamma camera may be interfaced to a dedicated nuclear medicine computer which will allow computational, as well as visual analysis of the resulting data. In non-imaging studies either the patient or samples from the patient (e.g. plasma samples) are counted by external counting equipment, and information about the uptake and/or clearance of a given radiopharmaceutical obtained.

Nuclear medicine investigations are easily carried out in any patient whether adult or child although suitable adjustments to the amount of radioactivity administered must be made in children (see chapter 27). Where absolutely necessary clinically such tests can even by performed in pregnant patients or lactating mothers. In such cases the lowest possible activity of radiopharmaceutical should be used and suitable instructions given to the mother about interrupting or discontinuing breast feeding as appropriate (see chapter 27). This chapter describes some of the more commonly performed nuclear medicine investigations, both imaging and non-imaging; it is not intended as a comprehensive review of all such techniques nor does it cover all radiopharmaceuticals, particularly the newer ones, which are described elsewhere (see chapter 25). The activities of isotopes quoted are the maximum doses recommended by the Administration of Radioactive Substances Advisory Committee [ARSAC] for administration to adults; in practice activities lower than those quoted are usually administered.

Radiopharmaceuticals are usually administered by simple intravenous (IV) injection. However, in some instances when information about blood flow to an organ is required the patient is positioned with the gamma camera (interfaced to a computer) over the area of interest, and data acquired whilst the patient is being injected with a fast IV bolus technique which ensures that the radiopharmaceutical reaches the target organ as a compact bolus.

21.2 IMAGING STUDIES

21.2.1 Bone Scans

The isotope bone scan is widely used in the investigation of skeletal problems (Table 1) and is probably the commonest nuclear medicine investigation performed. No specific patient preparation is necessary prior to the IV injection of a Tc-99m-labelled-bone-seeking radiopharmaceutical (Table 2). The patient then waits for 3–4 hours before images of

TABLE 1
Skeletal problems which can be diagnosed by isotope bone scanning

Metastatic disease
Osteomyelitis
Metabolic bone disease
Paget's disease
Fractures
Primary bone tumours
Avascular necrosis
Loose/infected joint prosthesis

TABLE 2
Some commonly used bone seeking radiopharmaceuticals

Radiopharmaceutical	*Activity*
Tc-99m Methylene diphosphonate (MDP)	500–600 MBq
Tc-99m Hydroxymeythylene disphosphonate (HMDP)	500–600 MBq

the whole skeleton are obtained (either as multiple overlapping gamma camera views or as a whole body bone scan in both anterior and posterior projections). The labelled diphosphonate is actively taken up by the skeleton, and non-skeletal tracer is excreted in the urine. The patient is therefore asked to drink two pints of water between the injection and scan, and frequent bladder emptying is encouraged to minimise radiation dose to the bladder.

Tc-99m diphosphonate is absorbed onto hydroxyapatite crystals at sites of new bone formation and the amount of osseous uptake is proportional to the metabolic activity of the bone. Thus in normal circumstances (Figure 1) areas of high stress (e.g. the sacro-iliac joints, Figure 1) or active growth appear "hotter" or blacker than less active adjacent areas. Abnormalities on a bone scan usually appear as hot spots as a result of increased bone formation in the diseased

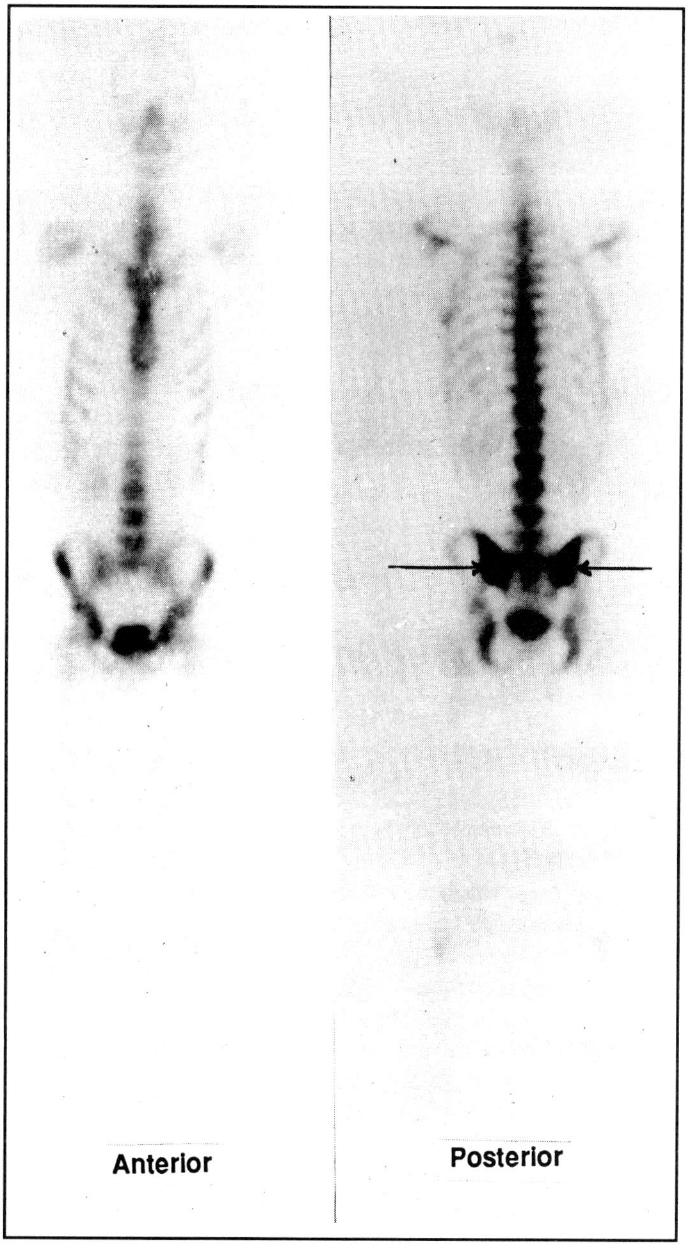

Figure 1. Normal 99m Tc-MDP whole body bone scan, anterior and posterior 4 hr views. Images taken with a gamma camera in scanning mode. Note the normal high uptake in the sacroiliac joints (arrows) where the weight of the axial skeleton is transmitted to the pelvis.

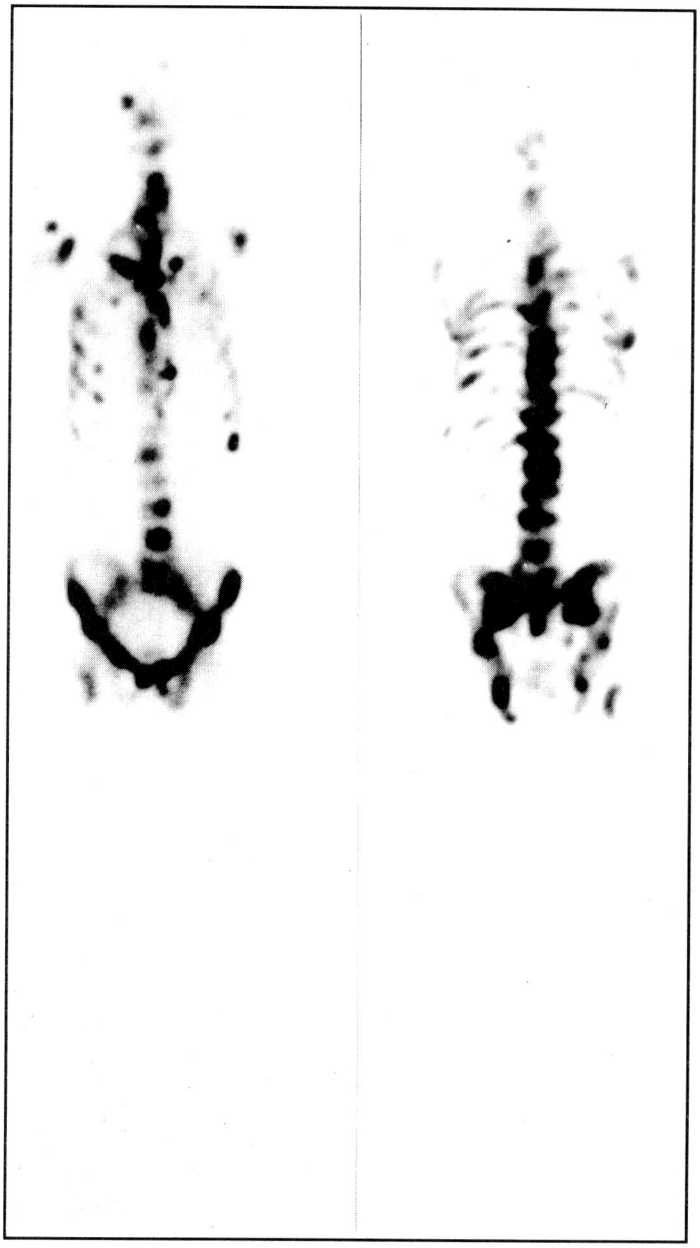

Figure 2. 99mTc-MDP bone scan (anterior and posterior 4 hr images) showing multiple bone metastases (black areas) throughout the skeleton in a patient with prostatic carcinoma.

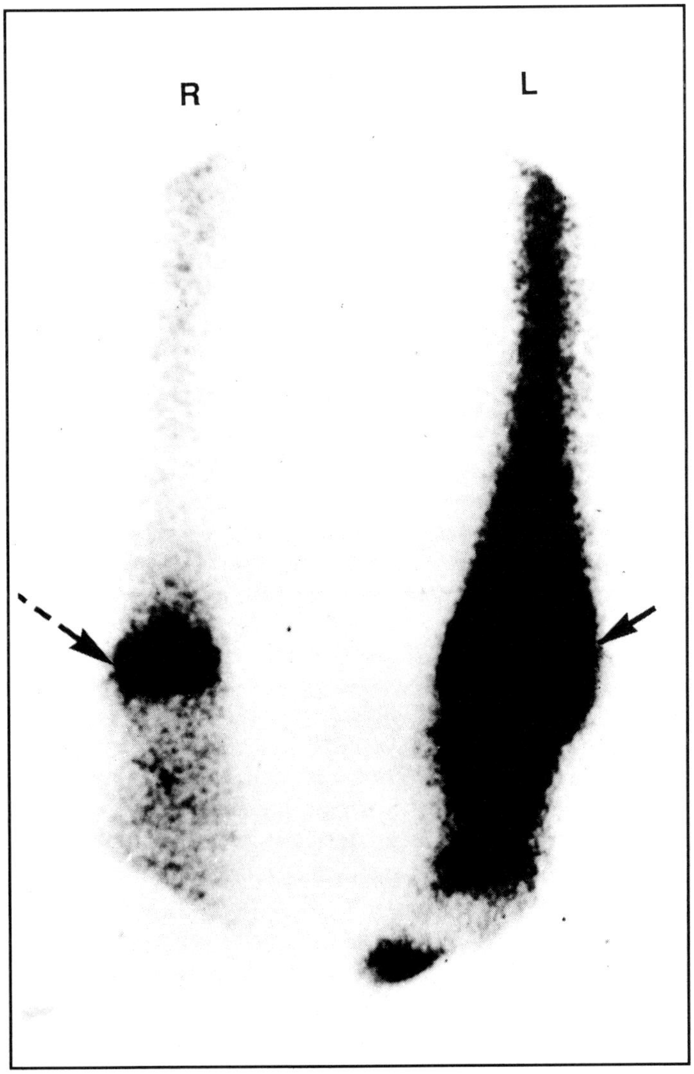

Figure 3. 99m-Tc-MDP bone scan; anterior 4 hr image of the lower limbs in a 14 year old girl with osteomyelitis of the distal left tibia (solid arrow). Note the high uptake in the normal epiphyseal growth plate in the distal right tibia (broken arrow).

sites (Figures 2 and 3) although occasionally cold (photon deficient) areas may be seen if the bone is avascular or there is a lot of bone destruction.

In certain circumstances (e.g. infection or avascular necrosis) additional clinical information can be obtained by performing a three phase bone scan, where the injection is given as a fast bolus and flow data acquired. A blood pool image of the affected areas is also taken at 1–2 mins after injection, when the radiopharmaceutical is still in the vascular space as well as the standard four hour bone images.

21.2.2 Brain Scans

The number of isotope brain scans carried out has fallen in recent years because of the advent of computerised tomography; however, isotope brain scanning still has a role to play and can be used in diagnosing many conditions (Table 3). Several different radiopharmaceuticals can be used for brain scans (Table 4) and all are suitable for clinical purposes. If Tc-99m pertechnetate is used the patient is given oral potassium perchlorate 1 hour before the scan; this blocks uptake of the radiopharmaceutical by the choroid plexus, thus improving image quality. The thyroid is also blocked, reducing radiation dose to this organ. Neither of the other two radiopharmaceuticals listed are taken up specifically by the choroid plexus and thyroid and no patient preparation is therefore necessary.

TABLE 3
Clinical conditions which can be diagnosed by brain scanning

Cerebrovascular disease
Cerebral abscess
Chronic subdural haematoma
Cerebral tumours (primary or secondary)
Encephalites

TABLE 4
Some commonly used radiopharmaceuticals for brain scanning

Radiopharmaceutical	*Activity*
Tc-99m pertechnetate	500 MBq
Tc-99m diethylenetriamine penta-acetic acid (DTPA)	500 MBq
Tc-99m glucoheptonate	500 MBq

A fast IV bolus injection is given with the patient positioned under the gamma camera. Anterior dynamic images of the head and neck are acquired for 1 min. at the time of injection, thus providing useful information about flow in the carotid and middle cerebral arteries (Fig. 4). Static brain images in the anterior, posterior and both lateral projections are then taken 1 hour after injection.

Under normal circumstances radiopharmaceuticals do not cross the "blood-brain barrier" and the brain therefore appears to be "cold", while structures which still contain circulating radiopharmaceutical appear to be "hot" (Fig. 5). When there is cerebral pathology, capillaries which are more permeable than normal are usually found in the abnormal area, allowing the radiopharmaceutical to accumulate at this site which then appears as a hot spot on the scan images (Fig. 6).

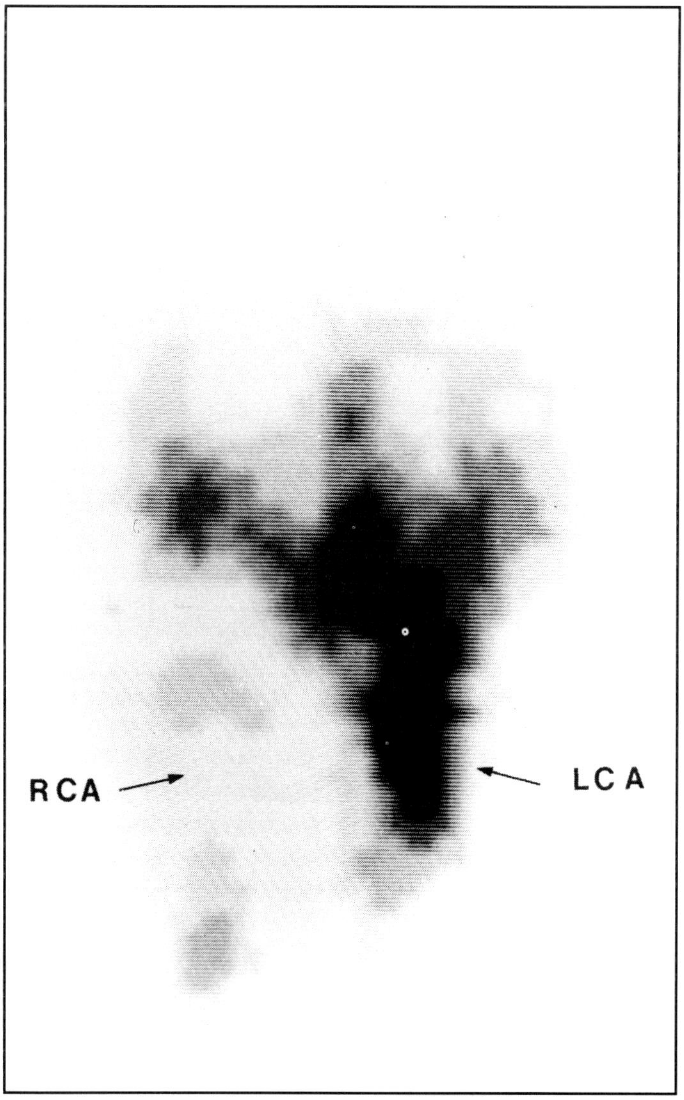

Figure 4. Dynamic flow image of the anterior neck and head after injection of Tc-99m pertechnetate for brain imaging. There is normal flow in the left carotid (LCA) and middle cerebral arteries. There is stenosis of the right carotid artery (RCA).

21.2.3 Thyroid Scans

Several different radiopharmaceuticals can be used for isotope thyroid imaging (Table 5) and for assessing thyroid activity by quantifying thyroid uptake of radiopharmaceuticals (Table 6). Uptake of the radiopharmaceuticals listed in Table 5 is impaired if the patient has been on thyroxine or iodine-containing medication or has received IV iodinated contrast (e.g. for kidney X-rays) in the 6 weeks before the isotope study. Uptake of radioactive iodine compounds (but not Tc-99m pertechnetate) is also reduced if the patient is on antithyroid medication (e.g. carbimazole or propylthiouracil). It is therefore essential to take an appropriate drugs history from the patient before embarking on a thyroid scan.

TABLE 5
Some commonly used radiopharmaceuticals for thyroid scanning

Radiopharmaceutical	*Activity*
Tc-99m pertechnetate	80 MBq
I-123 (sodium iodide)	20 MBq
I-131 (sodium iodide) in patients with thyroid carcinoma	400 MBq

TABLE 6
Radiopharmaceuticals used for quantitative assessment of thyroid function

Radiopharmaceutical	*Activity*
I-123 (sodium iodide)	2 MBq
I-131 (sodium iodide)	0.2 MBq

A choice must then be made about which radiopharmaceutical to use. Tc-99m pertechnetate is usually preferred unless there is a specific indication for a radioactive iodine scan (see Table 7), as Tc-99m pertechnetate is readily available and results in a lower radiation dose to the patient. Anterior and right and left anterior oblique views of the neck are obtained 20 minutes after IV injection of Tc-99m pertechnetate or 4 hours after oral IV administration of I-123.

TABLE 7
Clinical indications for thyroid scintigraphy

Radiopharmaceutical	*Clinical indication*
Tc-99m pertechnetate	? functional status of palpable thyroid nodule ? multinodular goitre ? retrosternal goitre ? assessment of thyroid prior to I-131 treatment for thyrotoxicosis
I-123 (sodium iodide)	as above if Tc-99m pertechnetate scan not diagnostic ? ectopic thyroid tissue
I-131 (sodium iodide)	? residual tissue after "total" thyroidectomy for thyroid carcinoma ? functioning metastases from thyroid carcinoma

In the normal thyroid there is symmetrical tracer uptake throughout both lobes of the thyroid (Figure 7). Thyroid nodules may be either non-functional (and appear as a cold

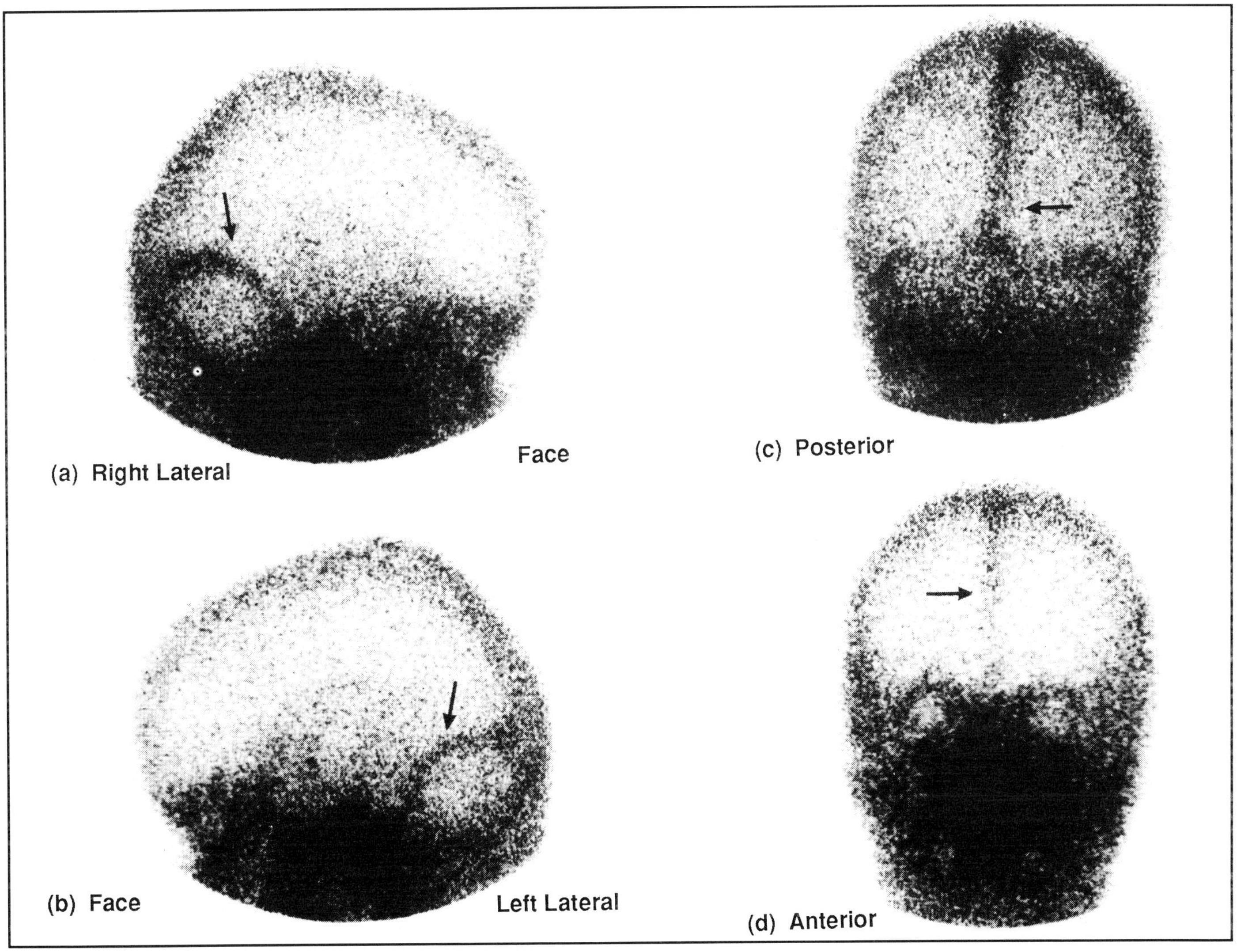

Figure 5. Tc-99m pertechnetate brain scan (1 hr images). Note the normal venous structures ((a), (b), transverse sinus; (c), (d) sagittal sinus).

defect, Figure 8) or functional (where they show the same or increased tracer uptake compared to the normal tissue).

Ectopic thyroid tissue may be seen anywhere in the neck, from the back of the tongue (Figure 9) down to the retrosternal region, reflecting the migration of the thyroid during foetal development.

In patients with thyroid carcinoma, whole body scans can be performed 3 days after oral administration of I-131 to detect residual thyroid tissue in the neck or functioning metastases elsewhere.

In addition to imaging the thyroid, radioactive iodine can be used to quantify thyroid activity (Table 6). Thyroid uptake of iodine can be measured by a probe counter positioned over the thyroid 2–24 hours after oral I-123 or I-131 administration. The counts in the thyroid are then compared with the counts in a known standard and the percentage uptake of iodine calculated. Such measurements can be invaluable in differentiating between thyroiditis (where uptake is low) and thyrotoxicosis (where uptake is high) in patients who have raised serum thyroxine levels. This technique is also used in the assessment of thyrotoxic patients prior to treating them with therapeutic I-131.

21.2.4 Lung Scans

Lung scans are commonly used to diagnose pulmonary emboli and to assess regional pulmonary function prior to thoracic surgery. They can also be used to diagnose inhalation of a foreign body. Lung scintigraphy is usually performed as two procedures, a ventilation study and a perfusion study, and it is often necessary to compare the patterns of ventilation and perfusion in the same patient to reach an accurate diagnosis.

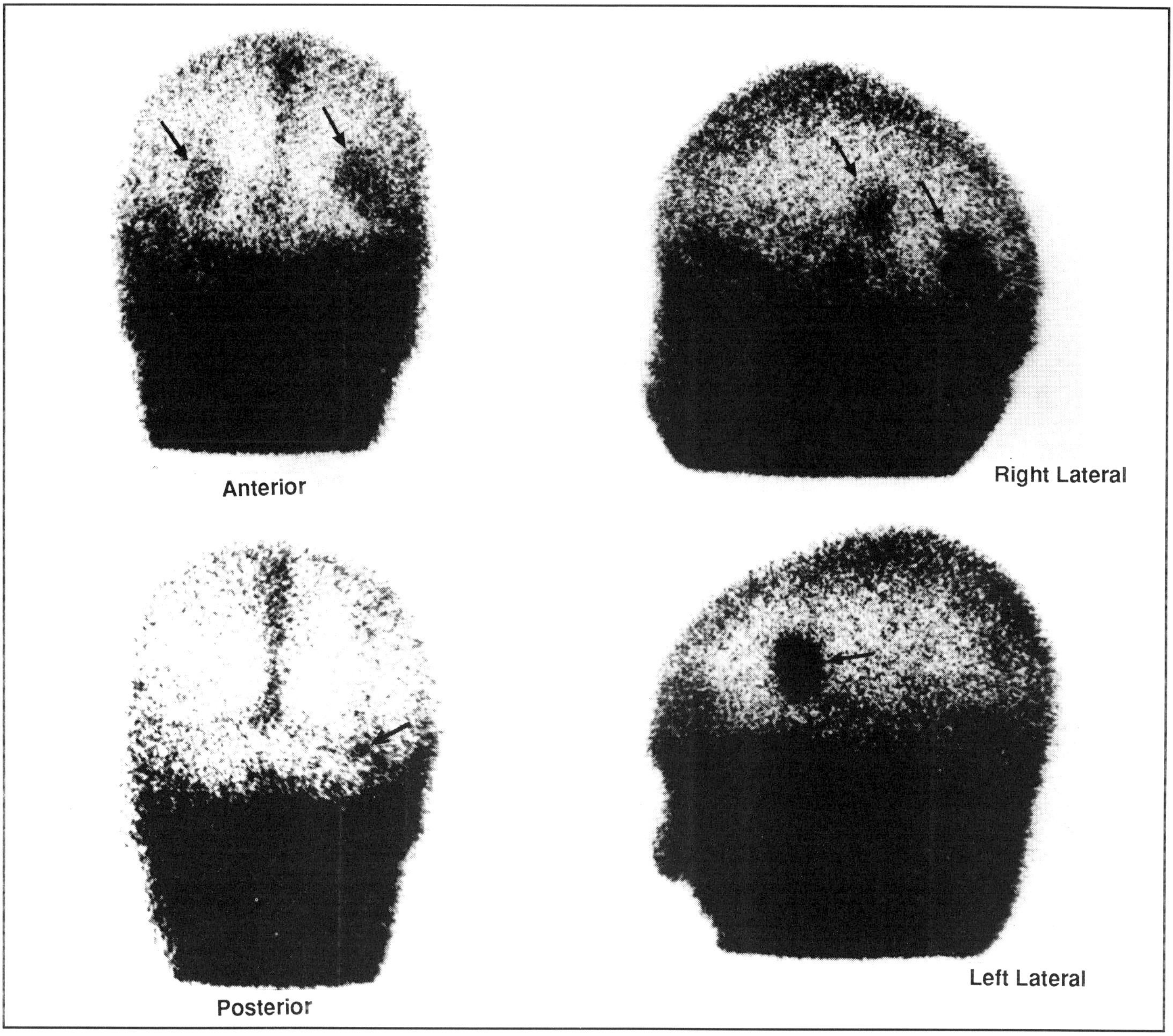

Figure 6. Tc-99m DTPA brain scan (1 hr images) showing multiple cerebral metastases (arrows) in both cerebral hemispheres in a patient with bronchial carcinoma.

TABLE 8
Some Commonly used radiopharmaceuticals for lung ventilation studies

Radiopharmaceutical	*Activity*
Tc-99m diethylenetriamine penta-acetic acetic (DTPA) aerosol	80 MBq
Xenon-133 (Xe-133)	400 MBq per litre (rebreathed for 300 seconds)
Krypton-81m (Kr-81m)	3600 MBq secs

21.2.4.1 Perfusion Scan

The patient is injected intravenously with 100 MBq Tc-99m microspheres or macroaggregates of albumin (MAA). The labelled albumin then lodges in some of the small pulmonary capillaries, and the distribution can be imaged. Scintigrams of the lungs are obtained in multiple projections (usually anterior, posterior, both laterals and both posterior obliques) to show the perfusion in all areas of the lung. In a normal patient, perfusion tends to be relatively lower in the lung apices, gradually increasing towards the lower zones (Figure 10). In patients with pulmonary emboli multiple segmental

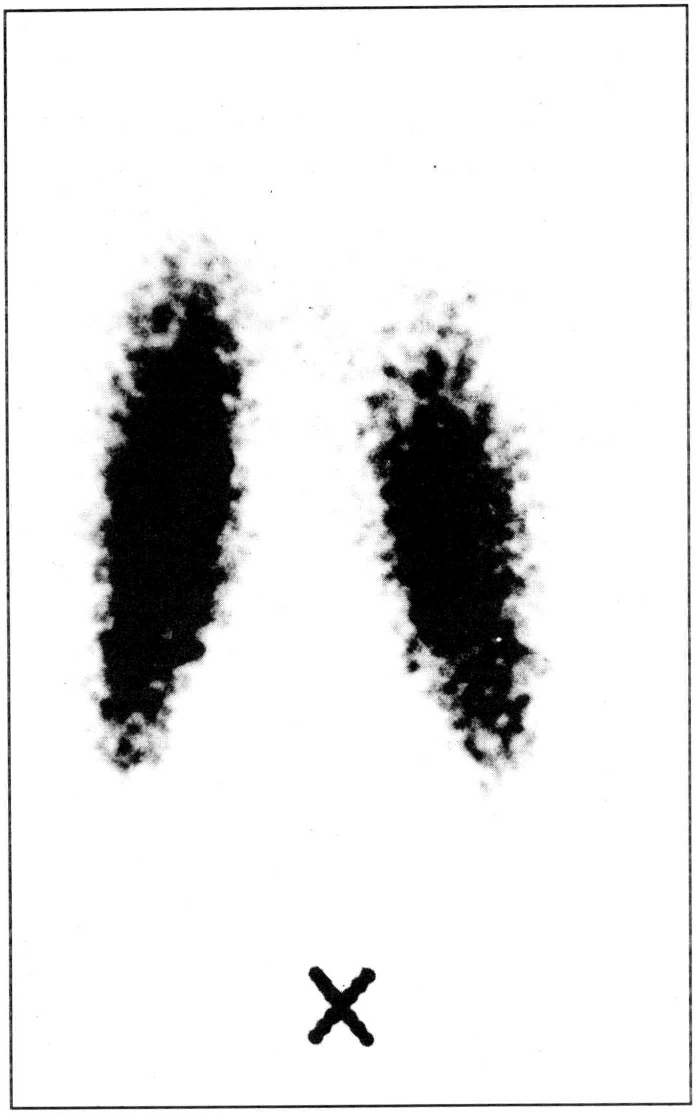

Figure 7. Normal Tc-99m pertechnetate thyroid scan (anterior view at 20 min.) showing the two normal lobes. The thyroid cartilage is marked with a cross.

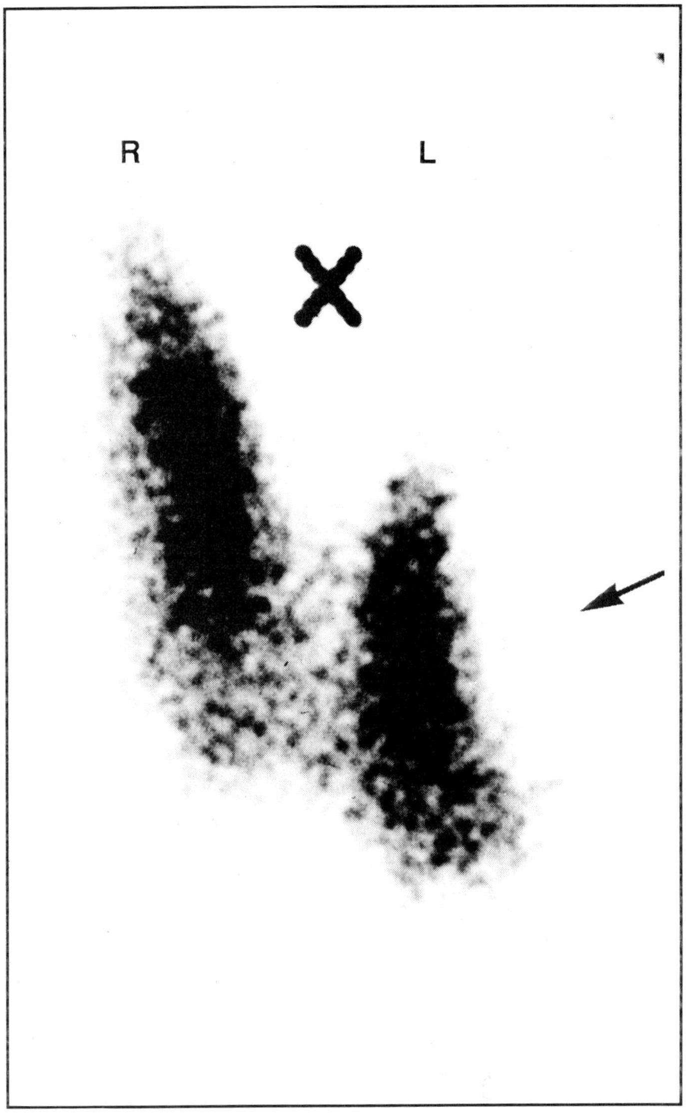

Figure 8. Tc-99m pertechnetate thyroid scan in a patient with a solitary non-functioning thyroid nodule in the left lobe (arrow). The right lobe is normal.

cold perfusion defects are usually seen (Figure 11); such patients usually have a normal ventilation scan.

21.2.4.2 Ventilation Scan

Depending on the radiopharmaceutical used for the ventilation scan, this can be performed either before or after the perfusion scan. Xe-133 images are obtained whilst the patient rebreathes the radioactive gas ("wash-in" and "equilibration" images) and then while they exhale the gas ("wash-out" images). Because of the time this takes, Xe-133 images are usually obtained in only one projection. Kr-81m images can be obtained in all six projections with the patient inhaling the gas during each image. If Tc-99m DTPA aerosol or Tc-99m 'Technegas' is used, multiple images in different projections can be obtained after the patient has inhaled the aerosol. In normal patients ventilation mirrors the distribution of perfusion (Figure 12). Any regional reductions in ventilation, e.g. due to infection or other pathologies, will result in a cold defect (Figure 13); this may be matched with a similar perfusion defect. As already mentioned patients with pulmonary emboli will have a normal ventilation scan, but an abnormal perfusion study.

21.2.5 Liver/Spleen Scans

Isotope liver/spleen scans can be useful in a variety of clinical conditions (Table 9). Information about liver blood flow can be obtained by acquiring computer data at the time of a fast IV bolus injection of the radiopharmaceutical. Any of the Tc-99m labelled colloid preparations can be used, e.g. albumin, tin colloid etc. (administered activity 80 MBq). The labelled colloid is phagocytosed by the reticuloendothelial cells which form the framework of the liver and spleen and is also taken up to a lesser extent by similar cells in the bone marrow. The relative uptake by liver, spleen and bone marrow will be determined to a small extent by the particle size of the colloid used.

Static upper abdominal images (anterior, posterior, right and left laterals) are obtained 20 minutes after injection to ensure adequate views of both liver and spleen. The exposure of the X-ray film is set so that only the liver and spleen are visualised. Bone marrow is not seen under normal

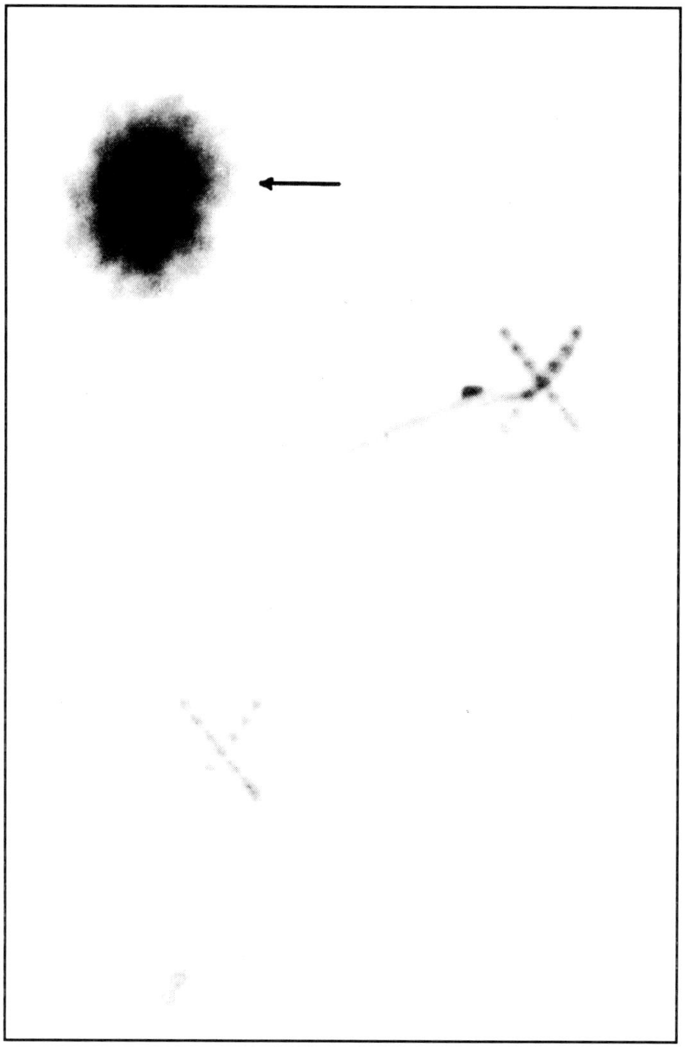

Figure 9. I-123 scan of lower face and neck (lateral 4 hr image) showing uptake in a lingual thyroid (arrow). No thyroid tissue is present in the normal thyroid site. The chin and neck outlines are drawn and the crosses mark the chin (upper cross) and thyroid cartilage (lower cross).

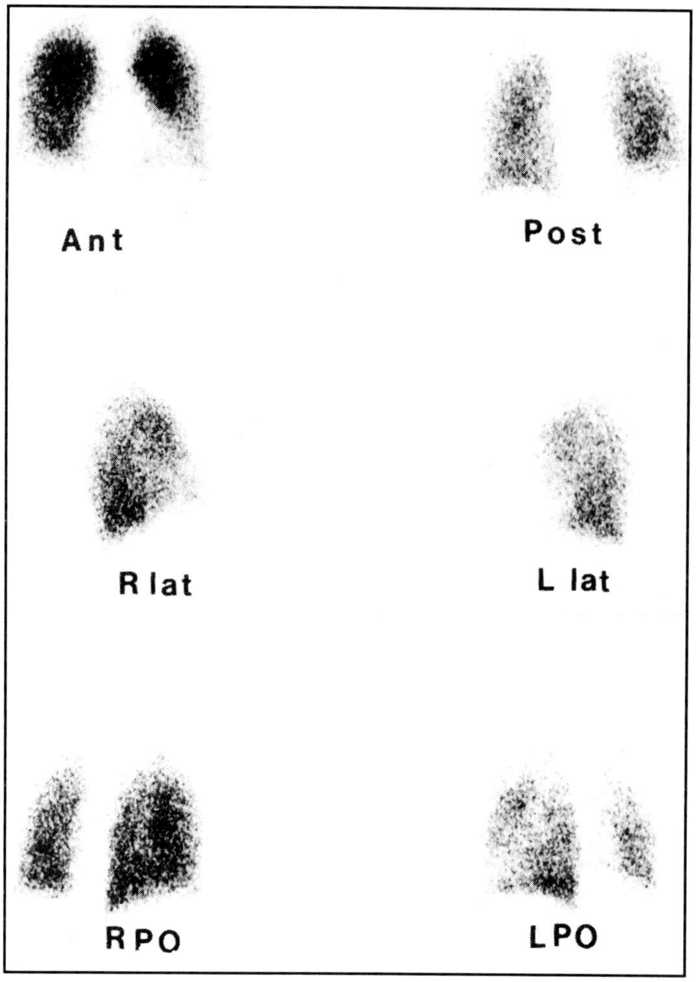

Figure 10. Tc-99m-MAA perfusion lung scan showing normal distribution throughout both lungs. The heart and mediastinum appear as a photon deficient area (on the anterior view). LPO and RPO refer to left and right posterior oblique.

TABLE 9
Clinical conditions which can be detected on liver/spleen scans

Parenchymal liver disease
Cirrhosis
Hepatic metastases
Hepatic/splenic cysts
Hepatic/splenic abscesses
Hepatic/splenic trauma
Hepatic/splenic infarcts
Transplant assessment

circumstances. In healthy patients the liver is more clearly seen on the anterior and the spleen on the posterior view (Fig 14) and both organs show fairly uniform tracer uptake. When there is focal liver pathology, abnormalities appear as cold defects (Figure 15). In the presence of diffuse liver

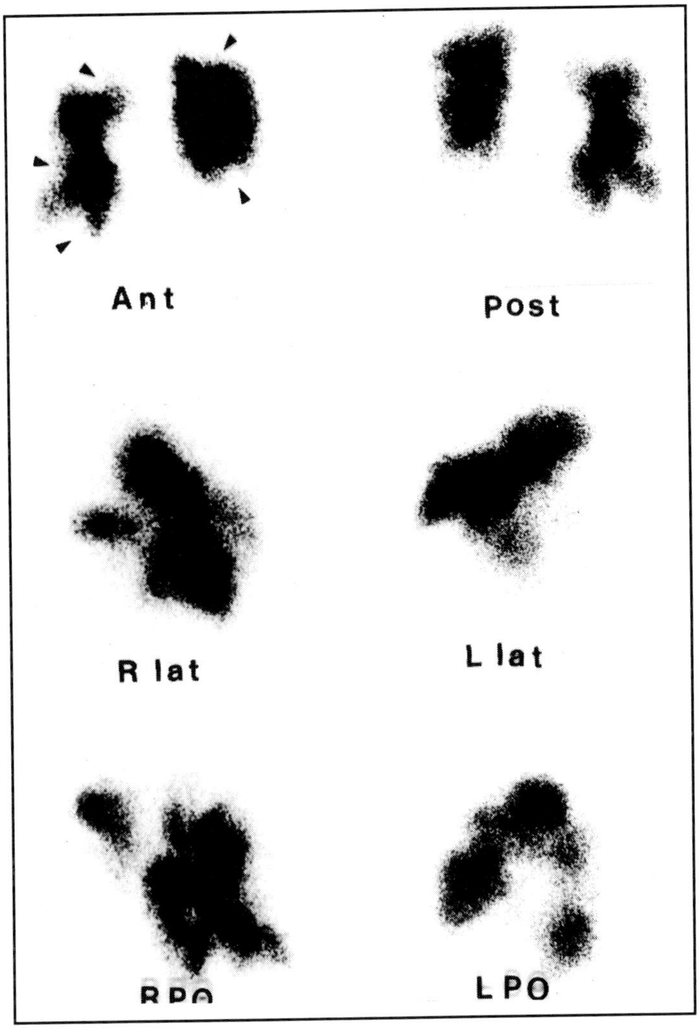

Figure 11. Several cold defects are seen in all views (marked with arrow heads on anterior view) of this Tc-99m MAA lung scan. These abnormalities are the result of pulmonary emboli. The ventilation lung scan in this patient was normal.

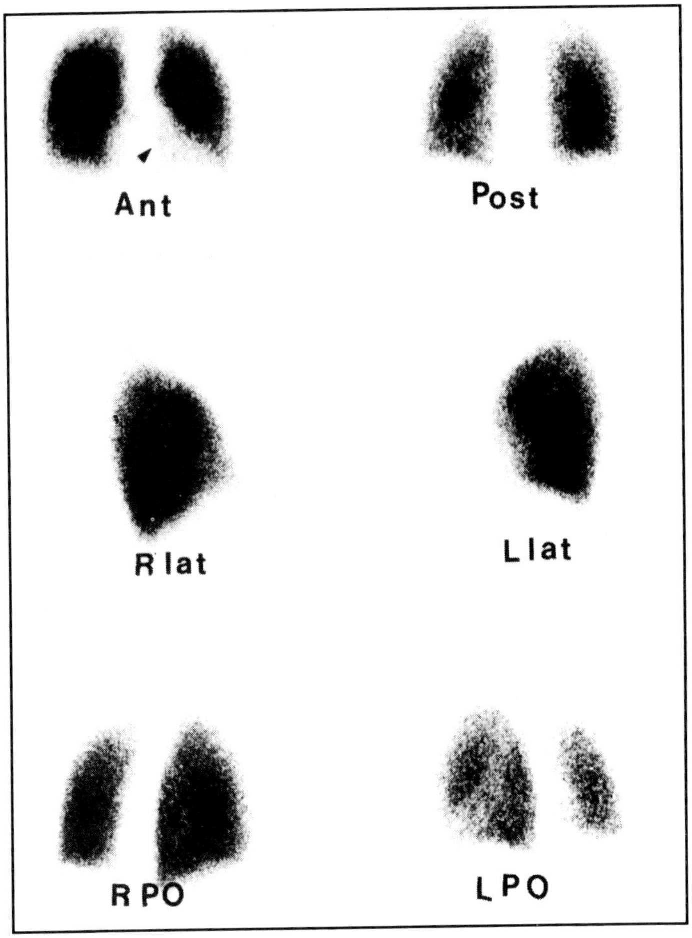

Figure 12. Normal Tc-99m DTPA aerosol ventilation lung scan showing a similar distribution of tracer of that of the patient's normal perfusion study (Figure 10).

disease, there may be very poor tracer uptake by the liver, and the spleen and bone marrow may then show higher uptake of the radiopharmaceutical (Figure 16).

21.2.6 Bone Marrow Scans

By using one of the smaller sized colloids (e.g. Tc-99m nano-colloid) a greater activity of isotope (400 MBq) and altering the intensity of the x-ray images useful information about the distribution of the bone marrow in the ribs, spine, pelvis, skull and long bones can be obtained. Images of all these areas (and liver and spleen if indicated) are obtained one hour after IV injection of the radiopharmaceutical and will give information about the extent of normal bone marrow (which will take up tracer) and the presence of diseased bone marrow (which appears as cold defects) in patients with tumour deposits in the marrow, myelofibrosis or marrow aplasia.

21.2.7 Hepatobiliary Scans

Information about the biliary tree and bile outflow can be obtained by performing a hepatobiliary scan using one of the Tc-99m iminodiacetate compounds (e.g. Tc-99m HIDA, Tc-99m EHIDA etc.). These radiopharmaceuticals are taken up by the hepatocytes in the liver and are then excreted in the bile via the biliary tree and gall bladder into the

TABLE 10
Clinical conditions which can be diagnosed by hepatobiliary scans

Acute cholecystitis
Bile duct obstruction
Biliary leak (fistula)
Dueodeno-gastric bile reflux
Afferent loop obstruction (after gastric surgery)
Choledochal cyst

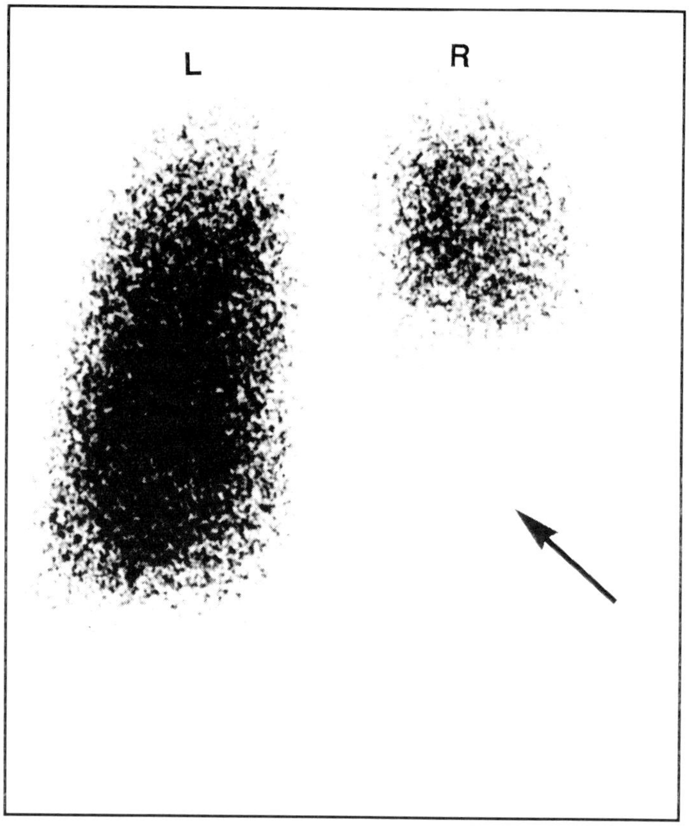

Figure 13. Tc-99m DTPA aerosol ventilation lung scan (posterior view) showing absence of ventilation in the right middle and lower lobes (arrow) due to an inhaled foreign body blocking the right immediate bronchus.

duodenum (Figure 17). The patient is required to fast for at least 4 hours prior to IV administration of 75–150 MBq Tc-99m HIDA and timed imaged are then obtained at 20 mins intervals until a normal pattern is seen or all the radiopharmaceutical has been cleared from the hepatocytes (this takes about 1–2 hours in normal circumstances). Hepatobiliary scans can be used to diagnose many clinical problems (Table 10), but are probably most commonly used in the diagnosis of acute cholecystitis (Figure 18) where the gallbladder is not visualised because inflammation of the cystic duct prevents localisation of the radiopharmaceutical in that area.

21.2.8 Kidney Scans

There are two main types of kidney scan, those which provide information about relative function of the kidneys and urine outflow, known as renograms (using the radiopharmaceuticals listed in Table 11) and those which demonstrate functioning renal parenchyma (Tc-99m dimercaptosuccinic acid (DMSA) scans).

In the half hour prior to a renogram the patient is hydrated with 1 litre of fluid to stimulate urine flow. The patient is then positioned with either a computer-linked gamma camera or probe system posteriorly over the kidneys and data is acquired while the patient is given a fast IV bolus of radiopharmaceutical and for 30 mins. thereafter. The rate of arrival of the bolus in the kidneys gives information about renal blood flow and the rate of uptake and subsequent

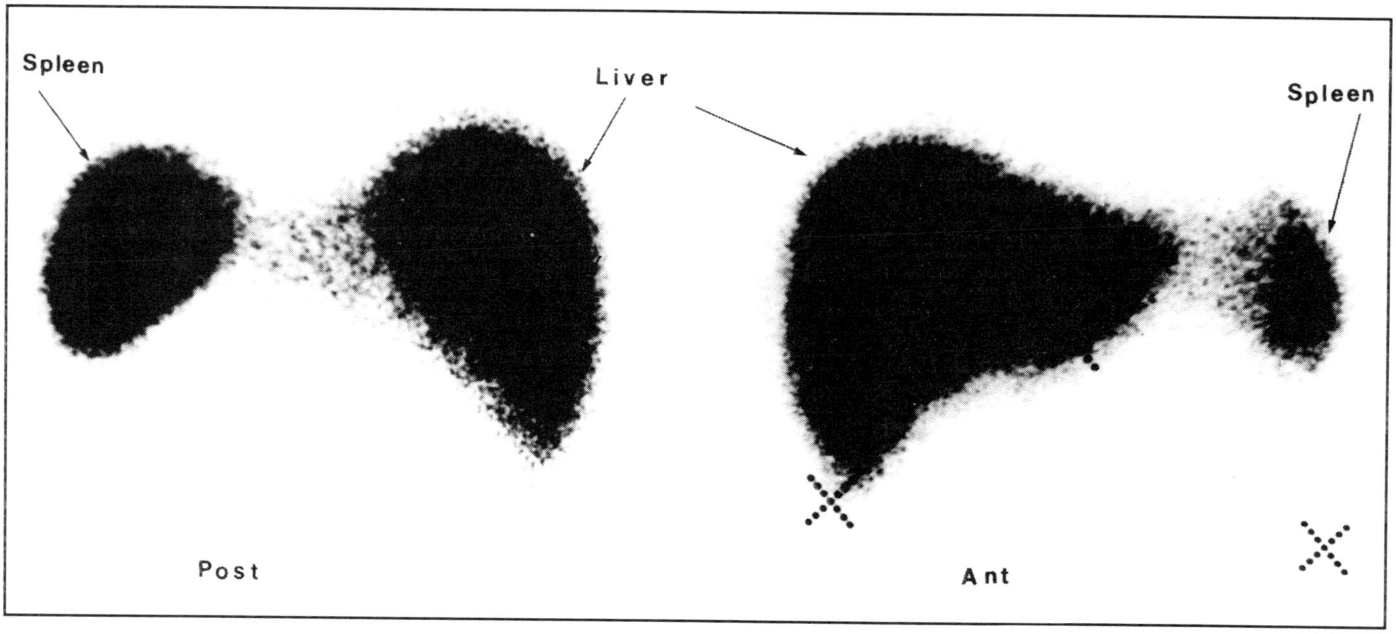

Figure 14. Normal Tc-99m-colloid scan of liver and spleen (anterior and posterior views). The crosses mark the xiphisterum (midline) and rib margins.

TABLE 11
Some commonly used radiopharmaceuticals for dynamic renal imaging

Radiopharmaceutical	*Activity*
Tc-99m diethylenetriamine penta-acetic acid (DTPA)	300 MBq
Tc-99m glucoheptonate	300 MBq
I-123 orthoiodohippurate (OIH)(imaging)	20 MBq
I-123 orthoiodohippurate (probe)	2 MBq
I-131 orthoiodohippurate (probe)	2 MBq
Tc-99m MAG3	75 MBq

excretion of the radiopharmaceutical by glomerular filtration and tubular secretion (OIH). This provides information about relative renal function and the patency of the pelvic calyceal systems and ureters and is useful in many clinical situations (see Table 12). DTPA is excreted by glomerular filtration only; both OIH and MAG3 are excreted by glomerular filtration and tubular secretion although the extraction efficiency is greatest with OIH. Gamma camera images using Tc-99m DTPA, Tc-99m MAG3 and I-123 OIH provide a visual display of the kidneys and collecting systems as shown in Figures 19 and 20. Computer analysis can be used to provide outflow curves as shown in Figure 21. Probe renography (using I-131-OIH or a low activity of 123-I-OIH) results only in uptake and outflow curves without the images. In some instances a patient may have an unusually large renal collecting system which gradually accumulates tracer and may appear obstructed even when there is no functional obstruction present. This can be detected by giving the patient intravenous frusemide during the study to increase the urine outflow rate and so "washout" the radiopharmaceutical from a non-obstructed but dilated system. In a truly obstructed kidney the excretion curve will continue to rise despite frusemide administration.

TABLE 12
Conditions which can be diagnosed by renography

Outflow obstruction
Renal artery stenosis
Renal transplant assessment
Vesico-ureteric reflux
Non-perfused kidneys

At the end of the dynamic phase of renography, a micturing cystogram can be performed to test the integrity of the vesico-ureteric junction. The patient is asked to empty the bladder while still in position in front of the gamma camera. If vesico-ureteric reflux is present tracer will be seen going back up the ureter and may even reflux into the kidney.

A Tc-99m DSMA scan is carried out in a rather different way. No prehydration is necessary. The patient is given a simple IV injection of 80 MBq Tc-99m DMSA and images are taken 2–4 hours later in the posterior and both posterior

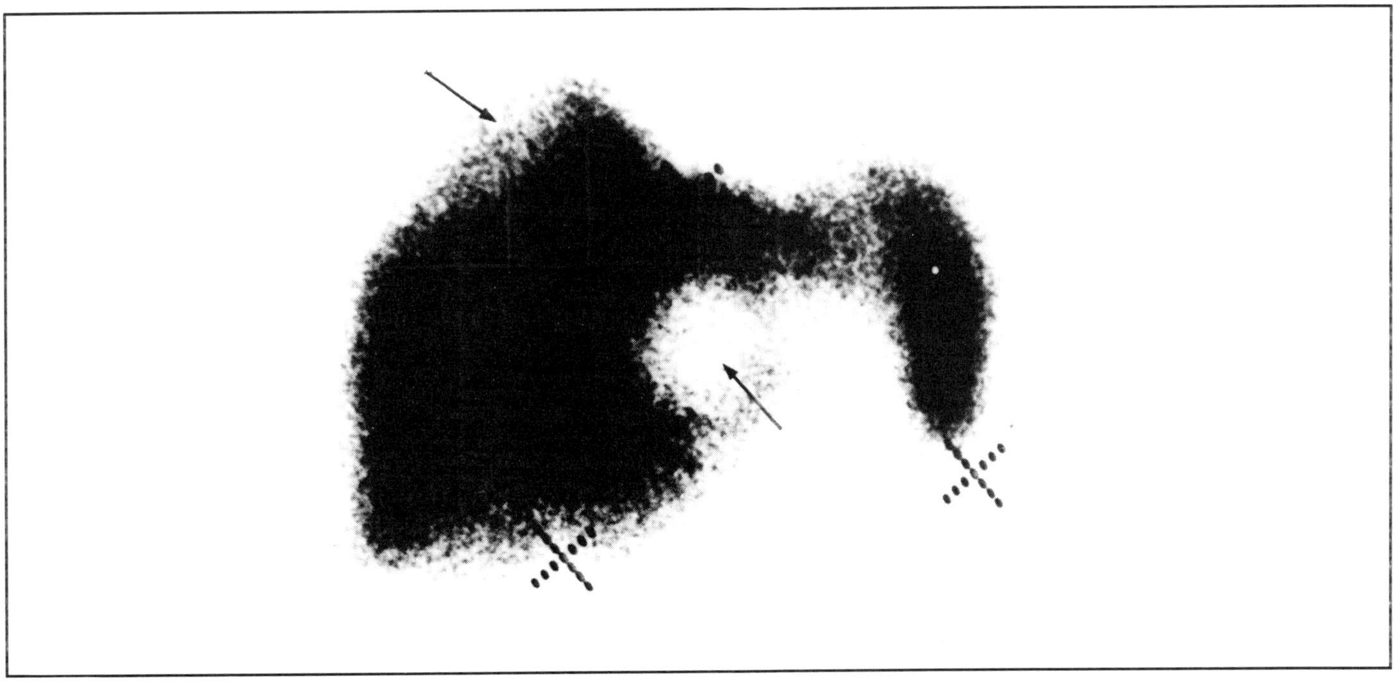

Figure 15. Tc-99m-colloid scan of the liver and spleen (anterior view) showing filling defects (arrows) in the liver due to metastases in a patient with ovarian carcinoma.

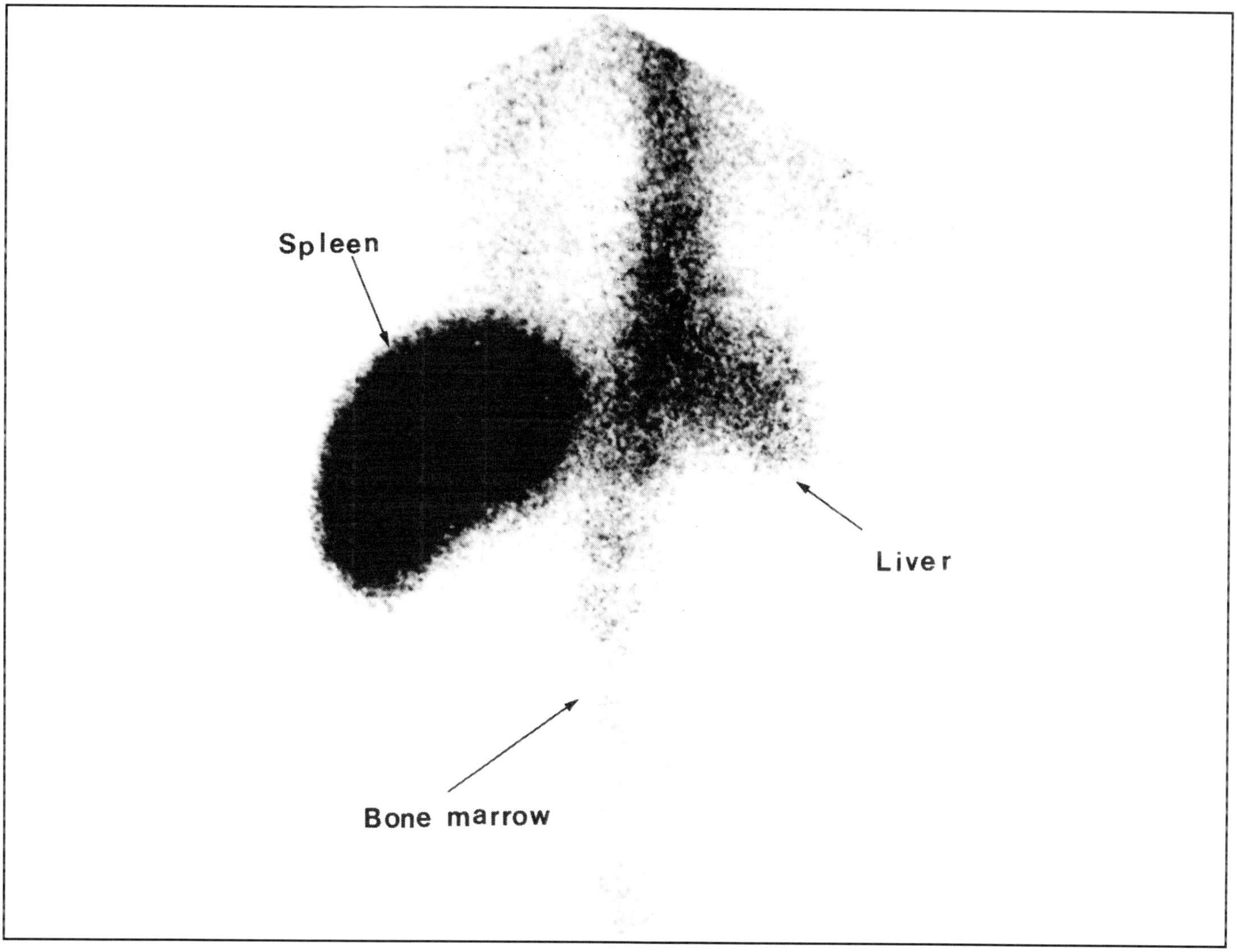

Figure 16. Tc-99m-colloid scan of the liver and spleen (anterior view) showing filling defects (arrows) in the liver due to metastases in a patient with ovarian carcinoma.

oblique projections (Figure 22). The radiopharmaceutical is taken up by the cells in the renal tubules and can be useful in a variety of clinical conditions (see Table 13).

TABLE 13
Conditions which can be diagnosed using ^{99m}Tc-DMSA

Renal scarring (due to urinary tract infections)
Space occupying lesions (e.g. cysts, tumours)
Renal trauma
Renal function

Any of the above renal scans may be used to calculate the relative contribution of each kidney to total renal function.

21.2.9 Adrenal Scans

The adrenal gland is composed of two parts, the inner medulla which is responsible for producing adrenalin and noradrenalin, and the outer cortex which secretes the gluco- and mineralo-corticoids.

Functional tumours of the adrenal medulla (phaeochromocytomas) can be localised on I-131 or 123-I metaiodobenzylguanidine (MIBG) scans, as abnormal tissue takes up the radiopharmaceutical and appears as a "hot" spot. The normal adrenal medulla is not visualised. Patients undergoing labelled-MIBG scans are pretreated 24 hours before and for four days after the scan with potassium iodide to block thyroid uptake of any free radioactive iodine which may be present in the radiopharmaceutical preparation. The radiopharmaceutical is given by slow intravenous injection (400

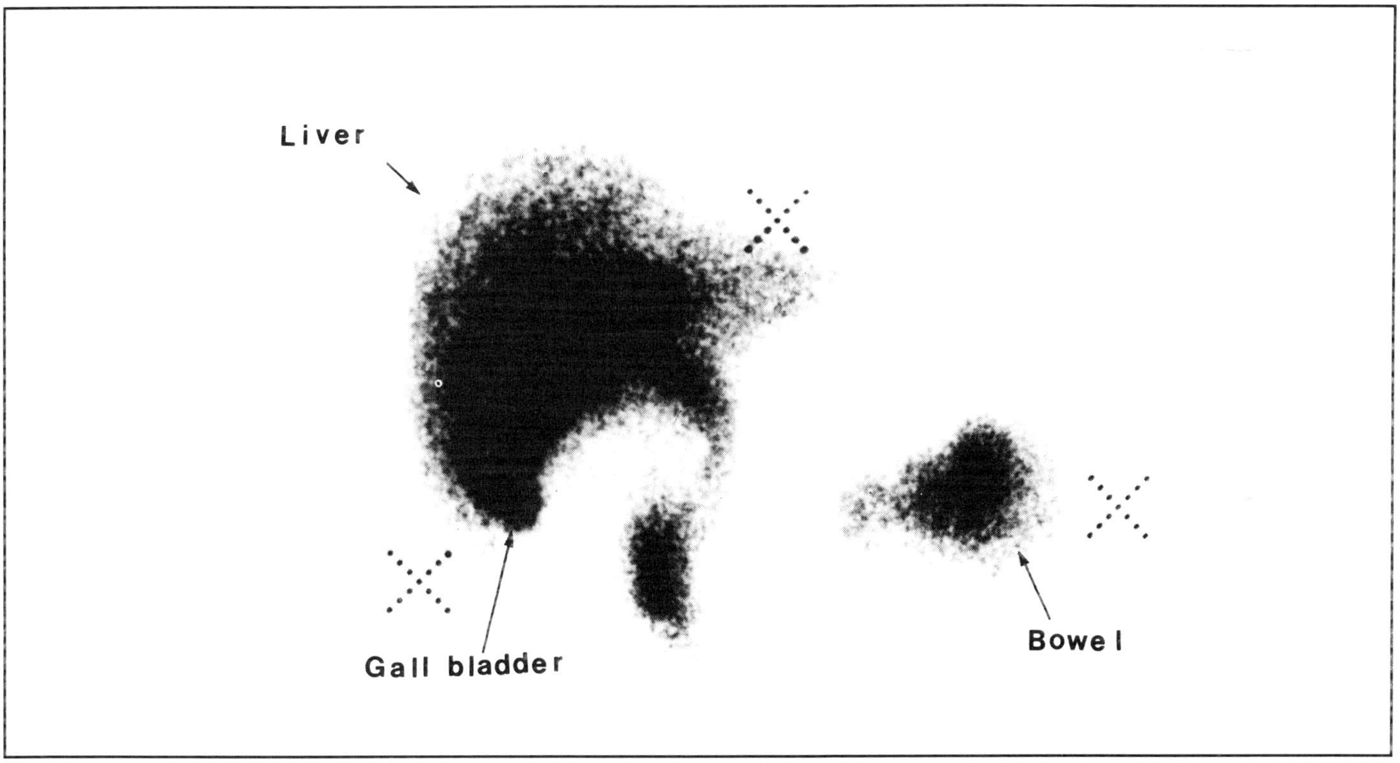

Figure 17. Anterior upper abdominal view 20 mins. after injection of Tc-99m EHIDA showing a normal pattern with tracer uptake in the liver and gallbladder and secreted into bowel. The crosses mark xiphisternum (mid-line) and lower rib margins.

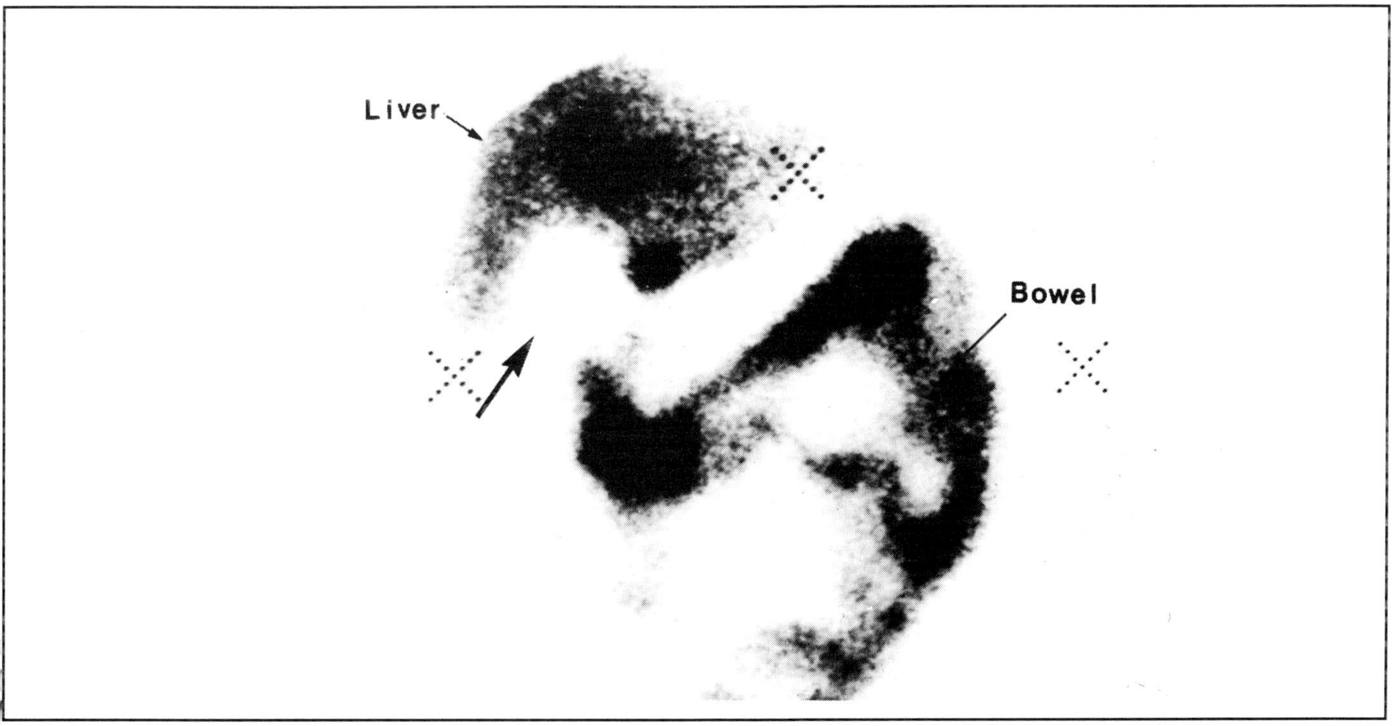

Figure 18. Anterior upper abdominal view 1½ hrs. after injection of Tc-99m EHIDA showing some tracer in the liver and a lot in the bowel. The gallbladder is not visualised (photon deficient area, arrowed) as this patient had acute cholecystitis. Xiphisternum and rib markers as before.

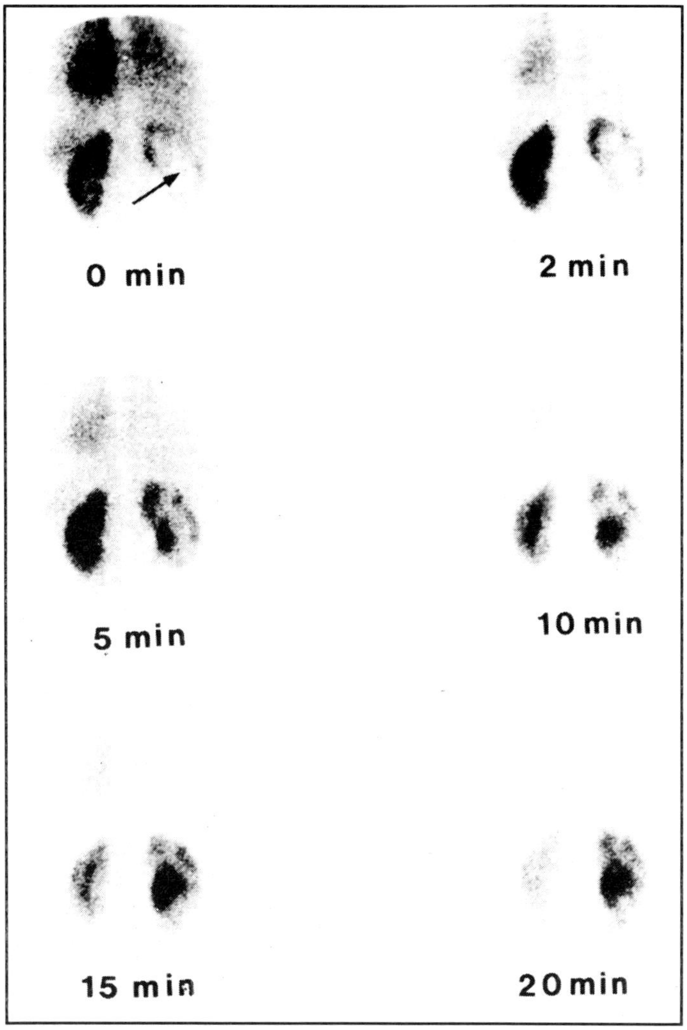

Figure 19. Timed posterior images taken during a dynamic Tc-99m DTPA kidney scan. The left kidney shows a normal excretion pattern. The obstructed right kidney shows an initial negative pyelogram (arrows) with slow accumulation of tracer in the right collecting system and ureter; the obstruction was due to a stricture at the lower end of the right ureter.

MBq 123-I MIBG, 20 MBq I-131 MIBG) and posterior and both lateral images of the adrenal areas obtained 24, 48 and 72 hours later. Whole body scans can also be obtained if there is any possibility of an ectopic phaechromocytoma lying outside the adrenals. Uptake of the radiopharmaceutical by a phaechromocytoma may be blocked by certain drugs (reserpine, cimetidine and tricyclic anti-depressants) and so a careful drug history should be taken before the scan is initiated.

The adrenal cortex secrete cortisol, aldosterone and adrenal androgens. In patients with excess cortisol production the adrenal overactivity may be primary (Cushing's syndrome due to an adenoma or, less commonly, carcinoma) or secondary, where there is bilateral adrenal hyperplasia as a result of hypersecretion of pituitary or ectopic adrenocorticotrophic hormone. Excess aldosterone production can be due to a benign adenoma (Conn's syndrome) or bilateral adrenal hyperplasia. The appropriate therapy will depend on the type of adrenal overactivity that is present, and isotope scans using radiolabelled cholesterol may help to determine this.

For an adrenal scan the patient is given an intravenous injection of 8 MBq 75-selenonorcholesterol and computerised scan images (posterior and both laterals) of the adrenal areas obtained seven and fourteen days later. In addition to visual analysis, adrenal uptake of radiopharmaceutical as a percentage of the injected dose, is also measured and it is therefore necessary to measure the syringe containing the radiopharmaceutical both before and after injection.

Normal adrenal glands will take up a very small amount of the injected radiolabelled cholesterol. If bilateral adrenal hyperplasia is present, both glands will show increased uptake. Patients with Cushing's syndrome show increased uptake in the adenoma with suppressed uptake in normal adrenal tissue. In Conn's syndrome the adenoma appears "hot" and the remaining adrenal tissue shows normal uptake.

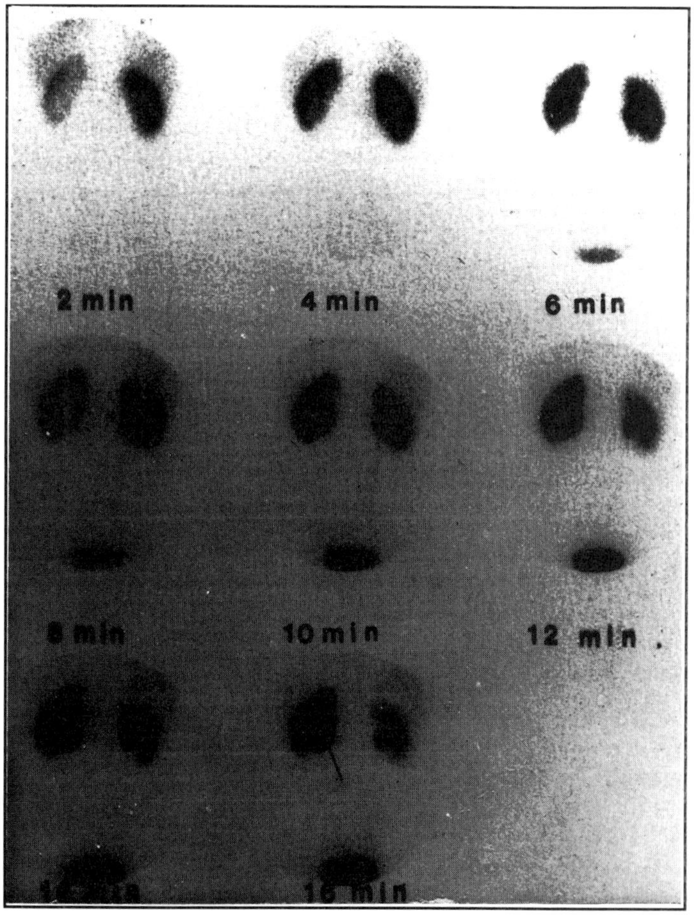

Figure 20. Timed posterior images of a Tc-99m MAG3 scan. The right kidney shows a normal excretion pattern whilst the left kidney shows obstruction.

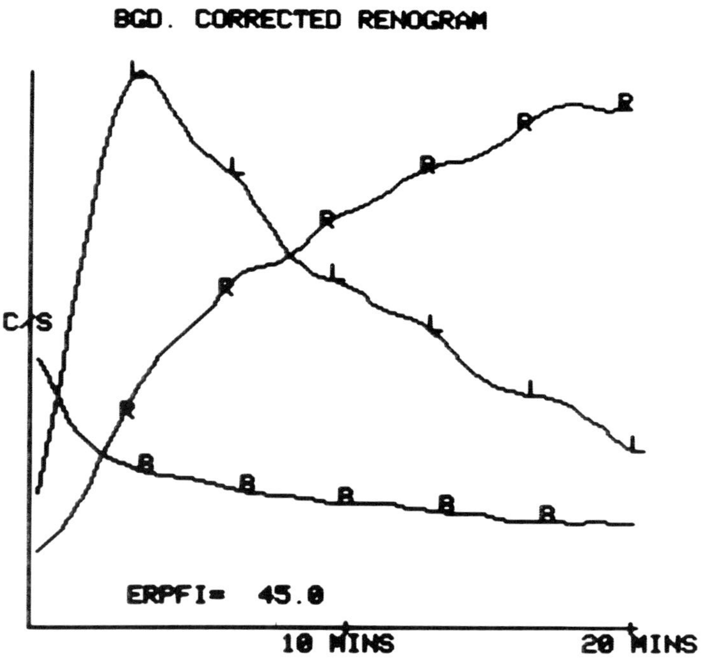

Figure 21. Computer curves from the kidney scan in Figure 19 showing the amount of activity in the kidneys (y-axis) plotted against time (x-axis). There is a normal outflow curve on the left and a rising obstructed outflow curve on the right.

"hot" and the remaining adrenal tissue shows normal uptake. Normal uptake may be suppressed by treating the patient with oral dexamethasone for seven days before and fourteen days during the scan. Uptake in an adrenal carcinoma may be low, normal or increased.

21.2.10 Heart Scans

Heart scans are usually performed to provide either functional information about left ventricular contraction (using a gated blood pool study) or to determine the perfusion of the myocardium, especially the left ventricle, in patients suspected of having heart disease.

In gated blood pool studies, the patient's own red blood cells are labelled with 800 MBq Tc-99m pertechnetate (see chapters 6 and 7). The patient is then attached to an electrocardiograph (ECG) monitor which is also connected to a computer interfaced to the gamma camera. The patient's heart is then imaged in the anterior and left anterior oblique (LAO) prejections while the patient is at rest, followed by LAO images while the patient is stressing the heart by supine bicycle exercise (this is carefully done under the supervision of a cardiologist).

Each time the heart contracts, radiolabelled blood is ejected from the right and left ventricles. The computer data is analysed with reference to the ECG tracing (each cardiac cycle being divided up into short intervals), and the contours of the ventricles at end-systole (when the ventricles are fully contracted) and end-diastole (when they are full relaxed) are obtained (Fig. 23). The recorded counts within these regions, after suitable background subtraction, allows calculation of left ventricular ejection fraction, and visual assessment of left ventricular wall motion is also possible. The data can also be presented as a cine display, giving a dynamic representation of ventricular contraction. Analysis of the timing (phase) and amplitude of contraction of the ventricular muscle will provide further information about the myocardium.

Ischaemic myocardium may appear normal at rest, but will show impaired wall motion with a fall in ejection fraction on exercise (Figure 24). Scarred myocardium may show decreased wall motion both at rest and on exercise.

Myocardial perfusion scans provide information about blood flow to the different parts of the ventricle and are invaluable in assessing patients with ischaemic heart disease. Such scans are usually performed in two parts, the initial stress study and the later redistribution study. The patient is exercised to their maximal capacity using either a bicycle ergometer or a treadmill (this is done under ECG control by a cardiologist). When patients are at peak exercise they are given an intravenous injection of 80 MBq Thallous-201 chloride, and the heart is then imaged in the anterior, lateral and LAO projections to allow good visualisation of the whole of the left ventricle.

Exercise increases blood flow to the myocardium via the coronary arteries and under normal circumstances fairly uniform tracer uptake is seen in the left ventricle (Figure 25). If there is narrowing or occlusion of a coronary artery then blood flow through the diseased vessel cannot be increased sufficiently during exercise and the ischaemic area of myocardium shows less tracer uptake than the surrounding normal muscle (Figure 26).

The patient is rescanned 4 hours after injection to provide information about the redistribution of tracer under normal, non-stressed conditions. Ischaemic muscle, which still has some blood supply, appears normal on the redistribution image, whereas infarcted muscle continues to show less tracer uptake than the surrounding normal myocardium.

An alternative approach to looking at myocardial perfusion is to use one of the Tc^{99m} labelled isonitriles (Tc^{99m} methoxyisobutylisonitrile [MIBI] is the most commonly used). Tc^{99m} MIBI combines the superior imaging characteristics of Tc^{99m} (resulting in potentially clearer images and better tomographic studies) with relatively stable tracer uptake and little redistribution after exercise, allowing a longer imaging time where appropriate. The slow redistribution means that separate rest and exercise studies need to be performed (on

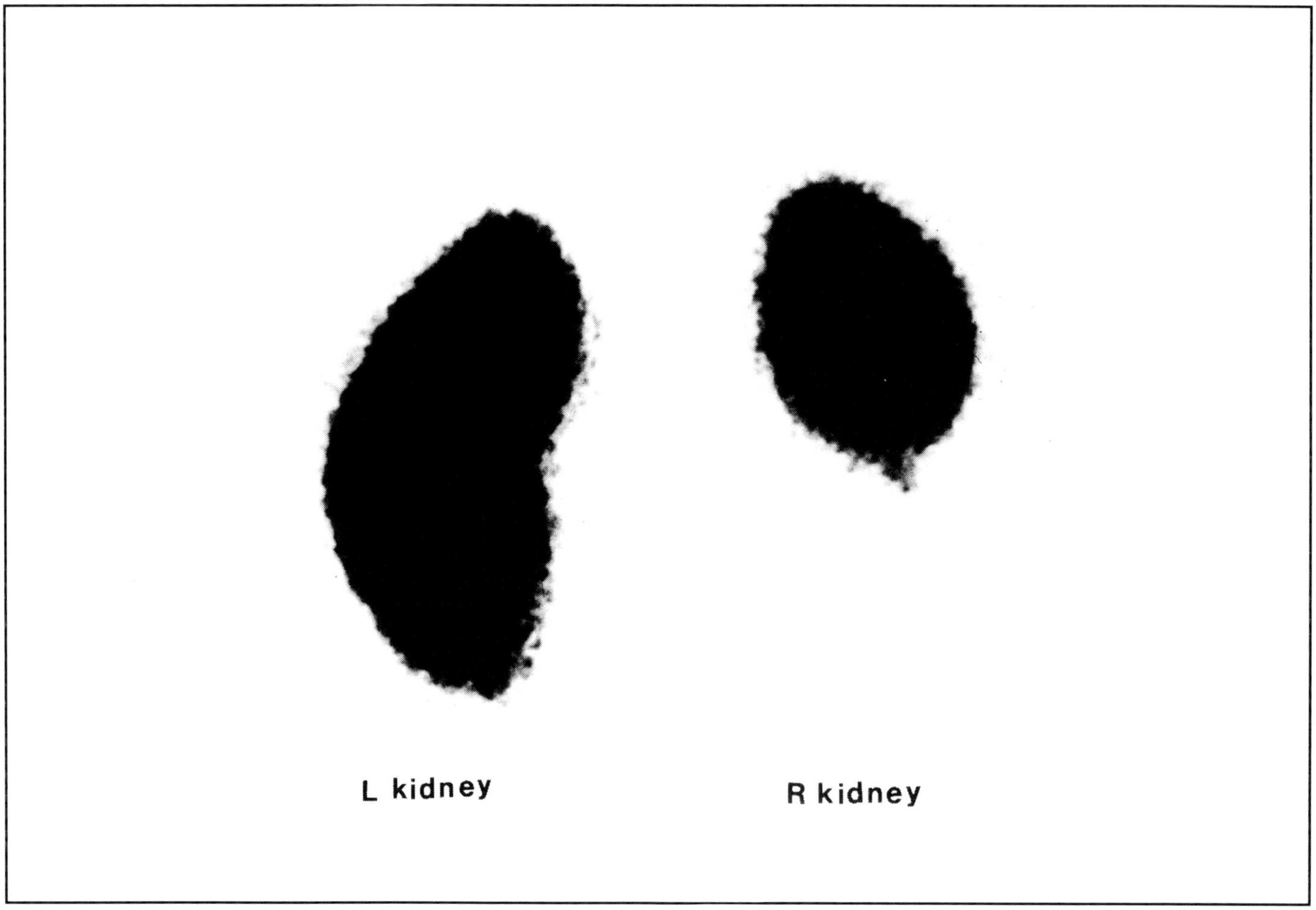

Figure 22. Posterior view of the kidneys taken 4 hrs. after injection of Tc-99m DMSA. The left kidney is normal. The right kidney shows absence of function in the lower pole as a result of trauma.

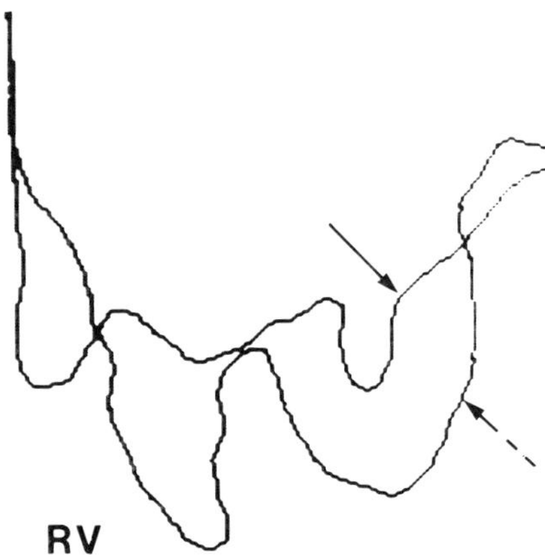

Figure 23. Cardiac gated blood pool study using Tc-99m-labelled red blood cells showing the outlines of the left ventricle at end of systole (broken arrow), and end diastole (solid arrow). Data was collected in the left anterior oblique projection and the scintigram shows normal left ventricular wall motion. The right ventricle (RV) contours are also seen.

the same or different days) using a total administered activity of up to 600 MBq Tc^{99m}MIBI over the two studies.

Tc^{99m}MIBI has also been used to assess the severity of disease in patients with peripheral vascular disease (PVD). Patients with PVD show reduced leg muscle uptake of Tc^{99m}MIBI; the more severe the PVD, the lower the muscle uptake.

21.2.11 Tumour Imaging

Many radiopharmaceuticals are taken up by a variety of tumours, and serendipity may play a role in tumour imaging, e.g. a primary bronchial carcinoma may take up Tc-99m diphosphonate and appear on a bone scan being performed for investigation of skeletal metastases. However, some radiopharmaceuticals can be used specifically to try and identify a suspected tumour.

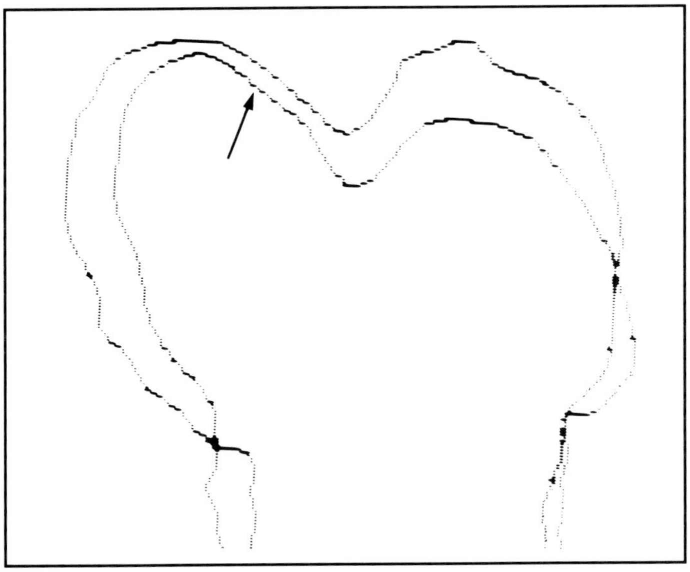

Figure 24. Cardiac gated blood pool study (exercise study) using Tc-99m-labelled red blood cells showing impaired wall motion in the septum (arrow) during systole in the LAO projection. This was caused by myocardial ischaemia due to atheroma in the left anterior descending coronary artery.

The use of I-131 for detecting thyroid metastases and the radiopharmaceuticals used for imaging adrenal tumours have been discussed above. In addition to detecting phaeochromocytoma, labelled-MIBG can also be used to detect tumours arising in other tissues derived from neural crest cells, e.g. medullary cardinoma of the thyroid neuroblastoma, carcinoid tumours, etc. The imaging protocol is similar to that for detecting phaeochromocytoma and whole body images are obtained as discussed earlier.

Gallium-67 (67-Ga) citrate is taken up nonspecifically by many primary and secondary tumours. Imaging of the area of interest takes place 48 hours after injection of 100–150 MBq 67-Ga. This radiopharmaceutical is perhaps most commonly used to detect hepatomas (primary liver tumours), but is also useful in assessing the extent of lymphomas.

A number of new radiopharmaceuticals have been used for tumour imaging, e.g. pentavalent Tc-99m dimercapto-succinic acid to detect medullary thyroid cardinoma and radio-labelled monoclonal antibodies to image ovarian and colonic tumours, and these are described elsewhere (see Chapter 8).

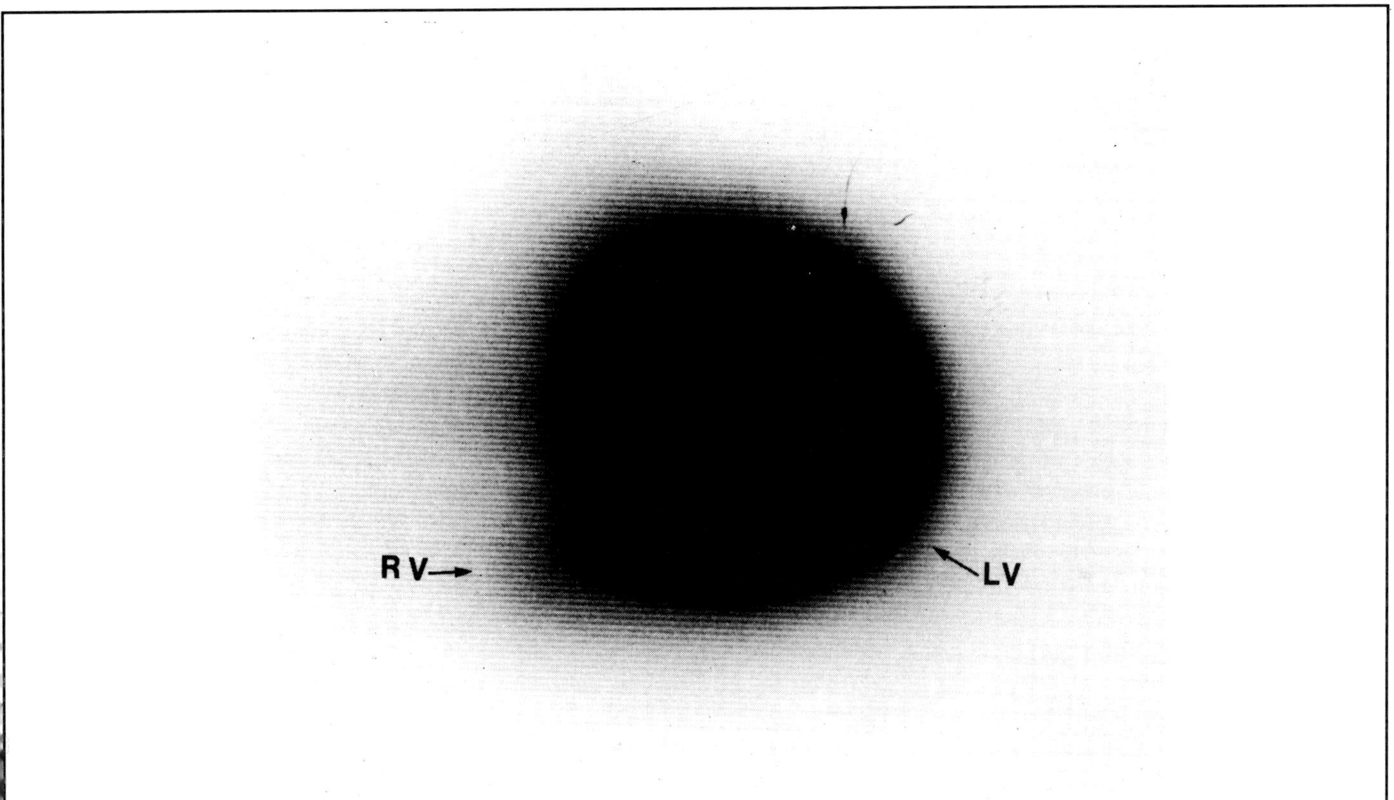

Figure 25. Normal exercise TL-201 scan of the heart in left anterior oblique (LAO) projection showing symmetrical uptake of tracer throughout the left ventricle (LV). The right ventricle (RV) is also very faintly visualised.

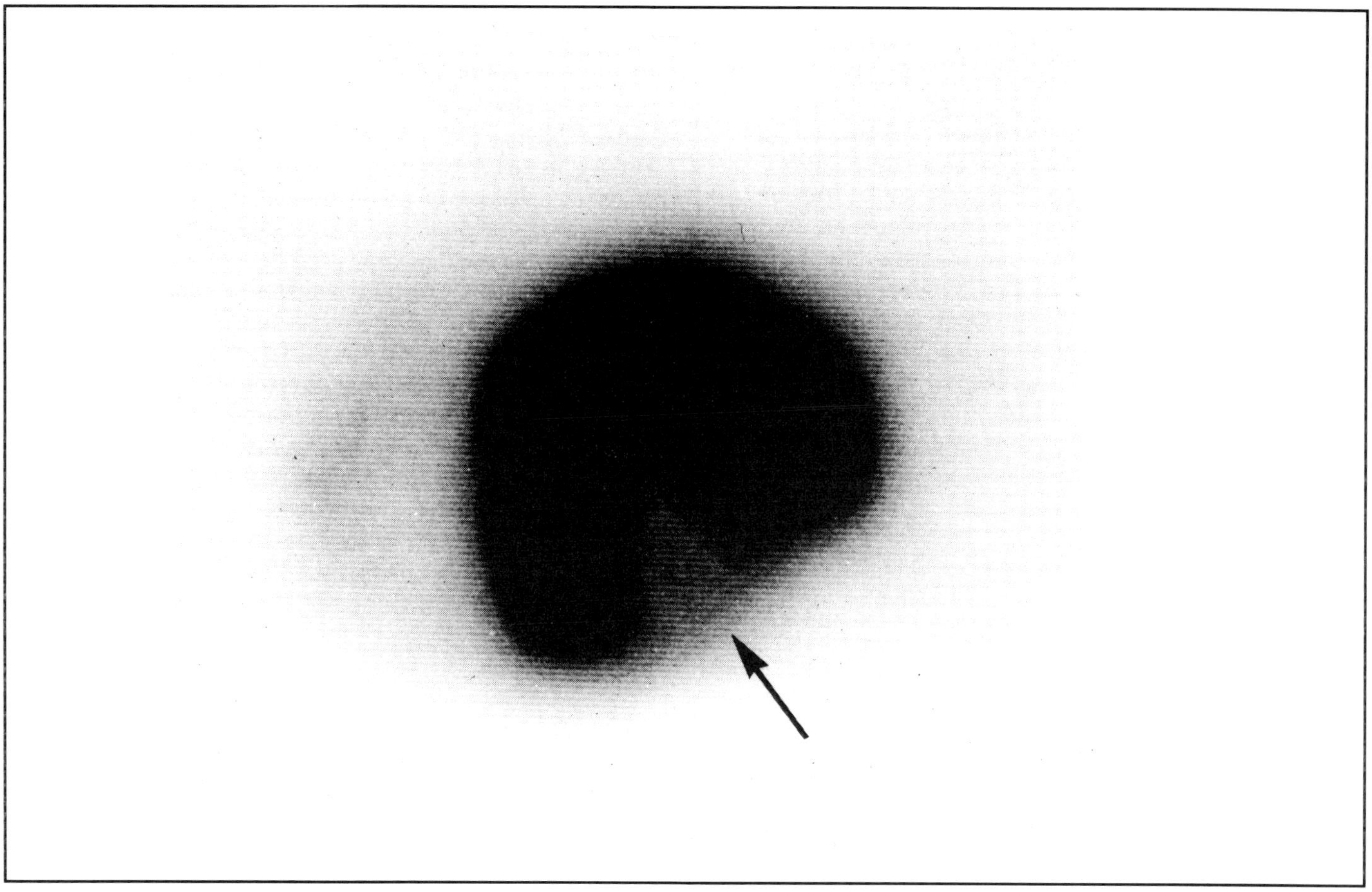

Figure 26. Exercise TL-201 scan of the heart in LAO projection showing decreased uptake in the infero apical area of the LV. This was present both on the exercise and redistribution images and was due to an old myocardial infarct.

21.2.12 Acute Gastrointestinal Blood Loss Scans

In the majority of patients admitted with a history of acute gastrointestinal bleeding, the cause of the blood loss is quickly diagnosed, e.g. by endoscopy. However, in a small percentage of patients the bleeding site may remain undetected despite extensive investigations. In this situation a nuclear medicine scan may be invaluable to localise the bleeding site.

A Tc-99m labelled red blood cell scan is the most useful test, particularly where the bleeding is thought to be intermittent. The patients's own red blood cells are labelled with 400 MBq Tc-99m (see Chapters 6 and 7). Once the labelled cells have been reinjected, frequent anterior abdominal images are taken at regular intervals to try and determine the bleeding site. Imaging can continue for up to 24 hours if necessary.

The labelled RBC are normally contained in the vascular compartment allowing visualisation of the great vessels, liver, spleen and kidneys (Fig. 25). The radiopharmaceutical is also excreted by the kidneys and appears in the bladder.

When bleeding occurs an abnormal collection Tc-99m-RBC is seen at the bleeding site (Figure 27). Frequent images are necessary to localise the exact site of blood loss as labelled RBC entering the bowel lumen will eventually pass into distal bowel loops.

21.2.13 Meckel's Scan

A Meckel's diverticulum is a small diverticulum in the terminal ileum which is present in about 2% of the population. It may contain gastric mucosa which can ulcerate and result in abdominal pain or gastrointestinal bleeding and may require surgical removal.

Tc-99m pertechnetate is taken up by normal gastric mucosa and will also accumulate in ectopic gastric mucosa in a Meckel's diverticulum. The patient is fasted overnight before the scan and is then injected intravenously with 400

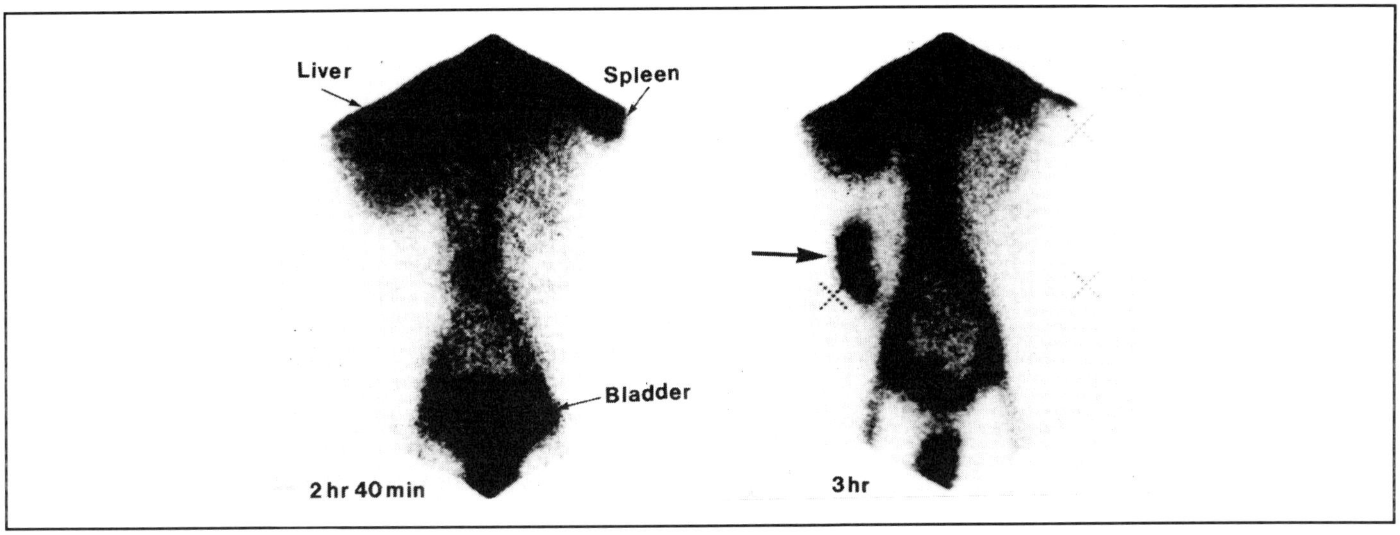

Figure 27. Anterior abdominal images 2 hrs. 40 mins., and 3 hrs. after injection of Tc-99m-labelled red blood cells. Normal image at 2 hrs. 40 mins. showing liver, spleen, great vessels (aorta and inferior vena cava) and bladder. By 3 hrs. there is also abnormal activity in the right iliac fossa due to a bleeding site in the caecum (arrow).

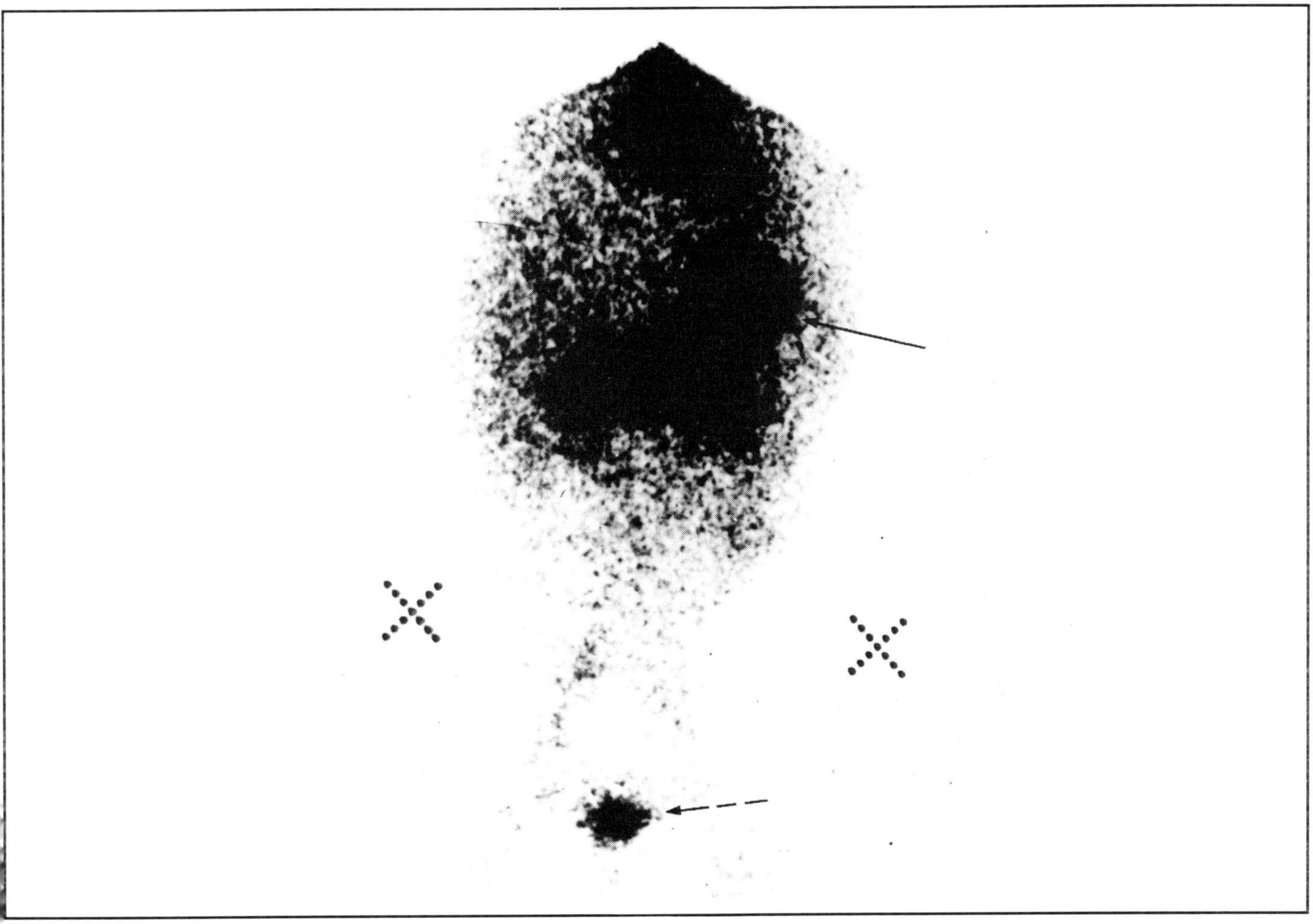

Figure 28. Anterior abdominal image 30 mins. after injection of Tc-99m pertechnetate. Note normal stomach and bladder activity. There is no evidence of an ectopic gastric mucosa. The crosses mark the (solid arrow) iliac crests (dashed arrow).

MBq Tc-99m pertechnetate. Images are then obtained at 15 min. interval for 1 hour.

In normal individuals the stomach is seen, the kidney may be visualised and activity is excreted in the urine (Figure 28). The radiopharmaceutical is also present in gastric secretions and may start to pass into proximal small bowel. A Meckel's diverticulum shows up as an abnormal focal accumulation of radiopharmaceutical which appears at the same time as the stomach (Figure 29).

In some centres patients are treated with oral cimetidine for 48 hours before a Meckel's scan to try to minimise gastric secretion of tracer and enhance uptake in the ectopic gastric mucosa.

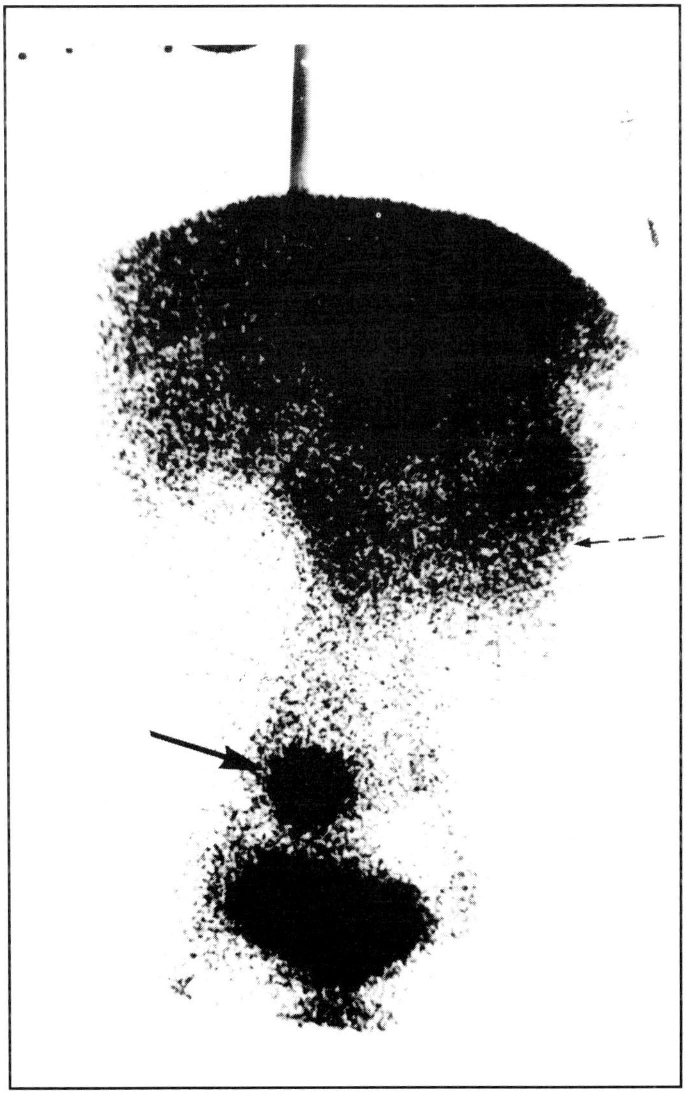

Figure 29. Anterior abdominal image 45 mins. after injection of Tc-99m pertechnetate. There is normal stomach uptake with activity passing distally into the proximal small bowel (broken arrow). Also visualised is an intense area of isotope uptake in an ectopic mucosa in a Meckel's diverticulum above the bladder (solid arrow).

21.2.14 Infection/Inflammation Imaging

Three radiopharmaceuticals are commonly used in the diagnosis of infective and inflammatory disorders; gallium-67 citrate, indium-111 leucocytes and Tc-99m HMPAO leucocytes. Labelled-WBC scans can be carried out in departments with appropriate labelling facilities. The patient's own leucocytes are labelled with up to 40 MBq of ^{111}Indium (^{111}In) or with 200 MBq Tc^{99m} hexamethylpropylene amine oxime (HMPAO) (see chapter 7 for details of cell labelling). The labelled WBC are then reinjected into the patient, and the area of interest imaged at the appropriate time. If the scan is being done to diagnose inflammatory bowel disease, e.g. ulcerative colitis or Crohn's disease, then early images (at approx. 3 hrs. with indium-WBC or ½ hr. and 2–3 hrs. with Tc^{99m}HMPAO-WBC) should be obtained (and a lower activity of indium injected). If the scan is being used to localise a site of suspected sepsis, then later images (up to 24 hrs.) are generally necessary with indium-WBC but may not be required with Tc^{99m}HMPAO-WBC.

In a normal patient indium-WBC are seen in the liver, spleen and bone marrow (figure 30) at both 3 and 24 hrs. Any abnormal area, e.g. inflamed bowel (figure 31) or localised sepsis (figure 32) will appear as an abnormal region of increased indium-WBC uptake.

If sepsis in or around the liver is suspected, a special "subtraction" scan should be obtained. In this instance the patient has a ^{99m}Tc-colloid scan performed in addition to the ^{111}In-WBC scan. Computer subtraction of the two images will then detect any hepatic abscess, as this will show positive uptake of ^{111}In-WBC, but appear as a cold defect on ^{99m}Tc-colloid scan.

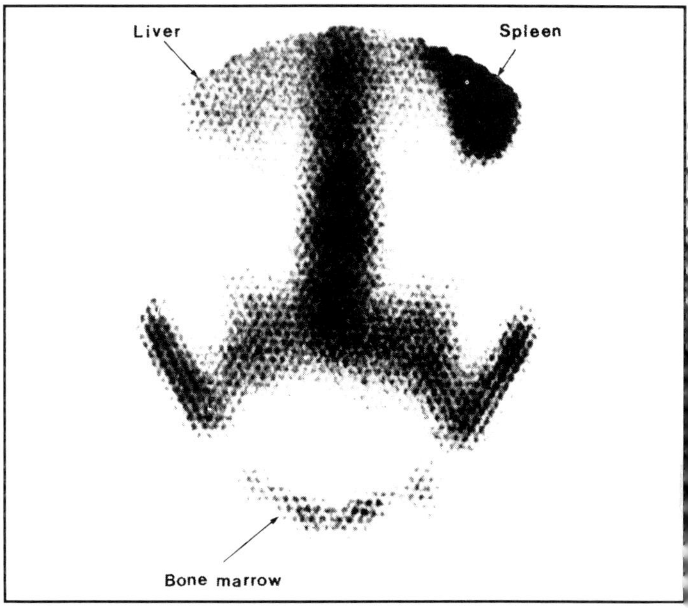

Figure 30. Anterior abdominal image 3 hrs. after injection of In-111 labelled white blood cells. Normal tracer uptake is seen in the liver, spleen and bone marrow.

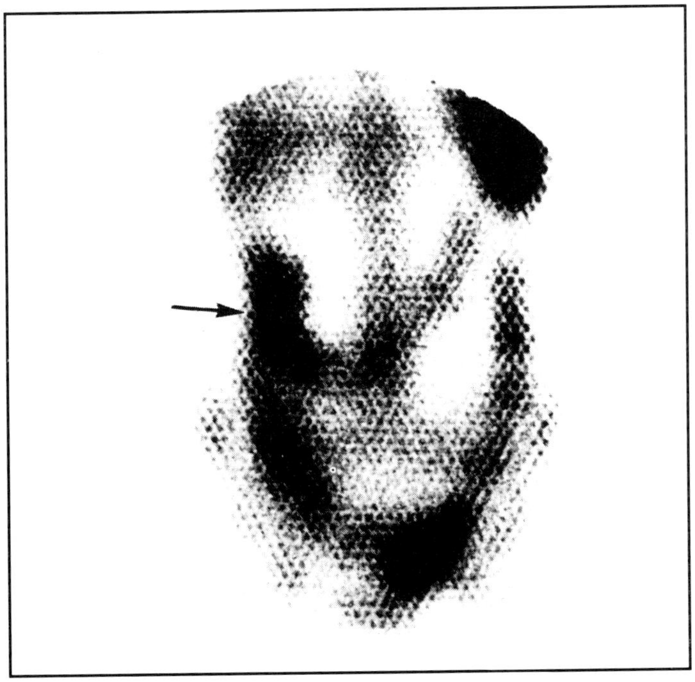

Figure 31. Anterior abdominal view 3 hrs. after injection of In-111 labelled white blood cells showing abnormal uptake throughout the whole of the inflamed colon in a patient with pancolitis (arrow).

In normal patients Tc^{99m}HMPAO-WBC are seen in liver, spleen, bone marrow, and blood pool. There is also urinary excretion of tracer and so bladder and often kidneys are visualised (figure 33a). By about 3 hrs. post-injection biliary excretion also occurs and non-specific bowel activity may therefore be seen from 3 hrs. onwards (figure 33b).

The relative advantages and disadvantages of the two different WBC labels are summarised in Tables 14 and 15.

TABLE 14
^{111}In-WBC labelling

Advantages	*Disadvantages*
Longer imaging	Increased dose
Less non-specific activity	Later imaging
Less vascular activity	Availability

TABLE 15
Tc^{99m}HMPAO labelling

Advantages	*Disadvantages*
Earlier imaging	Renal/biliary activity
Decreased dose	Vascular activity
Easy availability	Limited imaging

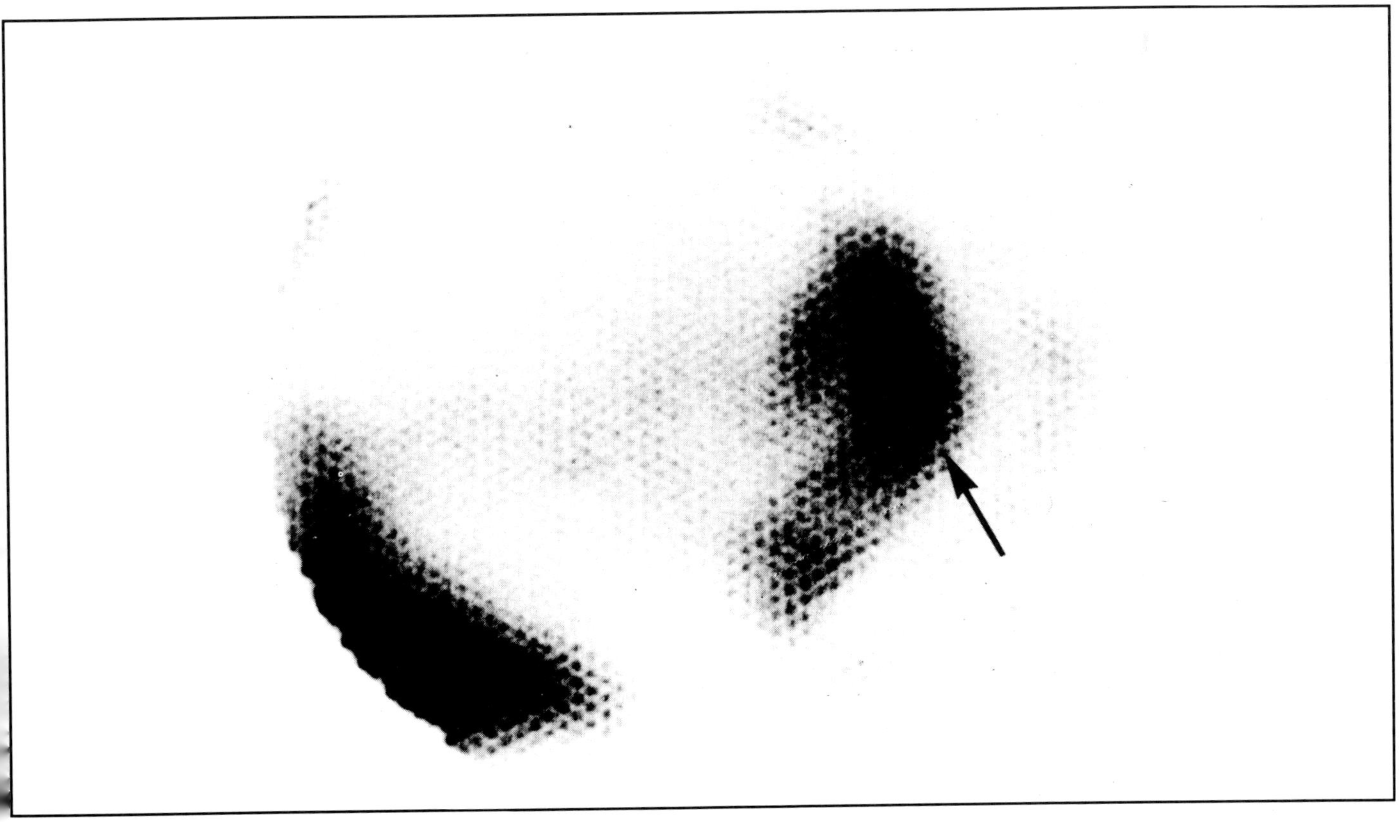

Figure 32. Anterior view of the abdomen 22 hrs. after injection of In-111 labelled white blood cells showing extensive pelvic sepsis resulting in abnormal tracer accumulation (arrow).

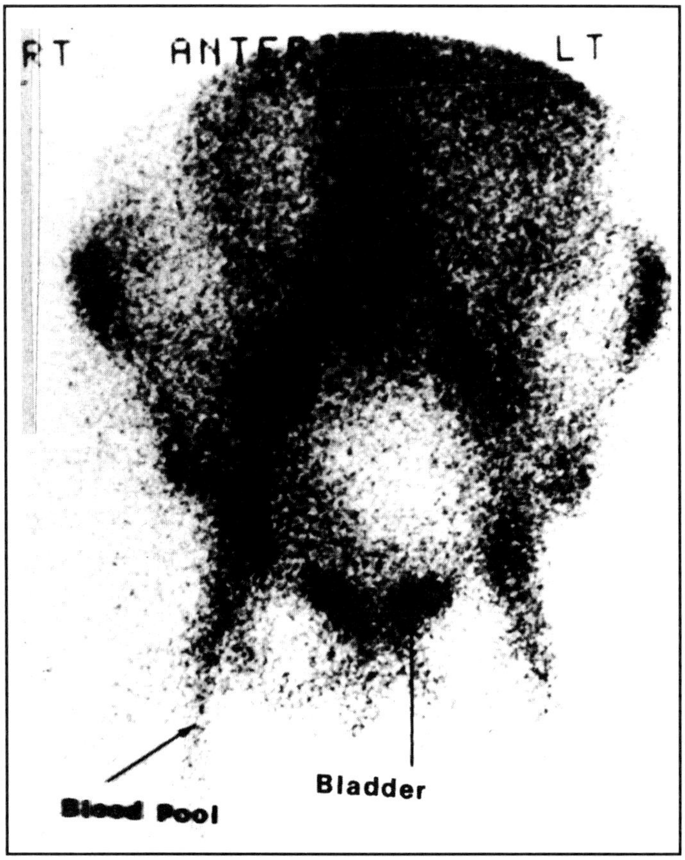

Figure 33(a). Scan of Tc-99m HMPAO leucocytes showing normal uptake in liver, spleen, bone marrow and blood pool.

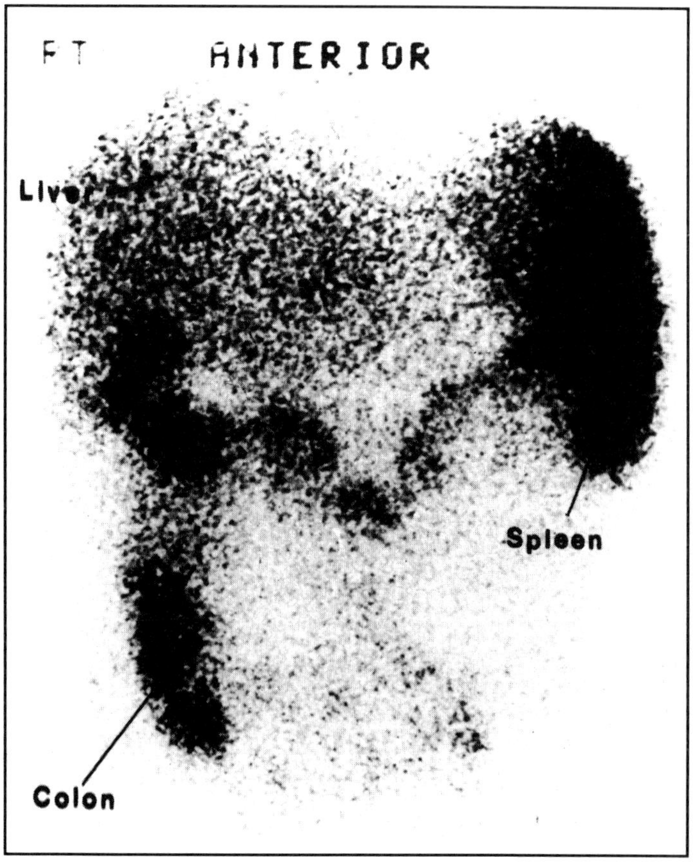

Figure 33(b). 3 hour scan of Tc-99m HMPAO leucocytes showing liver, spleen, and non-specific bowel activity.

The choice of label will depend on the clinical problem and on local expertise.

^{67}Ga citrate can be used to detect inflammatory conditions, e.g. sarcoidosis, as well as chronic sepsis (particularly around an infected joint prosthesis, figure 34) and the neoplastic conditions already discussed above. The imaging protocol is the same as for suspected neoplasms, i.e. images 48 hrs. after intravenous injection of ^{67}Ga. Unfortunately ^{67}Ga is also taken up in normal bowel which rather limits it's use for abdominal imaging.

21.3. NON-IMAGING STUDIES

Thyroid and adrenal uptake measurements and probe renography have been described above under the appropriate imaging section.

21.3.1. Vitamin B12 Absorption

Vitamin B12 is one of the many factors required for the production of normal blood cells. Deficiency of this vitamin will result in megaloblastic anaemia. Vitamin B12 is absorbed in the terminal ileum, but it can only be absorbed when it is bound to intrinsic factor, a protein secreted by the gastric parietal cells. In patients with megaloblastic anaemia it is often important to measure vitamin B12 absorption and determine whether any malabsorption of the vitamin is due to a lack of intrinsic factor.

Vitamin B12 contains cobalt and can therefore be labelled with one of the radioactive isotopes of cobalt (Co). When vitamin B12 has been absorbed from the intestine some of it will then be excreted in the urine. By administering a known amount of radioactive B12 and then measuring its urinary excretion over the next 24 hours a measurement of Vitamin B12 absorption can be made (known as the Schilling test).

It is often valuable to measure B12 absorption both with and without intrinsic factor. It is therefore usual to perform a dual isotope absorption study. Vitamin B12 is labelled with Co-58 and vitamin B12 bound to instrinsic factor (IF) labelled with Co-57. The patient attends the department after an overnight fast and receives 2 capsules containing the above radiopharmaceuticals (0.04 MBq of the appropriate isotope in each capsule) and continues fasting for a further 2 hours. They are also given an intramuscular injection of non-

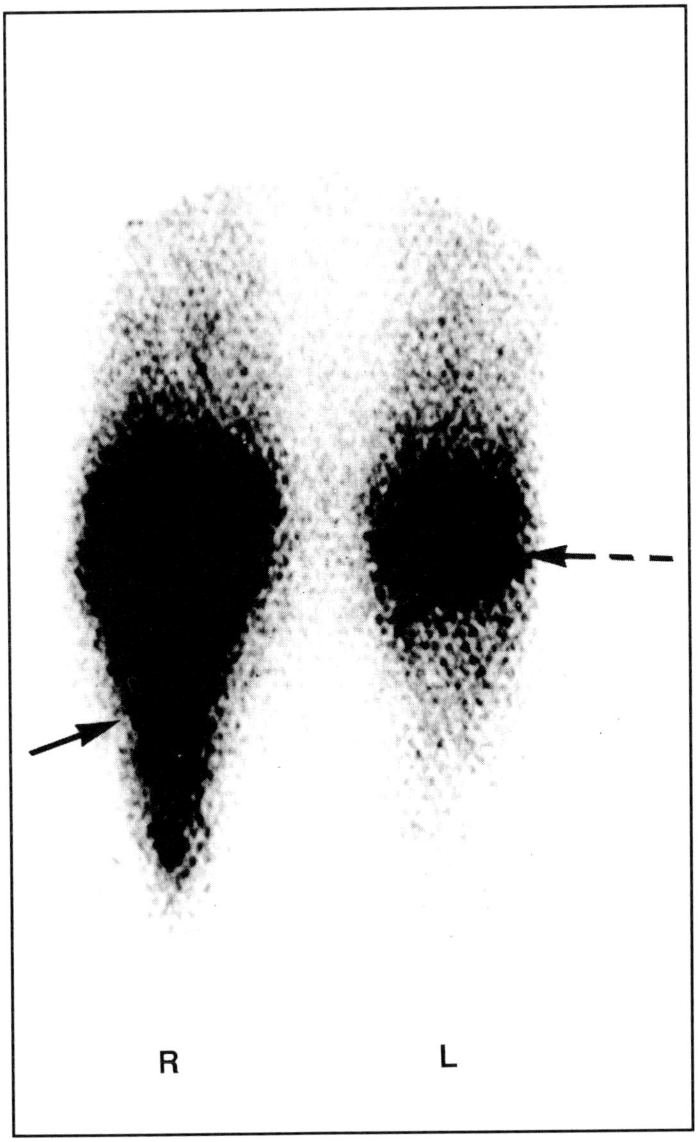

Figure 34. Anterior image of the knees 48 hrs. after injection of Ga-67 (broken arrow) and abnormal uptake around an infected tibial component of a right knee replacement (solid arrow).

radioactive vitamin B12 to ensure urinary excretion of some of the radio-labelled B12. The patient is then asked to collect all the urine for 24 hours (or for 48 hours if they have renal impairment) and the amount of each isotope in the urine is calculated as a percentage of the ingested activity.

In patients with pernicious anaemia (in which there is a lack of intrinsic factor) the absorption, and consequently excretion, of B12 which is not bound to intrinsic factor (i.e. Co-58 B12) is low, but that of B12 bound to intrinsic factor (i.e. Co-57 B12) is usually normal. If there is malabsorption of vitamin B12 due to other pathology diseases of the terminal ileum (Crohn's disease, etc.), then urinary excretion of both Co-57 and Co-58 will be low.

An alternative approach to measurement of vitamin B12 absorption is to measure the amount of radio-labelled vitamin B12 retained in the body 3 days after ingestion of the radiopharmaceutical. This requires a whole body counter and is therefore less widely used than the Schilling test.

21.3.2 Bile Salt Absorption Test

Bile salts are important in the emulsification and absorption of fats. They are synthesised and conjugated in the liver and are then excreted in the bile, via the gallbladder into the deodenum. Under normal circumstances they are largely reabsorbed from the terminal ileum and are then extracted from the portal blood by the liver and recirculated into the bowel; this is known as the entero-hepatic circulation. Measurement of bile salt absorption can thus provide information about the entero-hepatic circulation, particularly ileal function. Malabsorption of bile salts causes diarrhoea as bile salts are colonic irritants.

To measure bile salt absorption the patient takes an oral preparation of a synthetic bile salt, the taurine conjugate of homocholic acid labelled with selenium-75 (75-SeHCAT). This is taken as a capsule containing 0.04 MBq of the radiopharmaceutical (this radiopharmaceutical is not included in the current ARSAC list).

The patient is then counted in a whole body counter immediately after taking the capsule and 7 djays later. The percentage of retained bile salt can then be calculated. Patients with diseases of the terminal ileum, e.g. Crohn's disease, will have a low retention of SeHCAT-75 as the bile salt is malabsorbed and is excreted in the faeces instead of being recirculated.

21.3.3 Bile Acid Breath Test

Small intestinal bacterial overgrowth may occur in a variety of clinical conditions, e.g. blind loop syndrome, and small intestinal diverticulosis, and can result in many different symptoms such as diarrhoea, malabsorption, etc. Bacterial overgrowth will result in the deconjugation of bile salts, and this can be measured by performing a bile acid breath test.

The patient fasts overnight before the test and then receives an oral dose of 0.4 MBq Carbon-14 (C-14)-glycocholic acid, followed by an oral test meal to stimulate bile secretion. The C-14-glycocholic acid is deconjugated if there is bacterial overgrowth, and the C-14 is absorbed from the intestine and exhaled as C-14 carbon dioxide (CO_2-14). The patient is therefore asked to blow into a tube containing a material which absorbs CO_2 at hourly intervals for 4 hours. The amount of CO_2-14 exhaled can then be measured by counting the tubes in a scintillation counter. The patient rests during the study and is allowed to drink fluids once the test is under way.

Under normal circumstances very little CO_2-14 is exhaled, but if bacterial overgrowth is present in the small intestine, the amount of exhaled CO_2-14 is increased.

21.3.4 Red Cell Volume Measurement

Red cell volume measurements are of value in the diagnosis of polycythaemia. Measurement of red cell volume depends on the dilution principle. A known volume of the patient's red blood cells are labelled usually with Chromium-51 (Cr-51) or occasionally with Tc-99m (see chapter 12 for details of cell labelling). The labelled RBC are then reinjected into the patient (see Table 16 for administered activity) and the labelled-RBC allowed to mix with the circulating blood. It is important that the volume and activity of the injected cells are accurately recorded (a standard is also prepared from the labelled-RBC). A blood sample is then taken from the patient 10–60 minutes later (a later sample is occasionally necessary in patients with marked splenomegaly or congestive cardiac failure to ensure adequate mixing). The red cell volume can then be calculated from the relationship between the administered activity to the specific activity of the blood sample. The activities of the standard and the blood sample are measured in a scintillation counter. The red cell volume is expressed as mls/kg (with reference to the patient's ideal weight).

TABLE 16
Radiopharmaceuticals Used to Determine Red Cell Volume

Radiopharmaceutical	*Activity*
Cr-51 labelled red blood cells	0.8 MBq
Tc-99m labelled red blood cells	2 MBq

The red cell volume is increased in patients with polycythaemia and decreased in those with anaemia.

21.3.5 Plasma Volume Measurement

Measurement of red cell volume is often combined with measurement of plasma volume. This again depends on the dilution principle. The patient is injected with a known volume and activity (0.2 MBq) of 125-I labelled albumin. Blood samples are taken at 10, 20, and 30 minutes. Several samples are taken to allow a correction to be made for slow clearance of albumin from the plasma. The plasma volume is then calculated in a similar manner to red cell volume and is again expressed as mls/kg (with reference to the patient's weight).

Measurements of the plasma volume helps to differentiate those patients with true polycythaemia from those with apparent polycythaemia due to contraction of the plasma volume.

21.3.6 Measurement of Glomerular Filtration Rate (GFR)

The degree of renal impairment in patients with renal disease can be determined by measuring GRF. This is usually done by measuring creatinine clearance (over a 24 hour period) which relies on an accurate and complete urine collection. This is impracticable in some patients and an alternative approach is to measure the clearance of radiolabelled ethylene diamine tetra acetic acid (EDTA). EDTA is distributed in the plasma and extra-cellular fluid and is cleared from there by glomerular filtration in the kidneys. The patient is injected with a known volume and activity (3 MBq) of Chromium-51—EDTA and blood samples taken 2, 3 and 4 hours later. The blood samples and a standard of the injected material are counted in a scintillation counter. The rate of clearance of the radiopharmaceutical from the blood provides a measurement of GFR. This simple test can be repeated as necessary to monitor the patient's renal function.

21.3.7 Measurement of Gastrointestinal Blood Loss

Iron deficiency anaemia is a relatively common condition. It may be caused by chronic gastrointestinal (GI) bleeding (e.g. from a peptic ulcer, colonic neoplasm, etc.). If the bleeding is very slow, the patient may be unaware of it and it may occasionally be necessary to quantify the GI blood loss to determine whether this is the cause of the patient's anaemia. This can be done by labelling some of the patient's red blood cells with 4 MBq chromium-51 (see Chapters 6 and 7) and measuring the excretion of the Cr-51-RBC in the stools.

The labelled RBC are then reinjected into the patient and a blood sample taken 15 minutes and 7 days later. The patient is asked to collect their stools for 7 days. The amount of GI blood loss can then be calculated by counting the stool and blood samples and a standard of the labelled-RBC in a scintillation counter.

This test will measure the amount of gastrointestinal blood loss in mls per day, but will not determine the site of the blood loss as the administered activity is too low to allow images to be obtained.

21.4 CONCLUSION

This chapter has, hopefully, demonstrated the scope of nuclear medicine investigations, and the wide variety of clinical situations where such techniques may be of value. It is, of necessity, a brief introduction to clinical nuclear medicine rather than a comprehensive review of the topic. Those interested in finding out more about the investigations already described and learning about those which have not been mentioned are referred to the list below for further reading.

REFERENCES

Notes for guidance on the administration of radioactive substances to persons for purposes of diagnosis, treatment or research. Administration of Radioactive Substances Advisory Committee (ARSAC) (July 1988)

FURTHER READING

Essentials of Nuclear Medicine—M.V. Merrick Churchill Livingson, Edinburgh. (1984)

Clinical Nuclear Medicine Ed. M.N. Maisey, K.E. Britton, D.L. Gilday—Chapman and Hall, London. (1983)

Nuclear Medicine; a clinical introduction. M. Maisey—Update Books. London (1980)

Freeman and Johnson's Clinical Radionuclide Imaging, Ed. L.M. Freeman-Grune and Stratton Inc. Orlando. (1984)

Seminars in Nuclear Medicine Vols. 1–18, (1971–1988).

Chapter 22

Therapeutic Applications of Radiopharmaceuticals

D.T. Murray and T.E. Hilditch

22.1 INTRODUCTION

The use of radiopharmaceuticals to deliver therapeutic doses of ionising radiation to disease sites in the body dates back more than half a century. A variety of radionuclides have been exploited for their therapeutic potential (Table 1). Therapies such as ^{131}I-sodium iodide for the treatment of thyroid disorders and ^{32}P-sodium phosphate for myeloproliferative disease are well established. Other therapeutic radiopharmaceuticals have been introduced over this same period but it is only in the last decade that several more have found a place in routine therapy. Falling into this latter category are ^{131}I-metaiodo-benzylguanidine (MIBG) for treatment of neuroendocrine tumours and ^{89}Sr-chloride for pain control in bone metastases, an application which was first recognised some fifty years ago, but was largely overlooked until recently.

Although conventional radiotherapy plays a vital role in the treatment of cancer, it has no direct effect on occult secondary tumours outwith the treated area. In contrast, systemic administration of a radiopharmaceutical, which is designed to be taken up selectively by diseased tissue, offers the opportunity of treating widely disseminated disease, the object being to irradiate the diseased sites but at the same time spare normal tissue.

During the last decade there has been renewed interest in therapeutic application of radiopharmaceuticals, mainly due to the development of a range of new carrier molecules which can target radionuclides more selectively to the disease site and also due to wider availability of radionuclides with desired physical properties. There is every indication that in the future more extensive use will be made of therapeutic radiopharmaceuticals, perhaps realising more of the early hopes for this form of treatment.

22.2 FACTORS DETERMINING THE EFFECTIVENESS OF RADIONUCLIDE THERAPY

Several factors have a bearing on the effectiveness of radionuclide therapy, not the least of which is delivery of the radionuclide to the site of disease (the target) whilst minimising its concentration in normal tissue. It is important that once in the target, the emissions from the decay of the radionuclide irradiate only tissues within the target area. For example gamma radiation is undesirable since it contributes little to therapeutic effectiveness but augments the irradiation of non-target tissues. The emissions from some radionuclides are better for treating bulk disease, but other radionuclides are more effective for the treatment of small volume disease (e.g. micrometastases), because of the very short range of the radiation. An important factor is the relative sensitivity of the target to the low dose rate delivered by radionuclide therapy, as against the high dose rate irradiation of conventional radiotherapy.

22.1.1 Choice of Radiopharmaceutical

The ideal physical and biological properties of a radiopharmaceutical intended for therapy should be such that a large absorbed dose of radiation is received by the tumour, or diseased tissue, with minimal dose to normal tissues. This requires the use of an appropriate radionuclide, administered in a chemical form, and by a route of administration, which will allow selective uptake in target tissue in sufficient concentration to elicit a therapeutic response.

22.2.1.1 Choice of radionuclide

Ideal radionuclides for therapy are those with an abundance of non-penetrating radiations (charged particles) and lack of penetrating radiations (gamma or X-rays). When these radionuclides are taken up selectively by the target, their energy is deposited within a relatively small volume, determined by the range of the particles emitted, while surrounding normal tissue is spared. Different types of particle have different ranges, different levels of linear energy transfer (LET) and relative biological effectiveness (RBE). The type of particle emission required for specific applications will depend on the microdistribution of the radionuclide within the target sites. Although any gamma-ray emissions present will add to irradiation of non-target tissues, a small amount in the energy range 100–200 keV is useful for scintigraphic imaging, thus allowing the distribution of radionuclide in target and non-target areas to be visualised. A tracer amount of the radiopharmaceutical can be used therefore to obtain kinetic and dosimetric information prior to therapy.

Radionuclides which are considered suitable for therapy may be divided into three categories, i.e. beta-particle emitters, alpha particle emitters, and Auger and Coster-Kronig electron emitters. The physical characteristics of the most commonly used therapeutic radionuclides, along with others whose use is in various stages of development, are listed in Table 1. Most of the radionuclides in routine use are beta emitters. Beta particles are of low LET and their RBE is unity. The path length is quite variable, ranging from 1.0 mm for the beta particles of ^{169}Er, to 12.0 mm for those of ^{90}Y. Nevertheless, the range of beta particles is considerably greater than the diameter of a typical cell (5–20 μm), and thus the whole cell and surrounding cells are irradiated. Beta particles are not necessarily optimal for the treatment of microscopic disease (< 1.0 mm diameter). In this case alpha particles with their high LET and high RBE are theoretically more effective, their high LET limiting the ability of cells to repair damage.

Alpha particles deposit their energy over short distances (range 40–80 μm for 5–8 MeV particles), and relatively few alpha particles compared to beta particles are required for cell inactivation. Very little of the emitted energy will escape from microscopic disease containing an alpha emitting radionuclide. On the other hand, a disadvantage of alpha emitters is that they require to be taken up by most of the cancer cells in a tumour, or by their near neighbours, for the whole tumour to be irradiated. The application of alpha emitters in clinical radionuclide therapy is still at the experimental stage and it may be that the additional precautions for safe handling and for administration to patients will impede progress. Auger electrons have a shorter range than alpha particles (the dominant Auger electrons from ^{125}I have a range of 10nm) and, if the radionuclide is incorporated within the cell nucleus, most of the energy will be deposited therein, thus destroying cellular DNA. In this case their toxicity is similar to that of high LET alpha particles. The cytotoxicity of an Auger electron emitter will be much less if the radionuclide is attached only to the surface of the target cell or is present within the cytoplasm. Therapeutic radiopharmaceuticals based on Auger-emitters require incorporation of the radionuclide into the entire tumour cell population. Thus methods of selective guidance to target cells and subsequent introduction of these radionuclides into the cell nuclei require to be developed. Whilst ^{125}I has been used in radionuclide therapy, further exploratory work will be required before Auger emitters become more widely used.

The time course of irradiation of a target is related to both physical half-life and biological turnover. In selecting an appropriate radionuclide, consideration must be given to the rate of localisation and the turnover of the radiopharmaceutical in the target tissue relative to its residence time in normal tissue. If the radiopharmaceutical localises slowly in the tumour but the half-life of the radionuclide is short, most of the radionuclide will have decayed by the time it reaches its target, thus delivering the majority of the dose to non-target organs. If on the other hand, the half-life of the radionuclide is long and the radiopharmaceutical is metabolised rapidly in the target, this could also lead to less than optimal target to non-target absorbed dose ratio. A further consideration, from the point of view of clinical applicability, is that the half-life of the radionuclide should be sufficiently long to make supply and use of it a practical proposition.

The chemical nature of the radionuclide dictates the types of carrier molecule to which it may be attached. In developing successful therapeutic agents, methods of attaching radionuclides to tumour specific agents need to be explored. The formed complex requires to be stable and retain receptor specificity. When the complex is eventually metabolised, the sites and rates of any redistribution of radioactivity will depend on the chemical nature of the radionuclide, if it becomes completely dissociated from the complex.

22.2.1.2. Pharmaceutical and physiological factors

Factors which influence localisation of radioactivity in tissues include the chemical and physical nature of the radiopharmaceutical and the route of its administration. Many normal physiological processes will also affect the biodistribution and clearance of the radiopharmaceutical, as may any underlying pathology or concomitant drug use. Following systemic administration of a radiopharmaceutical, the resulting biodistribution in the patient is determined by a number of factors, including the degree to which the substance is diluted in the body and transported into cells, the location and blood supply to cells that have an affinity for the substance and the manner in which the substance is metabolised and eliminated from the body. Several methods which circumvent a number of these physiological

TABLE 1
Radionuclides Used in Therapy

Radionuclide	*Half-life*	*$E_\beta$max (MeV)*	*Max Range*
^{90}Y (beta)	2.67d	2.28	12.0mm
^{188}Re ,,	17.00h	2.11	10.8mm
^{32}P ,,	14.30d	1.71	8.7mm
^{89}Sr ,,	50.50d	1.49	8.0mm
^{165}Dy ,,	2.33h	1.29	6.4mm
^{186}Re ,,	3.77d	1.08	5.0mm
^{198}Au ,,	2.70d	0.96	4.4mm
^{153} ,,	1.95d	0.81	3.0mm
^{131}I ,,	8.04d	0.61	2.4mm
^{169}Er ,,	9.40d	0.34	1.0mm
^{125}I (Auger)	60.30d	0.40 (keV)*	10.0nm
		*$E\alpha$ mean (MeV)***	
^{212}Bi (alpha)	1.00h	7.8	70.0μm
^{211}At ,,	7.20h	6.8	65.μm

d = days h = hours
*most abundant Auger electron
**mean of parent and daughter alpha particles
(adapted from Hoefnagel (1991)).

processes have been proposed to produce better targeting and hence higher radiation doses to the target tissue. These include intra-arterial and intra-cavitary administration, as well as direct injection of radiopharmaceuticals into solid tumours (Bierwaltes *et al.,* 1985).

Radiopharmaceuticals exhibit a variety of chemical and physical properties and several different mechanisms are exploited for localisation in target tissues. It is possible to incorporate radionuclides into the DNA of the cell nucleus, as is the case with radiolabelled nucleotides. Some radiopharmaceuticals gain intracellular entry via specific metabolic pathways while others can target intracellular receptors. Agents such as radiolabelled antibodies and somatostatin analogues attach themselves to the tumour cell surface by extracellular receptor mechanisms. Other therapeutic agents are brought into the close vicinity of target cells by exploiting natural processes (e.g. irradiation of thyroid cells by radioiodine stored in intrafollicular colloid), while others achieve this by local or regional administration into arteries or cavities.

The distribution of the radiopharmaceuticals can be altered by the concomitant use of drugs. Some drugs with known effects on biodistribution are used deliberately to enhance the uptake of radiopharmaceuticals in target tissue, such as the use of nifedipine to enhance uptake of ^{131}I-MIBG (Blake *et al.,* 1988). Other drugs, including non-prescription products can adversely affect radiopharmaceutical uptake. In these situations it is necessary to discontinue the use of such preparations prior to therapy (Solanki *et al.,* 1992).

22.2.2 Radiosensitivity of Diseased and Normal Tissue

Diseased tissues differ greatly in their response to external beam irradiation and this is probably also true of radionuclide therapy. Radiotherapy achieves its principal effects on both tumours and normal tissues by sterilisation of proliferating cells. This is thought to result from damage to cellular DNA caused by ionising radiation, especially the production of double strand breaks.

22.2.2.1 Diseased tissues

The biological mechanisms underlying individual tumour response are complex and not fully understood. However, some of the most important factors may be intrinsic cellular radiosensitivity, cellular repair, repopulation kinetics and tumour hypoxia (Hall, 1988). There are marked differences in the radiosensitivities of cells from particular tumour types; cells from neuroblastoma and lymphoma are characteristically sensitive, cells from melanoma and from brain tumours such as gliomas are more resistant. The molecular basis of these differences is not understood. Cells also differ in their ability to repair sub-lethal DNA damage caused by radiation. These differences exist for external beam irradiation, but may be even more important for radionuclide therapy, for which the dose rate is usually low, providing opportunities for cellular repair. Repopulation of the tumour during therapy by cells that have survived undamaged may be an important mechanism in external beam irradiation, for which a course of therapy typically lasts several weeks. The time-scale of treatment in radionuclide therapy depends both on the radionuclide half-life and on the kinetics of clearance of the radiopharmaceuticals. However, most of the dose will usually be delivered over a few days rather than a few weeks. This provides less opportunity for cellular repopulation during therapy, so this factor will probably be less important for radionuclide therapy than for external beam irradiation.

The importance of hypoxia in radiobiology has been known for many years. Irradiated cells not only experience DNA damage from direct ionisation but also from the action of free radicals which are produced by ionising events close to DNA. Oxygen acts to "fix" radical damage to DNA, so hypoxic conditions are radioprotective. An important variable in this is the rate of reoxygenation during therapy. Cells that were formerly hypoxic may become oxic once more, as the tumour shrinks during therapy, so making the treatment more effective. Reoxygenation takes time and the short time scale of radionuclide therapy could mean that hypoxia is more of a problem for this modality. In that case, it is possible that the efficiency of radionuclide therapy could be improved by administration of hypoxic cell radiosensitisers or the newer bioreductive agents which are selective in the killing of hypoxic cells (Workman, 1992).

22.2.2.2 Normal tissues

In radiotherapy, the principal adverse effects, i.e. those which limit the treatment which can be given, are due to functional impairment of normal tissues. This largely results from radiation sterilisation of dividing cells in the tissue. It is the inability of radiation sterilised stem cells to provide replacements for differentiated cells, that are lost by natural processes, which underlies most clinical radiation syndromes. From this, it is apparent that the time from irradiation to the observation of functional impairment is largely governed by the kinetics of cell renewal in the tissue. For the epithelium of the gastrointestinal tract, for example, which normally has a high rate of cell loss and a need for rapid renewal, irradiation results in clinical symptoms within only a few days. For the epithelium of the skin and the blood forming tissues of the bone marrow, it usually takes a few weeks for radiation effects to be expressed in the form of functional impairment.

Some tissues however, have very low rates of cell loss and therefore a long latency period (months or years) can elapse between irradiation and the appearance of overt tissue damage. This is true of the brain and spinal cord and the vascular endothelium which makes up blood vessels. It is important that rapidity of appearance of symptoms should not be confused with the radiosensitivity of a tissue, i.e. what dose it may tolerate without experiencing irreversible injury. The central nervous system, for example, is a "late-responding" organ system which typically takes many months for serious radiation injuries to appear. It is, however, quite radiosensitive, and must be protected from receiving high doses of radiation, which could be tolerated by some other organs (e.g. skin) which nevertheless express their injury more quickly.

The tissues likely to be injured by radiopharmaceutical therapy depend on the distribution and pharmacokinetics of the radionuclide as well as the tissue radiosensitivity. In most clinical experience to date, it has been the haemopoietic bone marrow which has been most affected by radionuclide therapy, for example, in ^{131}I-MIBG treatment of neuroendocrine tumours (Fielding *et al.,* 1991). Bone marrow depression occurs at whole body doses of greater than 2–3Gy and this is usually the treatment limiting consideration. In certain cases, it is possible this restriction could be overcome by use of bone marrow transplantation or administration of haemopoietic growth factors. Apart from marrow, appreciable radiation doses may be delivered to the liver as a result of free or bound radionuclide being sequestered there, or to the urinary bladder for radiopharmaceuticals that are excreted via the kidneys. The tolerance doses in these cases are, however, likely to be greater than 20Gy (Wheldon and O'Donoghue, 1990; Fielding *et al.,* 1991). Whilst doses of this magnitude to organs such as the liver and urinary bladder are not normally exceeded with the activities of radionuclide administered at present, the situation would change if methods of overcoming bone marrow depression were introduced.

22.3 CLINICAL APPLICATIONS

Many different radiopharmaceuticals have been applied clinically in the treatment of various malignant and benign conditions over the past 50 years. However, a considerable number of the reported applications have been of an exploratory nature on a small number of patients and relatively few radiopharmaceuticals have been evaluated adequately. The net result is that only a small number of radiopharmaceuticals have been developed on a commercial basis and have become established as routine therapeutic agents. Falling into this category are ^{131}I-iodide for thyroid disorders, ^{32}P-phosphate for blood disorders, ^{89}Sr-chloride for pain control in metastatic bone disease, ^{131}I-MIBG for neuroendocrine tumours and ^{90}Y or ^{32}P-colloids for intracavitary therapy (which have replaced the formerly used ^{198}Au-colloid). These and other reported radiopharmaceuticals are considered here.

Several of the treatments can be given on an out-patient basis but precautions must be taken to minimise exposure of personnel coming in contact with the patient. Other treatments fall into the category of high activity therapy, for which the patient requires to be hospitalised. A special treatment facility for exclusive use of the patient is required and staff instructed accordingly about necessary precautions, with the added complication that very young children are sometimes treated with therapeutic radiopharmaceuticals. Adequate measures must be in place to prevent radioactive contamination and to dispose of radioactive waste. For full details of the radiological protection measures to be taken, reference should be made to the relevant guidance documents; in the UK these are produced by the National Radiological Protection Board (NRPB, 1988).

2.3.1 Radioiodine Treatment of Hyperthyroidism

Dietary iodine is an essential requirement for the synthesis of thyroid hormones and as a consequence, a large proportion of the body's iodine is concentrated in the thyroid gland. Since the turnover of this iodine is slow compared to iodine in the blood and other parts of the body, administration of radioactive iodine (^{131}I) results in highly selective irradiation of the thyroid gland. Although most of the intra-thyroidal iodine is stored within the colloid of the thyroid follicles, the range of the beta emission from ^{131}I (Table 1) is such that the follicular cells surrounding the colloid are irradiated. Therefore administration of an appropriate quantity of the radionuclide inhibits the function of the gland, as is required for the treatment of hyperthyroidism.

Iodine-131 is used extensively throughout the world for the treatment of hyperthyroidism, being first used for this purpose in the 1940's. Upon oral administration of the radionuclide approximately 60% of the radioactivity is taken up by the overactive gland. In some countries, particularly the USA, it is the treatment of choice for most patients (Farrar and Toft, 1991). The principal disadvantage of radioiodine therapy is the high incidence of early (within the first year) and late hypothyroidism,making it necessary to monitor patients adequately after treatment. Although there is a theoretical possibility of radiation induced cancer or genetic defects there is no substantial evidence to support this on the basis of several large follow-up studies conducted over the past 20 years or so (Holm *et al.,* 1991; Farrar and Toft 1991; Reiners, 1990). As a consequence, treatment is no longer restricted to older patients, with adolescents, and even children, now being treated with radioiodine (Hamburger, 1985).

Pregnancy is an absolute contra-indication, since radioiodine passes across the placental barrier, and so in treating women of child-bearing age, the clinician must ensure that the patient is not pregnant. Furthermore because of the slow turnover of radioiodine, pregnancy should be avoided within the first 4 months after therapy. Radioiodine is excreted in the maternal milk and thus breast-feeding must be discontinued before radioiodine is given. Uptake of radioiodine into the gland will be inhibited if the patient has recently received large quantities of stable iodine, e.g. as in radiological contrast media.

22.3.1.1 Dosage of ^{131}I-iodide

With regard to the dosage of ^{131}I there is wide variation in current practice (Clarke, 1991), but in the UK the limit for out-patient treatment is 800 MBq (NRPB, 1988) and therefore doses are usually kept below that value. It is usual to render the patient euthyroid with antithyroid drug therapy before radioiodine treatment. In some centres ablative doses, 550 MBq upwards, are advocated as a method of achieving early remission of the disease, linked to effective follow-up to ensure adequate supervision and treatment of the resultant hypothyroidism. Another approach is to give smaller doses, repeated if necessary, with the object of rendering as many patients as possible euthyroid. Some endocrinologists adopt a more rigorous approach with the object of achieving a specific concentration of ^{131}I in the gland or specific radiation dose to the gland. However this requires estimation of gland weight in addition to measurement of ^{131}I uptake (and effective half-life in the gland) using a pre-treatment tracer dose. There is reason for believing that patients with large goitres and severe disease tend to require greater doses than those with little or no goitre and mild symptoms. Patients with toxic nodular goitre generally require larger doses. Administered activities of 150-200 MBq are the lower end of the dosage range and with these there is a lower incidence (20%) of early hypothyroidism, but at the expense of a lower cure rate (30% remain hyperthyroid). With greater administered activities (370 MBq upwards) less than 10% will remain hyperthyroid, but up to 60% will develop early hypothyroidism (Reiners, 1990). Late incidence of hypothyroidism, occurring in 2–3% of treated patients per year over a lifetime, does not appear to be dependent on the activity administered. No matter the dosage regimen chosen, there is a necessity for regular lifetime follow-up to check against recurrence of hyperthyroidism, or the onset of hypothyroidism, or non-compliance with hormone replacement therapy.

22.3.1.2 Practical details

Radioiodine in the form of sodium ^{131}I-iodide is available for oral use in liquid or capsule form, the amount of stable iodine being less than 1μg. With capsules there is no risk of spillage at administration but, on the other hand, some patients may have difficulty in swallowing a capsule and so liquid may be preferred. When the radioiodine is given in liquid form it is advisable to have means whereby the patient can drink from the vial without having to remove the seal. It is prudent to have the patient sign a consent to treatment form because of the risk of inducing hypothyroidism which can be considered as a significant side-effect. It is important, also, to ensure that the patient has no difficulty in swallowing and is unlikely to vomit, so as to avoid a contamination incident. Radioiodine may be given intravenously if circumstances preclude oral administration.

In the UK, patients may be treated on an out-patient basis if the administered activity is kept below 800 MBq. However, they cannot travel home by public transport if the administered activity is greater than 400 MBq and must use private transport. They are advised to stay off work and avoid close contact with other adults at home, until residual body activity falls below 150 MBq. With regard to contact with children, the restrictions are more severe in that they are advised to avoid non-essential contact with them until body activity falls below 30 MBq (NRPB, 1988). The turnover of radioiodine is such that for doses of up to 400 MBq the patient need not stay off work for more than 5 days. However, resumption of normal contact with children may have to be delayed for up to 19 days. For greater administered doses of radioiodine the period of restriction is longer (Hilditch *et al.,* 1991). An instruction card should be given to the patient detailing the restrictions and their duration. Patients in the UK requiring doses greater than 800 MBq, are required to be hospitalised but in a room with facilities for exclusive use of the patient. Staff caring for the patient must take adequate precautions. If a patient requires treatment for hyperthyroidism but is in hospital for other reasons, they will require to be nursed in a similar facility if the administered activity is 400 MBq or greater.

Treatment of hyperthyroidism with radioiodine is effective, and relatively inexpensive, but the administered activities and characteristics of ^{131}I are such that due care and attention requires to be paid to the radiological protection of persons coming in contact with the treated patients.

22.3.2 Radioiodine Treatment of Thyroid Carcinoma

Radioiodine has been used for several decades in the treatment of differentiated thyroid carcinoma, a tumour which metastasises to bone, lungs and other soft tissue (Beierwaltes *et al.,* 1984). However, it is slow growing and the prognosis is relatively good, allowing long term follow-up of treated patients. Malignant thyroid tumours usually appear as cold areas in a radioiodine image of the gland. Radionuclide imaging for evidence of spread at this stage is usually of no value, as any metastases which are present, like the primary tumour, do not as a rule, concentrate iodine to any great extent. However, after thyroidectomy (usually total) or an ablative dose of ^{131}I, when normal thyroid tissue has been removed, differentiated carcinomas (follicular or papillary) and their metastases usually take up iodine after a period of a few weeks, due to stimulation by high levels of thyroid stimulating hormone. The uptake of the functioning tumours is usually sufficiently great (about 0.1%/g average) for them to be destroyed by acceptable doses of radioiodine. Response to therapy can be assessed by repeating radionuclide imaging with radioiodine and, if necessary, further therapeutic doses of ^{131}I given until there is no longer evidence of tumour uptake. Up to 5 or 6 treatment doses of ^{131}I may be required in advanced or resistant cases. Several large follow-up studies have shown that side effects and long-term complications do not constitute a significant problem with this form of therapy (Clarke, 1991; Hoefnagel, 1991).

22.3.2.1 Dosage of ^{131}I-iodide

For ablation of normal thyroid tissue there is fairly wide variation in the doses administered (Maxon *et al.,* 1992a). In some patients ablation can be achieved with doses as low as 1110 MBq, but a dose of 3700 MBq will achieve successful ablation in all cases. Once thyroid ablation has taken place the patient will become hypothyroid and will require hormone replacement therapy (thyroxine). However before radionuclide imaging or radioiodine therapy is repeated, the patient will require to discontinue thyroxine therapy 4–6 weeks before, in order not to suppress radiodine uptake. Thyroxine may be replaced with triiodothyronine which has a shorter biological turnover and need only be discontinued 1–2 weeks before therapy (Maxon *et al.,* 1992a). For treatment of residual tumour and metastases, the dose is usually 7400 MBq.

22.3.2.2 Practical details

Treatment of thyroid carcinoma with radioiodine falls into the category of high-activity therapy, requiring the patient to be nursed in a specially designated room with toilet and bathroom facilities for the patient's exclusive use. Care must be taken to minimise contamination because radioiodine is excreted in urine, faeces, sweat and saliva. Any patient-related procedures which are not urgent should be postponed for as long as possible after administration of the dose, to take full advantage of the reduction in body activity by decay and excretion. Radioiodine is available in liquid or capsule form and is administered in exactly the same way, and with the same precautions, as in the treatment of hyperthyroidism.

Once the dose has been administered, it is good practice to monitor body activity on a daily basis by placing a radiation dose rate meter at a reproducible distance from the patient and noting the reduction in dose rate. In the case of ablation therapy, the turnover of radioiodine is such that it takes 4–5 days before body activity reduces to less than 800 MBq, at which time the patient may leave hospital. With doses given to treat residual tumour and metastases, the turnover of radioiodine is faster and sometimes the patient can return home in 2–3 days.

As with radioiodine treatment for hyperthyroidism, the patients are required to take certain precautions on leaving hospital in order to reduce irradiation of persons with whom they come in contact. The periods of restriction at home depend on the predicted time course of whole body activity, but are generally less than for radioiodine treated hyperthyroid patients, because of more rapid turnover of the radioiodine.

22.3.3 Treatment of Neuroendocrine Tumours

Metaiodo-benzylguanidine is similar in structure to the adrenergic neuron blocker guanethidine and the neurotransmitter noradrenaline. Due to this structural similarity, it is taken up by the adrenal medulla and other tissues with rich sympathetic innervation but unlike noradrenaline it is not metabolised and is largely excreted unchanged in the urine (Solanki *et al.,* 1992). Iodine-131-MIBG was initially investigated as a means of locating phaeochromocytomas (Shapiro *et al.,*

1985), but it was also found to be taken up by other neuro-endocrine tumours, including neuroblastoma, carcinoid tumours, non-secreting paragangliomas and medullary carcinoma of the thyroid. It has been used therapeutically for the treatment of all thcse tumours (Hoefnagel, 1991). Some preliminary work has also been undertaken with ^{125}I-MIBG, which is more effective in destroying micrometastases (Hoefnagel, 1991), but at present most patients are treated with ^{131}I-MIBG. The new agent pentavalent ^{186}Re(V)-DMSA may prove to be an alternative to ^{131}I-MIBG in the treatment of medullary carcinoma of the thyroid (Clarke *et al.*, 1990).

Not all tumours concentrate ^{131}I-MIBG for reasons that are not yet clear and, before therapeutic use of the material is considered, it is essential to perform diagnostic radionuclide imaging first with a tracer dose. Occassionally however, sites of uptake only become apparent on radionuclide imaging following a therapeutic dose, due to much greater accumulated counts and therefore improved statistical quality of the images. Experience in the treatment of neuroendocrine tumours with ^{131}I-MIBG has been accumulating over the past ten years. It is evident that not all tumours respond to this type of therapy, even with relatively good uptake, but on the other hand there are cases where the effect of ^{131}I-MIBG has been sufficiently great to achieve reduction in tumour volume and regression of the disease. A limiting factor is the radiation dose to the bone marrow which restricts the quantity of ^{131}I-MIBG than can be administered (Fielding *et al.*, 1991). It is likely that tumouricidal radiation doses could be delivered with greater administered activities, but with irreversible damage to the bone marrow and perhaps also to the liver. Newer techniques where ^{131}I-MIBG therapy is combined with whole body irradiation and bone marrow rescue (Wheldon *et al.*, 1988), are currently being investigated as a means of treating childhood neuroblastoma.

Upon intravenous administration, ^{131}I-MIBG is distributed throughout most tissues of the body but by 24 hours there is some concentration of radioactivity in the salivary glands, liver and myocardium. Iodine-131-MIBG is mostly excreted via the kidneys so there is also concentration of radioactivity in the urinary bladder. The colon may also be visualised due to a small amount of excretion via the gastrointestinal tract. Any tumour tissue with active MIBG uptake will be visible at 24 hours. There is likely to be thyroid uptake, due to release of free iodine, if the gland has not already been blocked by pharmacological quantities of iodine.

22.3.3.1 Dosage of ^{131}I-MIBG

For adults, the treatment dose of ^{131}I-MIBG requires to be at least 3700 MBq. A typical dose is 7400 MBq but single doses of up to 1200 MBq have been given. If necessary, the treatment may be repeated after a delay of a few months. Administered activities of these magnitudes may cause temporary reduction in white blood cell count. In childhood neuroblastoma, the approach tends to be more aggressive due to the rapidly proliferating nature of the disease. The administered activity is determined by the limit set for the whole body radiation dose to the patient. A limit of 2Gy is not untypical. To give a radiation dose of this magnitude requires administered activities of 4000–12000 MBq for body weights of 10–30kg (Fielding *et al.*, 1991).

22.3.3.2 Practical details

The patient's thyroid must be blocked by the administration of potassium iodate (170mg per day for adults), commencing one day before treatment and continuing for at least 3 weeks afterwards. It is essential that the patient's renal function has not been severely impaired by any previous nephrotoxic chemotherapy, as this could inhibit excretion of the ^{131}I and thereby significantly increase the whole body and bone marrow radiation dose. The patient should be well hydrated in order to improve excretion of MIBG not taken up by the tumour. It is also important that the patient has good bowel motility to avoid unnecessary accumulation of radionuclide in the gastro-intestinal tract. Certain drugs are known to inhibit the uptake of MIBG by tumour tissue and these should be discontinued 1–2 weeks before MIBG therapy. The classes of drugs which interfere with MIBG uptake include tricyclic antidepressants, antihypertensives, calcium channel blocking drugs and sympathomimetics, including nasal decongestants containing phenylpropanolamine (Solanki *et al* 1992).

Iodine-31-MIBG treatment falls into the category of high activity therapy and, as with ^{131}I therapy for thyroid carcinoma, the patient is required to be nursed in a room with separate facilities. The ^{131}I-MIBG is given by slow intravenous infusion over a period of 60 min with the patient's blood pressure being monitored during the infusion, and for 1–2 hours after it ceases, as there is a possibility that MIBG may displace noradrenaline from the storage granules, precipitating hypertension. Any other nursing procedures which are not urgent should be postponed for as long as possible to minimise radiation exposure of staff caring for the patient. The main route of excretion is via the kidneys and care has to be taken to limit spread of contamination.

As with ^{131}I therapy for thyroid carcinoma the reduction in total body activity can be monitored with the use of a radiation dose rate meter. Clearance of ^{131}I-MIBG from the whole body can be described by two main exponential components. Nearly 50% is cleared within the first 24 hours, but the remainder is cleared more slowly with an effective half period of some 30 hours. In practice, a typical patient can be discharged from hospital in less than 1 week, provided precautions are taken at home to minimise exposure of other persons, as in ^{131}I therapy for thyroid carcinoma.

22.3.4 Treatment of Bone Tumours

Bone metastases are a common finding in patients suffering from cancers of the prostate, breast and lungs, and in these patients control of bone pain is a significant clinical problem. External beam radiotherapy, in combination with analgesic drugs, remains the mainstay of treatment (Campa and Payne, 1992) but the proportion of the body that can be treated is limited. In patients with breast and prostate carcinoma, however, bony metastases are usually multiple, and often widespread, and in theory the systemic administration of a suitable therapeutic radiopharmaceutical offers the opportunity of a more specific and less toxic method of treating disseminated disease.

The development of effective radiopharmaceutical therapy for the palliation and treatment of bone metastases has long been a challenge in nuclear medicine. Ideally the radiopharmaceutical compound should accumulate in the metastatic lesion, but not in normal bone. Some tumours such as thyroid carcinoma and neuroblastoma, which may metastasize to bone, can be treated with tumour specific therapies, i.e ^{131}I-iodide ^{131}I-MIBG. However, the agents that are presently available for the vast majority of primary tumours that metastasise to bone, are unfortunately all bone-seeking substances and thereby irradiate bone marrow. Four beta emitting radionuclides, in a variety of chemical forms, have been used for treatment of bone metastases: ^{32}P, ^{89}Sr, and the newer agents ^{186}Re and ^{153}Sm (Lewington, 1993). Phosphorus-32 and ^{89}Sr have relatively long half-lives, while ^{186}Re and ^{153}Sm have shorter half lives (Table 1) and the advantage of emitting suitable gamma rays allowing scintigraphic imaging and means of quantifying uptake for dosimetric purposes. There is little hard evidence to show that any of these radionuclides alter the course of the disease, their action is principally palliative, i.e. reducing pain and maintaining mobility of the patient.

22.3.4.1 Phosphorus-32

Phosphorus-32 (Table 1) has been used in a variety of chemical forms to treat bone metastases, with a considerable number of clinical trials having been reported. Silberstein *et al.*, (1992) reviewed the literature on the clinical use of ^{32}P-orthophosphate alone or in combination with androgen or parathyroid hormone (PTH), in an attempt to increase tumour uptake. Efficacy was demonstrated for the treatment of pain in 84% of 322 breast cancer patients and 77% of 444 prostate cancer patients. The data, however did not suggest that any particular ^{32}P regimen is superior to another. The authors point to a number of major flaws in these studies, including the complete lack of placebo controlled trials. Other ^{32}P compounds have been used over the years including ^{32}P-polymetaphosphate and ^{32}P-pyrophosphate. Both these compounds are hydrolysed by phosphatases in-vivo to orthophosphate and it is therefore not surprising that no clinical advantage could be shown for these compounds (Harbert, 1987). Diphosphonates on the other hand have an enzyme-resistant P—C—P bond and hence a much longer biologic half-life on bone, following chemisorption. Although ^{32}P-hydroxyethylidene-diphosphonate was shown to have better biodistribution properties in rats, clinical studies in 5 patients were disappointing (Potsaid *et al.*, 1978). Phosphorus-32 would not now be considered to be the first choice therapy for bone metastases due to the myelotoxicity of the radionuclide in ionic form (because of its uptake not only in bone but in bone marrow) and its relatively low tumour to normal bone uptake ratio. Other radionuclides are less toxic and are taken up by bone metastases to a greater extent (Lewington, 1993).

22.3.4.2 Strontium-89

The therapeutic potential of ^{89}Sr for systemic therapy of bony metastases was first recognised by Pecher in 1941, but is only now becoming an important treatment in palliation of bone pain. The long physical half-life of ^{89}Sr (Table 1) allows relatively long duration of irradiation of the lesions. Metastatic lesions concentrate up to 25 times more ^{89}Sr than normal bone and the turnover of the radionuclide can be slower, thus enhancing the target to non-target dose ratio.

Robinson *et al.*, (1992) reviewed their experience with ^{89}Sr-chloride in almost 500 patients. When treated with doses of 1.48 MBq/kg the overall response rate, in terms of pain relief, for patients with bone metastases from prostate cancer was 79% and from breast cancer was 83%. They concluded that there is a threshold level of approx 1.11 MBq/kg before the treatment becomes effective, with the ideal dose in the range 1.48–2.22 MBq/kg. In a multicentre study, an overall response rate of 79% was seen in 117 patients with painful metastases from prostatic carcinoma (Laing *et al.*, 1991). In this study the authors noted a transient pain flair in the first 48 hours in some patients but the onset of pain relief generally occurred 10 to 20 days after administration of ^{89}Sr, and continued for an average of 6 months therafter. There was an average reduction of 30% in platelet count, the nadir occurring 6 weeks after therapy. Strontium-89-chloride is now being used in many centres as an effective means of pain relief in patients suffering from widespread bony metastases.

22.3.4.3 Rhenium-186-(tin)hydroxyethylidene diphosphonate (Sn-HEDP)

Rhenium-186 is a medium energy beta emitter (Table 1) and also emits a 137keV gamma ray, suitable for scintigraphic imaging. The physical half-life is 3.77 days which is adequate from the availability point of view, but not so long that it presents a problem with disposal. Most of the reported experience has been with the ^{186}Re diphosphonate compound, ^{186}Re-Sn-HEDP.

Maxon *et al.*, (1992b) reported their initial experience using ^{186}Re-Sn-HEDP. A single intravenous dose of the approximately 1295 MBq resulted in significant reduction in pain in 33 of 43 patients (77%) with cancer of breast and prostate. Approx 10% of the injections were followed by a transient increase in pain within 2–3 days of injection which subsided within a week of onset. Clinically significant pain relief occurred within 2 weeks in 75% of the patients responding to an initial injection, with a median time of onset of one week. The average duration of pain relief was 5 weeks although the period of follow-up was limited. Decreases in white blood cells were observed, but these were considered to be clinically unimportant. The efficacy of a single injection of ^{186}Re-(Sn)-HEDP was also evaluated by this group, using a double blind crossover comparison with placebo. The new rhenium compound resulted in significantly greater pain relief than placebo (Maxon *et al.*, 1991). A number of patients have received two administrations and these have been well tolerated (Maxon *et al.*, 1992b).

22.3.4.4 Samarium-153-ethylenediamine-tetramethylene phosphonic acid (EDTMP)

Samarium-153 is a beta emitting radiolanthanide with a half-life of 1.95 days (Table 1). It also emits a 107keV gamma ray, suitable for scintigraphic imaging. The compound that has been most widely researched is ^{153}Sm-EDTMP. Early bio-distribution studies with this agent in animals showed that most of the activity is found in bone, with bone lesions concentrating up to 17 times more than normal bone. In a dose escalation study, Farhangi *et al.*, (1992) evaluated ^{153}Sm-EDTMP in a group of 22 patients given between 7.4 and 37 MBq/kg. Due to the small numbers of patients and the diversity of their neoplasms, no clear dose response relationhip could be established. Sixty-five percent of the patients experienced pain relief, with the decrease in pain lasting for an average period of 3.8 months. Myelotoxicity was mild and transient. However further work is required to determine whether pain relief is due to the irradiation or the physiological effect of the EDTMP (Holmes, 1992).

Because of the short half-life of the radionuclide, and hence short period irradiation, ^{153}Sm-EDTMP has been postulated as a treatment for primary bone tumours. Since osteogenic sarcomas and other primary tumours exhibit markedly increased metabolic rate, this will lead to fast turnover of any targeted radiopharmaceutical. Therefore in such tumours ^{153}Sm, and for that matter ^{186}Rh compounds, may offer theoretical advantages over ^{89}Sr (Lattimer *et al.*, 1990).

22.3.4.5 Practical details for ^{89}Sr therapy

Strontium-89 is available commercially in the form of strontium chloride in isotonic saline for intravenous administration. The long physical half-life makes availability and supply fairly straightforward. Administered activities of 150-200 MBq are typical. At this dosage there is no external radiation hazard to other persons from the Bremsstrahlung radiation emanating from the patient. It is prudent, however, to use a perspex shielded syringe when administering the radiopharmaceutical because the beta radiation is sufficiently energetic to penetrate the walls of a syringe, thus leading to unnecessary finger exposure. Treatment can be given on an out-patient basis but it should be remembered that the patient remains radioactive for many weeks afterwards. Particular care should be taken to avoid contamination from radioactive urine over the first 5 days, especially in the case of patients with prostatic cancer, who could well have incontinence problems.

22.3.5 Treatment of Myeloproliferative Disease

Phosphorus-32 (Table 1) has been used for more than 50 years in the treatment of a variety of haematological disorders. Following intravenous injection, ^{32}P as the phosphate ion, is concentrated selectively by rapidly proliferating tissue and there is also bone uptake. In this way a significant radiation dose is delivered to the bone marrow and results in growth retardation of the haemopoeitic cell lines.

The primary application of ^{32}P is its role in the treatment of polycythaemia rubra vera. In this condition there is an abnormal increase in the number of red cells in the circulation. Symptoms are often widespread and nonspecific resulting from increased blood viscosity and if the disease is left untreated the prognosis is poor. However, treatment with phlebotomy, radioactive phosphorus or chemotherapy all result in significant increase in life expectancy (Silberstein et al., 1979). Without therapy, median survival in polycythaemia vera is as short as 1.5 years. However after therapy with ^{32}P or chemotherapeutic agents, the survival time is increased markedly (median 13–16 years). The most common cause of death in patients with polycythaemia vera managed with ^{32}P or chemotherapy are cardiovascular complications including haemorrhage (30–50%), myelofibrosis with myeloid metaplasia (10–20%) and acute myelogenous leukaemia (10–20%) (Wasserman *et al.*, 1981).

The efficacy of ^{32}P therapy as against other treatment for polycythaemia vera has been studied fairly extensively. A prospective study carried out by the European Organisation for Research on Treatment of Cancer (EORTC, 1981), comparing ^{32}P with busulphan chemotherapy in 293 patients, suggests the busulphan treatment to be superior. Although there were a similar number of patients who died of acute leukaemia in each treatment group, there were significantly more deaths due to vascular complications in patients treated with ^{32}P (18%) as against busulphan (5%).

In contrast, a long term follow up study carried out by the Polycythaemia Vera Study Group was unable to demonstrate survival differences between different therapies at 10 years (Berk *et al.,* 1981). In this study, 431 patients were randomised into three groups receiving phlebotomy alone, or ^{32}P or chlorambucil with phlebotomy as required. Deaths due to acute leukaemia were 1% for phlebotomy, and 6% for ^{32}P. The figure for chlorambucil was 11% and as a result treatment with this agent has been discontinued. With all chemotherapeutic agents, it is essential to perform regular blood counts to assess effectiveness of therapy and compliance with treatment. For that reason, ^{32}P remains the agent of choice in patients who are likely to be unreliable in returning for follow-up blood counts, or in taking medications regularly.

22.3.5.1 Dosage of ^{32}P and practical details

Phosphorus-32 sodium phosphate is supplied in isotonic saline, ready for intravenous administration. As with other high energy beta emitters the radionuclide is given using a perspex shielded syringe, to reduce unnecessary finger exposure. The usual treatment dose is 1.9–3.7 MBq/kg body weight with an upper limit of 185 MBq. For administered activities of this magnitude, there is no external hazard to other persons from Bremsstrahlung emanating from the patient. Patients are usually treated on an out-patient basis and after treatment their blood count is measured at 3 months. If there is no improvement the treatment may be repeated. Patients can experience variable periods of remission, ranging from several months to several years.

22.3.6 Intracavitary Therapy

Direct intracavitary administration is a means of delivering radiopharmaceuticals in high concentration to tumours that are spread out over the serosal linings of cavities and to tumour cells present in malignant effusions. In order to minimise leakage of the radionuclide from the cavity, it is usually given in the form of a radiocolloid. Even so, a proportion of the radionuclide will reach the bloodstream by lymphatic drainage, and by leakage of ionic radionuclide, as the colloid is degraded, thus irradiating non-target tissues. Intracavitary therapy is applied to the peritoneal, pleural and pericardial cavities as well as to cystic brain tumours and to the spinal canal. A non-cancer application of this method, is the intra-articular injection of radiocolloid to treat inflammatory joint disorders.

Colloidal ^{198}Au was formerly the most widely used agent, but the radionuclide emits unwanted gamma radiation, leading to unnecessary exposure of non-target tissue within the patient, and of other personnel. The agents of choice are now ^{32}P and ^{90}Y-colloids, with perhaps radiolabelled antibodies having a wider role to play in the future. In general, it is difficult to assess the efficacy of this method of therapy in malignant conditions because the therapeutic effect may take some time to become manifest, during which time some patients may succumb to the disease. There is, therefore, a deatth of well reported data on large numbers of patients.

22.3.6.1 Treatment of intra-peritoneal metastases

Ovarian cancer is a disease where the whole peritoneal cavity is at risk from metastatic spread. A major problem is the presence of sub-clinical tumour deposits and intraperitoneal administration of radiocolloid is used in an attempt to destroy such micrometastases. Much of the recent published work relates to the use of ^{32}P-chromic phosphate colloid, administered in doses of 370–740 MBq, although ^{90}Y-colloidal silicate is an acceptable alternative. The agent is instilled via an indwelling catheter mixed with 500–1000 ml saline. A practical problem is that distribution of the radiocolloid within the peritoneal cavity can often be irregular and localised, if precautions are not taken (Boye *et al.* 1984). It is good practice to check catheter placement and the procedure for instillation by administering a diagnostic dose of ^{99m}Tc labelled colloid, prior to the therapeutic procedure. In terms of efficacy, the evidence in support of radiocolloid therapy is largely circumstantial (Harbert, 1987). There is a need for well controlled studies to assess the effectiveness of ^{32}P-colloid over other treatment modalities (Rosenhiem *et al.,* 1979). In one small study of 29 patients with minimal residual disease, reported by Varia *et al.,* (1988), 17 were treated with ^{32}P-colloid with or without chemotherapy, and 12 by chemotherapy alone. The 4-year survival rates were 59% and 22% respectively, thus indicating that ^{32}P therapy may contribute to controlling intraperitoneal disease.

One of the obvious problems with ^{32}P-colloid therapy is that radiation is delivered indiscriminately to both normal and tumour tissue within the peritoneal cavity. This can result in scarring of the omentum, with formation of adhesions as well as increased friability of the bowel wall. Tumour specific radiolabelled antibodies may well provide the opportunity of better targeting of the radionuclide. Some preliminary studies with therapeutic quantities (up to 925 MBq) ^{90}Y labelled antibodies have been undertaken, but there is indication that uptake of free ^{90}Y, leading to bone marrow toxicity, could be a problem (Stewart *et al.,* 1990).

22.3.6.2 Treatment of malignant effusions

The main aim of radiopharmaceutical therapy is to reduce fluid accumulation in the serosal cavities of the peritoneum, pleura and pericardium, produced by the dissemination of a variety of cancers. A successful response is usually defined as cessation or reduction in the rate of fluid production.

The tumours chiefly responsible for increased production of peritoneal fluid are ovarian, renal and gastrointestinal cancers. Treatment with intraperitoneal colloids takes effect only after about 3 months and therefore candidates for this form of therapy should have a life expectancy longer than this period of time. Card *et al.*, (1960), reported improvement in 53% of more than 2000 patients given ^{198}Au-colloid and also observed a similar response in a group of 222 patients given ^{32}P-colloid. More recently, Jackson and Blosser (1981), obtained a response rate of 85% using ^{32}P-colloid in patients surviving 3 months or longer, the administered activity being 555 MBq.

Cancers that most commonly give rise to malignant pleural effusions are breast, lung and ovarian carcinomas and lymphomas. Treatment with colloidal ^{198}Au, ^{32}P and ^{90}Y has been reported to be effective in 50–76% of patients (Harbert, 1987). In one of the more recent studies Jackson and Blosser (1981), used ^{32}P-colloid (370 MBq) in 115 patients with malignant pleural effusion. Therapy was successful in 75% of patients who survived three months or longer, but since most of the patients did not survive that length of time, the overall response rate was only 28%. Pectasides *et al.*, (1986), in some preliminary studies, administered up to 2220 MBq ^{131}I labelled antibody for treatment of pleural effusions with 7 out of 10 patients showing good response.

There are only a few reports in the literature with regard to the use of radiopharmaceutical therapy for the treatment of malignant pericardial effusions. Experience in a total of 39 patients treated with 185 MBq ^{32}P-colloid suggests a 71–91% success rate (Harbert, 1987). The use of 740–1110 MBq ^{131}I labelled monoclonal antibody in 3 patients has been reported by Pectasides *et al.*, (1986).

22.3.6.3 Intracystic therapy

There are several reports in the literature regarding the treatment of cystic brain tumours by intracavitary administration of radiocolloid. This type of treatment is most commonly applied to cystic craniopharyngiomas, a benign brain tumour, which has a peak incidence between the ages of 5 and 15 years. Most patients referred for radiocolloid therapy are either patients who have been treated by total surgical excision but who develop recurrence, or patients treated with partial excision followed by external beam radiotherapy, but who develop recurrences. Three different radiocolloids have been used, namely colloids of ^{90}Y, ^{32}P and ^{186}Re, the dosage given being dependent on cyst volume (Pollack *et al.*, 1988). The object is to deliver 200–300Gy to the wall of the cyst. In practice this means administered activities of several hundred MBq for ^{32}P and ^{90}Y (Strauss *et al.*, 1982) and up to 1800 MBq for ^{186}Re (Askienazy *et al.*, 1990). Two of the more recent reports are from Strauss *et al.* (1982) who administered ^{90}Y-colloid and Pollack *et al.* (1988) who administered ^{32}P-colloid. In all, a total of 27 patients were treated. Of these, 20 were followed up using computerised tomography to assess cyst volume with 17 having radiological evidence of cyst regression.

22.3.6.4 Intrathecal therapy

Intrathecal administration of a radiocolloid is used as a substitute for external beam therapy in the treatment of childhood meningeal leukaemia. The use of ^{32}P-colloid, in doses of 111MBq, has been reported by Sackmann Muriel *et al.* (1976) and the use of ^{198}Au-colloid, in doses of 55–185MBq by Metz *et al.* (1982). In the former study, 32 patients received either multiple doses of chemotherapy or multiple doses of ^{32}P-colloid. There was no significant difference in duration of remission between the two therapies, but there were fewer and less side effects with the ^{32}P. Metz *et al.*, (1982) treated 23 children using a single dose of ^{198}Au-colloid with an outcome somewhat better than that experienced with chemotherapy (Harbert, 1987).

22.3.6.5 Radionuclide synovectomy

In severe cases of chronic rheumatoid arthritis where medical therapy has been unsuccessful, surgical removal of the inflamed joint lining (synovectomy) has been shown to provide symptomatic relief lasting from 2–5 years (Davis and Chinol, 1989). An alternative to surgical synovectomy is the intra-articular injection of chemicals or radiocolloid. However, with chemical synovectomy, concerns have been expressed about systemic toxicity and local injury to articular cartilage. Hence the useful role of radiocolloids in the management of chronic synovitis. The radiocolloids most frequently used have been those of ^{90}Y and ^{198}Au, whereas ^{169}Er, ^{186}Re and ^{32}P-colloids, and ^{165}Dy-ferric hydroxide macroaggregates, have been used less often. At present the most commonly used radiocolloid is that of ^{90}Y (Spooren *et al.*, 1985). In theory it is possible to select the optimum radionuclide for the specific joint and synovial thickness (Hoefnagel, 1991): ^{32}P and ^{90}Y-colloids (high energy beta emitters) being best for large joints and thick synovia (knee joints), ^{186}Re-colloids (medium energy beta emitter) being best for ankles, shoulders, elbows and wrists; ^{169}Er (a low energy beta emitter) being best for small joints such as the digital joints. Whilst this approach is desirable, the practical application thereof depends a great deal on the commercial availability of the radiocolloid.

A significant problem in radiocolloid synovectomy is leakage of radioactivity from the joint space either by lymphatic clearance of the colloid or as a result of the radionuclide being dissociated from the colloid (Davis and Chinol, 1989). The problem of leakage can be minimised by choosing colloid of the correct size, a smaller particle showing a greater degree of leakage. A size of 2–5μm would seem to be desirable but in fact the particle size of commercial preparations can be as low as 0.1μm. A further measure is to immobilise the treated joint for 48 hours after administration of the radiocolloid. Finally, choosing a radionuclide with a short half-life minimises the radiation dose to non-target tissue arising from leaked radioactivity.

Experience with ^{90}Y-colloid has shown it to be superior to saline, osmic acid and several steroids for the treatment of chronic synovitis (Winfield and Gumpel, 1979). When compared with surgical synovectomy, there is little difference in outcome after a period of 2 years (Gumpel and Roles, 1975). However some 28% of patients fail to improve, or experience only transient improvement, following radiocolloid synovectomy but a proportion of these may benefit from further treatment (Winfield and Gumpel, 1979).

In practice the technique is fairly straightforward but care has to be taken to avoid spillage of the radiocolloid and to reduce finger tip exposure by using a shielded syringe. Typical doses of ^{90}Y-colloid are 278 MBq for knee joints and 185 MBq for the ankles and shoulders. Steroid is given through the same needle, after the radiocolloid, not only to flush the needle but also to reduce any chemical synovitis from the colloidal material. The joint is immobilised for a period of 48 hours and it is usual practice to hospitalise the patient for at least 24 hours. On leaving hospital the patient should avoid contact with children until body radioactivity falls to 100 MBq, i.e. for a period not exceeding 4 days from the time of treatment.

22.3.7 Regional use of therapeutic radiopharmaceuticals

The use of the arterial route to deliver radioactive formulations which preferentially lodge in arterioles or capillaries of tumours has long been seen as an attractive method of therapy. Over the past 30 years a number of radionuclides including ^{90}Y and ^{32}P have been labelled to a variety of particulate carriers, which in the main have been microspheres. These preparations have been administered regionally to treat tumours resident in liver, lung, kidney, tongue, spleen and soft tissue tumours of the extremities. However, despite this lengthy experience the technique has not become established in routine therapy. When the technique was first introduced clinically the results were discouraging. This lack of success was due to poor delivery to the tumour but developments in arteriographic techniques now allow more precise delivery of radionuclide to target tissue. Early studies also suffered the problems of biodegradation of the particle and leaching of free radionuclide. These problems have been largely overcome and stable preparations are now available (Ehrhardt and Day, 1987).

Most clinical experience with intra-arterial microspheres has been gained in the treatment of metastases to the liver which are known to derive their blood supply predominantly from the hepatic artery. In two studies, Ariel and Padula (1978 & 1982), used ^{90}Y labelled microspheres (3.7–5.5 GBq) together with chemotherapy in more than 100 patients with liver tumours arising from colo-rectal cancer, and reported average survivals of 26 and 31 months. These figures compare favourably with average survival figures of 6–12 months in patients treated using alternative methods (Harbert, 1987). Hepatic artery scintigraphy with ^{99m}Tc-macroaggregated albumin has become an essential aid to verify the correct positioning of the arterial catheter, also to quantify arteriovenous shunt to the lungs and to assess tumour to normal liver ratios just prior to radioactive particle therapy (Ziesmann *et al.*, 1984). Other clinical studies using activated ^{90}Y-glass microspheres (Herba *et al.*, 1988), and ^{90}Y-resin microspheres (Roeslar *et al.*, 1990) have been carried out with some limited success in the treatment of liver tumours. It would appear from most of these studies that the best clinical results are obtained in those patients with small tumours that are well perfused.

In addition to particulate agents, there has been interest in the intra-arterial use of tumour specific materials. The observation that oil-based contrast material was selectively retained in tumour vessels as well as in tumour cells, has led to the use of ^{131}I-lipiodol in hepatocellular carcinoma (HCC) (Yumoto *et al.*, 1985). In a short term study by Park *et al.* (1987), ^{131}I-labelled lipiodol was administered intra-arterially to patients suffering from HCC. Doses ranged from 74–4810 MBq, depending on tumour volume. The majority of the 47 patients studied showed symptomatic improvements as well as disappearance of ascites and shrinkage of tumour volume. In another study Bretagne *et al.* (1988), treated a total of 23 patients with HCC or hepatic metastases. Doses of ^{131}I-lipiodol ranged from 888–2220 MBq injected into the hepatic artery with 4 patients receiving 2 treatments and 1 patient 3 treatments. The HCC patients in this series responded well to therapy and tumour size was reduced in those cases where follow-up was possible. However, results in patients with hepatic metastases were disappointing.

The selectivity of intra-arterial radioactivity to the tumour may be increased by the use of vasoactive agents. Unlike normal blood vessels those supplying tumours are immature, possessing neither smooth muscle nor an adrenergic nerve supply and are therefore unable to respond to arterio-constrictors (Häfstrom *et al.*, 1980). In a tracer study using radiolabelled microspheres, angiotensin II was used to modify the pattern of arterial blood flow in patients with liver metastases, to produce an increase in tumour to normal ratio by a factor of 3 (Goldberg *et al.*, 1990). The use of such agents might therefore enhance delivery of arterially administered substances to tumours.

22.3.8 Radiolabelled Antibodies (Radioimmunotherapy)

The advent of hybridoma technology brought with it increased expectation that antibodies could provide the vehicle for specifically targeting and destroying malignant disease. A variety of techniques for preparing suitable antibodies and labelling these with radionuclides have been developed (Perkins and Pimm, 1991). Clinical experience to date has largely been confined to the use of antibodies as in-vivo diagnostic agents in radioimmunoscintigraphy (RIS). A vast number of studies have been undertaken with a host of different monoclonal antibodies (MAbs) or their fragments. These have been radiolabelled with a range of different radionuclides and have been used in a variety of patient studies. No generalisation of RIS as a technique can be made, since experience varies considerably with a range of reported sensitivities and specificities. The accumulation of radiolabelled MAbs is in most cases very low (typically 0.001–0.01%/g) and is associated with relatively short retention times which limits their usefulness for therapeutic purposes. There are many factors leading to low antibody uptake at target sites which include technical problems during preparation, such as low antibody purification efficiency and loss of immunoreactivity resulting from damage incurred in the radiolabelling process. Other problems encountered are alterations in antigen expression by the tumour, effects of dilution after in-vivo administration, shedding of antigen into the circulation and the induction of human antimouse antibody response.

No controlled studies comparing radioimmunotherapy with other cancer treatments have been published. Most studies reported so far have been of an exploratory nature in patients with nonresectable cancers. These studies include the use of radiolabelled antibodies given intravenously in a variety of tumour types including Hodgkin's disease, leukaemia, lymphoma, hepatoma, melanoma and neuroblastoma. Hoefnagel (1991), has summarised several reported studies. Of 203 patients given one of a number of MAbs labelled with ^{131}I, 12 had complete remissions while 61 had partial remissions of disease. There is evidence to suggest that although partial and transient response can be achieved in certain solid tumours, it is the lymphoproliferative malignancies which tend to be more responsive to radioimmunotherapy (Goldenberg, 1992).

In certain conditions, regional or intracavitary administration of radiolabelled antibodies might be more appropriate and it is possible this could lead to increased tumour uptake at sites of localised disease. Hoefnagel (1991) has reviewed the results from several different studies in which therapy doses of radiolabelled antibodies had been administered intraperitoneally. Of 76 patients with ovarian and colon carcinoma, 5 had complete remissions while 15 had partial remissions. Although percentage uptakes per gram of tumour tissue still tend to be quite low (less than 0.019%), some encouraging clinical responses have been obtained, especially in patients with limited disease (Stewart *et al.* 1988). Pectasides *et al.*, (1986), reported the use of ^{131}I-labelled MAbs in the treatment of malignant pericardial and pleural effusions. No fluid re-accumulation was seen in 77% of the effusions, the effect of treatment lasting for periods ranging between 3 and 18 months. Radiolabelled antibodies have also been administered intrathecally. An example of this is the study carried out by Lashford *et al.*, (1988), in which objective responses were obtained in 4 of the 5 patients treated with ^{131}I labelled MAbs.

Techniques for increasing the concentration of antibodies in target tissue must be developed for radioimmunotherapy to become more effective. In addition to physical methods of selective delivery, such as intra-arterial and intracavitary administration, antibodies with improved selectivity must be found. Such developments could come from the use of "pancarcinoma" antibodies such as 88BV59 (DeJager *et al.*, 1991) or through the use of chimeric MAbs (Hardman *et al.*, 1989) and human MAbs (Haisma *et al.*, 1990). Better kinetics and distribution of antibodies may be achieved through the use of genetically engineered antibody fragments such as single domain antibody fragments (dAbs) (Ward *et al.*, 1989). Additionally, substitution of ^{131}I with other beta emitters such as ^{90}Y and ^{186}Re (Table 1), may lead to delivery of higher radiation doses to the tumour sites. Other radionuclides including there alpha emitters ^{211}As and ^{212}Bi (Knapp and Lau, 1990) and the generator produced beta emitter ^{188}Re (Griffiths *et al.*, 1991) (Table 1) may provide even more effective treatment.

CONTRIBUTORS

For the section on Radiosensitivity we are grateful to:

Dr Tom Wheldon,
Department of Radiation Oncology,
C.R.C. Beatson Laboratories,
Garscube Estate,
Glasgow.

REFERENCES

Ariel I.M. and Padula G. (1978). *Treatment of symptomatic metastatic cancer to the liver from primary colon and rectal cancer by the intra-arterial administration of chemotherapy and radioactive isotopes.* J. Surg. Oncol., **10**, 327–336.

Ariel I.M. and Padula G. (1982). *Treatment of asymptomatic metastatic cancer to the liver from primary colon and rectal cancer by the intra-arterial administration of chemotherapy and radioactive isotopes.* J. Surg. Oncol., **20**, 151–156.

Askienazy S. *et al.* (1990). *Colloidal 186Re in the endocavitary irradiation of cystic craniopharyngiomas.* Eur. J. Nucl. Med., **16**, S143.

Beierwaltes W.H. *et al.* (1984). *An analysis of "ablation of thyroid remnants with I-131 in 511 patients from 1947–1984: experience at University of Michigan.* J. Nucl. Med., **25**, 1287–1293.

Beierwaltes W.H. (1985). *Horizons in radionuclide therapy.* J. Nucl. Med., **26**, 421–427.

Berk P.D. *et al.* (1981). *Increased incidence of acute leukemia in polycythemia vera associated with chlorambucil therapy.* N. Eng. J. Med., **304**, 441–447.

Blake G.M. *et al.*, (1986). *Sr-89 therapy: Strontium kinetics in disseminated carcinoma of the prostate.* Eur. J. Nucl. Med., **12**, 447–454.

Blake G.M. *et al.* (1988). *Modification by nifedipine of ^{131}I-meta-iodobenzyl-guanidine kinetics in malignant phaeochromocytoma.* Eur. J. Nucl. Med., **14**, 345–348.

Boye E. *et al.* (1984). *Whole body distribution of radioactivity after intraperitoneal administration of ^{32}P colloids.* Br. J. Radiol., **57**, 395–402.

Bretagne J-F *et al.* (1988). *Hepatic artery injection of I-131-labeled lipiodol.* Radiology, **168**, 547–550.

Campa J.A. III and Payne R. (1992). *The management of intractable bone pain: A clinician's perspective.* Sem. Nucl. Med., XXII, **1**, 3–10.

Card R.Y. *et al.* (1960). *Summary of ten years of the use of radioactive colloids in intracavitary therapy.* J. Nucl. Med., **1**, 195–201.

Clarke S.E.M. *et al.* (1990). *Re-186-V-DMSA: a new radiopharmaceutical for therapy of medullary carcinoma of the thyroid.* Eur. J. Nucl. Med., **16**, S70.

Clarke S.E.M. (1991). *Radionuclide therapy of the thyroid.* Eur. J. Nucl. Med., **18**, 984–991.

Davis M.A. and Chinol M. (1989). *Radiopharmaceuticals for radiation synovectomy: evaluation of two yttrium-90 particulate agents.* J. Nucl. Med., **30**, 1047–1055.

DeJager R.L. *et al.* (1991). *Radioimmunodetection of colorectal carcinoma with Tc-99m-labeled human IgG antibody: 88BV59-1. Phase I clinical trial.* Proc. Am. Assoc. Cancer Res., **32**, 184–203.

Ehrhardt G.J. and Day D.E. (1987). *Therapeutic use of ^{90}Y microspheres.* Int. J. Rad. Appl. Instrum. [B], **14**, 233–242.

European Organisation for Research on Treatment of Cancer (EORTC), "Leukemia and Hematosarcoma" Cooperative Group (1981). *Treatment of polycythemia vera by radiophosphorus or busulphan: a randomized trial.* Br. J. Cancer, **44**, 75–80.

Farhangi M. *et al.* (1992). *^{153}Sm-EDTMP, a radio-therapeutic agent for palliative treatment of metastatic bone cancer pain.* J. Nucl. Med., **33**, 1451–1458.

Farrar J.J. and Toft A.D. (1991). *Iodine-131 treatment of hyperthyroidism: current issues. Clin. Endocrinol.*, **35**, 207–212.

Fielding S.L. *et al.* (1991). *Dosimetry of iodine 131 metaiodobenzylguanidine for treatment of resistant neuroblastoma: results of a UK study.* Eur. J. Nucl. Med., **18**, 308–316.

Goldberg J.A. *et al.* (1991). *The use of angiotensin II as a potential method of targeting cytotoxic microspheres in patients with intrahepatic tumour.* Br. J. Cancer, **63**, 308–310.

Goldenberg D.M. (1992). *Radioimmunotherapy of cancer: Arming the missiles.* J. Nucl. Med., **33**, 1110–1112.

Griffith G.L. *et al.* (1991). *Direct radiolabeling of monoclonal antibodies with generator produced rhenium-188 for radioimmunotherapy: labeling and animal biodistribution studies.* Cancer Res., **51**, 4594–4602.

Gumpel J.M. and Roles N.C. (1975). *A controlled trial of intra-articular radiocolloids versus surgical synovectomy in persistent synovitis.* Lancet, **1**, 488–489.

Häfstrom L. *et al.* (1980). *Effects of catecholamines on cardiovascular response and blood flow distribution to normal tissue and liver tumours in rats.* Cancer Res., **40**, 481–485.

Haisma H.J. *et al.* (1990). *Human IgM monoclonal antibody 16.88: pharmacokinetics and distribution in mouse and man.* Br. J. Cancer, **62** (Suppl A), 40–43.

Hall E.J. (1988). *Radiobiology for the Radiologist. 3rd edition.* Lippincott, Philadelphia.

Hamburger J.I. (1985). *Management of hyperthyroidism in children and adolescents.* J. Clin. Endocrinol. Metab., **60**, 1019–1024.

Harbert J.C. (1987). *Nuclear Medicine Therapy.* Thieme Medical Publishers, Inc., New York.

Hardman N. *et al.* (1989). *Generation of a recombinant mouse-human chimaeric monoclonal antibody directed against human carcinoembryonic antigen.* Int. J. Cancer, **44**, 424–433.

Herba M.J. *et al.* (1988). *Hepatic malignancies: Improved treatment with intra-arterial Y-90.* Radiology, **169**, 311–314.

Hilditch T.E. *et al.* (1991). *Radiological protection guidance for radioactive patients—new data for therapeutic* ^{131}I. Nucl. Med. Commun., **12**, 485–495.

Hoefnagel C.A. (1991). *Radionuclide therapy revisited.* Eur. J. Nucl. Med., **18**, 408–431.

Holm L.E. *et al.* (1991). *Cancer risk after iodine-131 therapy for hyperthyroidism.* J. Natl. Cancer Inst., **83**, 1072–1077.

Jackson G.L. and Blosser N.M. (1981). *Intracavitary chromic phosphate (^{32}P) colloidal suspension therapy.* Cancer, **48**, 2596–2598.

Knapp R.C. and Lau C.C. (1990). *Monoclonal antibodies and radioimmunoconjugates; keeping feasibility at centre stage.* J. Clin. Oncol., **8**, 1938–1940.

Laing A.H. *et al.* (1991). *Strontium-89 chloride for pain palliation in prostatic skeletal malignancy.* Br. J. Radiol. **64** (765), 816–822.

Lashford L.S. *et al.* (1988). *A pilot study of ^{131}I monoclonal antibodies in the therapy of leptomeningeal tumors.* Cancer, **61**, 857–868.

Lattimer J.C. *et al.* (1990). *Clinical and clinicopathologic effects of samarium-153-EDTMP administered intravenously in normal dogs.* J. Nucl. Med., **32**, 1316–1325.

Lewington V.J. (1993). *Targeted radionuclide therapy for bone metastses.* Eur. J. Nucl. Med., **20**, 66–74.

Maxon H.R. *et al.* (1991). *Re-186(Sn)-HEDP for the treatment of osseous metastases: Results of a double-blind crossover comparison with placebo.* J. Nucl. Med., **32**, 1877–1881.

Maxon H.R. *et al.* (1992a). *Radioiodine-131 therapy for well differentiated thyroid cancer—a quantitative radiation dosimetric approach: outcome and validation in 85 patients.* J. Nucl. Med., **33**, 1132–1136.

Maxon H.R. *et al.* (1992b). *Rhenium-186 hydroxyethylidene diphosphonate for the treatment of painful osseous metastases.* Sem. Nucl. Med., XXII, **1**, 33–40.

Metz O. *et al.* (1982). *Meningosis prophylaxis with intrathecal ^{198}Au-colloid and methotrexate in childhood acute lyphocytic leukaemia.* Cancer, **49**, 224–228.

National Radiological Protection Board (NRPB) (1988). *Guidance notes for the protection of persons against ionising radiations arising from medical and dental use.* Her Majesty's Stationery Office, London.

Park C.H. *et al.* (1987). *Treatment of hepatocellular carcinoma (HCC) with radiolabeled Lipiodol: a preliminary report.* Nucl. Med. Commun., **8**, 1075–1087.

Pectasides D. *et al.* (1986). *Antibody-guided irradiation of malignant pleural and pericardial effusions.* Br. J. Cancer, **53**, 727–732.

Perkins A.C. and Pimm M.V. (1991). *Immunoscintigraphy: Practical Aspects and Clinical Applications.* Wiley Liss publishers.

Pollack I.F. *et al.* (1988). *Stereotaxic intracavitary irradiation for cystic craniopharyngiomas.* J. Neurosurg., **68**, 227–233.

Potsaid M.S. *et al.* (1978). *(^{32}P) diphosphonate dose determination in patients with bone metastases from prostate carcinoma.* J. Nucl. Med., **19**, 98–104.

Reiners C. (1990). *"Radioiodine therapy of Graves disease" pp 226–239. In* "The Various Types of Hyperthyroidism" Ed. D. Reinwein and P.C. Scriba, Urban & Schwarzenberg, Munich-Vienna-Baltimore.

Robinson R.G. (1992). *Radionuclide therapy of intractable bone pain: Emphasis on strontium-89.* Sem. Nucl. Med., **16**, 439.

Roeslar H. *et al.* (1990). *Superselective ^{90}Y-resin embolization therapy of solid tumors.* Eur. J. Nucl. Med., **16**, 439.

Rosenheim N.B. *et al.* (1979). *Radiocolloids in the treatment of ovarian cancer.* Obstet. Gynecol Surv., **34**, 708.

Sackmann Muriel F. *et al.* (1976). *Remission maintenance therapy for meningeal leukaemia intrathecal methotrexate and dexamethasone versus intrathecal craniospinal irradiation and with a radiocolloid.* Br. J. Haematol. **33**, 119–127.

Shapiro B. *et al.* (1985). *Iodine-131 metaiodo-benzyguanidine for the location of suspected phaeochromocytoma: experience in 400 cases.* J. Nucl. Med., **26**, 576–585.

Silberstein E.B. *et al.* (1992). *Phosphorus-32 radiopharmaceuticals for the treatment of painful osseous metastases.* Semin. Nuc. Med., XXII, **1**, 17–27.

Silberstein E.B. (1979). *Radionuclide therapy of hematologic disorders.* Semin. Nucl. Med., **IX**, 100–107.

Solanki K.K. *et al.* (1992). *A pharmacological guide to medicines which interfere with the biodistribution of radiolabelled metaiodo-benylguanidine (MIBG).* Nucl. Med. Commun., **13**, 513–521.

Spooren P.F.M.J. *et al.* (1985). *Synovectomy of the knee with ^{90}Y.* Eur. J. Nucl. Med., **10**, 441–445.

Stewart J.S.W. *et al.* (1988). *Intraperitoneal ^{131}I- and ^{90}Y-labelled monoclonal antibodies for ovarian cancer: Pharmacokinetics and normal tissue dosimetry.* Int. J. Cancer Suppl., **3**, 71–76.

Stewart J.S.W. *et al.* (1990). *Intraperitoneal yttrium-90-labelled monoclonal antibody in ovarian cancer.* J. Clin. Oncol., **8**, 1941–1950.

Strauss L. *et al.* (1982). *Radioisotope therapy of cystic craniopharyngiomas.* Int. J. Radiat. Oncol. Biol. Phys., **8**, 1581–1585.

Varia M. *et al.* (1988). *Intraperitoneal chromic phosphate therapy after second-look laporotomy for ovarian cancer.* Cancer **61**, 919–927.

Ward E. *et al.* (1989). *Binding activities of a repertoire of single immunoglobulin variable domains secreted from Escherichia coli.* Nature, **341**, 544–546.

Wasserman L.R. *et al.* (1981). *Influence of therapy in causes of death in polycythemia vera.* Trans. Assoc. Am. Physicians, **94**, 30–38.

Wheldon T.E. and O'Donoghue J.A. (1990). *The radiobiology of targeted radiotherapy.* Int. J. Radiat. Biol., **58**, 1–21.

Wheldon T.E. *et al.* (1988). *Strategies for systemic radiotherapy of micrometastases using antibody targeted ^{131}I.* Radiother. Oncol., **11**, 133–142.

Winfield J. and Gumpel J.M. (1979). *An evaluation of repeat intra-articular injections of yttrium-90 colloids in persistent synovitis of the knee.* Ann. Rheum. Dis., **38**, 145–147.

Workman P. (1992). *Bioreductive mechanisms.* Int. J. Radiat. Oncol., Biol. and Phys., **22**, 631–637.

Yumoto Y. *et al.* (1985). *Hepatocellular carcinoma detected by iodized oil.* Radiology, **154**, 19–24.

Ziessman H.A. *et al.* (1984). *Hepatic arterial perfusion scintigraphy with Tc-99m MAA.* Radiology, **152**, 167–172.

Chapter 23

Adverse Reactions and Untoward Events Associated with the Use of Radiopharmaceuticals

D.H. Keeling

23.1 INTRODUCTION

For many centuries, the golden rule governing medications was that they should do no harm – *primum non nocere* – and not a lot was seriously expected of genuine efficacy beyond what faith and hope could achieve. It is only in comparatively recent times with the scientific study of disease and its treatment that potent and biologically active medicines have come into widespread use but this in turn has led to the maxim that unless a drug is capable of doing some harm, it is unlikely to do much good. Experience has shown there is much truth in this.

The series of disasters culminating in the thalidomide experience prompted many nations to introduce legislation covering drug safety though there was still less regulatory concern regarding efficacy. In the United Kingdom it was not until the Medicines Act of 1968 that the three separate factors of safety, quality and efficacy were brought together. Many countries in Europe and North America as well as Australia and Japan started national reporting schemes for adverse reactions during the 1960's – some meeting with more success than others (Griffin 1987). This era also saw the first widespread use of radiopharmaceuticals. Many, principally due to labelling with short-lived radionuclides, were of necessity produced 'in house' often using materials not always available in pharmaceutical grade. The national schemes were designed to cover the larger field of therapeutic medicines and rather assumed that quality assurance rested with the commercial sources. Radiopharmaceuticals therefore frequently fell outside the scope of these schemes and their use by a small specialist group of hospital doctors not usually involved with therapeutic drugs did not help. It was scarcely surprising that little or no useful feedback to nuclear medicine came from these national schems. This, together with the subsequent recognition that occasional reactions to radiopharmaceuticals did indeed occur led a number of national professional bodies to organise their own schemes (see Keeling, 1986) – rather as radiologists had done with X-ray contrast reactions (Ansell, 1987).

23.2 DEFINITIONS

Radiopharmaceuticals are almost invariably administered in very small (chemical) quantities and on only one or two occasions to any individual. Definitions of adverse reactions to therapeutic drugs cannot be used for radiopharmaceuticals without slight modification. Diagnostic agents make up the majority of radiopharmaceuticals and no therapeutic or pharmacological effects are looked for – but then there are also therapeutic radiopharmaceuticals. Do these require a separate definition? Misadministrations and maladministrations are again separate issues, though equally unfortunate from the recipient's point of view (NCRP Comm. 7). Cordova *et al.* (1986) have reviewed this question in some detail and propose a composite definition:

1. The reaction is an unexpected or unusual and undesirable clinical manifestation resulting from the administration of the radiopharmaceutical.
2. The reaction is associated with the vehicle carrying the radiation and not with the radiation itself.
3. The reaction does not result from an overdose which is more properly classified as maladministration.
4. The reaction is not a result of injury caused by poor injection technique.

Many would agree with this strict definition of an adverse reaction due to the acute pharmacological effects of administration of a radiopharmaceutical though the exclusion of any early radiation effects is arbitrary. The definition of 'overdose' is not always clear-cut either for the pharmaceutical or its radioactive label. It is often impossible to tell whether any single acute 'reaction' to administration of a radiopharmaceutical is due to one of the materials injected, or to the injection technique—or a combination of both. The outcome of clumsy injection technique probably depends as much on the patient's constitution as on the operator's skill—or lack of it. From the patient's point of view and from that of the responsible physician, these other factors are no less relevant and need not be less important. Perhaps, to avoid fruitless controversy, it is better to use the term 'adverse reaction' in its strict pharmacological definition as given above and to group these other problems as 'untoward effects'.

Some have suggested that failure of a normal expected radiopharmaceutical behaviour should also be classified as an untoward effect. However, decisions about this would of necessity be subjective and in many cases it would be unclear whether the problem lay with the formulation of the radiopharmaceutical, with its pharmacokinetics or with the patient's own biochemistry. In some cases more than one of these factors would be operating and it does not seem helpful to bring in problems of reliability of a pharmaceutical or technique to the question of adverse reaction and untoward effect. These matters have been more fully discussed by Lazarus and Maisey (1987).

As the range of nuclear medicine investigations diversifies, there has been an increase in the use of other medicines as part or preparation for these studies. Cardiac stress studies and renal blood flow and autonomic control typify these newer procedures and each brings its own potential hazards, to which may be added the fear and anxiety of the patient with attendant vasomotor changes. These factors are not considered here, but are no less relevant for the safety of the patient.

23.3 CLASSIFICATION

Classifications of adverse drug reactions have been proposed under such various headings as over-dosage, intolerance, side-effects, secondary effects, idiosyncracy and hypersensitivity.

The widely used scheme of Rawlings and Thompson (1981) attempts to divide adverse reactions into just two varieties. Type A is dose related and represents an exaggerated but otherwise normal response to the pharmaceutical. These are reactions occurring in subjects at the extreme of the dose-response curve for pharmacological effect and are essentially predictable, relatively common but rarely serious. If large enough doses of the material were administered, they would occur in most subjects. The threshold for such reactions may be lowered by illness, increased absorption, alteration in protein binding or metabolism or by delayed excretion. Some of these effects may be exacerbated by interaction with other drugs. Effects due to transient high blood levels following rapid injection, avoidable by slower infusion could also be considered Type A effects, as would many examples of 'toxicity' of drugs.

The Type B reactions are aberrant effects, unexpected and unpredictable from the known normal pharmacology of the drug and not clearly dose related. They are usually rare events but can be serious. This group would include the immunological and pharmacogenetic mechanisms of adverse reactions. The former would include the hypersensitivity phenomena including anaphylaxis, immune complex reactions with complement activation and the occasional serum sickness type effect which may show fever, polyarthralgia, urticaria or macular erythematous rashes. Patients may be genetically predisposed to immunological reaction, but pharmacognetic problems, as exemplified by the precipitation of acute porphyria by certain drugs, have not been recognised amongst radiopharmaceutical reactions.

23.4 RADIATION EFFECTS

The administration of a radiopharmaceutical to a patient inevitably results in some radiation dose to that patient. Therapeutic radiopharmaceuticals not infrequently show potential for 'untoward events' such as the sudden release of thyroid hormones which may occur when radioablation of substantial amounts of thyroid tissue is undertaken; this can be anticipated and treated with antithyroid medication and beta blockade. The use of sialogogues will lessen the danger of radiation sialadenitis, a side effect which otherwise increases with repeated large doses of I-131 for thyroid cancer. A significant proportion of thyroid cancer patients, treated with I-131, develop nausea and may vomit in the following 12 to 24 hours. It is not always avoidable by intravenous administration and is probably due to local acute radiation effects in the gastro-intestinal tract. Here enterochromaffin cells release 5-hydroxy tryptamine which, via vagal stimulation, can trigger the vomiting centre in the brain stem. Dopamine antagonists such as metoclopramide are useful, but selective 5-hydroxy tryptamine receptor antagonists such as ondansetron would be preferable. The cost of these newer drugs should be more than offset by the saving in radionuclide costs from repeat treatment, time saved by effective patient treatment and not least, the avoidance of contamination of hospital rooms etc.

Great care is needed in the selection of patients for treatment of widespread marrow malignancy with Sr-89, Sm-153 or P-32 or the combined effect of the disease plus radiation may lead to bone marrow failure. Y-90 silicate colloid used for radiosynovectomy can, rarely, cause a transient synovitis with acute effusion, even in the absence of any obvious bleeding into the joint space. The silicate colloid preparation is rather alkaline and this may be the cause, but the possibility of pyogenic arthritis will often lead to a need for repeat arthrocentesis for diagnostic purposes.

Even diagnostic radiopharmaceuticals have been incriminated as causing radiation damage. (Shapiro, Pillay and Cox 1987) when clearance is delayed. Some of these possible extravasation effects can be classified as misadministration though part of the problem may lie in the patient's reaction and other therapy. All this is in addition to the long term potential for somatic or genetic damage (Sarker *et al.* 1976; Edmonds and Smith 1986) though with most modern diagnostic radiopharmaceuticals, this risk seems extremely small but must always be borne in mind whenever a nuclear medicine technique is undertaken. Knowledge of these 'untoward effects' with radiopharmaceuticals may be clinically valuable.

23.5 PHARMACOLOGY OF HYPERSENSITIVE REACTIONS

The mechanisms of allergic or hypersensitive reactions to radiopharmaceuticals should theoretically correspond to the general groupings of hypersensitivity reactions classified by Coombs & Gill Types I to IV. (Grahame-Smith and Aronson 1992). Type I is the immediate hypersensitivity reaction or anaphylaxis. These usually present with urticaria or angiooedema, asthma – from trivial wheezing to severe bronchospasm – and anaphylactic shock. Type II cytotoxic reactions occur when a circulating antibody interacts with the radiopharmaceutical hapten fixed to a protein cell membrane constituent to form an antigen antibody complex which then activates complement. Type III reactions involve immune complex deposition in tissues, again with complement activation and damage to capillary endothelium: serum docknes is the name still used for many examples of this reaction. Type IV cell mediated reactions are a form of delayed hypersensitivity exemplified by contact dermatitis.

In practice, whilst it may be desirable to classify reactions ultimately on this pharmacological basis, drug reactions occur in less clear-cut clinical syndromes with fever, rigors, nausea and a variety of rashes including urticarial and erythematous eruptions, cutaneous vasculitis and chest and loin pain. Respiratory problems with dyspnoea and varying degrees of bronchial constriction are certainly seen as are vasomotor problems with hypotension. These in turn can lead to faintness, loss of consciousness, epileptiform movements or precipitation of true epilepsy.

23.5.1 Skin Reactions

Skin eruptions are the commonest forms of adverse reaction to therapeutic drugs and can often be classified into the Types I to IV described above (Bruinsma, 1986; Wintroub, Stern *et al.* 1987; Felix and Smith 1991). For radiopharmaceuticals, with their very short exposure and small quantity administered, a more limited clinical picture is seen. Thus no cases of exfoliative dermatitis, bullous eruptions, changes in pigmentation, lichenoid or fixed drug eruptions have been described, but toxic erythema, pruritis, 'hives', urticaria and erythema multiforme-like states are well recognised and cutaneous vasculitis and purpura occur. All these are Type B (Rawlings & Thompson) – bizarre, unpredictable (in the first instance) and apparently due to hypersensitivity.

Urticaria, angioedema and pruritis can develop within minutes of radiopharmaceutical administration. The maculopapular and 'morbilliform' rashes of toxic erythema, well known with methylene diphosphonate, usually come on within a few hours and may last several days. Treatment with a non-sedative H_1 blocking antihistamine such as terfenadine 60 mg b.d. or cetirizine 10 mg orally for two days is usually successful in alleviating symptoms. Cutaneous vasculitis is occasionally noted but over a longer time scale – many days. The blood disorders relating to marrow suppression, frequently a serious problem with therapeutic drugs, have not been described with diagnostic radiopharmaceuticals.

23.5.2 Anaphylactic Shock

This uncommon manifestation of allergy is the most serious with fatal potential. It is a systemic reaction which occurs as a result of a massive immunoglobulin (usually IgE) triggered response with release of bioactive agents. A variety of substances such as proteins, polysaccharides and simple organic chemicals can act as the antigen to induce the hypersensitivity. (Bochner & Lichtenstein 1991; Brueton *et al.* 1991). Most radiopharmaceuticals are small molecules or even inorganic chemicals and presumably act as haptens in association with native protein; in practice an initial sensitising exposure to the material is often not found. The B lymphocyte produced antibodies circulate to become fixed to the surface of mast cells and basophils and their site of tissue location will effect the subsequent manifestation of the anaphylactic reaction. Reaction with antigen results in the immediate release of histamine, kinins, leukotrienes and other bioactive autacoids and can rapidly lead to collapse, coma and death. With some radiopharmaceuticals, this chain of reaction is not seen, though the end result is the same and classified, therefore, as 'anaphylactoid' reaction. The main effects are thought to be due to local histamine release (Laurence and Bennett, 1992). Since anti-histamines (either H_1 or H_2 type) are competitive inhibitors of histamine, they are much more effective when used before histamine release. Reversal of the effects of histamine release are more readily achieved clinically by physiological antagonism by adrenaline which is the first line of treatment in life threatening allergic reactions. In severely collapsed patients, subcutaneous and even intra muscular injection of adrenaline may be ineffective and the intravenous route can be used, at suitable dilution, but cardiac arrest facilities should be on hand. Adrenaline will also be absorbed from the lungs and, in extreme emergency, can be given by intra-tracheal injection, or inhalation. Glucocorticoids have numerous effects which interfere with immune reactions. However, they take some time to act and although intravenous hydrocortisone is generally recommended in severe anaphylaxis it is by no means clear how effective this is in the critical acute phase; much the same is true for parenterally administered H_1 antihistamines which are almost always used. Restoration of blood volume and pressure is vital, as is adequate oxygenation. The airway may be compromised by glottic or laryngeal oedema and early intubation may be required to avoid emergency tracheostomy (Guyton, 1976; Keeling, 1988).

23.5.3 Vasovagal Reactions

The vasomotor centre in the medulla is a diffuse area of the reticular formation extending from the floor of the fourth ventricle up towards the pyramids. Connecting nerve fibres run to all the dorsal and upper lumbar segments with the sympathetic nervous system and control vasoconstrictor tone in the arterioles and hence peripheral resistance and blood pressure. The centre receives afferents from higher centres in the brain as well as from the aortic arch body and the carotid sinuses, sensitive to both blood pressure and chemoreceptor stimulation, and is directly responsive to changes in blood O_2 and CO_2 levels. Excessive vagal activity slowing the heart is mainly due to separate direct stimulation of the cardioinhibitory centre.

Vasomotor syncope is responsible for simple faints where the cause is primarily from higher cerebral centres. The loss of consciousness is due to sudden hypotension and cerebral anoxia from widespread vasodilatation and bradycardia with resulting marked drop in the cardiac output. Whilst certain subjects are more liable to suffer fainting attacks, fear and anxiety undoubtedly contribute to this problem. Neurogenic release of adrenaline may additionally predispose to cardiac arythmias with attendant complications and cardiac arrests have been documented in just this situation.

23.5.4 Other Hypersensitivity and Undefined Effects

Reaction to intravenous injection per se is common and not confined to the obviously nervous anxious patient. Difficulties in entering the vein lumen will prolong discomfort and extravasation of blood or radiopharmaceutical cause additional pain. Local discomfort may also be exacerbated by rapid injection, excessive volume, irritant chemicals, unduly high or low temperatures or unphysiological osmolarity. These conditions will also produce transient high blood levels which may effect chemo and osmo-receptors in the heart and major vessels and have a passing effect on the central nervous system itself. A radiopharmaceutical given as a single bolus injection in one second will reach the lung capillaries at a concentration approximately 170 times that of the ultimate circulation equilibrium level. Since so many radiopharmaceuticals rapidly diffuse into the extracellular space, the equilibrium blood levels are further reduced and a fast i.v. bolus can pass the lungs and reach sensitive centres at a concentration of the order of 500 times that calculated for its ultimate volume of distribution. Many radiopharmaceuticals show binding with plasma proteins and are less pharmacologically active in this form but in the first few seconds, before mixing is complete, free radiopharmaceutical levels will be high. Other medications such as non-steroidal anti-inflammatory drugs which bind strongly with albumin may reduce available binding sites for 'acidic' radiopharmaceuticals. For 'basic' radiopharmaceuticals lipoproteins play a more important role and levels are reduced in pregnancy and patients on the contraceptive pill. It is not uncommon for patients to note the transient high concentration as a strange or unpleasant taste in the mouth; many patients mention this immediately after i.v. injection of the myocardial imaging agent 2-methoxy isobutyl isonitrile (MIBI), and the anxious patient will appreciate being forewarned. The use of central venous lines for administration of (i.v.) radiopharmaceutical doses – not infrequently accompanied by badly bruised or thrombosed peripheral veins – brings two factors into play. The first is the high concentration possible in the central circulation of radiopharmaceutical noted above and another is loss of dose in the lumen or onto the wall of the central line, or the 'labelling' of small platelet thrombi not infrequently dislodged from their ends by the bolus of fluid.

Untoward effects due to intravenous injection have been recognised for many years. A well-documented example (Hald *et al.* 1988) occurred when, unknown to the healthy young male subject, the injection was only the control – normal saline. He became pale and dizzy at three minutes with a blood pressure of 69/45mm Hg, the heart rate dropped slightly with a weak pulse and the E.C.G. showed absence of the P-wave, interpreted as SA-block with nodal rhythm. In addition minor changes in several coagulation parameters were noted, possibly secondary to pressor amine output.

In practice it may be very difficult to differentiate between adverse reaction to a radiopharmaceutical and a vasovagal reaction from higher centres to the procedure. Histamine and several kinins produce marked vasodilatation and some immunological reactions therefore show marked vasomotor abnormalities.

The plasma substitutes dextran, gelatine, polyvinyl pyrolidone (PVP) and heta-starch have been variously used in nuclear medicine for a number of years. Several commercial kit preparations for technetium radiopharmaceuticals also contain poloxamers. Dextran and methyl cellulose compounds can be used as sedimentation aids in the separation of blood cell fractions prior to labelling. Reactions (Black *et* al. 1975) have been reported where sufficient of the sedimentation agent has either been carried through the labelling process or has been added again in supernatent plasma for the final resuspension. The presence of the sedimentation agent in the final preparation is unwanted and proper technique and methodology should see that the possibility does not arise. Of the plasma volume substitutes, hetastarch seems the safest in terms of unwanted side effects, but all available colloid volume substitutes carry a risk of anaphylactoid reaction (Ring and Messmer, 1977) and even human serum albumin is not free from life-threatening anaphylactoid reactions.

The introduction of radio-labelled antibodies or their fragments for scintigraphic investigations and therapy brings with it the obvious possibility of foreign protein reactions including anaphylaxis. Monoclonal antibodies and their fragments are produced in hybridoma cultures involving malignant myeloma cells and sensitised lymphocytes from animals – usually mice. The tissue cultures are known to contain animal viruses though measures are taken during production and purification to separate and inactivate any living particles.

At present relatively few mono (or poly) clonal antibody reactions have been reported to national schemes but in many centres, patients with a history of allergy to foreign protein or atopy are considered unsuitable and furthermore, where an intradermal skin test has been used to detect hypersensitivity, patients showing a positive reaction have not been further investigated. This may well have avoided some potentially serious reactions though doubts have been raised about the wisdom of prior intradermal injection. A negative skin test result does not preclude the possibility of anaphylaxis and there is evidence to suggest this route may be a more potent method of sensitizing patients than the intravenous route used for the investigation proper. One principle role of immunoscintigraphy is for the detection of recurrent malignant disease with the repeated use of an antibody for serial imaging. The induction of the patient's own antibodies to the imaging agent – usually mouse protein – is common and not often indicated by the preliminary skin test. Such human anti-mouse antibodies (HAMA) can and do affect scan quality though they are not necessarily associated with clinical symptoms (Perkins *et al.* 1988). They can also interfere with the serum assay of tumour markers such as CA125 (Sykes *et al.* 1990).

Most reporting schemes including the present U.K. radiopharmaceutical system have noted a higher proportion of patients with atopic histories including hay fever, asthma or food allergies. In particular those exhibiting hypersensitivity reactions to other (therapeutic) drugs seem more likely to produce problems with certain radiopharmaceuticals. However, the probability is still too low for it to be of any useful clinical guidance; indeed the likelihood of hypersensitive reaction in patients with known circulating antibodies is not clear cut. This would correspond with the well known immunological enigma that not all patients showing an immunological response to an allergen develop symptomatic allergy – hypersensitivity – to the antigen. It is likely that the immunological reaction which can be demonstrated by laboratory techniques is, in some cases, irrelevant but refinements in technique and new understanding may lead to better predictions.

23.6 PYROGENS

Pyrogens are certain proteins and polysaccharides produced by the metabolism or breakdown of micro organisms. They are soluble and hence not removed by ultra-filtration and being heat stable, unaltered by autoclave sterilization. The commonest are endotoxin products of bacterial metabolism and can be introduced into radiopharmaceuticals in many ways. Although certain exchange columns are commercially available which claim to remove pyrogens, the only reliable technique is to ensure that radiopharmaceuticals start and finish pyrogen-free. The use of tested water, glassware air sterilized at 175° for two hours and pharmaceutical quality chemicals should avoid the introduction of pyrogens but in nuclear medicine a number of the starting materials for radiopharmaceutical production have not been available in guaranteed pyrogen-free form. Fortunately the small volumes of most radiopharmaceutical injections means that even by the intravenous route, symptoms are unlikely but special care is required for the intra-thecal route. The introduction of radionuclide cisternography and localisation of CSF leaks into clinical practice was followed by a high incidence of aseptic meningitis due to pyrogens. All the materials involved had passed the standard pharmacopoeial rabbit test for pyrogens and were sterile. The cases were not even confined to a single type of radiopharmaceutical, both iodine and technetium labelled albumin preparations, colloids and chelated compounds were involved. The demonstration by Cooper and Harbert (1975) using the limulus amoebocyte test demonstrated bacterial endotoxin at levels insufficient to be detected by the standard method (approximately one thousandfold less sensitive). Phosphate buffers or exchange resins were contaminated and although subsequent dilution reduced the pyrogen levels below those detected by the usual methods, intrathecal injection in man caused severe meningism. Awareness of the problem has greatly reduced the incidence of this untoward effect – no cases have been reported in the U.K. system for several years though in the U.S.A., six cases were reported in 1987 (which were the majority of the serious reactions requiring hospitalisation). It is important to differentiate between pyrogen induced meningitis and the meningism and headache associated with altered CSF pressure or bleeding following cisternal or lumbar puncture.

23.7 STERILITY

All centres producing in-house radiopharmaceuticals should check sterility with random tests of their products. In some countries it may be deemed necessary, for legal reasons, to check each preparation. If radiopharmaceuticals are produced by a reliable aseptic technique using suitable starting materials, there is little opportunity for micro-organisms to gain access (Sorensen, Kristensen & Frandsen, 1977) and less for their multiplication because of the short interval between preparation and use. Radiopharmaceuticals vary considerably as growth media for micro-organisms. Some discourage bacterial growth whilst in others, only very limited multiplication occurs, as demonstrated by Abra, Bell and Horton, 1980. Because of this, sterility testing long after the possible contamination of the radiopharmaceutical with micro-organisms, is of limited value. The result of deliberate inoculation of bacteria into non-radioactive radiopharmaceuticals ranges from death, through bare survival to active growth, and in the presence of usual levels of radioactivity, most bacteria die or barely survive. This was well demonstrated by Brown and Baker (1986) and meaningful tests of sterility must therefore take place very shortly after preparation, without awaiting radioactive decay. Soluble and colloidal radiopharmaceuticals could be tested by ultrafiltration, microbial contamination being retained on the filter and separated from radioactive materials and separately cultured. For particulate preparations, dilution into larger volumes of a suitable broth growth medium would be more convenient. Unfortunately these techniques with radioactive materials do make for handling difficulties and are often unwelcome in hospital microbiological departments. A practical solution is for all radiopharmaceutical types to be randomly tested by inoculation into a larger volume of growth media. This is incubated in a shielded container in the nuclear medicine pharmacy and passed to the microbiology department when sufficiently decayed. A fuller discussion is to be found elsewhere in this book (Chapter 12). Despite this, lack of sterility has not been reported as a cause of adverse reaction or untoward effect in radiopharmaceuticals in the U.K. for many years. This does not of course mean that 100% of all preparations have been sterile.

23.8 REPORTING SCHEMES

Adverse reactions to radiopharmaceuticals are rare events and it was early appreciated that to get significant numbers of reports, schemes would have to be organised on a large scale, preferably national. Such schemes are in operation in North America, the United Kingdom and twelve European countries (which, with others, contribute to an overall European scheme), Japan and Australia. Reporting schemes vary from country to country. Some define adverse reactions closely and thus look only for relatively acute pharmacological reaction and would therefore not include mal-administration, overdosage or radiation effects. Others with a pharmacy bias are also interested in problems in packaging, labelling, generator efficiency, contaminants and aberrations of in vivo behaviour.

Radiopharmaceutical problems in Japan are monitored by the Radiopharmaceutical Safety Sub-committee of the Japanese Radioisotope Association who have well over 600 reports on file since 1975.

The U.S. scheme has been altered slightly in recent years and uses a single double sided form for adverse reactions and radiopharmaceutical defects. The same is now true in the U.K. and it is hoped the other European countries in the EANM scheme will adopt this basic format, with reports collected by national professional society representatives before entry into the European scheme. The interpretation of cause:effect relationship remains a problem but criteria do exist to help here and larger numbers assist this with earlier recognition of patterns of reaction. The United Kingdom scheme not only solicits information on any possible adverse reaction even where the cause and effect relationship is questionable but also looks for other untoward effects or possible (shorter-term) problems with radiation.

In the U.K., there have been two separate schemes but these now share a single report form. The organisation of the national scheme is sponsored by the professional bodies involved, namely the British Nuclear Medicine Society, the Royal College of Radiologists, the Radiopharmacy group of the British Nuclear Medicine Society, the Hospital Physicists Association and the British Institute of Radiology and the British Nuclear Medicine Society provide the forum for collection. All adverse reaction reports are passed to the medical assessor (currently the present author). Pharmaceutical defect reports are dealt with by a radiopharmacist (Dr. S. Hesslewood) who also collates the European scheme reports. A new Drug Defect Reporting Form is currently under review.

The U.K. proforma (Figure 1) asks for relatively few details as long and involved forms discourage reporting, particularly if some details are not available. The number of reports is not large and the assessors, apart from acknowledging the reports, can contact informants for further particulars.

No direct involvement of a licencing or regulatory authority arises, but reports are in turn passed to the Committee on Safety of Medicines at the U.K. Department of Health for inclusion in the national computer bank of reports. Apart from contributing to the general knowledge about reactions, this could also bring useful feedback to nuclear medicine if some (non-radioactive) material or excipient were found to be a potential problem.

Details are also passed to the European Reporting Scheme, sponsored by the Committee on Radiopharmaceuticals of the

Confidential

Details will not be disclosed to any person without the express permission of the person submitting this report, but all reports are "banked" with your National Adverse Reaction Scheme and the European Reporting Scheme.

REPORT OF AN ADVERSE REACTION ATTRIBUTED TO A RADIOPHARMACEUTICAL

1 Patient . . . . Initials . . . . Hosp No . . . .

Age . . . . Sex . . . . Date of Study . . . .

Nature of Study . . . .

. . . .

Clinical Diagnosis . . . .

2 **Radiopharmaceutical** Radionuclide . . . . Chemical Form . . . .

Brief details of materials, sources, preparation and storage . . . .

. . . .

. . . .

. . . .

Has a commercial manufacturer been informed ? **Yes/No**

3 **Nature of Reaction** Timing, symptoms and clinical observations . . . .

. . . .

. . . .

. . . .

. . . .

Has the patient any known allergies etc ? . . . .

4 Other medications currently or recently taken . . . .

. . . .

5 Treatment of the Reaction. Drugs and Resuscitative measures required . . . .

. . . .

. . . .

. . . .

6 Can you estimate the frequency of this reaction ? . . . .

7 Any other comments . . . .

. . . .

. . . .

Signed . . . . Name . . . .

Address . . . .

. . . .

Please return this completed form to your National Scheme Co-ordinator at the address shown opposite, marked "Confidential".

Figure 1

European Association of Nuclear Medicine. This wider scheme is an attempt to gather sufficient numbers of reports, despite a very low incidence. Results to date (Kristensen, 1992) suggest that individual reporting on a European scale is not yet workable, and it is only the few European countries with successful national schemes which contribute useful data. Efforts are currently being made to help countries which do not yet contribute to build up their own national schemes. The European Assessor till 1991 was Dr. K. Kristensen who has kindly provided a twelve year assessment (Table 1) of the commoner reports, but the data is unduly influenced by the U.K. contribution.

TABLE 1
European Reaction Report Data 1979–1990
Radiopharmaceuticals with more the 5 reports

	Type of Adverse Reaction				
	Allergic	*Vasovagal*	*Local*	*Other*	*Total*
Tc99m Radiopharmaceuticals					
Albumin Microcolloid	11	5	1	0	17
Albumin Microspheres	3	3	0	1	7
MAA	9	2	1	3	15
DTPA	9	34	0	2	45
MDP	23	15	1	13	52
RBC Label	5	3	0	2	10
HMDP	2	3	0	1	6
Colloids	12	2	2	4	20
DMSA	4	0	0	1	5
Mag3	0	5	0	1	6
Total	78	72	5	28	183
Non-Tc99m Radiopharmaceuticals					
I123 MIBG	3	2	0	12	17
I131 MIBG	2	1	0	2	5
I131/Se75 Cholesterol	10	0	0	0	10
I123/I131 Hippuran	4	1	0	1	6
Ga67 Citrate	4	0	0	3	7
T1201 Chloride	1	0	1	3	5
Total	24	4	1	21	50

Total of all reports = 311. **Overall Total = 233.**
From data kindly supplied by Dr. K. Kristensen.

23.9 INTERPRETATION OF REPORTS

A true causal relationship between the administration of a radiopharmaceutical and the reaction observed is very difficult to prove in many cases. (Rhodes and Wagner, 1974). The data recorded on the adverse report forms is limited, necessarily subjective and the patient is commonly on other drugs which may not be completely listed. Cordova, Hladik and Rhodes (1984) detail an algorithm which attempts to objectively assess the probability of causal relationship. Reviewing 277 cases, they rated only 17% as "definitely" due to the radiopharmaceutical though a further 40% were 'probably' so. 36% were 'possible' and just 7% 'unlikely' due to the radiopharmaceutical.

Most of the reactions were, as noted by others, of an allergic nature and the limited spectrum of clinical presentations is in no way unique to radiopharmaceuticals. Timing and the establishment of a recognisable pattern of reaction to an individual radiopharmaceutical provide the best pointers.

23.10 RESULTS OF REPORTING SCHEMES

Following sporadic case reports in the literature and doubtless rather more remembered but unreported problems, the Society of Nuclear Medicine in the U.S.A. sponsored the first survey of adverse reactions to radiopharmaceuticals in 1970 and Atkins *et al.* published their early results in 1972. A total of 142 cases were noted with the largest group involving colloidal preparations of Tc-99m and In-113m. A relatively high incidence following the use of intrathecal preparations was evident at that early date. Since that time, results from the North American experience have been published (Ford *et al.* 1978; Rhodes and Cordova; 1980, Cordova *et al.* 1982; Atkins, 1986) and note an apparent decrease in incidence, though this was felt to be less due to improved radiopharmaceutical quality than to reduced reporting of minor problems. At the same time, similar problems were being noted in nuclear medicine practice in the United Kingdom and the professional bodies involved set up a joint reporting scheme with the first report, including a backlog of earlier problems, published by E. Williams in 1974. This drew attention to a relatively high incidence of severe reactions, including some fatal, following the use of ferric hydroxide precipitate used as a lung scanning agent, coprecipitated with In-113m. Although the incidence seemed to vary between different producers, no satisfactory method of reliable prevention or treatment (Keeling 1979) was found and advice was given that this material no longer be used.

Japanese data up to and including 1989 is available when 22 adverse reports were received from just over 900,000 radiopharmaceutical doses. The data in Table 2 is collated from the decade 1980 to 1989 and taken from the 12th report of the Radioisotope Safety Sub-committee which appeared in the Japanese medical literature. Some details were made

TABLE 2
Japanese Reaction Report Data 1978–1989

Tc99m Radiopharmaceuticals	*1978–1981*		*1982–1985*		*1986–1989*	
	No.	*%*	*No.*	*%*	*No.*	*%*
DTPA	13	50	10	38	17	41
DTPA/HSA	0	0	0	0	1	2
HSA	1	4	1	4	0	0
MAA	1	4	1	4	1	2
Microspheres	0	0	0	0	1	2
PYP/RBC	4	15	8	31	9	22
EHDP	1	4	0	0	0	0
MDP	3	12	4	15	5	12
HMDP	0	0	0	0	1	2
Colloids	1	4	2	8	2	5
Other	2	8	0	0	4	10
Total	26		26		41	

27% of reactions 1978–1989 Total = 93
46% of reactions 1986–1989

Non Tc99m Radiopharmaceuticals	*1978–1981*		*1982–1985*		*1986–1989*	
	No.	*%*	*No.*	*%*	*No.*	*%*
I131 Hippuran	54	46	46	52	19	39
I131 Adosterol	49	42	31	35	22	45
Se75 Cholesterols	1	1	4	5	0	0
Ga67 Citrate	4	3	6	7	3	6
TI201 Chloride	0	0	0	0	2	4
In111 DTPA	7	6	1	1	0	0
I131 Therapy	0	0	0	0	1	2
I131 Diagnostic	2	2	0	0	0	0
Other	1	1	0	0	2	4
Total	118		88		49	

73% of reactions 1978–1989 Total = 255
54% of reactions 1986–1989 **Overall Total = 348**

From data kindly supplied by Professor Y. Sasaki.

available courtesy of the Chairman, Professor Y. Sasaki and some notable differences are immediately obvious compared to the U.K. and European experience. A large number and a relatively high incidence of reports is seen to radiocholesterol radiopharmaceuticals, principally I-131 Adosterol (methylnorcholesterol). I-131 hippuran with 98 reports – 34% of the total—shows an incidence figure approximately one reaction per 5,500 doses. Also notable are the 12 reports attributed to Gallium-67 citrate though with 135,000 doses used in 1989 alone, the incidence figure is under 1:50,000 doses. Technetium radiopharmaceuticals over this decade make up only 29% of the total. The small number of reports attributed to the diphosphonates is in contrast with Western European data. The U.K. experience did not suggest any one particular commercial source was associated with higher incidence reactions and though the Japanese data probably largely reflects Japanese produced radiopharmaceuticals, the interpretation up to now has been that it is the diphosphonate itself and not other excipients which is associated with skin reactions etc.

There have been many changes in the types and formulation of technetium radiopharmaceuticals used, reflected in the varying pattern of adverse reactions (Sampson and Keeling, 1982; Keeling, 1984; Keeling and Sampson, 1984; Keeling 1987; Keeling 1991). A full early summary by Shani *et al.* (1976) was more clinical in emphasis and classified reactions according to the target organ or system involved rather than radionuclide or pharmaceutical.

Table 3 contains data from the U.K. reporting series for the last 12 years from 1981 to 1992 inclusive. Divided into three periods of four years, the changing incidence pattern for some groups of radiopharmaceuticals is seen.

TABLE 3
U.K. Reaction Report Data 1981–1992

Tc99m Radiopharmaceuticals	*1981–1984*		*1985–1988*		*1989–1992*	
	No.	*%*	*No.*	*%*	*No.*	*%*
Bone and RBC agents (a)	17	46	30	39	37	39
Colloids (b)	7	19	8	10	0	0
Albumin particulates (b)	3	8	8	10	9	9
DTPA	8	22	24	31	17	18
Others	2	5	7	9	32	34
Total	37		77		95	

(a) All phosphate and phosphonate compounds.
(b) Albumin macroaggregates, microspheres, millimicrospheres and colloids are classed as 'Albumin particulates'. Total = 209

Non Tc99m Radiopharmaceuticals	*1981–1984*		*1985–1988*		*1989–1992*	
	No.	*%*	*No.*	*%*	*No.*	*%*
I123 Iodide	0	0	1	6	1	6
I131 Iodide	0	0	0	0	3	17
I123 Hippuran	1	13	2	13	0	0
I131 Hippuran	1	13	0	0	0	0
I123 MIBG	0	0	4	25	9	50
I131 MIBG	0	0	2	13	0	0
Ga67 Citrate	1	13	2	13	0	0
Se75 Cholesterol	0	0	1	6	0	0
In111 DTPA Intrathecal	1	13	0	0	0	0
All Other	4	50	4	25	5	28
Total	8		16		18	

Total = 42
Overall Total = 251

23.10.1 Colloids

Reactions from colloids in use for imaging the liver and spleen via their reticuloendothelial cell uptake were prominent but are no longer a major group. Almost all the variety of colloids described have in turn featured in reports though it is uncertain whether any particular physico-chemical form is more liable to reaction but the U.K. series does include a considerable number involving antimony sulphide colloid. The reactions have primarily involved vasomotor problems with malaise, pulse changes and lowered blood pressure. Cutaneous reactions have been relatively rare (Table 4). The majority have been relatively mild requiring no specific treatment but a small number have been serious and one fatal reaction occurred in a severely debilitated patient.

TABLE 4
Tc99m Colloids 1975–1992
28 cases/341 = 8% of total

10	Vasomotor signs/symptoms: flush, faint, bradycardia and hypotension.
9	Dyspnoea, chest/back pain.
7	Malaise, nausea, vomiting
6	Skin rash, itching
3	cases excluded as causally related some patients appear under more than one heading.

23.10.2 Albumin Particulates

These were introduced for lung perfusion scanning and occasional adverse reactions were noted. Quality control of particulate size was a particular problem in the early in-house preparation of macro-aggregates of albumin and several reactions appeared to be primarily haemodynamic following probable overdosage though the problem may have been compounded by a grossly reduced pulmonary capillary bed with pulmonary hypertension (Dworkin, Smith and Bull, 1966; J. Williams, 1974; Vincent, 1968). Bliek and Bachynski (1971) reported a more complex reaction following the administration of I-131 macroaggregates and Lugols iodine. Several reactions, however, were recognised as being of a hypersensitive nature and following the introduction of albumin microspheres the incidence of this particular problem seemed to increase, particularly in the U.S.A. where Littenberg (1975) first noted an undoubted anaphylactoid reaction to albumin microspheres. As can be seen from Table 3, this has been a minor problem in the U.K. series to date though again microspheres and millimicrospheres account for a higher proportion of adverse reactions than the general pattern of use in the U.K. would suggest. Macroaggregates, microspheres and the colloidal forms of albumin are mainly

TABLE 5
Tc99m Albumin Preparations 1975–1992
27 cases/341 = 8% of total

2	Late fatalities after MAA and DTPA, probably unrelated and due to disease.
1	Fatality immediately after intracoronary injection of MAA.
1	Cardiac arrest – resuscitated.
1	Albumin in solution – delayed sensitivity type.
6	Albumin colloids – mostly prompt anaphylaxis.
5	Microspheres – allergic type reactions.
15	Macroaggregates, some vasomotor symptoms – mostly allergic phenomena.

associated with hypersensitive-type reactions and Table 5 summarises recent U.K. experience. Of particular interest is the occurrence in recent years of cases of severe anaphylactic shock following the use of one form of albumin colloid, whereas other commercially available forms have been related to only minor problems. The preparation which has recently caused fatal anaphylactic reactions abroad contains, in addition to albumin colloid and soluble albumin, methylene diphosphonate. This material in its own right as a bone scanning agent is associated with a relatively high incidence of cutaneous reactions (vide infra).

23.10.3 Phosphates/Phosphonates

The first successful Tc-99m radiopharmaceuticals for bone scanning used polyphosphates and these caused relatively few problems. Pyrophosphate is still incriminated in very few reactions in the U.K., contrasting with Japanese experience (Tables 2 and 6). Ethane hydroxy-diphosphonate (EHDP) was rarely associated with reactions and to this day is used (in unlabelled form) in much larger doses in the treatment of Paget's disease and other diseases causing soft tissue calcification. Methylene diphosphonate (MDP) and HMDP are the most widely used radiopharmaceuticals for this purpose and account for the great majority of reactions, but bone scanning is the commonest single nuclear medicine investigation in the U.K. (Wall *et al.* 1985). Although the present author and Hoving, Roosjen and Brouwers, 1988, have noted vague early complaints including headaches in approximately 1% of all patients questioned, the commonest reported problem has been an irritative maculopapular or morbiliform rash, coming on several hours after injection and lasting up to 3–4 days. The rash appearance is non-specific and forms of toxic erythema are the commonest cutaneous drug reaction noted worldwide with all therapeutic drugs. Ramos-Gabatin *et al.* (1986), demonstrated by skin tests that one subject, sensitive to MDP and HMDP, could be safely given pyrophosphate. Occasionally the skin reaction to the

TABLE 6
Tc99m Bone and RBC Agents 1975–1992
74 cases/341 = 22% of total

PYP – 2 cases
2 Skin rashes.

HMDP – 16 cases
4 Vasomotor.
13 Allergic signs with skin reactions; 4 principally local to i.v. site. One late polyarthralgia.

MDP – 56 cases
13 Vasomotor; including faints and neurological signs. One case V.F.; resuscitated.
45 Allergic type with erythematous and urticarial rashes commonly.
Some localised near injection site. May appear up to 48 hours later.
Malaise, nausea and vomitting quite common, occasional rigor, often delayed for several hours.

Some patients appear under more than one heading.

diphosphonates is urticarial with a distribution still mainly confined to the trunk. A smaller proportion of cases involve a symptomatic drop in blood pressure shortly after injection and less commonly, the skin reaction is more severe, longer lasting and shows signs typical of cutaneous vasculitis (eg. Elliott *et al.* 1988). A late polyarthralgia has also been reported suggestive of a serum sickness type of reaction.

23.10.4 Diethylene-Triamine Penta-Acetate

The widespread use of technetium DTPA, mostly for renal studies, has brought with it a small incidence of vasomotor problems. Signs and symptoms of falling blood pressure predominate quite often resulting in loss of consciousness. Table 7 shows recent U.K. experience. Evidence of an immunological process such as skin reaction or bronchospasm is most unusual but recently cases have been reported following inhalation of Tc-DTPA aerosol. In one case, a typical erythematous skin rash appeared within 10–15 minutes of nebulisation and in another abroad, a subject with a history of asthma developed very acute severe bronchospasm and died within a matter of minutes, despite intensive efforts at resuscitation.

TABLE 7
Tc99m DTPA 1975–1992
49 cases/341 = 14% of total

5 Aerosol cases – remainder i.v.
3 Fatalities – all aerosol, only 1 questionably related (other 2 probably unrelated – see MAA).
Almost all cases showed vasomotor signs and symptoms; pulse changes hypotension and faints (some with transient neurological signs).
Allergic reactions such as skin rashes and bronchospasm noted in 6 cases only (2 aerosol, 4 i.v.).

A series of very serious problems developed following the intrathecal injection of Tc.DTPA in what turned out to be, strictly speaking, misformulation accidents (Verbruggen *et al.* 1982). Almost all the commercially available kits for the in-house production of Tc-DTPA contain the mixed calcium/sodium salt of DTPA. These, carefully prepared, have not been associated with undue problems, but one source supplied the pentasodium salt, though the difference was not clearly marked on the package, or apparently appreciated by the users. This form is capable of gross chelation of C.S.F. calcium and magnesium, causing gradual onset of severe neurological signs and several cases of permanent saddle anaesthesia and loss of sphincter control were reported and it may have been responsible for at least one fatality.

Although not an adverse reaction or even untoward effect as defined previously, the use of the reporting schemes to collect, collate and then publicise the problem should hopefully not only prevent further examples, but is a useful warning to be extremely vigilant when using a radiopharmaceutical in a new formulation, or administration via a novel route. The intrathecal route is particularly sensitive to contaminants, overdosage and apparently minor misformulations.

D.T.P.A. is used, as the gadolinium chelate, in much larger doses as i.v. 'contrast' in magnetic resonance imaging and trials have shown approximately 1% incidence of unwanted concomitant symptoms such as headache, nausea and vomiting but saline placebo injections produced similar types and numbers of problems. Urticaria was reported in 14% and focal convulsions in a similar percentage, though only in patients with cerebral tumours or a history of epilepsy (Niendorf, 1988).

23.10.5 Other Radiopharmaceuticals

Apart from these four main groups of radiopharmaceuticals, there has always been a small number from the wide range of other radiopharmaceuticals in use which have made up a miscellaneous group (Table 3) accounting for approximately one quarter of all reports. Experience in the U.S.A. and the U.K. include four minor groupings. Radioiodinated hippuran preparations have always featured in small numbers in published series of reports and have been predominantly of vasomotor type. The adrenocortical imaging agents of cholesterol labelled with radio-iodine or selenium have also featured in small numbers though the infrequency of their use points to quite a high incidence of reaction: Japanese experience has also confirmed these. Ga-67 gallium citrate has continued to provide a few reports—predominantly typical erythematous skin reactions clinically indistinguishable from other toxic erythemas. Although strictly a non-physiological element, it is interesting to note that a typical dose contains only 250 ng of elemental gallium. Radioiodinated metaiodobenzylguanidine (mIBG) used for adrenal medullary studies and visualisation of other neuroepithelial tumours has been associated with a number of reactions. This material is pharmacologically active and not a few reports would seem to be of Type A reactions, probably due to transient high blood levels following the use of low specific activity material, high dosage or unduly rapid injection.

23.11 INCIDENCE

No absolute figures for the incidence of adverse reactions and untoward effects due to radiopharmaceuticals are available apart from some Japanese data and more details are awaited. All schemes admit to considerable under-reporting particularly with respect to mild reactions requiring little or no active treatment. An estimate in the U.K. suggested that only 10% of cases were reported with the inevitable bias to the more obvious and serious cases. The rising number of reports in the U.K. is thought to be due to two main factors. The first is the ever increasing number of nuclear medicine procedures undertaken each year. Secondly the reporting scheme has been getting more widespread support which in turn has allowed publication in journals and at scientific meetings of the collected and collated results so that the attendant publicity has itself led to more support for the scheme. It is still estimated that the reports cover barely 15% of the true incidence.

Reactions occurring well after the administration of a radiopharmaceutical stand an increased likelihood of being missed or blamed on other factors. The nature of the reaction itself may not suggest a causal relationship with the radiopharmaceutical study and even immediate vasomotor reactions may be thought due to the injection procedure, anxiety or preparation for the investigation.

Two Nuclear Medicine departments under the author's care in the South West of England were surveyed in some detail for a period of five years to try and include all reactions including trivial ones. Eight reactions were noted—a figure of approximately 1 per 4,000 administrations. Serving a population of very close to three quarters of a million people, this implies a nationwide total of about 550 reports for the five years—more than ten times higher than those actually received.

The original United Kingdom report of Williams, E. (1974) suggests that sulphur colloid reactions showed an incidence of 1 in 250 and for albumin macroaggregates, figures varied considerably from different centres with an approximate mean of 1 in 36! Whilst these figures undoubtedly reflect early problems in quality control with preparation made entirely "in house", all subsequent figures have shown a much lower incidence. In the U.S. the incidence of reactions has been quoted as 1 to 6 per 100,000 and a figure of 3 per 100,000 was reported in the U.K. (Abra *et al.* 1980b) thought these figures are quoted as excluding the most minor problems. Personal experience suggested that Tc.99m antimony sulphide colloids produce problems, mostly very minor, approximately once per thousand injections. Serious reactions are at least ten times less common, and fatalities quite exceptional.

All those involved in nuclear medicine should be encouraged to report reactions and untoward events associated with the use of radiopharmaceuticals so that problems can be identified early and clinicians forewarned. In this way, even if trouble cannot be avoided, at least the recognition and prompt treatment of reactions can be expedited, to the great benefit of our patients.

REFERENCES

Abra R.M., Bell N.D.S. and Horton P.W. (1980a). *The growth of microorganisms in some parenteral radiopharmaceuticals.* Int. J. Pharmaceutics., **5**, 187–193.

Abra R.M., Bell N.D.S., Horton P.W. and McCarthy T.M. (1980b). *A survey of radiopharmaceutical manufacture in U.K. Hospitals.* J. Clin. Hosp. Pharmacy, **5**, 11–20.

Atkins H.L. (1986). *Reported adverse reactions to radiopharmaceuticals remain low in 1984.* J. Nucl. Med. **27**, p. 327.

Atkins H.L., Hauser W., Richards P. and Klopper J. (1972). *Adverse Reactions to Radiopharmaceuticals.* J. Nucl. Med., **13**, pp. 232–233.

Ansell G. (1987). *Contrast Media and Urography. In* Complications in Diagnostic Imaging. 2nd Edition. p. 1. Ed by Ansell, G. and Wilkins, R.A., Blackwell Scientific Publications, Oxford.

Bliek A.J. and Bachynski J.E. (1971). *Two severe reactions following a pulmonary scan in a patient with idiopathic pulmonary haemosiderosis.* J. Nucl. Med. **12**, pp. 90–92.

Black L., Menard F.J.R.R., Beadle G.G. and Pay T.W.F. (1975). *Hypersensitivity in cattle after foot and mouth disease vaccination: response to hydroxypropyl methylcellulose.* J. Hyg. Camb., **75**, pp. 79–87.

Bockner B.S. and Lichtenstein L.M. (1991). *Anaphylaxis.* N. Engl. J. Med., **324**, pp. 1785–1790.

Brown S. and Baker M.H. (1986). *The sterility testing of dispensed radiopharmaceuticals.* Nucl. Med. Communications., **7**, pp. 327–336.

Brueton M.J., Lortan J.E., Morgan D.J.R. and Sutters C.A. (1991). *Management of Anaphylaxis.* Hospital Update, **17**, pp. 386–398.

Bruinsma W. (1986). *Skin Reactions. In* Monitoring for Drug Safety. 2nd Edition, pp. 357–361. Ed by: W.H.W. Inman. M.T.P. Press Ltd., Lancaster.

Cooper J.F. and Harbert J.C. (1975). *Endotoxin as a cause of aseptic meningitis after radionuclide cisternography.* J. Nucl. Med. **16**, pp. 809–813.

Cordova M.A., Hladik W.B. and Rhodes B.A. (1984). *Validation and characterisation of adverse reactions to radiopharmaceuticals.* Non-invasive Med. Imaging. **1**, pp. 17–24.

Cordova M.A., Hladik W.B., Rhodes B.A. and Atkins H.L. (1986). *Adverse reactions associated with radiopharmaceuticals. In* Essentials of Nuclear Medicine Science. Ed by: Hladik W.B., Sabra G.P. and Study K.T. pp. 303–320. Baltimore: Williams and Wilkins.

Cordova M.A., Rhodes B.A., Atkins H.L., Glenn H.J., Hoogland D.R. and Solomon A.C. (1982). *Adverse Reactions to Radiopharmaceuticals.* J. Nucl. Med., **23**, pp. 550–551.

Dworkin H.J., Smith J.R. and Bull F.E. (1966). *A reaction following administration of macroaggregated albumin for a lung scan.* Am. J. Roentgenol, **98**, pp. 427–433.

Edmonds C.J. and Smith T. (1986). *The long-term hazards of the treatment of thyroid cancer with radioiodine.* Brit. J. Radiol, **59**, pp. 45–51.

Elliott A.T., Murray T., Mackie R.M. and Hunter J.A. (1988). *Severe reaction to diphosphonate: implications for treatment of Paget's disease.* Brit. Med. J., **297**, pp. 592–593.

Felix R.H. and Smith A.G. (1991). *'Skin Disorders' Chap. 17. pp. 514–534. In* Textbook of Adverse Drug Reactions 4th Edition. Ed by Davies D.M. Oxford University Press, Oxford.

Ford L., Shroff A., Benson W., Atkins H. and Rhodes B.A. (1978). *S.N.M. Drug Problems Reporting System.* J. Nucl. Med., **19**, pp. 116–117.

Grahame-Smith D.G. and Aronson J.K. (1992). *Oxford Textbook of Clinical Pharmacology and Drug Therapy.* 2nd Edition, Oxford Medical Publications.

Griffin J.P. (1987). *Adverse drug reaction monitoring in 16 countries. In* Adverse Drug Reactions. pp. 87–88. Ed by Mann R.D., Parthenon Publishing.

Guyton A.C. (1991). *Circulatory Shock and Physiology of its Treatment. In* Textbook of Medical Physiology, 8th Edition. pp. 263–271. W.B. Saunders, Philadelphia.

Halde J.K., Jakobsen J.A., Andrew E. and Stormoken H. (1988). *Adverse reactions to contrast media: related to medium or procedure? Observations on a case.* Brit. J. Radiol. **61**, pp. 337–338.

Hoving J., Roosjen J.N. and Brouwers J.R.B.J. (1988). *Adverse reactions to Technetium-99m methylene diphosphonate.* J. Nucl. Med. **29**, pp. 1302–1303.

Keeling D.H. (1979). *Side effects associated with the use of radiopharmaceuticals. In* Drug Toxicity. pp. 285–295. Ed by Gorrod J.W. Taylor and Francis Ltd., London.

Keeling D.H. (1984). *Adverse reactions to radiopharmaceuticals. In* Safety and Efficacy of Radiopharmaceuticals. pp. 240–250. Ed by Kristensen K. and Norbygaard E. Martinus Nijhoff, The Hague.

Keeling D.H. (1986). *Radiopharmaceuticals. In* Monitoring for Drug Safety. 2nd Edition, pp. 349–356. Edited by W.H.W. Inman, M.T.P. Press Ltd., Lancaster.

Keeling D.H. (1987). *Problems with Radiopharmaceuticals.* Radiology Now, **4**, pp. 44–45.

Keeling D.H. (1988). *Editorial: Clinical emergencies in the Nuclear Medicine Department.* Nuc. Med. Communications. **9**, pp. 259–261.

Keeling D.H. (1991). *Recent Experience with Radiopharmaceuticals and other Drug Reactions and Untoward Events in Nuclear Medicine. In* Nuclear Medicine, The State of the Art of Nuclear Medicine in Europe. pp. 100–102. ed. Schmidt, H.A.E. and Van der Schoot. Shattauer, Stuttgart.

Keeling D.H. and Sampson C.B. (1984). *Adverse reactions to radiopharmaceuticals. U.K. 1977–1983.* Brit. J. Radiol., **57**, pp. 1091–1096.

Kristensen K. (1992). *European system for reporting adverse reactions and drug defects. Eighth report: 1990 EANM Newsletter. P. A11 Ninth report: 1991 EANM Newsletter. pp. A10–11.* Eur. J. Nucl. Med. **19**.

Laurence D.R. and Bennett P.N. (1992). *Histamine and Histamine H1 and H2 receptor antagonists. In* Clinical Pharmacology 7th Edition, pp. 507–510. Churchill Livingstone. Edinburgh.

Lazarus C.R. and Maisey M.N. (1987). *Radioisotope Techniques. In* Complications in Diagnostic Imaging. 2nd Edition, pp. 373–390. Ed by Ansell G. and Wilkins R.A. Blackwell Scientific Publications, Oxford.

Littenberg R.L. (1975). *Anaphylactoid reaction to human albumin microspheres.* J. Nucl. Med., **16**, pp. 236–237.

NCRP Commentary No. 7 (1991). *Misadministration of Radioactive material in Medicine: Scientific background.* Bethesda.

Niendorf H.P. (1988). *Tolerance and safety of Gd-DTPA in 7000 patients: a review. Diagnostic Imaging International.* Supplement. Nov. 1988, pp. 16–17.

Perkins A.C., Pimm M.V. and Powell M.C. (1988). *The implications of patient antibody response for the clinical usefulness of immunoscintigraphy.* Nucl. Med. Communications. **9**, pp. 273–282.

Ramos-Gabatin A., Orzel J.A., Maloney T.R., Murnane J.E. and Borchert R.D. (1986). *Severe systemic reaction to diphosphonate bone imaging agents: skin testing to predict allergic response and a safe alternative agent.* J. Nucl. Med. **27**, pp. 1432–1435.

Rawlins MD. and Thompson J.W. (1991). *Mechanisms of adverse drug reactions. In Textbook of Adverse Drug Reactions. 4th Edition. pp. 18–45.* Ed by Davies, D.M. Oxford University Press, Oxford.

Rhodes B.A. and Cordova M.A. (1980). *Adverse Reactions to Radiopharmaceuticals: Incidence in 1978 and associated symptoms.* J. Nucl. Med. **21**, pp. 1107–1110.

Rhodes B.A. and Wagner H.N. (1974). *Adverse Reactions to Radiopharmaceuticals.* J. Nucl. Med. **15**, 213–214.

Ring J. and Messmer K. (1977). *Incidence and severity of anaphylactoid reactions to colloid volume substitutes.* Lancet. i. 466–469.

Sampson C.B. and Keeling D.H. (1982). *Adverse reactions to radiopharmaceuticals: follow up survey in the U.K.* Annual Scientific Meeting. Brit. Nuc. Med. Soc. London, 1982.

Sarker S.D., Beierwaltes W.H., Gill S.P. and Cowley B.J. (1976). *Subsequent fertility and birth histories of children and adolescents treated with I-131 for thyroid cancer.* J. Nucl. Med., **17**, 460–464.

Shani J., Atkins H.L. and Wolf W. (1976). *Adverse reactions to radiopharmaceuticals.* Sem. in Nuc. Med. **6**, 305–328.

Shapiro B., Pillay M. and Cox P.H. (1987). *Dosimetric consequences of interstitial extravasation following i.v. administration of a radiopharmaceutical.* Eur. J. Nucl. Med. **12**, 522–523.

Sorensen K., Kristensen K. and Frandsen P. (1977). *Microbial contamination of radionuclide generators.* Eur. J. Nucl. Med. **2**, 105–107.

Sykes C.J., Jager W. and Noujaim A.A. (1980). *In* Advances in Radiopharmacology pp. 243–252. Ed. Maddalena, D.J. *et al.*, Woolongong.

Verbruggen A., de Roo M., Dewit P., Guelinckx P. and Dom R. (1982). *Complications after intrathecal administration of Tc-99m DTPA. In* Progress in Radiopharmacology. Pt.III, p. 223–235. Ed by P. Cox. Martinus Nyhoff, The Hague.

Vincent W.R. (1968). *Fatality immediately following rapid infusion of macroaggregates of Tc.99m albumin (MAA) for lung scan.* Radiology., **91**, 1181–1184.

Wall B.F., Hillier M.C., Kendall G.M. and Shields R.A. (1985). *Nuclear Medicine activity in the United Kingdom (1982)* Brit. J. Radiol. **58**, 125–130.

Williams E.S. (1974). *Adverse Reactions to radiopharmaceuticals: a preliminary survey in the United Kingdom.* Brit. J. Radiol. **47**, 54–59.
Williams J.O. (1974). *Death following injection of lung scanning agent in a case of pulmonary hypertension.* Brit. J. Radiol. **47**, 61–63.
Wintroub B.U., Stern R.S. and Arndt K.A. (1987). *Cutaneous Reactions to Drugs. In* Dermatology in General Medicine. 3rd Edition. p. 1353. Ed by Fitzpatrick T.B., *et al.,* McGraw Hill, New York.

Chapter 24

Dosimetric Aspects

M. Pillay

24.1 INTRODUCTION

Dosimetry is aimed at the protection of individuals, their offspring, and ultimately, mankind as a whole against the detrimental effects of radiation, while at the same time, permitting the use of radioactive material for diagnoses and treatment. The medical use of radiation (x-rays, radiotherapy and nuclear medicine), contributes to about 12% of all radiation dose to the public. It is, therefore, important to consider the dosimetric aspects of administerd radiopharmaceuticals with the view of minimising the radiation dose to patients as well as personnel.

The increasing awareness in radiation safety should be critically considered in terms of its potential benefit in diagnoses and/or therapy. With this objective, the International Commission on Radiological Protection (ICRP) has suggested the following guidelines for dose limitation:

(i) Procedures should only be introduced if they offer a net positive benefit.

(ii) Accounting for the risk/benefit and socio-economic factors, all exposures should be kept As Low As Reasonably Achievable (ALARA).

(iii) The dose equivalents limits for the various procedures as described by the ICRP should not be exceeded.

This chapter describes the most important internal dosimetric aspects related to the use of radionuclides in nuclear medical procedures which are generally applicable to diagnostic patient investigation, accidental internal contamination and radionuclide therapy. The radiation dose rates to personnel from external radiation sources is also discussed.

24.1.1 Ionising Radiation

Ionising radiation is a collective term for high energy electromagnetic waves produced by charged or non-charged atomic particles. All these radiations produce ionisation along their natural path by releasing one or more electrons of an atom and leaving behind a positively charged ion. This energy deposition is the prime contributor to absorbed dose. The range of electromagnetic forces useful for diagnoses and therapy fall on either side of the visible spectrum (Figure 1). The origins of ionising radiation are varied and could find infancy in the cosmos, from naturally occuring radioactive elements in the earth's crust (radon), and from man-made machines (x-ray and television tubes, linear accelerators) (Table 1).

Table 1
Estimate of the Various Contributions to the Annual Effective Dose Equivalent from Natural Sources Based on 8 hours Outdoors and 16 hours Indoors; and from Medical Applications Averaged per capita.

Natural Sources	*mSv/year*	
Cosmic radiation	0.3	
Earth's crust	0.2	
Building material	0.5	
Inhalation of radon & thoron	0.9	
Contribution of K-40, C-14, U-238, Th-232	0.5	
Total Natural sources	2.4	
Medical Sources		
Radiology		1.0
Nuclear Medicine		0.1
Total Medical		1.1

In 1982 the United Nations Scientific Committee on the Effects of Atomic Radiation (UNSCEAR) reported variations of doserates of 1-10mGy per year due to natural radioactivity in the earth's crust. The atmosphere attenuates some of the cosmic radiation resulting in a 0,3 mGy annual contribution at sea level to about 0,8 mGy at 2 km height. The mean dose to the general public in the U.K. is approximately 2.5 mSv and 3.6 mSv in the USA.

The most important types of radiation for dosimetric considerations are the alpha and beta particles, gamma and x-rays, internal conversion electrons, Auger electrons, and indirectly, neutrons.

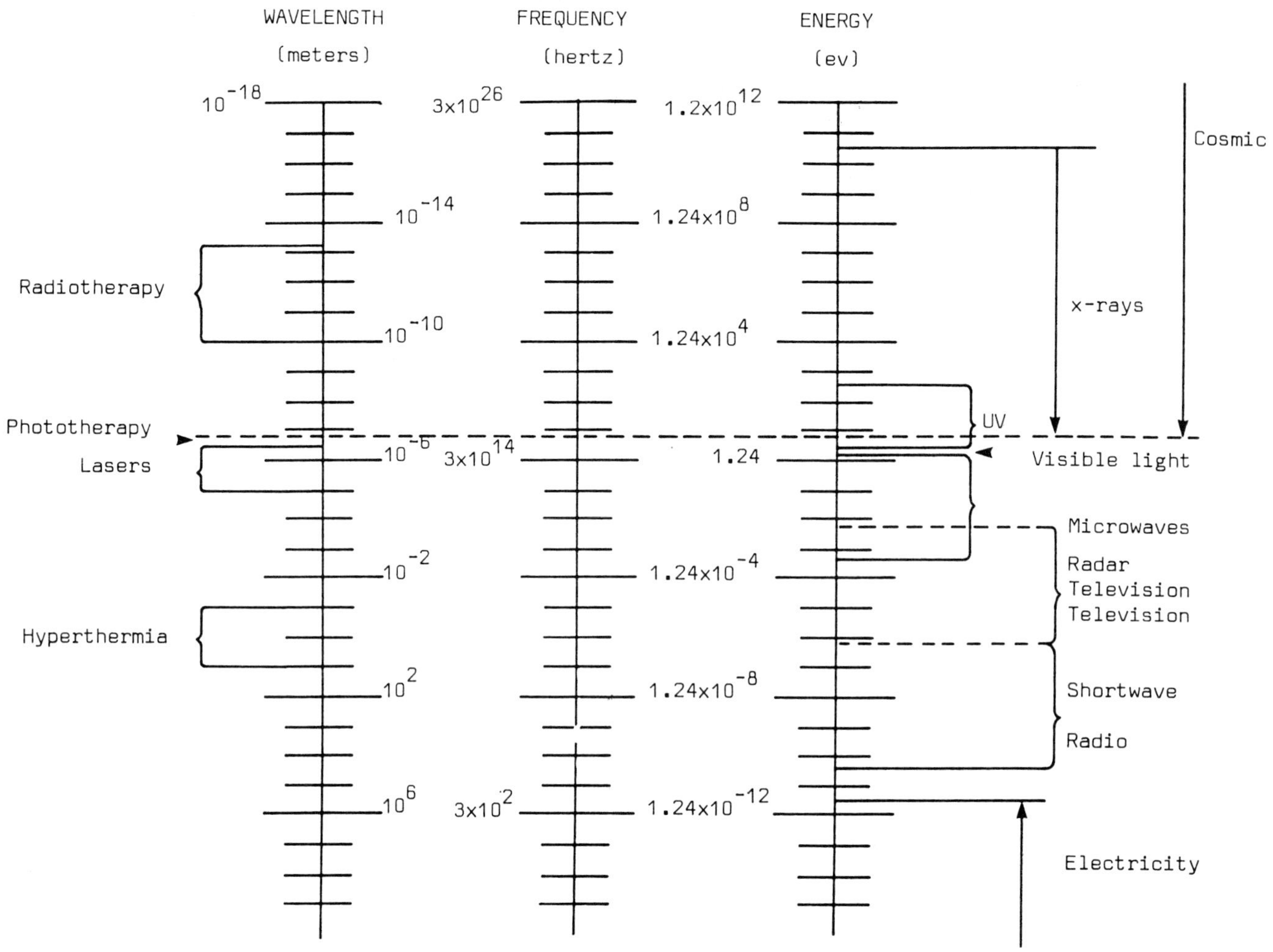

Figure 1. Electromagnetic Spectrum: relation of wavelength, frequency and energy and the ranges useful for medical applications.

(i) Alpha radiation is produced by heavily charged particles primarily from high atomic mass elements such as uranium and thorium. Their ionisation potential is extremely high but they have limited penetrability of only a few millimeters (about 0,04 mm in tissue).

(ii) Beta radiation originates from the atomic nucleus by conversion of neutrons to protons (negative beta), or the conversion of protons to neutrons (positive beta or positron). The positive beta has the equivalent weight of an electron but is of opposite charge. The ground state of the positron is reached by annihilation, and is the process by which its mass is converted to energy with the emission of electromagnetic radiation. Beta radiation has a high ionising potential. Their penetration is dependent on their mean energy and is in the region of 0,1–10 mm in tissue.
The beta emitting radionuclides are useful in radionuclide therapy (Table 2).

(iii) Gamma radiation originates in the atomic nucleus and results from the absorption of energy producing an isomeric state. The excited nucleus tends to its original resting state by producing a photon or internal conversion electron.

(iv) X-rays are the result of acceleration or deceleration of electrons.
The ionising effect of gamma and x-rays are small since they have a high penetration ability which is in the order of meters, dependent on their energies.

(v) Internal conversion and/or Auger electrons are a direct result of isomeric transition in which the nucleus gives its energy off to an orbiting electron which is in turn ejected from its orbit and referred to as the conversion electron. This event creates a vacancy in the shell from which the electron has been ejected and to reach stability, an electron from an outer shell will fill this vacancy and at the same time give off its excess energy in the form of characteristic x-rays or will transfer this energy directly to another orbiting electron (Auger electron), resulting in a second electron emission. The ionizing potential of these emissions are a few millimeters in tissue. The alpha, beta and conversion electron radiations are the highest contributors to radiation absorbed dose.

(vi) Neutron radiation has no direct ionisation ability but can produce indirect ionisation. Its penetration potential is many meters.

The estimation of the electron range is complex and requires knowledge of the beta ray spectral data and point dose kernels of the radionuclide. As a rule of thumb the range in water may be approximated by the following relationship for monoenergies between 0.05 to 6 MeV.

$$\text{max. range (mm)} = (5.30 * E_{max}) - \exp(E_{max}/3)$$

where

E_{max} = maximum beta energy

24.1.2 Radiation Measurement

The measurement of radiation is dependent on the type of radiation and whether measurements are to be carried out for environmental contamination (Bq cm^{-2}) or for personal dose estimation (Sv hr^{-1}).

The ionisation chambers, Geiger Muller counters and various scintillation and solid state detectors are commonly used for environmental contamination detection and dose rate measurements.

For personal radiation control, the thermoluminescient dosimeter (TLD), film badge or pocket model ionisation chambers could be used.

24.2 BIOLOGICAL EFFECTS OF RADIATION

The result of exposure to ionising radiation could manifest in the development of cancers, cataracts (somatic), and chromosomal (hereditary) disorders. Stochastic effects are those effects related to the likelihood of occurrence as a function of dose, without a threshold. In contrast, the severity of a deterministic (non-stochastic) effect is dose related and therefore, has a threshold, hence the application of sufficiently low dose-equivalent limits aimed at a low threshold and subsequently the prevention of deterministic effects.

The observations on the biological effects of radiation have largely been made on populations at high risk, viz., personnel at nuclear reactor establishments and radiological workers in industry. The exposures considered in these groups were generally high, in the order of tens of Sieverts per year. Nevertheless, from a radiation hygiene point of view, a risk exists irrespective of the dose. Hence the introduction of the ALARA (As Low As Reasonably Achievable) principle which also accounts for the virtual impossibility of reaching zero dose in the working environment.

The risk attributed to a given dose and its effects are referred to as the dose-response relationship. Because of the

Table 2
Radionuclides Useful in Radioimmunotherapy

Nuclide	*Gamma-ray energy (MeV)*	*Max β energy (MeV)*	*Mean electron energy (MeV)*	*Max electron range (mm) (in tissue)*	*Half life (days)*
I-131	0.364	0.340 0.610	0.360	2.5	8.03
P-32	–	1.71	0.695	8.4	14.3
Y-90	–	2.2	0.934	11	2.7
Dy-165	0.095	1.29	0.318	6	0.01
Au-198	0.412	0.960	0.400	4.5	2.7
Re-186	0.137	0.930 1.070	0.400	5	3.7
Re-188	0.155	1.960 2.120	0.650	10.6	0.29
Er-169		0.340	0.100	1.2	9.5
Sr-89		1.46	0.47	7	52.7
At-211	0.687	5.87α 7.45α		<0.1	0.3
Bi-212	0.3–1.8	6.05α 6.09α + a range of 6		<0.1	0.04

complexity of this relationship, the ICRP has recommended a linear exrapolation of risk obtained at high doses. There are radiobiological grounds for this assumption. However, even if the dose-response is highly sigmoid, the linear extrapolation will overestimate the risk and make the actual risk at low doses lower than may be implied.

24.2.1 Acute Effects

These arise from absorbed doses in the order of several Gray (Gy) and normally produce symptoms within a few hours to days of the exposure. A total body dose of 3–5 Gy is considered to be lethal, i.e a dose from which 50% of the exposed population will eventually die from the bone marrow syndrome. Individual organs can, however, tolerate a much higher dose before acute symptoms arise. Acute effects from absorbed doses of $<0,5$ Gy have not yet been reported. A dose of 15 Gy produces damage to the central nervous system and death within 1–5 days and 5–15 Gy produces gastrointestinal and respiratory damage with death ensuing within 10–20 days.

24.2.2 Late (Chronic) Effects

The chronic effects could manifest years following exposure to radiation, and usually present in the form of leukemia or cancer. In terms of risk the minimum latent period for development of leukemia is considered to be two years and for other malignant tumours, greater than 10 years. The study of cancer induction is based on experimental data on laboratory animals, cell cultures, atomic bomb survivors and follow up studies on radiotherapy patients.

24.2.3 Genetic (Hereditary) Effects

Exposure to the reproductive organs of the male or female may produce irreversible mutations in the reproductive cells which finally partake in the propagation of the species. Subsequent generations carrying these defective chromosomes will show variable hereditary deficiencies. The results of animal studies show a large percentage of foetuses with chromosomal aberrations due to irradiation, aborting spontaneously.

Since every form and level of radiation carries with it a risk, and chromosome changes have only been studied in animals, we must assume that for genetic changes to occur, no dose limit exists. However, the positive effects of low doses should not be lightly discounted. Mankind has for generations been exposed to low doses of naturally occurring radiations.

24.2.4 The Risk During Pregnancy

This risk includes that of tumour to the mother as well as the undesired effects to the foetus which can generally be divided into three stages;

(1) up to 8 days following conception-total destruction of the embryo and spontaneous abortion. This risk is estimated at 1 per Sievert, i.e. 100% at 1 Sv.

(2) 9–15 days following conception is considered the greatest risk period, since severe mental and physical malformation can take place due to the high rate of cell division (mitosis), —this risk is magnified by the uncertainty of pregnancy during this period. The risk during this period is estimated at 50% per Sv.

(3) 8–15 weeks small doses may cause general reduction in the I.Q. of children in the order of about 30 I.Q. points per Sv.

(4) the exposure to the foetus 16 weeks following conception could result in growth disorders as well as the induction of leukemia and tumor. The risk for these disorders is probably greater in this period than exposure following birth and is estimated at approximately 2% per Sv.

The risk of fatal childhood cancer due to a constant prenatal exposure is estimated at 2.8×10^{-2} Sv^{-1}.

24.3 DEFINITIONS AND UNITS

To understand and perform simple absorbed dose calculations, it is necessary to be acquainted with the general definitions and units which are common to these estimations. For complete derivations the reader is referred to the relevant MIRD and ICRU publications listed at the end of this chapter.

24.3.1 Absorbed Dose (D)

The absorbed radiation dose (D) is the total energy absorbed per unit mass of tissue, i.e. the total energy absorbed per gram of tissue, and is expressed as the Rad (Radiation absorbed dose) or Gray (Gy).

$$\text{Absorbed dose} = \text{Gray (Gy)}$$

$$1\,\text{Gy} = 1\ \text{Jkg}^{-1} = 0.01\ \text{Rad}\ (100\ \text{Gy} = 1\ \text{Rad}).$$

24.3.2 Radiation Dose Rate (dD/dt)

The radiation dose rate is the amount of energy absorbed per unit time per gram of tissue and is measured in Gray per minute, hour or days.

24.3.3 Equivalent Dose (H)

The equivalent dose is the mean absorbed dose, rather than at a point, over a tissue or organ and defined numerically as the product of the absorbed dose (D), effects of exposure under various conditions determined by the radiation weighting factor (w_R). The radiation weighting factor describes the quality of the radiation in terms of its type and energy and is equivalent to the linear energy transfer.

$$H_T = \Sigma w_R \cdot D_{T,R} \text{ Sieverts } (1 \text{ Sv} = 100 \text{ rem})$$

where

$D_{T,R}$ = mean absorbed dose over tissue or organ T from radiation R.

The equivalent dose attempts at correction for factors affecting the biological effects of radiation which is not only affected by absorbed dose, but also by the energy of the primary radiation, type of radiation and dose rate.

The ICRP recommended values of w_R to be unity for medical diagnostic work with x-rays or gamma rays. Thus, for practical purposes, the equivalent dose is numerically equal to the absorbed dose in Gy.

24.3.4 Effective Dose (E)

The effective dose considers the radiosensitivity of the various organs and tissues. Tissue weighting factors are introduced to determine the contribution to stochastic effects associated with uniform exposure of several tissues to ionising radiation (Tables 3 and 4).

Table 3
Tissue Weighting Factors w_T, for the Estimation of Effective Dose, E, for Stochastic Effects, and the Associated Risk Factors.

Organ (tissue)	w_T	*Risk Factor Stoch. fatal Ca.* 10^{-4} Sv^{-1}	*Severe genetic effects* 10^{-4} Sv^{-1}
Breast	0.05	*20	
Bladder	0.05	30	
Bone cortical	0.03	5	
Bone marrow	0.12	50	
Colon	0.12	85	
Liver	0.05	15	
Lung	0.12	85	
Gonads	0.20	10	100
Stomach	0.12	110	
Skin	0.01	2	
Thyroid	0.05	8	
Oesophagus		30	
Ovary		10	
Remainder	0.30	**50	

The risk factors refer to the population as a whole. For workers the factors are approximately 20% lower.

*mean of male and female.

**refers to the adrenals, brain, upper large intestine, small intestine, kidney, muscle, pancreas, spleen, thymus and uterus.

TABLE 4
The following recommended dose limit applies to radiological workers and the public

	Occupational	*Public*
Effective dose	20mSv per year (mean over 5 years)	1 mSv in a year
Annual equivalent dose in:		
lens of eye	150 mSv	15 mSv
the skin	500 mSv	50 mSv
hand & feet	500 mSv	—

The effective dose is the sum of weighted equivalent doses in all the tissues and organs of the body measured in sieverts.

$$E = \Sigma w_T \,.\, H_T \text{ (i.e. the sum of all organs)}$$

Thus, the estimated whole body dose H_T carries with it the same risk of fatal cancer or genetic effect as the sum of all organ doses, E.

24.3.5 Other dosimetric quantities

24.3.5.1 Committed equivalent dose, $H_T(\tau)$ is the cumulative equivalent dose rate over a period of time (τ) and considers the varying rate of equivalent doses in tissue.

τ = integration time in years following intake. By implication

τ = 50 years for adults and 70 years for children unless τ is specified.

24.3.5.2 Committed effective dose $E(\tau)$ is the cumulative effective dose rate over a period of time where τ is defined as above.

24.3.5.3 Collective equivalent dose, S_T and *collective effective dose, S,* relate to the exposure of groups or populations and account for the number of people exposed to a source and expressed as the product of the mean dose and number of individuals in the group.

The unit is the man sievert.

24.3.5.4 Environmental monitoring

For dose equivalents at a point in radiation protection, the following quantities are useful:

(a) Ambient dose equivalent H*(d) (for strongly penetrating radiation) is the dose equivalent that would be produced by a similar expanded field in the ICRU sphere at depth, d.
(b) Directional dose equivalent H′(d) (for weakly penetrating radiation) is the dose equivalent that would be produced in the ICRU sphere at depth d, in a specified direction.

The whole body limit (1) is similar to the earlier dose equivalent of 5 rem per year ($W_{whole\ body} = 1$).

The annual dose limit for occupational exposure should not exceed 50 mSv in any single year. For the public, a higher annual exposure may be acceptable provided the mean exposure over 5 years is not in excess of 1mSv.

The weighting factors have been derived from risk factors in the populations exposed to radiation opposed to those not exposed.

24.3.6 Linear Energy Transfer (LET)

The energy loss (deposition) per unit distance can vary from 0.2 kev m^{-1} for fast electrons to 1000 kev m^{-1} for alpha particles and recoil protons. The measure of this energy deposition (ionisation) along the track of the ionising particle is referred to as the linear energy transfer (LET).

24.3.7 Specific Energy (z)

This is defined as the energy absorbed per unit mass in a small volume, e.g. within the volume of a cell nucleus. For example, consider a group of cells exposed to background radiation for one year (approximately 1 mGy of low LET radiation), then, for approx. 65% of the cell nuclei, z = 0. For the remainder of cells, z will vary a few orders of magnitude with a mean of approximately 3mGy.

In summary, the absorbed dose is dependent on:

(a) the magnitude of the dose (MBq)
(b) type and energy of the radiation (radiation weighting factor)
(c) distribution of the dose within the body (tissue weighting factor), and
(d) distribution of the dose in time (dose rate)

24.3.8 Relative Biological Effectiveness (RBE)

The RBE expresses the concept that different types of radiation have different effects on biological systems. The introduction of a z would not be of importance if the biological effects of the radiation were the same for all radiation types so that the mean specific energy, z, for a given volume would then be numerically equal to the absorbed dose (D), in which case the biological effects would not be dependent on the LET. However, this is not true in practice. The RBE of a given radiation type, i, relative to 200 kev x-rays (low LET), is expressed as the dose relation Dl/Di, where Dl and Di are the absorbed doses required to produce the same biological effects.

The RBE for gamma radiation is equivalent to 0.8, and for high LET radiation the RBE is >1. The dose effects, and thus, the RBE are dependent on the dose rate (dD/dt). The RBE is not only dependent on the type of radiation, but also on the dose effect in question, in contrast to the quality factor, Q (dose equivalent factor), which is a mean RBE for all effects and only applicable to low doses in the evaluation of risk following exposure.

24.4 PARAMETERS REQUIRED FOR INTERNAL DOSE CALCULATIONS

Unlike radiological investigations where internal absorbed doses are extrapolated from dose estimations to the skin, nuclear medical investigations require the knowledge of the physical as well as biokinetic data of the radiopharmaceutical in question. The biological parameters are related to the radiopharmaceutical, its biodistribution, retention and clearance from the different organs and tissues of the body. The physical parameters are those related to the inherent properties of the radionuclide such as decay half-time, types of radiation and number of nuclear transformations.

The physical and biological T½ are combined to give an effective T½. The Biological T½ is generally determined experimentally so that the T½ effective is mathematically expressed as:

$$T_{1/2\,eff} = (T_{1/2\,p} \times T_{1/2\,b})/(T_{1/2\,b})$$

24.4.1 General Formulation

The mean absorbed radiation dose (D) to a specific organ and for a specific radiopharmaceutical can be expressed as the sum of the non-penetrating and penetrating radiation components within the target as well as the penetrating radiation distributed in the remainder of the body:
where,

D	= mean absorbed dose in target (T) within a specific time interval (t)
A	= mean cumulated activity in μCi (Mbq) for time (t)
A_{wb}	= mean cumulated activity (rad hour) in the remainder of the body (whole body)
M	= mass of target organ (grams)
Δ_{np}	= equilibrium dose constant for non-penetrating radiations
Δ_i	= equilibrium dose constant for penetrating radiations
$\phi_i(T \leftarrow S)$	= absorbed dose fraction due to self radiation in the target for penetrating radiation
$\phi_i(T \leftarrow wb)$	= absorbed fraction due to radiation distributed in the rest of the body for penetrating radiation.

$$D = (A/M)\Delta_{np} + (A/M)\Sigma_i\Delta_i\phi_i(T \leftarrow T) + (A_{wb}/M)\Sigma_i\Delta_i\phi_i(T \leftarrow wb) \quad (1)$$

24.4.2 Equilibrium Dose Constant (Δ)

$$\Delta = n \text{ (particles/nuclear transform.)} \times 1.332.3.10^{-8}\text{(nucl.transform./}\mu\text{Ci-h)} \times E\text{(MeV/particles)} \times 1.602 \times 10^{-8}\text{(g-rad/MeV)}.$$
$$= 2.13 \text{ nE g-rad/}\mu\text{Ci-hr.}$$

for the i-th type radiation:

$\Delta_i = 2.13\ n_iE_i$ g-rad/μCi-hr.
(where n = frequency of emissions.)

24.4.3 Absorbed Fraction (ϕ_i)

For particulate radiation (α, β, conversion electrons), as well as for x and γ-rays of energy less than 10 KeV, practically all emitted radiation is self absorbed within the volume of distribution for source volumes larger than 1 cm^3 and $\phi(T \leftarrow S) = 0$. When the source and targets are the same organ then $\phi_i = 1$. The absorbed fractions used in Tables 5a, 5b and 5c (for I-131) were derived from the MIRD tables (see further reading).

TABLE 5a
The Contribution of Non-penetrating and Penetrating Radiations for an Absorbed Dose of I-131.

Radiation		*Energy (MeV)*	Δ_i *(g-rad/μCi-h)*	ϕ_i	$\Delta_i\phi_i$ *(g-rad/μ-h)*
beta − 1		0.0691	0.0029	1	0.0029
beta − 2		0.0867	0.0012	1	0.0012
beta − 3		0.0964	0.0136	1	0.0136
beta − 4		0.1916	0.3666	1	0.3666
beta − 5		0.2839	0.0048	1	0.0048
beta − 6		0.0456	0.0033	1	0.0033
int.conv.e^-	K	0.0751	0.0007	1	0.0007
	L	0.0792	0.0002	1	0.0002
	M	0.1426	0.0001	1	0.0001
	K	0.2497	0.0012	1	0.0012
	K	0.2792	0.0002	1	0.0002
	L	0.3299	0.0103	1	0.0103
	K	0.3594	0.0017	1	0.0017
	M	0.3635	0.0006	1	0.0006
	K	0.6021	0.0003	1	0.0003
Auger e^-	KLL	0.0244	0.0002	1	0.0002
	KLX	0.0285	0.0001	1	0.0001
	LMM	0.0031	0.0003	1	0.0003
	MXY	0.0009	0.0002	1	0.0002
				Total	0.4085

TABLE 5b
The Contribution of Penetrating Radiations Within the Target to Absorbed Dose for I-131.

Radiation	*Energy (MeV)*	Δ_i *(g-rad/μCi-h)*	ϕ_i	$\Delta_i\phi_i$ *(g-rad/μCi-h)*
Gamma 1	0.0801	0.0044	0.016	0.00007
Gamma 2	0.1772	0.0011	0.017	0.00002
Gamma 3	0.2723	0.0003	0.0175	0.00001
Gamma 4	0.2843	0.0350	0.0175	0.00061
Gamma 5	0.3180	0.0007	0.018	0.00001
Gamma 6	0.3250	0.0002	0.018	0.00000
Gamma 7	0.3257	0.0025	0.018	0.00005
Gamma 8	0.3585	0.0001	0.018	0.00000
Gamma 9	0.3644	0.6366	0.018	0.01146
Gamma 10	0.4048	0.0005	0.018	0.00001
Gamma 11	0.5029	0.0031	0.018	0.00006
Gamma 12	0.6367	0.0886	0.018	0.00159
Gamma 13	0.6430	0.0020	0.018	0.00004
Gamma 14	0.7228	0.0267	0.018	0.00048
K-a-1-X	0.0297	0.0015	0.081	0.00012
K-a-2-X	0.0294	0.0008	0.081	0.00006
K-b-1-X	0.0336	0.0004	0.081	0.00003
K-b-2-X	0.0345	0.0001	0.081	0.00001
			Total	0.02038

TABLE 5c
The Contribution of Penetrating Radiations Outside the Target to Absorbed Dose for I-131.

Radiation	*Energy (MeV)*	Δ_i *(g-rad/μCi-h)*	ϕ_i	$\Delta_i\phi_i$ *(g-rad/μCi-h)*
Gamma 1	0.0801	0.0044	0.557	0.00245
Gamma 2	0.1772	0.0011	0.475	0.00052
Gamma 3	0.2723	0.0003	0.473	0.00014
Gamma 4	0.2843	0.0350	0.473	0.01656
Gamma 5	0.3180	0.0007	0.472	0.00033
Gamma 6	0.3250	0.0002	0.471	0.00009
Gamma 7	0.3257	0.0025	0.471	0.00118
Gamma 8	0.3585	0.0001	0.470	0.00005
Gamma 9	0.3644	0.6366	0.469	0.29857
Gamma 10	0.4048	0.0005	0.469	0.00023
Gamma 11	0.5029	0.0031	0.460	0.00143
Gamma 12	0.6367	0.0886	0.455	0.04031
Gamma 13	0.6430	0.0020	0.454	0.00091
Gamma 14	0.7228	0.0267	0.450	0.01202
K-a-1-X	0.0297	0.0015	0.956	0.00143
K-a-2-X	0.0294	0.0008	0.956	0.00076
K-b-1-X	0.0336	0.0004	0.940	0.00038
K-b-2-X	0.0345	0.0001	0.938	0.00009
			Total	0.37745

The absorbed fraction $\phi_i(T \leftarrow S)$ depends on:

(i) X or γ-ray energy
(ii) dimensions of the source and target organs
(iii) distance of the source from the target.

Generally, $\phi_i(T \leftarrow S) \leq 1$

The absorbed fraction is defined as:

$$\phi_i(T \leftarrow S) = \frac{\text{energy absorbed by target}}{\text{energy emitted by source}}$$

Total Dose (D)

D = sum of instantaneous dose rates (d) for the total period of interest

hence,

$$D = \phi \int_0^t d.dt$$

$$= \phi \int_0^t A\Sigma\Delta_i\phi_i \,.\, dt$$

The integrated activity, or cumulated activity, (A) becomes: $A = \phi_0^t$ A dt, which is also proportional to the number of clear transformations; A is dependent on the physical and biological T½ which are combined in the T½ (eff) such that,

$$A = \phi \int_0^t A_0^{e(-0.693/T½\,eff).t}\, dt$$

$$= 1.44\ T½(eff)\ A_0 \qquad (2)$$

where A_0 is the administered activity in mu. hence (1) may be rewritten:

$$D = [(A_0/M) \times 1.44 \times T½\,eff \times \Delta_{np}]$$
$$+ [(A_0/M \times \Sigma_i\Delta_i\phi_i(T \leftarrow S)]$$
$$+ [(A_0/M) \times \Sigma_i\Delta_i\phi_i(T \leftarrow wb)] \qquad (3)$$

The introduction of the 'S' factors by Snyder and colleagues have appreciably reduced the calculation procedures of absorbed radiation dose. The 'S' factor depends uniquely on the physical data for a given radionuclide, source and target organs (Table 6).

Using 'S' factors, (3) can further be reduced to:

$$D = A\ .\ S(T\ \ T) + A_{wb}(T \leftarrow wb) \qquad (4)$$

where,

$S(T \leftarrow T)$ = mean absorbed dose in target per unit commulated activity from radiation within the target itserlf (rad/μCi-h)

$S(T \leftarrow wb)$ = mean absorbed dose in target per cumulated activity for radiation outside the target (rad/μCi-h).

The estimation of absorbed dose is based on a number of assumptions and can, therefore, only be used as a guideline. The problems associated with dose estimation can briefly be categorised into 3 groups:

(i) Anthropomorphic reference man which is based on a standard weight of 70 Kg with finite organ dimensions in the shapes of ellipsoids, cyclinders, etc. (Fig. 2)
(ii) Biodistribution studies of radiopharmaceuticals which are extrapolated from small experimental animal data to man, so that absorbed dose estimates especially in children and the aged may show significant variations.
(iii) Finally, biokinetic data is seldom corrected for a disease state of the individual for whom absorbed dose is being estimated.

External Dose rate estimation:

Radiation from an external source may be estimated from the following relationship:

$$J_s = (\Gamma \times A)/d^2$$

where

Γ = gamma rate constant (table 9)

J_s = exposure at distance d from source

A = activity in Bq

example:

A radiation source of strength 370 MBq of Tc-99m at a distance of 1.5 metres will produce the following dose rate:

$$J_s = (0.0164 \times 370)/(1.5)^2$$
$$= 27\ \mu Sv\ hr^{-1}$$

Examples of internal dose estimation.

1. 2mCi Tc-99m MAA is administered to an adult of weight 70Kg.
   Assume that 95% of the activity is taken up in the lungs in its first pass and remains there for there with effective t½ of 6 hours.
   (Assume mass of the lungs to be 1000g).

   From Table 7. $\Sigma_i\Delta_i\phi_i = 0.08$

   activity in lungs = 0.95 × 2000 = 1900 mu
   weight of lungs = 1000g
   dose to lungs = (1900/1000) × 1.44 × 6h × 0.08
   = *1.3 rads (0.013 Gy)*
   equivalent dose = 0.013 *0.12
   = 0.0015 Sv

Table 6
An Extract from the MIRD Tables of 'S' Factors for Tc-99m for Various Source and Target Organs Based on Organ Masses of Reference Man.

Source target	*Bladder content* $(\times 10^{-7})$	*Kidneys* $(\times 10^{-7})$	*Liver* $(\times 10^{-7})$	*Lungs* $(\times 10^{-7})$	*Total Body* $(\times 10^{-7})$
Bladder wall	1600	2.8	1.6	0.36	23
Kidneys	2.6	1900	39	8.4	22
Liver	1.7	39	460	25	22
Lungs	0.24	8.5	25	520	20
Total body	19	22	22	20	20

Using 'S' factors (table 6)

$$D(\text{lung} \leftarrow \text{lung}) = 1900 \times 6 \times 1.44 \times 5.2 \times 10^{-5}$$
$$= \mathit{0.85\ rads\ (0.0085\ Gy)}$$

$$\text{equivalent dose} = 0.0085 * 0.12$$
$$= 0.001\ \text{Sv}$$

In both cases above, the remaining 5% of the dose is ignored since its contribution will be relatively small and therefore, ignored. The slight difference between the results obtained from the two approaches arise from the differences in the standard man use for 'S' factor and absorbed fraction estimation. A therapeutic application is as follows:-

2 Patient with a hyperactive thyroid nodule is referred for I^{131} therapy. Assume: that the patient has an uptake of 60%, weighs 70Kg, has a nodule mass of 20gm, and the receives a 15mCi therapy dose of I^{131}, the residence time in the gland is 6 hours i.e. and effective t½ of 6 hours, then

From table 5a

For non-penetrating radiations:

$$\Sigma_i \Delta_i \phi_i = 0.4085$$

Activity in gland = 0.6 × 15000 = 9000mu

$$\text{Dose to thyroid} = (9000/20\text{g}) \times 1.44 \times 6\ \text{h} \times 0.4085$$

$$= \mathit{1588.2\ rads\ (15.88\ Gy).}$$

From table 5b

For penetrating radiation within the nodule:

$$\Sigma_i \Delta_i \phi_i = 0.02038$$

$$\text{Dose to nodule} = (9000/20) \times 1.44 \times 6\ \text{h} \times 0.02038$$

$$= \mathit{79.2\ rads\ (0.79\ Gy)}$$

From table 5c

For penetrating radiation outside the nodule:

$$\Sigma_i \Delta_i \phi_i = 0.3775$$

Activity distributed in rest of body

= 15000 − 9000 = 6000 mu

Assume effective T½ in rest of body

= 18 hours

$$\text{Dose to nodule} = (6000/(70000 - 20)) \times 1.44 \times 18 \times 0.3775$$

$$= \mathit{0.84\ rads\ (0.0084\ Gy)}$$

hence, total dose to the nodule

$$= 15.88 + 0.79 + 0.0084\ \text{Gy}$$
$$= \mathit{16.68\ Gy}$$

$$\text{Equivalent dose} = 0.05 * 16.68$$
$$= 0.834\ \text{Sv}$$

As we can see from example 2, the radionuclides useful for therapeutic applications should have an abundance of non-penetrating radiation components to be able to impart sufficient energy to the target to achieve cell death. Table 4 shows some of the nuclides which could successfully be used for this purpose.

The special case of the infiltrated radiopharmaceutical injection:

The intravenous administration of radiopharmaceuticals carry a certain risk of extravasation at the site of the injection leading to high absorbed dose at the site of infiltration. There have been reports of radiation necrosis resulting from such accidental extravasation.

The estimate of a worst case radiation dose to tissue may be approached by the following equation:

$$D = 10^3 \times (A \times \Delta_{np})/(L \times V)\text{cGy} \qquad (1)$$

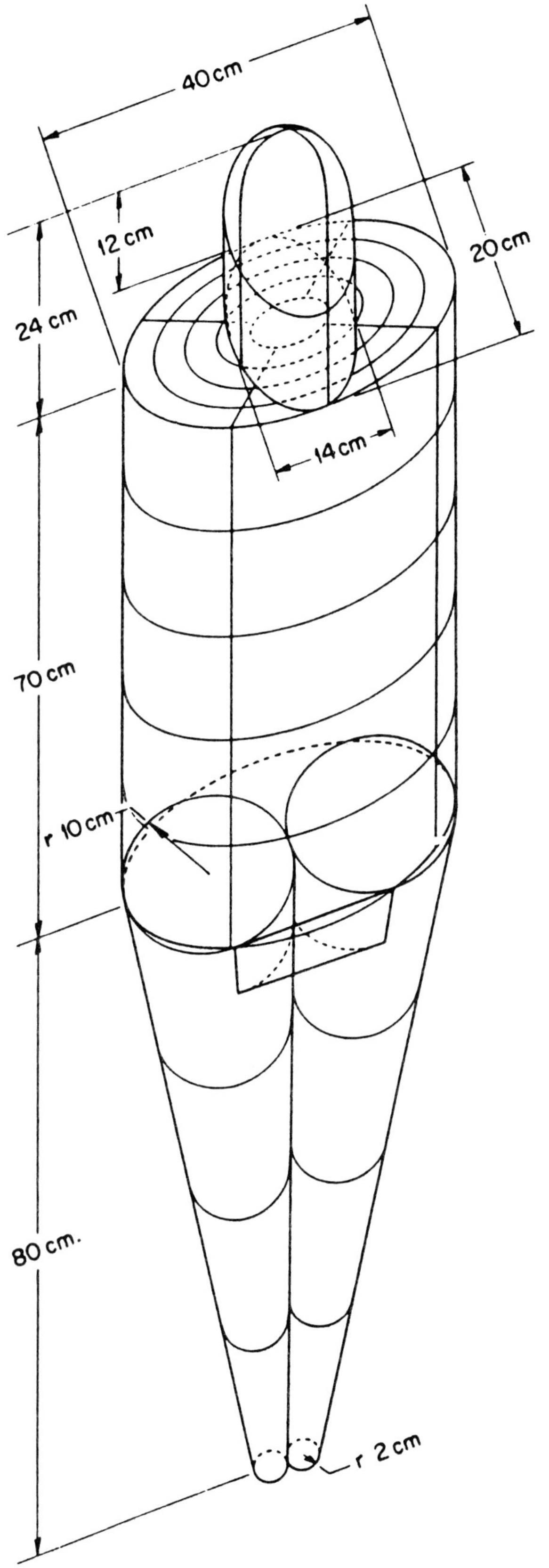

Figure 2. Reference Man showing the finite dimensions of the head, body and legs as used for the MIRD estimations.

Table 7.
Decay Table for Tc-99m. T½ = 6.03 hours

Radiation	N_i	E_i *(MeV)*	$\Delta_{i\,i}$	$\phi\phi_{i\,i}$	Δ
C_1-M int. conv. e^-	0.986	0.002	0.0035	1	0.004
$c_2 + c_3$ photons	0.883	0.140	0.2642	0.16	0.042
K int. conv. e^-	0.0088	0.1215	0.0022	1	0.022
L int. conv. e^-	0.012	0.138	0.0034	1	0.003
M int. conv. e^-	0.004	0.140	0.0011	1	0.001
K a_1 X-ray	0.044	0.0183	0.0017	1	0.002
K a_2 X-ray	0.022	0.0182	0.0003	0.88	0.003
K b X-ray	0.011	0.021	0.0004	0.87	–
KLL Auger electron	0.015	0.0154	0.0005	1	0.001
LMM Auger electron	0.109	0.0019	0.0004	1	–
MXY Auger electron	1.236	0.0004	0.0011	1	0.001
			$\Sigma_i\Delta_i\phi_i$		0.008

where,

Δ_{np} = equilibrium dose constant for non-penetrating radiation (The contribution of hard x-rays and gamma radiation to local dose can be neglected)
L = decay constant in hours
V = extravasated volume in ml. with a given activity, A

Eq. 1 can be rearranged as:

$$D = d \times a \text{ (cGy)} \qquad (2)$$

where,

d = specific dose factor
a = specific activity of the injection

$$d = 10_3 \times (\Delta_p/L) \text{ rad ml mCi}_{-1} \text{ (cGy ml 37 MBq}_{-1})$$

$Da = d \times a \times k$ cGy

where $k = Tm½ / t½$

Tm½ = measured half-time of clearance from infiltration site
t½ = physical half-life of radionuclide.

Assumption:

(1) the total tissue volume for local dose deposition (dose) is inversely proportional to the volume administered, taking a homogenous distribution of tissue and radiopharmaceutical = twice the volume of injection.

Table 8
d Values for Infiltrated Radiopharmaceuticals

Isotope	*d (cGy ml/MBq)*	*a(MBq/ml)*	*D cGY (rad)*
Ga-67	262.6	74	19430
Tc-99m	8.7	2220	19268
In-111	203.3	37	7521
I-123	31.0	74	2294
I-131	3081.4	37	114021
Tl-201	255.8	37	9465
F-18	36.5	370	1352

Table 9
Gamma Ray Constants Where the Mean Energy for an Ion Pair in Air is Taken as 33.7 eV and Associated Annual Limits on Intake

Nuclide	*T½*	*μSvm²h⁻¹ MBq⁻¹ (x10⁻³*	*ALI** MBq (μSv h⁻¹ at 1 metre*	
			Inhalation	*Ingestion*
K-40	1.28×10^9 y	21.92	6 (0.132)	4 (0.088)
K-42	12.44 h	37.13	50 (1.866)	50 (1.866)
Fe-52	8.275 h	112.75	40 (4.510)	10 (1.228)
Fe-59	44.53 d	171.17	5 (0.856)	10 (1.712)
Co-57	270.9 d	0.3822	30 (0.012)	90 (0.034)
Co-60	5.271 y	354.35	2 (0.709)	7 (2.481)
Ga-67	78.26 h	25.03	200 (5.006)	80 (2.002)
Ga-68	68.2 m	148.51	10 (1.485)	9 (1.337)
Mo-99	66.0 h	21.294	50 (1.065)	30 (0.639)
Tc-99m	6.02 h	16.598	2000 (33.196)	1000 (1.660)
In-111	2.83 d	55.419	100 (5.542)	50 (2.771)
In-113m	102 m	39.585	2000 (79.170)	900 (35.627)
I-123*	13.2 h	57.658	200 (11.532)	90 (5.189)
I-125*	60.14 d	36.145	2 (0.072)	1 (0.036)
I-131	8.04 d	57.876	1 (0.058)	0.8 (0.046)
Tl-200	26.1 h	149.60	200 (29.920)	100 (14.960)
Tl-201	3.03 d	2.1567	400 (0.863)	300 (0.647)
Tl-202	12.23 d	65.693	80 (5.263)	50 (3.290)

y = years; d = days; h = hours; m = minutes; s = seconds.
* Includes X-rays >11 keV.
** Annual Limits on Intake in Mbq (with estimated doserates at 1 metre distance).

Table 10 summarizes the absorbed dose estimates for common nuclear medical procedures, and where available, the absorbed dose to the critical organ, gonads and red bone marrow. A brief comparison of the effective dose equivalents between nuclear medicine and radiology are tabulated in Table 8.

The main differences in the factors contributing to absorbed dose in nuclear medicine and radiology are:

Nuclear medicine:

(1) Biodistribution of the radiopharmaceutical determines the organs and irradiation time;
(2) dose estimates are derived from physical data of radionuclides applied to reference man and laboratory animals;
(3) dose reports include source and target organ as well as all other organs of interest.

Radiology:

(1) Organ/s are only irradiated at time of investigation;
(2) doses received by internal organs are extrapolated from measured skin doses;
(3) reports normally include the skin dose, gonads and red bone marrow.

FURTHER READING

(1) Publications of the International Commission on Radiological Protection (ICRP).
  (a) Number 17 (1971) – Protection of the patient in radionuclide investigations.
  (b) Number 23 (1975) – Report on the task group on reference man.
  (c) Number 25 (1977a) – The handling, storage, use and disposal of unsealed radionuclides in hospitals and medical research establishments.
  (d) Number 26 (1977b) – Recommendations of the ICRP.
  (e) Number 27 (1977c)-Problems involved in developing an index of harm.
  (f) Number 28 (1978) – Statement from the 1978 Stockholm meeting of the ICRP.
  (g) Number 30 (1979) – Part 1-limits for intake of radionuclides by workers.
  (h) Number 52 (1987) – Protection of the patient in nuclear medicine.
  (i) Number 60 (1990) – 1990 Recommendations of the ICRP.
  (j) Number 61 (1190) – Annual limits on intake of radionuclides by workers based on the 1990 recommendations.
(2) Publications of the International Commission on Radiation Units and Measurements (ICRU).
  (a) Report 19 (1971) – Radiation quantities and units.
  (b) Supplement (1973) – Dose Equivalent.

Table 10
Typical Absorbed Dose Estimates from Nuclear Medical Procedures

Investigation and dose	*mCi*	*Total body*	*Critical organ*	*Gonads*	*R.B.M.*
Tc-99m					
Brain-Glucohept.	20	150 (1.5)	4500 (48) bladder	*55 (0.60)	120 (1.3)
Bone-MDP	10	≈ 100 (1.08)	1100 (12) bladder	180 (1.9)	–
Heart-HSA	15	–	750 (8.1) blood	300 (3.2)	300 (3.2)
Lung-MAA	2	≈ 30 (0.32)	1000 (10.8) lungs	*10 (0.11)	150 (1.6)
Liver-Colloid	4	60 (0.64)	1300 (14) liver	80 (0.86)	80 (0.86)
Gallbladder – HIDA	5	50 (0.54)	1600 (17.3) S.I.	*250 (2.08)	100 (1.1)
Kidneys – DMSA	2	8 (0.09)	≈ 1000 (10.8) kidneys	*37 (0.4)	70 (0.76)
– DTPA	2	20 (0.22)	76 (0.82) kidneys	*40 (0.37)	28 (0.30)
– MAG3	5	25 (0.27)	2350 (25.4) bladder	72 (0.77)	–
Thyroid – TcO_4	1	15 (0.16)	350 (3.78) thyroid	*15 (0.16)	22 (0.24)
I-131					
Thyroid uptake	0.005	13 (0.14)	15000 (160) thyroid	*6 (0.07)	–
I-123					
Renogram-hippuran	0.100	0.8 (0.009)	2 (0.02) kidneys	*2.2 (0.05)	–
Ga-67					
Tumor localisation	5	1300 (14.05)	4500 (48.65) L.I.	*1200 (6)	3000 (33)
TL-201					
Myocardium	2	480 (5.19)	293 (3.17) kidneys	600 (6.5)	500 (5.4)
In-111					
Myocardium antimyosin	2	1020 (11.03)	8800 (95) kidneys	*1100 (12)	1000 (11)

* mean male and female. ( ) = dose in Sv.

Table 11
Abridged Version of the Effective Dose Equivalents (e.d.q.) from Radiopharmaceutical and X-ray Investigations are Categorised by the W.H.O.

Nuclear Medicine Investigiation	*Radiopharm.*	*e.d.q. mSv/mBq*	*Radiology Investigation*	*e.d.q. mSv/film*
W.H.O. Category I.				
Lung	Kr-81m	0.01–0.03	Chest	0.034
Thyroid uptake	I-123 (oral)	0.17	Skull	0.05
Renography	I-123 Hippuran	0.017–0.035		
Renography	Tc-99m DTPA	0.005–0.009		
W.H.O. Category II.				
Thyroid image	$TcO_4$99m	0.011	IVU	0.54
Lung perfusion	Tc-99m MAA	0.012	Chest CT	0.37
Liver (RES)	Tc-99m Colloid	0.013	Cholecystog.	0.21
Thyroid uptake	I-131 (oral)	16.00	Thoracic spine	0.38
Bone	Tc-99m MDP	0.0067–0.011	Lumbar spine	0.65
			Pelvis	1.09
W.H.O. Category III.				
Static brain	$TcO_4$99m	0.11	Barium enema	0.91
Gated cardiac	Tc-99m RBC	0.007		
Mycoardium	Tl-201	0.093		
Abscess	Ga-67	0.1125		

(c) Report 25 (1976) – Conceptual basis for the determination of dose equivalent.
(d) Report 32 (1979) – Methods of assessment of absorbed dose in clinical use of radionuclides.
(e) Report 33 (1980) – Radiation quantities and units.
(f) Report 39 (1985) – Determination of dose equivalents resulting from external radiation sources.

(3) United Nations Scientific Committee on the effects of atomic radiation (UNSCEAR).
1977 – Sources and Effects of ionizing radiation.
1982 – Ionizing radiation: Sources and biological effects.
1988b – Sources, effects and risks of ionising radiation. Annex F.
Radiation carcinogenesis in man.

(4) World Health Organization (WHO).
(a) Technical report 591 (1976) – Nuclear Medicine.
(b) Technical report 611 (1977) – Use of ionizing radiation and radionuclides on human beings for medical research, training and non-medical purposes.

(5) Committee on the Biological Effects of Ionizing Radiation (BEIR).
Report III (1980) – The effects on populations of exposure to low levels of ionizing radiation. (National Academy Press, Washington).

(6) Publications of the Medical Internal Radiation Dose Committee (MIRD).
(a) Loevinger and Berman (1968) – A schema for absorbed dose calculations for biologically distributed radionuclides.
(b) Berger (1968) – Energy deposition in water by photons from isotropic sources.
(c) Brownell, Ellet and Reddy (1968) – Absorbed fractions for photon dosimetry.
(d) Dillman (1969) – Radionuclide decay schemes and nuclear parameters for use in radiation dose estimation – part I.
(e) Snyder, Ford, Warner and Fisher (1969) – Fractions for mono-energetic photon sources uniformly distributed in various organs of a heterogeneous phantom.
(f) Dillman (1969) – Radionuclide decay schemes and nuclear parameters for use in radiation dose estimation-part II.
(g) Berger (1971) – Distribution of absorbed dose around point sources of electrons and β-particles in water and other media.
(h) Ellet and Humes (1971) – Absorbed fraction for small volumes containing photon emitting radioactivity.

REFERENCES

Assisi A. and Poston J.W.(1987). *Comparison of measured and calculated internal absorbed doses in a heterogeneous phanton.* Phys. Med. Biol., **32**, **10**, 1245–1256.

Berger M.J. (1963). *Monte Carlo calculations of the penetration and diffusion of fast charged particles. Methods in computational physics volume 1.* Academic Press N.Y. pp. 135–215.

Broerse J.J. (1989). *Influence of physical factors in radiation carcinogenesis in experimental animals. In* Low dose radiation: Biological bases of risk assessment, pp 181–194.

Darby S.C., *et al.*, (1985). *A parallel analysis of cancer mortality among atomic bomb survivors and patients with ankylosing spondylitis given x-ray therapy.* J. Natl Cancer Inst. **75**, 1–21.

Fry R.J.M., *et al.*, (1987). *External radiation carcinogenesis.* Adv. Radiat. Biol. **13**, 31–89.

Hoop B. (1991). *The infiltrated radiopharmaceutical injection: risk considerations editorial.* JNM vol 32, no. **5**, 890–891.

Luckey T.D. (1982). *Physiological benefits from low levels of ionizing radiation.* Health Physics., **43**, **6**, 771–789.

Marks M.A. and Adelstein S.J. (1986). *Radiation doses from radionuclides administered for therapy.* Clinics in Oncology., **5**, **1**, 109–124.

NAS (1990). *Health effects of exposure to low levels of ionising radiation.* BEIR V Report. National Academy of Sciences. National Academy Press, Washington, DC.

Shapiro B., *et al.*, (1987). *Dosimetric consequences of insterstitial extravasation following I.V. administration of a radiopharmaceutical.* Eur. J. Nucl. Med. **12**, 522–523.

Upton A.C., *et al.*, *Radiation carcinogenesis.* Elsevier, New York.

Chapter 25

New Radiopharmaceuticals

P.H. Cox and S.J. Mather

25.1 INTRODUCTION

Despite the significant advances in morphological imaging, which have been made during the last decade, it remains a fact that pathological changes are often only detected after the disease has reached a fairly advanced stage. Pathophysiological alterations in organ function, on the other hand, usually occur and can be detected long before there is visual evidence of structural change.

Alterations in organ function frequently influence the biodistribution of radiopharmaceuticals and such changes are readily detectable on static scintigraphic images or in kinetic studies permitting the early detection of disease.

By selecting regions of interest on a planar scintigram or by means of single photon- or positron emission-tomographyit is possible to evaluate subregions of a given organ to identify foci of disease (Ott 1989). Despite the widespread use of nuclear medicine the exploitation of these possibilities has not been optimal. The development of positron emission tomography, which created the possibility to use labelled metabolites and many other carrier molecules, such as drugs, which could not otherwise have been labelled, has clearly demonstrated the potential of nuclear medicine to monitor subtle changes in metabolism.

This has, in turn, actively stimulated the development of more effective radiopharmaceuticals, analogous in some cases to positron emitters, but labelled with single photon emitters which have a wider application in clinical nuclear medicine and which are more economically viable.

The number of radionuclides is finite and relatively few are suitable for nuclear medicine because of various factors which combine to limit their usefulness such as

Radiation burden to the patient.
Radiation burden to personnel.
Detectability.
Reactivity (ability to form stable complexes with carrier molecules).
Availability.
Economic viability.

Within these limitations two groups of radionuclide emerge. The relatively short lived positron emitters and single gamma photon emitters of which the latter have until recently proved to meet the above criteria the best and are the most widely used.

When considering the possibilities to develop new radiopharmaceuticals it is both convenient and practical to consider these groups of nuclide separately. In both cases the biodistribution characteristics of the radiopharmaceutical are primarily determined by the nature of the carrier molecule. The choice of radionuclide will be limited by the possibilities for interaction with the carrier to form a stable compound without radically altering the biodistribution. The latter is the most difficult problem to overcome with single photon emitters.

25.2 POSITRON EMITTING RADIOPHARMACEUTICALS

The attraction of positron emitters are twofold, firstly the most readily available C-11,O-15,N-13 and F-18 are elements which are normal components of metabolites and many other potential carrier molecules. Consequently it is possible to label carriers, by synthesis, without alteration of their structure and biological behaviour. F-18 is a minor exception in that it is substituted for hydrogen whereby the labelled material may not follow the full metabolic pathway of the carrier.

Nevertheless a large number of natural metabolites, such as fatty acids, sugars, proteins, and amino acids have been produced and used with success to study the function of the heart, brain and tumours and how they are affected by disease and react to therapy (Ott, 1989) (Jacobson, 1988). Labelled drug molecules for the identification of receptor sites are also providing a wealth of original information.

The second advantage of positron emitters is the relatively high count rates which can be achieved and which, coupled with coincidence counting, enables high quality tomographic images to be produced.

The major problem is the high cost of producing the radionuclides and also of the scanning equipment. From the economic point of view PET will likely remain restricted to relatively few specialised centres with a limited number of satellite units around them using longer life products. The US Council on Scientific Affairs identified some 40 PET centres in 1988 whilst in Europe in 1989 there are 29 units in operation or being installed.

If the cost of the scanning apparatus could be reduced it would be possible to operate viable PET units without cyclotron facilities using generator produced radionuclides and pharmaceuticals labelled with F-18 or one of the other halogens.

25.3 SINGLE PHOTON EMITTING RADIOPHARMACEUTICALS

25.3.1 Technetium Complexes

There are a number of reasons why Technetium-99m remains the radionuclide of choice for in-vivo nuclear medical procedures. The favourable radiation characteristics, availability and relative cheapness are the major influences, but equally important is its chemical reactivity. The latter makes it possible to bind technetium to a variety of carrier molecules. Until recently this has mainly been realised by reducing technetium from pertechnetate to a lower valency form in the presence of a reducing agent, such as stannous tin ions, whereupon it forms coordination complexes with suitable carrier molecules.

In recent years, however, much attention has been paid to the synthesis of carrier molecules in which the technetium is incorporated into the carrier molecule structure to produce a stable molecule. The most successful examples to date have been Tc-HMPAO, which passes the blood brain barrier and has proved to be a useful agent to study cerebral and tumour blood flow, Tc-MAG3 a hippuran analogue for renal function studies and the isobutylnitrile complex to evaluate myocardial perfusion (Quang Sheng, 1988). Partly because of its lipophilicity HMPAO is also being propagated as a reagent to label blood cells without damaging their viability (McAfee 1987; Podreka 1987). At the same time several other novel methods, to label leucocytes, have also been proposed using technetium labelled antibodies against CEA (Joseph 1987) or technetium colloids (Mock, 1987). With respect to the development of novel cationic technetium compounds Deutsch (1987) has discussed in-vivo reactions which may occur to affect their biodistribution, (see also Chapters 3 and 18).

In the past the *in vivo* stability of technetium labelled proteins has greatly limited their value but recently the labelling methods developed by Schwartz (1988) for labelling antibodies appears to have surmounted this problem and may well pave the way for the widespread in vivo-use of technetium labelled antibodies and other peptide carrier molecules, (for fuller discussion see Chapter 8).

25.3.2 Generators

The requirement for a short lived radionuclide for blood pool studies either for organ perfusion or multiple first pass myocardial studies has stimulated much interest in the development of generator systems. The most successful to date has been the Rb-81/Kr-81m generator which has found widespread use for lung ventilation studies, particularly in Europe where the supply logistics are favourable to widespread distribution. This generator as also found to have a considerable potential for organ perfusion when the Krypton is eluted in solubilised form in 5% Glucose solution. This has been found to be particularly useful for selective coronary perfusion. The generator is only suited for continuous elution and cannot be used for bolus injections.

For the generation of bolus activity several generators have been proposed the first of which was the Mercury-197/Gold-198 generator. This generator has not received widespread acceptance because although the bolus generation is efficient the energy of the daughter element is too high for efficient counting with the thin crystal gamma cameras in common use so that high count rates could only be achieved using digital cameras or older thick crystal cameras. A further drawback is the constant requirement to elute at frequent intervals in order to keep the level of mercury breakthrough down to acceptable levels. This inevitably results in the accumulation of active fluid waste.

An alternative with considerable potential is the osmium iridium generator which has already been used with considerable success. The energy of iridium is better suited for modern gamma cameras, and is suited for paediatric use. This generator could have a wide field of application once it becomes readily available.

Recently the development of a Tungsten-178/Tantalum-178 generator has been described, (Lacyet al). Ta-178 has a half life of 9.3 min with a primary energy emission of 55 and 64 keV X-rays. The generator has a useful life of up to 30 days and therefore is of potential interest as clinical tool. For optimal detection however a multiwire gamma camera is required and therefore its further implementation is dependent upon developments in instrumentation.

25.4 GENERATOR SYSTEMS FOR P.E.T.

As we have mentioned earlier the development of Positron Emission Tomography as a routine nuclear medical procedure outside of specialised centres will be dependent upon considerable cost reductions both with respect to instrumentation and the production of radiopharmaceuticals.

The possibility of developing a positron camera which is economically viable would now appear to be feasible

(Scotanus, 1988) and much work has already been done to develop radiopharmaceuticals which are cyclotron independent. Appart from the potential of F-18 and other halogens to produce ready for use radiopharmaceuticals outside the hospital a number of useful Positron emitters can be made available as generator eluates.

Probably the most viable of these is the Germanium-68/Gallium-68 generator (Gleason 1960, Greene and Tucker 1961). This generator has the advantages that the daughter element has a short half life with a rapid build up to equilibrium enabling elutions to take place every 3–4 hours. The useful generator life is long, the half life of germanium is 275 days, which considerably reduces the cost.

Gallium-68 has a half life of 68 minutes which allows ample time to prepare labelled compounds and administer them to the patient. The reactivity of gallium, is such that a wide range of radiopharmaceuticals, analogous to technetium, can be prepared (Yano 1971, Cox 1987). Furthermore the propensity of Gallium for protein binding offers opportunities with respect to the labelling of tumour markers and other peptides.

The Strontium-82/Rubidium-82 generator has also been proposed as a potentially important system for the study of myocardial ischaemia and infarction (Yano, 1968). The short halflife of Rb-82 (1.5 min) would permit serial PET studies to be made at frequent intervals and at the same time the reagent could also prove to be useful in studying the perfusion of other organs such as the brain, (for further discussion on generators see Chapter 2).

25.5 NEW CARRIER MOLECULES

Several potentially important groups of carrier molecule are under investigation as potential radiopharmaceuticals which could be labelled with either single photon or positron emitters.

25.5.1 Monoclonal Antibodies

The development of monoclonal antibodies for the detection and accurate measurement of antigenic materials, such as hormones and tumour associated antigens, in serum and urine clearly demonstrated their potential as specific markers for the tissues producing the antigen. The problems of bulk production of highly purified antibody suitable for injection into humans have been largely solved but the products remain expensive which limits their use.

At the present time the majority of antibodies in vivo use are against tumour associated antigens. In most cases supplies are limited to selected centres and are not available for widespread clinical use. Nevertheless several have become available through commercial sources (ie: Anti-CEA, Anti-melanoma, OC-125 and Antimyosin) either as ready labelled injectable material labelled with I-131 or In-111 or as labelling kits for in house labelling with these radionuclides or with Technetium-99m.

A number of potentially interesting applications for labelled antibodies, unrelated to oncology, have been reported for the detection of myocardial infarcts and cardiac myopathy, deep venous thrombosis and for the selective *in vivo* labelling of granulocytes. There are many other possible areas of exploration, for instance in the detection of focal parasitic infection, where antibodies could be usefully employed.

In developed countries the introduction of monoclonal antibodies for in vivo use has been retarded by the stringent registration requirements which have been implemented, either through the National Drug Registration authorities or via the regulatory authorities for Blood Products. The control procedures involved are also costly and this is clearly influencing the rate of development of products suitable for clinical use.

When using labelled antibodies in vivo the whole antibody, usually an IgG, clears slowly from the blood so that optimal scanning times vary from 48 to 120 hours post injection, which prohibits the use of technetium as a label. There is, in all cases a considerable accumulation of activity in the liver, spleen, bone marrow and intestines which can give rise to problems of interpretation particularly in the case of abdominal lesions. The majority of antigens are cell surface antigens which are frequently shed leading to high blood retention due to binding to circulating antigen.

The problem of background activity has been partly solved by breaking down the IgG into fractions, by peptide digestion and isolating and labelling the antigen specific Fab^2 fraction. This reduces the non specific binding and also increases the rate of blood clearance and excretion of the labelled antibody. The more rapid reduction of background activity also reduces the waiting time before optimal target to background activity ratio's are obtained thus reopening the door for the use of Technetium as label.

As foreign protein monoclonal antibodies can give rise to Human Antimouse Antibody (HAMA) development in patients, these at best may lead to high tissue background activity but may also result in the development of severe allergic responses in follow up studies. In the case of IgG's the incidence of HAMA development is almost 100% whilst the Fab^2 fractions it is considerably less at around 50%. Tests for the presence of HAMA's in serum are now commercially available. many of these problems may be solved in the future by the development of chimeric and synthetic antibodies or by the use of adjuvants to reduce critical organ uptake.

The target to background activity ratios have in general been found to be low, in the region of 3 to 1, so that serial scintigrams and often single photon emission tomography are necessary to indentify diffuse lesions. It is also self evident that a considerable degree of expertise is required of the nuclear medical specialist. nevertheless good results are now regularly being reported and whilst it is clear that labelled in monoclonal antibodies are not going to be the 'Magic Bullet' that was hoped for they do have a useful role to fulfill.

The potential for using labelled antibodies as radiotherapeutic agents is limited by the availability of suitable nuclides and by the dose to the critical organ, usually the liver, which often precludes the administration of an effective dose to the tumour. Some useful results have been claimed using selective administration routes, such as intracavity, intra arterial, intrathecal and interstitial injection, to give a higher initial tumour exposure but these remain experimental at the present time.

To summarize there are a number of labelled antibodies which are available for routine use, as in vivo diagnostic agents, in selected groups of patients but the majority of reports to date refer to antibodies which are not readily available. Radiotherapy with labelled antibodies is clearly restricted to a few specialised centres and is in an early stage of development, (see also Chapter 8 and 22).

25.5.2 Drug Receptors and Peptide Hormones

A number of labelled compounds have been produced, primarily labelled with I-123, which localise in drug receptor sites related to dopamines, amphetamine and acetylcholine. Such compounds show great potential in evaluating the progression of disease. A review of these and other compounds has been produced by McAfee (1989).

Somatostatin is a naturally occurring 14-amino-acid peptide hormone which is widely present in the body and has a variety of biological functions (Wass, 1989). It is present in the hypothalamus and other areas of the central nervous system, in peripheral nerves, the gastrointestinal tract, placenta, retina, thymus and adrenal medulla. Its principal role appears to be as an inhibitor of pituitary growth hormone secretion. However it also inhibits the secretion of a large number of other hormones, notably TSH, ACTH, Gastrin, VIP and insulin. In normal tissues, the highest concentrations of somatostatin receptors are found in the brain, anterior pituitary, pancreas, gastrointestinal tract and adrenal gland. High expression of somatostatin receptors is also seen in a number of tumour types most frequently those arising from the pituitary and pancreas but also sometimes in more common tumours such as in breast and some types of lung cancer.

When somatostatin is administered exogenously to man it has a very short half-life in plasma (2–3 minutes) due to rapid excretion by both the liver and the kidney, and to breakdown by serum proteases. This short half-life would severely limit the scintigraphic application of this hormone. However the therapeutic potential of somatostatin has stimulated the development of a number of synthetic analogues which have more appropriate pharmacological profiles. The most widely used of these is octreotide, an octapeptide containing a number of D-amino acids which confer protease resistance on the molecule. Octreotide has a serum half-life of the order of 100 minutes. It has many of the actions of the parent hormone but appears to be more selective in its inhibitory actions. Octreotide is most widely used therapeutically to suppress growth hormone secretion in acromegaly. However it has also proved useful in alleviating the effects of hypersecretion of other hormones such as VIP and insulin from gastrointestinal tumours. Because of the expression of somatostatin receptors on a variety of cancers, the possibility exists of using radiolabelled molecules to localise these tumours.

Many tumours can be imaged with radiolabelled octreotide analogues (Krenning, 1992). However it is apparent that considerable differences exist between different tumour types. This phenomenon is due at least in part to the specificity of the targeting mechanism. Unlike other, non-specific means of imaging which are likely to identify any tumour mass, irrespective of pathology, positive localisation with radiolabelled octreotide will only occur if the tumour in question bears somatostatin receptors. Conventional measures of success in imaging such as sensitivity and accuracy need to be redefined when applied to tracers such as these. Thus, sensitivity needs to be defined in terms of the success of the technique in imaging receptor-bearing tumours. The difficulty lies in independently determining the receptor status of the tumours in question. Obtaining biopsy samples from many of these patients is difficult and many will be managed by pharmacological rather than surgical approaches.

An indirect assessment of the receptor status of a certain tumour type can be made by histochemical analysis of surgical or post-mortem samples from other patients. Reubi *et al* have examined the receptor status of several hundred human tumours in this way. As expected from the pharmacology of somatostatin, the highest levels of receptors are found in tumours of the pituitary and the pancreas although heterogeneity still exists between, for example, functioning and non-functioning pituitary adenomas and the different types of islet-cell carcinomas. A good correlation can be seen between the in-vitro receptor expression and the results obtained with imaging (Reubi, 1991).

Thus positive imaging with radiolabelled octreotide indicates the presence of somatostatin receptors on the tumour in question showing that we can in fact image function at a cellular level. Receptor status, of course, is more than either simply positive or negative and can exist as any point in a spectrum ranging from absolutely negative to abundant over-expression. A point will exist at which the density of expression will be insufficient for successful imaging and this threshold will be different for tumours of different size, different location and different depth and will also depend upon physicochemical parameters such as the affinity of the radiotracer, the radionuclide used for imaging, the dose of radioactivity used and the imaging protocol employed. A clear indication of this threshold is that despite our knowledge of the existence of somatostatin receptors in normal pancreas and adrenal glands for example, these organs are not routinely observed in images.

Clear differences can be observed in the pharmacokinetics of the octreotide labelled with different isotopes. I-123 labelled octreotide is cleared predominantly via the hepatobiliary tract and images taken greater than 30 minutes after administration show accumulation of radioactivity in the gall-bladder and the small intestine. I-111 labelled octreotide by contrast is cleared mainly via the kidneys and gastrointestinal accumulation of In-111 is seen only on images taken the day after injection. The ability of both radiopharmaceuticals to localise tumours within a few minutes of administration is a striking feature of these tracers. Some tumours can be imaged almost instantaneously and good tumour to blood contrast can often be observed within 10 minutes of injection.

These characteristics are in contrast to those observed when large molecules such as monoclonal antibodies are used for targeting. While the peptide hormones show rapid rates of blood clearance and prompt localisation, radio-labelled antibodies have much slower rates of blood clearance and localisation is normally seen only several hours after administration. Perhaps lessons can be learned frfom the success of Octreotide imaging when designing improved antibody-based tracers.

Both hormone and antibody have peptide structures and both are labelled using the same methodology – electrophilic substitution in the case of iodine and a bifunctional chelate of DTPA in the case of indium. The major difference between the two molecules is obviously that of size. Octreotide has a molecular weight of about 1000 daltons while antibodies are of the order of 150 kilodaltons. This supports the theory that a reduction in the size of antibody molecule would result in more rapid localisation. Fab and F(ab)'2 fragments of antibodies are still relatively large molecule with molecular weights of approximately 50 and 100 kilodaltons respectively. Recombinant DNA approaches have managed to produce smaller antigen binding fragments such as single domain (Dab) and single-chain Fv fragments with molecular weights of 15 and 25 kD. While such molecules are still 10–20 times larger than octreotide, it has been proposed that still smaller antibody fragments based upon minimum recognition units might be achieved.

An interesting finding arises from the comparison of the pharmacokinetics of iodine and indium labelled octreotide. While antibodies labelled with these two isotopes do show some differences in their biodistribution, these are relatively minor and relate more to the post-catabolic processing of radiolabelled metabolites than to differences in recognition of the antibody molecules themselves. Since Octreotide is such a small molecule, the decrease in lipophilicity conferred by the DTPA group is sufficient to radically alter the route of excretion of the molecule. This suggests that if targeting with very small antibody-like molecules can be achieved then it should be possible, with small changes in lipophilicity and molecular charge, to influence the route and rate of excretion to a greater extent than has been achieved with conventional antibodies and their fragments. The rapid pharmacokinetics of these compounds suggest that they could usefully be labeled with radionuclides with half-lives shorter than those of I-123 and In-111. The development of a technetium labelled native somatostatin has been reported (Cox 1992).

An important consideration for small molecules is that of binding affinity. The binding affinity of iodinated Tyr-^{11}-somatostatin and iodinated Tyr^{3}-octreotide have been reported as being similar at $K_D = 1.1$ nM and 1.5 nM respectively. In-111 D-Phe-DTPA-Octreotide has a reduced binding affinity – Bakker *et al* report that In-D-Phe-DTPA-Octreotide was approx 25 times less efficient that I-Tyr^{3}- octreotide in inhibiting receptor binding of radiolabelled octreotide. (Bakker, 1991) Thus even peptides with only moderate binding affinities can target effectively *in vivo*.

In size, octreotide must be approaching the smallest possible molecule that can have high affinity receptor interaction. The actual binding site consists of only 3 or 4 amino acids although these must be held in the correct secondary confirmation by the cyclic structure of the peptide. A widespread receptor interaction in man is mediated by the recognition of the 3-amino acid sequence – arginine-glycine-aspartic acid – (RGD). This peptide is a ligand for a subtype of the receptors known as 'integrins', a class of adhesion molecule which are ubiquitously distributed in mammalian tissues. One such receptor is carried on the surface of platelets and has been used as a target for a radiolabelled-RGD-peptide for *in-vivo* detection of platelet aggregation at sites of thrombosis. Knight *et al* have actually used a hybrid biomolecule which combines with RGD a portion of the metal binding protein metallothionein (Knight, 1990). The sequence – KCTCCA – efficiently binds technetium-99m and the combination results in a peptide which can both bind the radiolabel and interact with the receptor. Another small peptide employed in this way is melanocyte stimulating hormone (MSH) a 13-amino acid molecule which has been used, labelled with Indium-111 for the detection of melanoma. (Wraight, 1992)

If octreotide and the RGD peptides depict the smallest end of the molecular spectrum then the larget molecule so far employed in this way is probably Serum Amyloid P component (SAP). SAP is a normal constituent of human serum with a molecular weight of approximately 250,000 and an, as yet, undefined function. In the disease state amyloidosis, however, SAP become deposited in amyloid fibrils in affected organs. Hawkins *et al* have labelled SAP with radioiodine and shown that when injected into patients with systemic amyloidosis, the tracer targets with efficiently to the sites of amyloid deposition (Hawkins, 1990). This radiopharmaceutical provides a means of diagnosing and monitoring this disease with an ease and accuracy hitherto unavailable.

25.5.3 Therapeutic Agents

The introduction of organ specific, or tissue specific carrier molecules has greatly increased the potential for the use of radiopharmaceuticals to administer radiotherapy. In particular the use of monoclonal antibodies, and compounds binding to drug receptor sites have aroused much interest.

With all of these compounds the uptake in critical organs and the radiation dose to tissues around the target area poses a considerable problem (Langmuir, 1988). Attempts to surmount this problem by using more alternatives to Iodine-131 such as yttrium-90 or short lived alpha emitters such as bismuth-212 may provide an answer especially when combined with intracavity or intra arterial administration to provide a more direct route to the target tissue. (For further discussion see Chapter 22).

REFERENCES

Bakker W.H., Albert R., Bruns C. *et al.* (1991). *^{111}In-DTPA-D-Phe^{1})-Octreotide a potential radiopharmaceutical for imaging of somatostatin receptor-positive tumours: Synthesis, Radiolabelling and in-vitro validation.* Life Sci. **49**, 1583–1591.

Britton K.E. and Buraggi G.L. (1989). *A Brief Guide to the practice of radioimmunoscintigraphy and radioimmunotherapy in cancer.* Int. J. Biol. Markers., **4**, 106–118.

Cox P.H. (1987). *Gallium based Radio-pharmaceuticals. In:* Yearbook of Radio-pharmacy and Radiopharmacology. Ed: P.H. Cox. Gordon and Breach London. pp 171–184.

Cox P.H. (1992). *Technetium labelled Somatostatin a potential agent for* in vivo *tumour localisation.* Nuclear Medicine. Ed: Schmidt and Hofer, Schattauer Stuttgart, 589–592.

Deutsch E. and Hirth W. (1987). In vivo *organic chemistry of Technetium cations.* J. Nucl. Med., **28**, 1491–1500.

Gleason G.I. (1960). *A Positron Cow.* Int. J. Appl. Radiat. Isotopes., **3**, 90.

Greene M.W. and Tucker W.D. (1961). *An improved Gallium-68 cow.* Int. J. Appl. Radiat. Isotopes., **12**, 62.

Hawkins P.N., Lavender J.P. and Pepys M.B. (1990). *Evaluation of systemic amyloidosis by scintigraphy with 1231-labelled serum amyloid P component.* New. Eng. J. Med., **323**, 508–513.

Jacobsen H.G. (1988). *Cyclotrons and Radio-pharmaceuticals in Positron Emission Tomography.* J.A.M.A., **259**, 1854–1860.

Joseph K. *et al.* (1987). *In vivo labelling of Granulocytes using Technetium labelled monoclonal antibodies: first clinical results.* Nu Compact., **18**, 223–229.

Knight L.C., Radcliffe R., Kollman M. *et al.*, (1990). *Thrombus imaging with Tc-99m synthetic peptides reactive with activated platelets.* J. Nucl. Med. **31**, 757.

Krenning E.P., Bakker W.H., Kooiz P.P.M. *et al.* (1992). *Somatostatin receptor scintigraphy with indium-111 DTPA Phe-1 Octreotide in man: Metabolism, dosimetry and comparison with iodine-123-Tyr-3-Octreotide.* J. Nucl. Med., **33**, 652–658.

Lacy J.L. *et al.*, (1988). *An improved Tungsten-178/Tantalum-178 generator system for high volume clinical applications.* J. Nucl. Med., **29**, 1526–1538.

Langmuir V.K. and Sutherland R.M. (1988). *Dosimetry models for radioimmuno therapy.* Med. Phys., **15**, 867–873.

McAfee J.G. *et al.* (1987). *99m-Tc HMPAO for leucocyte labelling experimental comparison with 111-Indium Oxine in Dogs.* Eur. J. Nucl. Med., **13**, 353–357.

McAfee J.G. (1989). *Update on Radiopharmaceuticals.* Radiology., **17**, 1593–601.

Mock B.H. *et al.* (1987). *Leucocyte labelling with Technetium Tin Colloids.* J. Nucl. Med., **28**, 1471–1477.

Ott R.J. (1989). *Nuclear medicine in the 1990's: a quantitative physiological approach.* Brit. J. Radio 1., **62**, 421–432.

Podreka I. *et al* (1987). *Initial Experience with Technetium-99m HMPAO Brain SPECT.* J. Nucl. Med. **28**, 1657–1666.

Quang-Sheng Li *et al.*, (1988). *Technetium-99m methoxyisobutyll-sonitrile [RP30] for quantification of myocardial ischemia and reperfusion in Dogs.* J. Nucl. Med., **29**, 1539–1548.

Reubi J.C., Kvols L., Krenning E. and Lamberts S.W. (1991). *In vitro and in vivo detection of somatostatin receptors in human malignant tissues.* Acta. Oncol., **30**, 463–8.

Scotanus P. (1988). *A BaF2-MWPC gamma camera for positron emission tomography.* PhD Thesis University of Delft.

Sikora K. (1989). *Imaging with radiolabelled antibodies.* Clin. Radiol., **40**, 332–334.

Yano Y. (1971). *Preparation and control of 68-Ga radiopharmaceuticals. In:* Radiopharmaceuticals from generator produced radionuclides. IAEA Vienna. pp 117–125.

Yano Y and Anger H.O. (1968). *Visualisation of heart and kidneys in animals with ultrashort lived 82-Rubidium and the positron scintillation camera.* J. Nucl. Med., **9**, 412–415.

Wass J.A.H. (1989). *Somatostatin. In* Endocrinology ed. Leslie J. DeGroot. W.B. Saunders, London.

Wraight E.P., Bard D.R., Maughan T.S. *et al.*, (1992). *The use of a chelating derivtive of alpha melanocyte stimulating hormone for the clinical imaging of malignant melanoma.* Brit. J. Radiol. **65**, 112–118.

Chapter 26

Use of Radiopharmaceuticals in the Evaluation of Drug Formulations

J.G. Hardy

26.1 INTRODUCTION

Most pharmaceutical products are taken orally or by inhalation. These products may be designed to deliver drugs to specific sites or to release their active ingredients in a controlled manner. By incorporating an appropriate radiolabel into a formulation the distribution of the preparation can be monitored *in vivo* using a gamma camera.

Gamma scintigraphy is used extensively in the evaluation of pharmaceutical dosage forms (Davis *et al.,* 1992). For example, the technique can be used to confirm that enteric-coated tablets remain intact in the stomach. Additionally sites of drug absorption can be determined by combining gastrointestinal transit and pharmacokinetic data. Gamma scintigraphy has an important role in the optimisation of drug formulations for inhalation and in the assessment of inhaler devices. It is also used to monitor formulations administered by the nasal, opthalmic and rectal routes.

In general, the radiolabelling of drug formulations involves ther incorporation of a conventional radiopharmaceutical into the preparation. It is rarely possible to synthesize a drug molecule incorporating a gamma-emitting radionuclide suitable of imaging with a gamma camera. This chapter describes the methods employed for the radiolabelling of drug formulations. Examples are provided illustrating the applications of the technique.

26.2 ORAL DOSAGE FORMS

Radioactive tracers are incorporated into oral dosage forms in order to minitor gastrointestinal transit. In general, a radiolabel is required that is not absorbed from the stomach or intestines. The half-life of the radionuclide is also important. Studies of gastric emptying and small intestinal transit usually require monitoring periods of up to 10 hours, and technetium-99m may prove an appropriate radiolabel. For studies of longer duration, for example the monitoring of whole bowel transit when the imaging period may extend to 2 days or more, indium-111 is often the radionuclide of choice. The use of short-lived radionuclides, sich as technetium-99m, may be precluded by the time required to prepare the dosage form. Complex formulations may have to be prepared using specialised facilities remote from the study site. In such circumstances, it is generally more convenient to incorporate a non-radioactive tracer, such as samarium-152, into the formulation and subsequently to make the preparation radioactive by neutron activation.

26.2.1 Radiolabelling of Capsules and Tablets

26.2.1.1 Incorporation of radiopharmaceutical

Ion exchange resin in the form of beads 1–2 mm diameter can be labelled with pertechnetate or indium ions; the tracer remaining associated with the resin during transit through the gastrointestinal tract. Amberlite IRA-410 is a suitable resin for labelling with pertechnetate. A slurry is prepared of the resin in saline and sodium pertechnetate solution added. The resin is than dried in an oven at about 80°C. For indium labelling, a solution of indium chloride is added to a slurry of Amberlite IRP-69 in dilute hydrochloric acid.

The radiolabelled resin can be mixed with drug particles and loaded into capsules (Wilding *et al.,* 1991). Gamma camera imaging, following administration to volunteers, provides information on the time and position on drug release from the capsule, and of the extent of dispersion and the rate of transit through the gastrointestinal tract.

Radiolabelled tablets can be prepared by mixing radiolabelled resin powder with the tablet excipients prior to compression (Hardy *et al.,* 1987a). Typically, each tablet would contain only a few milligrams of resin. Standard *in vitro* tests can be undertaken to ensure that the addition of the resin powder does not affect the physical properties of the tablets.

Sustained-release tablets are intended to deliver drug at a predetermined rate. The incorporation of a soluble radiopharmaceutical into the tablet, the release of which matches that of the drug, facilitates monitoring of the *in vivo* behaviour of the formulation (Daly *et al.*, 1982). As with the resin, the radiopharmaceutical is added in powder form. It is necessary when undertaking such a study to carry out dissolution tests ensure that the release characteristics of the drug and radiopharmaceutical are the same. The radiopharmaceuticals most commonly employed in such studies are complexes of diethylenetriaminepentaacetic acid (DTPA) or one of the iminodiacetic acid derivatives.

The location of dispersed preparations can be established from the characteristic shapes of the stomach and colon. Determining the position of an intact dosage form may prove difficult, unless the preparation is taken with a radiolabelled drink to outline the anatomy. In such situations, the formulation is often radilabelled with indium-111 and the drink with Tc-99m DTPA (Hardy *et al.*, 1987a).

26.2.1.2 Labelling by neutron activation

The radiolabelling of solid dosage forms by neutron activation avoids the handling of radioactive materials during the preparation stages. The advantages of using this approach are:

no radioactive contamination of the production facilities
avoidance of the irradiation of staff during dosage form preparation
removal of time constraints imposed by radioactive decay
a single bath can be utilized during each phase of cross-over studies.

Radiolabelling by neutron activation involves the incorporation of a small quantity (typically 1–2 mg) of a non-radioactive tracer into each dose (Hardy *et al.*, 1991). The most useful tracers for the monitoring of oral dosage forms are samarium-152 and erbium-170 (Table 1). The nuclides are available as their oxides at >96% isotopic enrichment. The oxides are not absorbed from the gastrointestinal tract. Irradiation of a dosage form containing 2 mg Sm-152 samarium oxide for 4 minutes in a neutron flux of 10^{12} $cm^{-2}s^{-1}$ results in a radioactive content of 1 MBq samarium-153, 24 hours after removal from the nuclear reactor. Due to the lower neutron capture cross-section of erbium-170 and the shorter half-life erbium-171 compared with samarium-153, the corresponding irradiation time is 2 hours. Dual labelling of complex formulations, for example layered tablets, can be achieved by incorporating both samarium-152 and erbium-170 in appropriate quantities into the same preparation.

It is usual to undertake a trial irradiation of the standard dosage form prior to incorporation of the tracer. This enables quality control checks to be carried out to confirm that the irradiation procedure does not adverely affect the product and also to ensure that no unacceptable radioactive impurities are generated. The radioactive impurity most frequently encountered is sodium-24. When radiolabelling with samarium-153, the problem can be minimised by increasing the time between irradiation and dosing, thereby allowing the sodium-24 (half life 15 hours) to decay.

26.2.2 Radiolabelling of Liquid Preparations

Drug solutions for oral administration can be radiolabelled simply by the addition of Tc-99m DTPA. For the monitoring of suspensions, however, it is usual to radiolabel the particulate phase. This may be achieved by the addition of radiolabelled ion exchange powder of an appropriate particle size, or by the incorporation of a Tc-99m labelled colloid. Whenever possible, it is preferable to radiolabel the drug particles themselves.

26.2.2.1 Antacids

Alginic acid preparations are administered in order to protect the oesophagus against the reflux of gastric acid. These

Table 1
Tracers for radiolabelling by neutron activation

Stable nuclide	*Natural abundance (%)*	*Thermal neutron cross section* ($\times 10^{-24} cm^2$)	*Radionuclide*	*Half-life (h)*	*Principal photon energies (keV)*
Sm-152	27	216	Sm-153	47	103
Er-170	15	9	Er-171	7.5	296 308

preparations act by forming a raft that floats on the stomach contents and refluxes preferentially. The alginic acid readily combines with metal ions, such as indium or strontium, to form alginates. Administration of radiolabelled alginic acid preparation following a meal radiolabelled with a different radionuclide, for example technetium-99m, allows monitoring of the efficacy of the preparation (May *et al.,* 1984).

Many antacid preparations contain aluminium hydroxide. Radiolabelled aluminium hydroxide can be prepared by the coprecipitation of aluminium and indium hydroxides, by the addition of ammonia solution to a solution of aluminium and indium chlorides. The excess ammonia can be removed by washing the precipitate with water, and the precipitate added to the antacid preparation. The administration of radiolabelled antacids permits monitoring of the gastric residence of the formulations and can be usefully combined with studies of gastrointestinal pH.

26.2.2.2 Sucralfate

Sucralfate is used in the treatment of gastric and duodenal ulcers. It is a basic aluminium salt of sucrose sulphate and is believed to act by binding to exposed protein in the ulcer. The affinity between sucralfate and proteins has been exploited for radiolabelling purposes (Billinghurst *et al.,* 1989). The addition of Tc-99m labelled human serum albumin (Tc-99m HSA) to a sucralfate suspension results in the formation of Tc-99m labelled sucralfate that remains stable in the acid environment of the stomach. Radiolabelling can also be achieved by the reduction of Tc-99m pertechnetate with stannous ions in a sucralfate suspension (Billinghurst *et al.,* 1989). Following labelling by the pertechnetate reduction method the technetium remains bound to the sucralfate over a wider pH range. In acid conditions, however, the Tc-99m HSA label is more strongly bound to the sucralfate and is less likely to exchange with other components of the formulation. Technetium-99m labelled sucralfate can be used to compare different sucralfate formulations (Figure 1), in addition to its clinical applications in the detection of gastric ulcers.

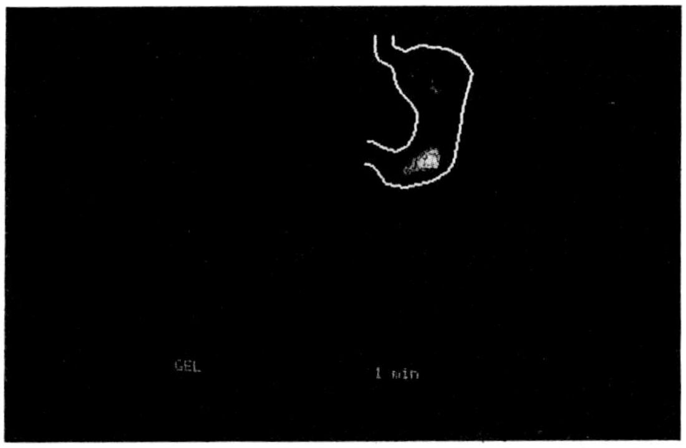

(a)

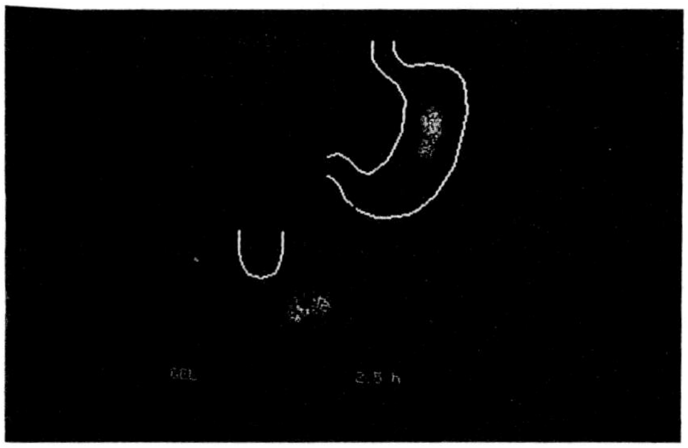

(b)

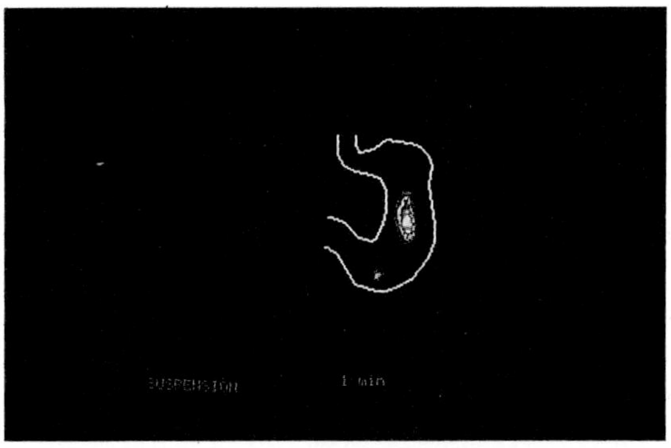

(c)

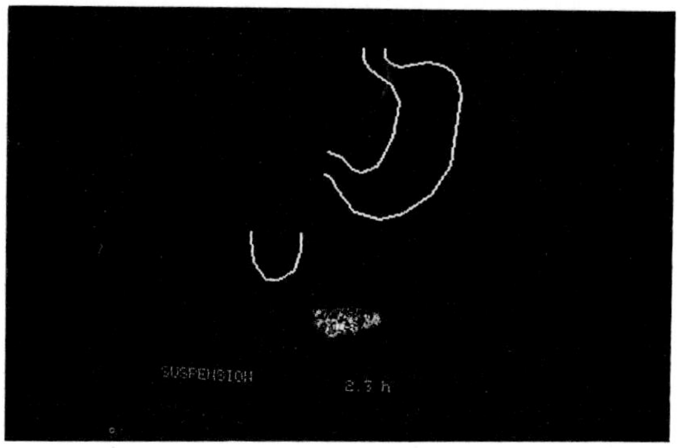

(d)

Figure 1 Enhanced retention of a Tc-99m labelled sucralfate gel in the stomach compared with a sucralfate suspension.

26.3 RECTAL FORMULATIONS

The main purpose of monitoring drug forfmulations following rectal administration is to assess the extent of spreading. This is of particular importance for drugs administered for their topical action, for example mesalzine in the treatment of ulcerative colitis. The preparations are of three types; solution and foam enemas and suppositories.

26.3.1 Radiolabelling of Enema Preparations

Most of retrograde spread of enema preparations tends to occur within the first 1–2 hours of dosing. Since dispersion is usually complete by 4 hours, technetium-99m generally proves to be an appropriate radiolabel (Hardy *et al.,* 1986).

Enema solutions can be readily labelled by the addition of Tc-99m DTPA solution. With foam enemas, however, it is important to ensure that the radiolabel becomes uniformly dispersed throughout the foam and that the addition of the tracer does not affect the stability of the product. Foam enemas are supplied in a canister fitted with a mixture of aqueous drug concentrate and propellent. Radiolabelling can be achieved by the addition into the canister of a small volume of Tc-99m DTPA solution via the valve. This technique should ensure that the foam generated is radiolabelled uniformly. This can be verified by sampling the foam and measuring the radioactivity per unit mass.

If the equipment for back filling into the canister is not available, it may be possible to radiolabel the foam by the incorporation of Tc-99m labelled ion exchange resin powder. Approximately 20–30 mg powder radiolabelled with 4 MBq technetium-99m is placed in the metering head or the applicator prior to dispensing the foam (Wood *et al.,* 1985). The extent of the mixing achieved will depend on the design of the system. The addition of small amounts of resin poweder by this technique does not, in general, affect the stability of the foam.

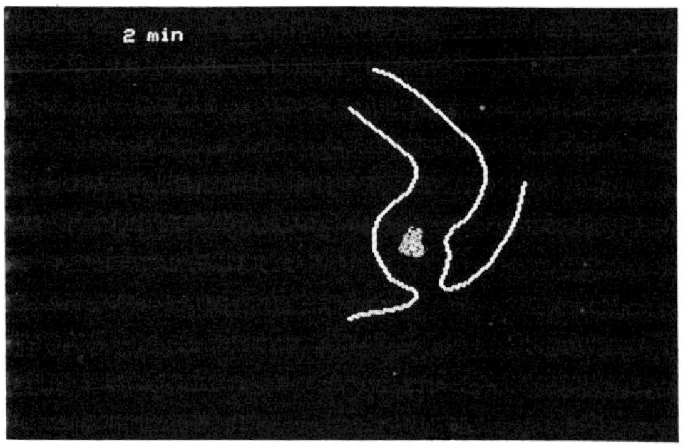

(a)

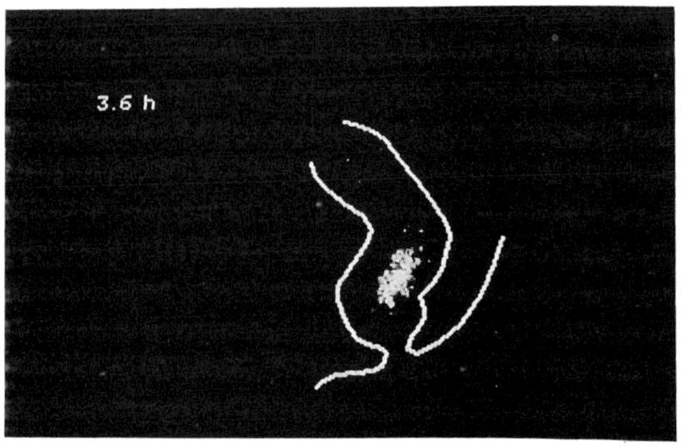

(b)

Figure 2. Spreading of an In-111 labelled suppository in the rectum.

26.3.2 Radiolabelling of Suppositories

Suppositories are radiolabelled by incorporating the tracer into the molten base prior to moulding. Ion exchange resin powder radiolabelled with technetium-99m or indium-111 can be used to simulate drug prticles distributed within the suppository. Figure 2 shows the spreading of a suppository containing 5 mg ion exchange resin powder radiolabelled with indium-111. Alternatively, Tc-99m DTPA or Tc-99m labelled hydroxymethyldiphosphonate can be added to represent a water soluble drug (Jay *et al.,* 1985). The lipid phase of suppository can be labelled by the addition of fatty acid radiolabelled with iodine-123. A combination of In-111 labelled particulate and I-123 labelled lipid, allows both phases of a suppository to be monitored simultaneously (Hardy *et al.,* 1987b).

26.4 OPHTHALMIC FORMULATIONS

Solutions of low viscosity are cleared rapidly from the eye via the lacrimal drainage system. Precorneal residence times of drugs can be enhanced by the administration of more viscous formulations (Zaki *et al.,* 1986). The effects of formulationon precorneal retention can be assessed by gamma scintigraphy.

Technetium-99m radiopharmaceuticals, such as DTPA and colloids, are commonly used as tracers. Typically, doses of 1 MBq technetium-99m in 10–50 μl of the preparation are applied to the eye. Viscosity enhancement can be achieved by the addition of polymers, such as polyvinyl alcohol, hydroxypropyl methyl cellulose or sodium hyaluronate. Similarly, technetium-99m compounds can be incorporated into gel and film preparations (Greaves *et al.,* et al., 1990).

26.5 FORMULATIONS FOR INHALATION

Pharmaceutical products for inhalajtion can be divided into three groups: nebuliser solutions; pressurised metered dose inhalers; and dry powder inhalers. A major factor influencing drug delivery to the lungs is particle size (Dolovich, 1991). Particles having a diameter greater than 5 μm are unlikely to penetrate into the lower airways. In general, less than 20% of the dose is deposited in the lungs. Gamma scintigraphy provides information concerning the sites and extent of drug deposition. Since it is rarely possible to label the drug molecule with a radionuclide suitable for imaging with a gamma camera, the tracer is unlikely to remain associated with the drug following deposition. Thus most studies are designed primarily to determine the proportion of the dose depositing in the lungs and the regional deposition pattern.

In addition to the assessment of specific drug formulations, gamma scintigraphy is used extensively in the evaluation of inhalation devices (Newman 1991). This includes the comparison of nebuliser systems and the assessment of novel dry powder inhalers. Many patients have difficulty in coordinating the firing of metered dose inhalers with inhalation and, therefore, receive only a fraction of the intended dose. Actuators have been produced that ensure that drug release from the canister coincides with inhalation. Additionally, a range of spacer devices for attachment to the actuator has been developed in an attempt to overcome the problem by reducing the need for precise coordination. Gamma scintigraphy plays an increasingly important role in the development of improved delivery devices.

26.5.1 Evaluation of Nebuliser Systems

Nebulisers are used widely to generate aerosols of drug solutions. The aerosol is produced either ultrasonically or by passing a jet of air through the device. Technetium-99m labelled DTPA solution is commonly used as the tracer. Following inhalation the radiopharmaceutical is either swallowed and passes through the gastrointestinal tract, or is absorbed from the lungs and excreted via the kidneys. Particulate tracers, such as colloidal serum albumin or tin colloid labelled with technetium-99m, can be added to represent drug suspensions and are cleared more slowly from the lungs. Technetium compounds can be incorporated into liposomes for pulmonary deposition. Hydrophilic tracers, such as Tc-99m DTPA, are associated with the aqueous phase of the liposomes and are retained in the lungs for longer than the free radiopharmaceuticals (Taylor and Newton, 1992).

Studies of aerosol deposition from nebulisers provide an aid to the selection of the most appropriate devices for use in particular circumstances. For example, the administration of inhaled pentamidine is associated with unpleasant side effects, which can be minimised by judicious selection of the delivery system (Thomas *et al.,* 1992). Figure 3 illustrates the difference in lung deposition following inhalation from a nebuliser generating relatively large aerosol particles and from one generating smaller particles.

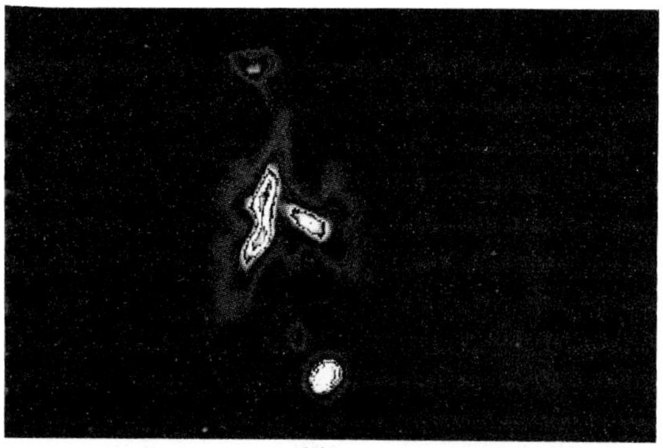

(a)

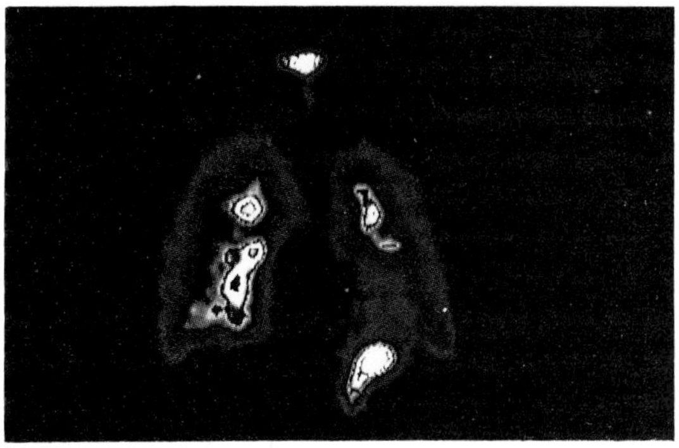

(b)

Figure 3. Central deposition of an aerosol in the lungs (a) compared with the more uniform distribution achieved with an aerosol of smaller particle size (b).

26.5.2 Radiolabelling of Pressurised Metered Dose Inhalers

Pressurised metered dose inhalers (MDIs) provide a convenient means of administering measured doses of drug. They comprise a canister fitted with a metering valve and are filled with, typically, 100–200 doses of the drug. The drug is usually in the form of a powder suspended in a chlorofluorocarbon propellant mixture, with an added surfactant such as sorbitan trioleate.

Drug deposition from MDIs can be monitored following radiolabelling of the drug particles with technetium-99m (O'Callaghan *et al.,* 1992). A simple procedure, applicable to a wide range of drug substances, involves the adsorption of Tc-99m-pertechnetate onto the drug particles. Sodium pertechnetate is extracted from saline into an organic solvent, such as butanone, and added to an empty MDI caniser. The solvent is evaporated to leave a coating of 1–2 GBq technetium-99m in the canister. The radiolabelled canister and a canister containing the drug formulation are cooled in liquid nitrogen. The metering valve is then removed from the drug-containing canister and the contents ransferred to the radiolabelled canister. A valve assembly is crimped on to the canister and the system checked for leaks in a water bath. Radiolabelling is completed by placing the canister in an ultrasonic bath for 10 minutes.

It is necessary to confirm that the radiolabelling has not affected the particle size distribution of the formulation and also that the distribution of the radiolabel reflects that of the drug. The validation can be carried out using a multistage impinger, such as an Andersen sampler. A non-radiolabelled MDI is actuated into the impinger and assays undertaken to determine the proportion of the drug deposited on each stage of the appararatus. The same experiment is carried out with a radiolabelled MDI and the distributions of both the drug and the radiolabel determined. In general, a close match can be expected between the three distributions. The good agreement between the mass of drug and the radioactivity probably reflects the rugosity of most drug particles. With smooth, regular particles relatively more radioactivity would be expected to be found on the stages collecting the smaller particles.

Lung deposition of drug particles from an MDI, in a healthy subject adopting a good inhaler technique, is typically 10–20%. Following administration, the radiolabel rapidly dissociates from the drug and is absorbed from the lungs. Thus imaging should be undertaken immediately after dosing.

The chlorofluorocarbon propellant of an MDI can be radiolabelled with a soluble radiopharmaceutical, such as Tc-99m-hexamethylpropyleneamine oxime, to represent a propellant soluble drug (Ashworth *et al.,* 1991). The tracer is extracted into trichlorofluoromethane and the solution added to an empty canister. The contents of a drug-containing canister are then added and a valve attached, using the same technique as for the particulate suspension. A relatively high lung deposition, of about 40%, can be achieved. This is probably a result of evaporation of the droplets during inhalation.

Metered dose inhalers currently rely on chlorofluorocarbons as propellants. As the production and use of these compounds is being phased out, alternative propellants are being sought (Newman, 1990). At the same time there is increasing attention being paid to the development of dry powder inhalers (Ganderton and Kassem, 1992).

26.5.3 Radiolabelling of Dry Powder Inhalers

Drug delivery from dry powder inhalers relies on the powder being withdrawn from the devicer during the inhalation procedure. The devices are loaded with the drug either in individual doses, for example in a capsule, or into a chamber from which individual doses are metered. The small size of the drug particles tends to affect adversely the flow properties of the powder. This problem can be overcome either by spheronisation, which involves aggregation of the particles, or by mixing the drug powder with carrier lactose powder having a larger particle size. The drug particles become re-dispersed during delivery from the device (Ganderton and Kassem, 1992).

The radiolabelling of the drug powder usually involves the adsorption of Tc-99m-pertechnetate on to the surface of the particles. The powder is best radiolabelled following spheronisation, since this reduces the handling of the radiolabelled material. When carrier is to be included, however, the drug powder should be radiolabelled before mixing. The labelling procedure involves the addition of a solution of the radiolabel in a solvent in which the drug powder is insoluble. Following drying, it is necessary to check that agglomeration of the particles has not occurred. As with the radiolabelling of MDIs, the procedure should be validated by impinger measurements.

There is an increasing interest in the potential of the inhalation route for drug administration. This is the case particularly for compounds such as polypeptides and proteins, that are currently given by injection. With such compounds it may be appropriate to radiolabel the molecules covalently with iodine-123. Alternatively, it may be possible to bind samarium-152 or erbium-170 to the molecules and to radiolabel powder formulations by neutron activation.

26.6 NASAL FORMULATIONS

Formulations deposited within the nasal cavity are cleared by mucociliary action and subsequently swallowed. Since the nasal cavity is readily accessible and the mucosa highly vascular, intranasal administration provides a convenient route for systemic drug delivery. Much attention has been directed towards devising methods for slowing the clearance to the stomach (Schipper *et al.,* 1991). Gamma scintigraphy is used widely to monitor preparations in the nasal cavity.

Many preparations are in the form of solutions for administration as sprays or drops (Hardy *et al.,* 1985). Such solutions can be radiolabelled with Tc-99m DTPA. A reduction in the rate of clearance can be achieved by the addition of polymers to the formulations (Pennington *et al.,* 1988). Microspheres of albumin, starch and dextran have been proposed as drug carriers for nasal administration (Illum *et al.,* 1987). These particles can be radiolabelled by the addition of Tc-99m pertechnetate solution to a suspension of the particles in stannous chloride solution. Other preparations are dosed from MDIs, or as powders, and these can be radiolabelled in the same way as the formulations intended for pulmonary drug delivery.

26.7 CONCLUSION

Gamma scintigraphy is being applied increasingly in the evaluation of drug formulations. Investigations are undertaken at all stages of product development, from initial feasibility studies to the assessment of the final products. The data generated are used widely in support of product licence applications.

Increasingly complex drug delivery systems are being developed. The radiolabelling of these products provide new challenges to tax the ingenuity of the chemist and radiopharmacist.

REFERENCES

Ashworth H.L., Wilson C.G., Sims E.E., Wotton P.K. and Hardy J.G. (1991). *Delivery of propellant soluble from a metered dose inhaler.* Thorax, **46**, 245–247.

Billinghurst M.W., Abrams D.N. and Lawson M.S. (1989). *Chemical aspects of labeling sucralfate with Tc-99m.* Journal of Nuclear Medicine, **30**, 523–530.

Daly P.B., Davis S.S., Frier M., Hardy J.G., Kennerley J.W. and Wilson C.G. (1982). *Scintigjraphic assessment of the in vivo dissolution of a sustained release tablet.* International Journal of Pharmaceutics, **10**, 17–24.

Davis S.S., Hardy J.G., Newman S.P. and Wilding I.R. (1992). *Gamma scintigraphy in the evaluation of pharmaceutical dosage forms.* European Journal of Nuclear Medicine, in press.

Dolovich M. (1991). *Clinical aspects of aerosol physics.* Respiratory Care, **36**, 931–938.

Ganderton D. and Kassem N.M. (1992). *Dry powder inhalers.* Advances in Pharmaceutical Sciences, **6**, 165–191.

Greaves J.L., Wilson C.G., Rozier A., Grove J. and Plazonnet B. (1990). *Scintigraphic assessment of an ophthalmic gelling vehicle in man and rabbit.* Current Eye Research, **9**, 415–420.

Hardy J.G., Lee S.W. and Wilson C.G. (1985). *Intranasal drug delivery by spray and drops.* Journal of Pharmacy and Pharmacology, **37**, 294–297.

Hardy J.G., Wood E., Clark A.G. and Reynolds J.R. (1986). *colonic motility and enema spreading.* European Journal of Nuclear Medicine, **12**, 176–178.

Hardy J.G., Healey J.N.C. and Reynolds J.R. (1987). *Evaluation of an enteric-coated delayed-release 5-aminosalicylic acid tablet in patients with inflammatory bowel disease.* Alimentary Pharmacology and Therapeutics, **1**, 273–280.

Hardy J.G., Feely L.C., Wood E. and Davis S.S. (1987b). *The application of gamma scintigraphy for the evaluation of the relative spreading of suppository bases in rectal hard gelatin capsules.* International Journal of Pharmaceutics, **38**, 103–108.

Hardy J.G., Lamont G.L., Evans D.F., Haga A.K. and Gamst O.N. (1991). *Evaluation of an enteric-coated naproxen pellet formulation.* Alimentary Pharmacology and Therapeutics, **5**, 69–75.

Illum L., Jorgensen H., Bisgaard H., Krogsgaard O. and Rossing N. (1987). *Bioadhesive microspheres as a potential nasal drug delivery system.* International Journal of Pharmaceutics, **39**, 189–199.

Jay M., Beihn R.M., Digenis G.A., DeLand F.H., Caldwell L. and Mlodozeniec A.R. (1985). *Disposition of radiolabelled suppositories in humans.* Journal of Pharmacy and Pharmacology, **37**, 266–268.

May H.A., Wilson C.G. and Hardy J.G. (1984). *Monitoring radiolabelled antacid preparations in the stomach.* International Journal of Pharmaceutics, **19**, 169–176.

Newman S.P. (1990). *Metered dose pressurized aerosols and the ozone layer.* European Respiratory Journal, **3**, 495–497.

Newman S.P., (1991). *Aerosol generators and delivery systems.* Respiratory Care, **36**, 939–951.

O'Callaghan C., Hardy J., Stammers J., Stephenson T.J. and Hull D. (1992). *Evaluation of techniques for delivery of steroids to lungs of neonates using a rabbit model.* Archives of Disease in Childhood, **67**, 20–24.

Pennington A.K., Ratcliffe J.H., Wilson C.G. and Hardy J.G. (1988). *The influence of solution viscosity on nasal spray deposition and clearance.* International Journal of Pharmaeutics, **43**, 221–224.

Schipper NG.M., Verhoef J.C. and Merkus F.W.H.M. (1991). *The nasal mucociliary clearance: relevance to nasal drug delivery.* Pharmaceutical Research, **8**, 807–814.

Taylor K.M.G. and Newton J.M. (1992). *Liposomes for controlled delivery of drugs to the lung.* Thorax, **47**, 257–259.

Thomas S.H.L., O'Doherty M.J., Page C.J., Nunan T.O. and Bateman N.T. (1991). *Which apparatus for inhaled pentamidine? A comparison of pulmonary deposition via eight nebulisers.* European Respiratory Journal, **4**, 616–622.

Wilding I.R., Hardy J.G., Maccari M., Ravelli V. and Davis S.S. (1991). *Scintigraphic and parhamcokinetic assessment of a multiparticulate sustained release formulation of diltiazem.* International Journal of Pharmaceutics, **76**, 133–143.

Wood E., Wilson C.G. and Hardy J.G. (1985). *The spreading of foam and solution enemas.* International Journal of Pharmaceutics, **25**, 191–197.

Zaki I., Fitzgerald P., Hardy J.G. and Wilson C.G. (1986). *A comparison of the effect of viscosity on the precorneal resisdence of solutions in rabbit and man.* Journal of Pharmacy and Pharmacology, **38**, 463–466.

Chapter 27

Paediatric Radiopharmacy

K. Evans

27.1 INTRODUCTION

Radiopharmaceuticals labelled with short lived radionuclides such as Tc-99m, Kr-81m, Tl-201, Ir-191m, and I-123 result in very low absorbed radiation doses and as radiopharmaceuticals are physiologically innocuous and can be given quite safely to children. However, it must be assumed that there are somatic and hereditary effects from even small amounts of absorbed radiation and this must be balanced against the possible benefits from the investigation (ICRP, 1977). New generations of gamma cameras offer higher spatial resolution and together with magnification techniques, examinations in small children and neonates are made much easier. Advances in computer analysis and the production of radiopharmaceuticals have created a large increase in nuclear medicine examinations, particularly in the evaluation of kidney function, radionuclide voiding cystography and in skeletal scintigraphy.

In administering radiopharmaceuticals to children, it is important to remember that rapidly growing tissues are generally more sensitive to ionizing radiations and that certain organs like the growing bone, take up radionuclides more avidly than those of adults. Also children under about one year have organ sizes in relation to the whole body, quite different from the older child or adult and most important, the radioactive dose is distributed into a smaller volume, so giving rise to a higher absorbed dose. Consequently the activity administered per kilogram of body weight or per square metre of body surface area, must be reduced so that the absorbed dose is similar to that of the adult. On the plus side, it is known that when radiation is absorbed in the body slowly (low—LET radiations), as in nuclear examinations, a certain amount of repair of damaged somatic and reproductive tissues can occur. However, it is generally accepted that the model used in calculating absorbed dose, is that the probability of an effect occurring from the ionizing radiation is proportional to the dose and that there is no repair and that there is no threshold value below which no effect occurs. Hence, the higher the dose the greater the probability of an effect occurring and that even very small absorbed doses of radiation can produce small immediate cellular damage or some later effect in life or the future generation.

The radiopharmaceutical dose administered to a child is normally based upon the adult dose reduced according to body weight or surface area. Below a certain weight or age it is necessary to have a minimum dose which is based on the smallest dose required which will give a satisfactory examination. This minimum dose is dependent on the sensitivity of the equipment, type of examination (dynamic or static) and the examination time.

The absorbed radiation dose in children not only varies with age and weight, but with physiological and pathological conditions. The biodistribution and kinetics of radiopharmaceuticals are also different from adults particularly in neonates. For example, neonates and infants have a higher uptake in bones, faster circulation times and washout of radioactive gases from lungs than older children and adults.

The gamma camera is the imaging system of choice in studying the paediatric patient because the child can be laid directly on top of the camera face so increasing the sensitivity and resolution of the system. The gamma camera has been of particular use in the study of children with bone and bone marrow diseases (Alavi *et al.,* 1974; Rosenfield, 1974; Gilday, 1976; Siddiqui *et al.,* 1979), renal disorders and radionuclide voiding cystography (Conway *et al.,* 1974; McDonald *et al.,* 1974; Pieretty *et al.,* 1974; Conway, 1976). It has been used extensively for rapid sequential visualisation of the heart and great vessels (Rosenthal, 1966; Mason *et al.,* 1968; Graham *et al.,* 1970). Ventilation and perfusion has been studied in children with lung diseases by Robinson *et al.,* 1969 and Alderson *et al.,* 1974a and 1974b). The gamma camera is also the system of choice in the study of biliary patency and function in the paediatric patient (Odell *et al.,* 1974; Butterman *et al.,* 1975; Majd *et al.,* 1981; Gerhold *et al.,* 1983) and has been used in the study of gastroesophagel reflux and gastric emptying (Signer, 1975; Heyman *et al.,* 1979; Herbat *et al.,* 1981; Rosen, 1984), Meckel's Diverticulum (Kerdmidas *et al.,* 1974; Wine *et al.,* 1974; Martin *et al.,* 1976; Tauscher *et al.,* 1978), the thyroid, (Clayton, 1978; Worm *et al.,* 1960; Heyman *et al.,* 1982; Wellington *et al.*, 1982), liver (Spencer, 1970; Treves, 1973; Rosenfield, 1974; Rosenthall, 1974), spleen (Walker, 1976; Fischer *et al.,* 1977;

Broker *et al.*, 1978; Ehrlich *et al.*, 1982), brain (Conway 1972; Golden, 1972; Hurley, 1972; Mishkin, 1972; Gates *et al.*, 1982), in the study of lacrimal drainage (Veirs, 1966; Rossomondo *et al.*, 1972; Hurwitz *et al.*, 1975a, 1975b) and in boys with testicular pain (Geirup *et al.*, 1975; Boedecker *et al.*, 1979; Kogan *et al.*, 1979; Valvo *et al.*, 1982). More recently, hexamethylpropyleneamineoxime labelled with Tc-99m (Tc-99m-HMPAO), which penetrates the blood brain barrier, has been used for paediatric brain studies (Denays *et al.*, 1990) and Tc-99m-mercaptoacetyltriglycine (Tc-99m-MAG3) has been used in the study of the kidneys (Gordon *et al.*, 1991). Metaiodobenzylguanidine (MIBG) labelled with I-123 and I-131 has been used to study and treat children with neuroblastomas (Mayes *et al.*, 1989).

Children are best examined recumbent and supine laying directly on the top of the camera face. A table (non-absorbent material) with a hole in the centre so that the camera face can be brought up flush with the table can be used to support the child's head and legs. The resolution and sensitivity is improved if the child can be studied in this way. *The supine position may impede drainage* in renal studies so the child should be asked to sit up or micturate and a further image taken in order to assess the drainage.

A pediatric collimator was developed by Scintronics Ltd for their gamma camera at the Hospital for Sick Children, Great Ormond Street, London. The collimator is 14.6 mm thick with a hole size of 1.18 mm, septal thickness 0.23 mm and has approximately 86,600 holes. The full width at half maximum of two line spread functions within the central field of view placed on the surface of the collimator is 1.9 mm. At 20 mm from the face of the collimator it is 3.9 mm and at 50 mm the FWHM is 6.6 mm. The camera with the paediatric collimator on, has an overall sensitivity of 138 c/s/MBq in a 20% window. The collimator was specially designed for technetium 99m and so for energies greater than about 150 kev, there is a 5% penetration.

Magnification is often important in neonates and infants and this can be achieved by the use of either a pinhole collimator or a converging collimator. The pinhole collimator has the best spatial resolution but has a non-uniform response to a flood field and a lower sensitivity, but is useful in scanning the thyroid and joints. In Perthes' disease the pinhole collimator is ideal for imaging the femoral epiphyses. The converging collimtor is more useful in dynamic studies as it provides magnification without lowering sensitivity, but it does not have as good a resolution as the pinhole collimator. In neonates and infants when sensitivity is more important than resolution, as in dynamic studies, *then the converging collimator should be used.*

When radioisotopes of iodine are used and the thyroid is not the organ of interest, then potassium perchlorate or Lugol's iodine should be administered to prevent unnecessary radiation dose to the thyroid. The normal dose of potassium perchlorate is 150 mg for children less than one year old, 300 mg for 1–4 year olds and 450 mg for 5 year olds and over. The dose is best given in liquid form in a soft drink, after the examination (usually of the gastrointestinal tract) as the potassium perchlorate could interfere with the test. If MIBG labelled with an iodine isotope is used, then Lugol's iodine is normally given (0.2 ml three times a day) for 5 days – 3 days before test and 2 days after. It is considered unnecessary to administer blocking agents to reduce radiation dose when Tc-99m labelled substances are used, including the chemical form pertechnetate.

Techniques described in this chapter do not attempt to give comprehensive details of the use of radiopharmaceuticals in paediatrics except in methods and techniques differing from those for adults. For a fully comprehensive description of the use of radiopharmaceuticals in paediatrics, readers are referred to the list for further reading.

27.2 ADMINISTERED DOSES

The dose of radiopharmaceuticals given to children for a given investigation will depend on whether body weight or surface area is used as the scaling factor to be applied to the adult dose. When the gamma camera is used, the photon flux density necessary for an adequate image is dependent on the square of linear dimension. This would suggest that a scaling factor based on surface area should be used when images are to be obtained as surface area is a function of the square of linear dimensions. In investigations involving body fluid measurements, the flux density necessary for adequate counts is dependent on the cube of linear dimensions. This would suggest that a scaling factor based on weight should be used as weight is a function of the cube of linear dimensions. Consequently, when images are to be obtained, the dose should be scaled down from the adult dose according to the surface area. When body fluids are to be measured *in vitro*, e.g. a blood or urine sample, then the dose should be scaled down according to body weight. As surface area is not a very convenient unit to obtain, it requires both height and weight and a pocket calculator, at the Hospital for Sick Children, London, the heights and weights of 100 children were measured and then surface areas calculated using the formula:

$$\text{Surface area } (\text{m}^2) = (\text{weight in kg})^{0.425} \times (\text{Height in cm})^{0.725} \times 0.00718 \quad (1)$$

(Dubois 1916)

The fraction of the adult dose to be administered was then obtained from a graph of the child's weight plotted against the child's surface area divided by 1.73 m^2 (the fraction of the adult dose). Table 1 was then obtained giving the fraction of adult dose to be used calculated from weight, based on the surface are a scaling factor. Hence using the table the appropriate scaling factor based on surface area, can be obtained from the weight of the child only.

TABLE 1
Fraction of Adult Dose Based on Surface Area Scaling Factor

Weight (kg)	*Fraction of adult dose*	*Weight (kg)*	*Fraction of adult dose*	*Weight (kg)*	*Fraction of adult dose*
3	0.1	26	0.56	50	0.88
4	0.14	28	0.58	52	0.90
6	0.19	30	0.62	54	0.91
8	0.23	32	0.65	56	0.92
10	0.27	34	0.68	58	0.93
12	0.32	36	0.71	60	0.95
14	0.36	38	0.73	62	0.96
16	0.40	40	0.76	64	0.97
18	0.44	42	0.78	66	0.98
20	0.46	44	0.80	68	0.99
22	0.50	46	0.82	70	1.00
24	0.53	48	0.85		

For calculation of average weight of child based on age see monogram (Appendix B)

Another formula for surface area is the one recommended by the DHSS (1979) based on weight alone:

$$\text{Surface area } (M^2) = 0.14 \times (\text{weight in kg})^{2/3} \qquad (2)$$

The International Commission on Radiological Protection (ICRP 1971) recommend that this formula be used to obtain the fraction of the adult dose when the surface area scaling factor is required. Table 2 is based on this formula and gives a result very similar to that obtained using formula 1.

TABLE 2
Fraction of Adult Dose Based on the Surface Area Formula Recommended by ICRP, 1971

Weight (kg)	*Surface area (m2)*	*Fraction of adult dose*
2	0.22	0.09
4	0.35	0.15
6	0.46	0.19
8	0.56	0.24
10	0.66	0.27
15	0.85	0.36
20	1.03	0.43
30	1.35	0.57
40	1.64	0.67
50	1.90	0.80
60	2.15	0.90
70	2.38	1.00

If the body weight scaling factor were used to obtain the fraction of the adult dose, then the dose administered would be lower particularly in smaller children. This scaling factor should only be used when body fluids are being measured when, if necessary, the samples can be counted for a longer time.

The administration of Radioactive Substances Advisory Committee (ARSAC), have listed the usual maximum dose administered to adults for a large number of investigations together with the effective dose equivalent in milliseiverts (DHSS, 1979 and 1988). Some of the more common investigations are listed in Table 3. In neonates and babies the use of the fraction of the adult dose would result in too small an administered dose and an entirely unsatisfactory study. Hence a minimum dose is normally used, based on experience of the equipment and type of investigation such that the desired diagnostic information is obtained. Table 3 also shows the minimum doses used at the Hospital for Sick Children, London. The fraction of adult doses and minimum doses are recommendations only and each centre should try to administer the lowest dose to obtain the desired diagnostic information even if it means varying the dose schedule depending on the equipment used. It may be of benefit on occasions to increase the dose for a problem child so that the test is over quicker and so minimising the error due to movement.

Sampson (1980) reported a number of dose schedules used in the USA. One such schedule is Clark's Rule which is based on body weight and the administered dose is given by the formula:

$$\text{Dose} = \frac{\text{Weight (lbs)} \times \text{Adult dose}}{150}$$

This would result in lower doses, particularly in younger children, compared with the surface area scaling factors and would be more appropriate for the measurement of body fluids.

Another schedule is Young's Rule which is based on the age of the children:

$$\text{Dose} = \frac{(\text{Age in years}) \times \text{Adult dose}}{\text{Age} + 12}$$

This rule roughly follows the surface area scaling factor between the ages of about 2 and 10 years and outside these limits it is closer to the body weight scaling factor. A modified version of Young's Rule is Webster's Rule (Webster *et al.*, 1974) which is:

$$\text{Dose} = \frac{(\text{Age in years} + 1) \times \text{Adult dose}}{\text{Age in years} + 7}$$

This rule follows the surface area scaling factor quite closely up to about the age of 10 years but after this age tends

TABLE 3
Some Commonly Used Radiopharmaceuticals and Minimum Doses Used at the Hospital for Sick Children, London

Radiopharmaceutical		*Investigation*	*Adult dose (MBq)*	*Min. dose (MBq)*
Tc99m	DMSA	Renal scan	100	20
Tc99m	DTPA	Dynamic renal scan	200	20
Tc99m	DTPA	Blood flow study	300	60
Tc99m	MAG3	Cystography	80	15
Tc99m	MAG3	Blood flow study	160	30
Tc99m	Pertechnetate	Direct cystography	20	20
Tc99m	Red cells	Ventricular function	500	80
Tc99m	MDP	Bone scan	500	40
Tc99m	MAA	Lung scan	80	10
Tc99m	Pertechnetate	Thyroid scan	80	10
Tc99m	HMPAO White cells	Infection/inflammation	200	40
Tc99m	HMPAO	Brain scan	500	100
Tc99m	Colloid	Liver/spleen scan	80	15
Tc99m	Colloid	Bone marrow scan	300	20
Tc99m	Rhenium Colloid	Lymphatic system	74 in each foot	
Tc99m	HIDA	Liver/biliary tract	150	20
Tc99m	Pertechnetate	Abdominal scan	75	15
Tc99m	Pertechnetate	Cardiac study	500	80
Tc99m	Colloid in milk	Gastric reflux	40	10
I123	MIBG	Neuroblastoma	<2yrs 110.	>2yrs 160
I123	MIBG	Adrenal tumour	80	35
I123	Iodide	Perchlorate discharge	2	1
Ga67		Infection	80	10
Cr51	EDTA	GFR	3	1
Cr51	Chloride	GI protein loss	4	1

to give a lower dose and is more like the body weight scaling factor.

Some ratios of organ to body weight in children are greater than the rates in adults particularly in babies. Table 4 shows body and organ weights in various ages. It can be seen from this table that ratios of the masses of the brain and liver to the whole body mass particularly, are larger than those of the adult. Consequently some institutions in the USA use a scaling factor based on the ratio of organ weight to whole body weight.

One formula used is:

$$\text{Dose} = \frac{(M_1)^{2/3} \times \text{adult dose}}{(M_2)^{2/3}}$$

where M_1 = Mass of paediatric body or target organ
M_2 = Mass of adult or target organ

When the body weight is applied to this formula it follows the surface area scaling factor as the surface area is approximately proportional to the body weight to the power two-thirds (equation 2). When the organ weight does not follow the growth curve pattern of the total body weight, the target organ mass is used and a more appropriate dose obtained. Other workers have calculated dose schedules based on the surface area scaling factor (Koenigsberg *et al.*, 1978).

27.3 PREPARATION OF DOSES AND DOCUMENTATION

Dispensing techniques in the paediatric radiopharmacy are similar to those for adults except that the doses and the volumes to be injected are smaller and may need to be diluted to obtain the minimum volume for injection (0.2 ml).

Individual doses can be prepared in evacuated vials labelled with patient's name, date, time, dose, radiopharmaceutical and volume to be injected; the individual vials taken to the gamma camera room and the doses drawn up by the

TABLE 4

Body and Organ Weights at Various Ages, Taken from Spector (1956) Keriakes (1971) ICRP (1975) Poston (1976) and NCRP (1983) (grammes)

Organ	*Newborn*	*1-year*	*5-year*	*10-year*	*15-year*	*Adult*
Brain	372	1005	1180	1355	1367	1451
Bladder wall	3	7	14	22	34	45
Intestines	32[a]	140[a]	301[a]	–	1265	1770
Kidney	19	68	116	179	230	284
Liver	110	300	608	896	1267	1809
Lungs	40	130	260	426	650	1000
Red marrow	40	150	400	600	950	1500
Yellow marrow	0	0	50	560	1500	1500
Ovaries	0.3	0.7	2	3.2	5	8
Pancreas	2.6	9	19	27	57	60
Skeleton	500	1600	2800	4573	8700	10500
Spleen	8.8	27	50	80	145	174
Stomach	5.9	27	52	88	118	150
Testes	0.8	1.5	1.6	1.9	16	37
Thyroid	1.0	2	5	8.8	13	20
Heart	20	47	86	140	209	298
Whole body	3990	10400	20000	32000	56980	70000

[a]Does not include contents for lower large intestine.

radiographer or doctor injecting the radiopharmaceutical. This method involves an extra transference of radiopharmaceutical carried out in a non-sterile area and the syringe also has to be labelled – another source of error. A better method now used at Great Ormond Street Hospital is to prepare individual doses directly into syringes which are labelled before they leave the radiopharmacy laboratory. The dose syringes are finally checked for the correct dose in an ionization chamber before being injected.

For investigations requiring an accurate volume to be injected, the doses are prepared in a vial, the vial is weighed, the appropriate required volume drawn up into a syringe and the vial reweighed to obtain the exact dose in the syringe. The dose is injected and the syringe flushed with saline or the patients own blood so that the exact dose injected is known. An accurate standard is obtained by weighing before and after the removal of the standard from the dose vial and diluting the standard in the usual way. Quantitative measurements can be made on subsequent biological samples by comparing the counts in the sample with those in the standard.

There are two documents produced at the Hospital for Sick Children, London during the preparation of radiopharmaceuticals, the patient elution record and the radiopharmaceutical production worksheet (Sampson, 1981). The elution record gives details of the generator used, date and time of elution, pH of eluate, sterility, patient's name, age and weight, dose to be given and the time of injection. This document also contains tables of the radiopharmaceutical doses, minimum doses and the fraction of the adult dose to be used for weights ranging from 3 kg to 70 kg. The dose required is calculated by the radiologist or physicist and checked by the radiopharmacist before dispensing.

The radiopharmaceutical production work sheet gives details of the drugs and chemicals used in the preparation. A decay chart for the radioisotope being used is included together with details of the patient, dose to be injected and injection time. This enables calculations to be made of the volumes to be injected at a particular time.

27.4 IMMOBILISATION OF CHILDREN

Most children need some form of physical restraint to help keep them in a fixed position. Even older children find it easier to keep still if they are supported at either side with sand bags. Smaller children are normally supported with sand bags held in position with velco straps fastened around their bodies. Care should be taken to avoid causing the child to become overheated. A policy of marking the monitor screen to detect any movement should be adopted. The air extracted bean bag is fine for immobilizing children but it does tend to frighten them, cause overheating and increases the distance between the patient and the collimator thus impairing resolution and sensitivity. The use of the evacuated bean bag has been discontinued at the Hospital for Sick Children, London.

27.5 SEDATION

In our experience at the Hospital for Sick Children, London only very rarely do children need sedation, but if it is necessary then aspiration and respiratory problems should be anticipated and the appropriate treatment should be available for use. Sedation can effect renal function (Vivian, 1983) and other quantitative measurements so sedation is actively discouraged. In dealing with children, staff should have a sympathetic approach and should not mislead the patient. They should explain what is going to happen in words appropriate to the child's understanding. It is important to gain the child's trust and to keep it once it is gained. The child can be distracted with toys, mobiles, pictures or their own image on the TV monitor. Cassettes with stories or music are useful in allaying the child's anxiety. A television or video cassette player placed within easy view of the patient could be a great help and comfort to the paediatric patient.

Children under 4 years of age undergoing bone or lung scans or in the case of a long investigation of a very frightened or overactive toddler, it may be better to administer a sedative. Trimeprazine (3 mg/kg) given orally is often adequate but sometimes has the opposite effect. A stronger sedative is nembutal (pentobarbitol sodium) 6 mg/kg <15 kg, 5 mg/kg >15 kg up to 100 mg, after which it increases more gradually. This is given 30 minutes before the injection and has a knockout effect rather than a calming efect. The child wakes within two hours. This is not recommended for neonates less than 2 months.

At the Hospital for Sick Children, London, Trimeprazine (4 mg/kg) is given orally 2 hours before the scan if the patient is over 8 years. Alternatively, Omnopon (0.4 mg/kg-maximum 15 mg) plus scopolamine (0.008 mg/kg) given intramuscularly one hour before the scan or if the child is between 3 months and 8 years, Droperidol (0.18 mg/kg) plus Vallergan (3 ml/kg). If the patient is less than 3 months and less than 5 kg, Peth-Co (0.06ml/kg). If the patient is less than 3 months and less than 5 kg, Peth-Co (0.06 ml/kg). If the patient is less than 3 months but greater than 5 kg. Peth-Co (0.08–0.1 ml/kg to a maximum of 1.5 ml) is given instramuscularly 45 minutes before the scan. If the patient is still very restless then Diazepam (0.5 mg/kg) is given intravenously. However Holloway *et al.,* (1982) has evaluated the use of Midazolam (Hynovel, Roche) 0.15–0.3 mg/kg, which is more widely available and has reported that it has a lower incidence of venous complications and a wider safety margin than Diazepam.

Parents are normally encouraged to be present at the investigation and normally they tend to have a calming effect on the child, although it has been known to have the opposite effect (Gilday, 1983) in which case the parents are asked to leave.

If neonates and infants are studied immediately after a feed they will often sleep through the investigation.

27.6 INJECTION TECHNIQUES

For intravenous injection of radiopharmaceuticals in paediatric patients, a butterfly needle and 3-way tap are invariably used at our hospital. The patient lies supine on top of the camera face and is immobilised if necessary. A site is chosen for the injection which is normally in the dorsum of the hand or foot as these veins are more visible and normally more accessible. A large vein can be chosen such as an antecubital vein if a rapid injection is needed. The butterfly is normally 23–25 gauge and when the vein is entered and blood is drawn, the butterfly is taped in position. Sterile saline is drawn into a 5 ml syringe and attached to the 3-way tap as is the syringe containing the dose. A final check is made to verify that the needle is still in place and the dose is injected followed immediately by the saline flush. For dynamic studies it is important to have a rapid injection of the dose which should be in a small volume (0.2–1.0 ml).

27.7 ORGAN DEPTH CORRECTIONS

Corrections for tissue attenuation have to be made when quantitative estimations of organ uptake of radionuclides are to be made. In children the estimation of depth of organs is particularly important as organ depth can vary enormously depending on the size of the patient. For instance, kidney depth can vary between 2 cm in the neonate to 7 or 8 cm in the largest of the paediatric patients. A 1-cm error in depth estimation of the kidney can lead to a 11.5% error in the uptake value (Kelly, 1987).

There are two main methods of estimating depth; (1) from a lateral image taken with a gamma camera using a small radioactive source to mark the skin and; (2) depth estimations from a formula. Measurements from lateral images are subject to a number of difficulties; (1) the plane of the patient's back must be exactly perpendicular to the camera face, otherwise parallax errors will occur; (2) the patient must remain in the same position for the lateral image otherwise the organ may move to a different depth; even moving the arms out of the field of view may cause arching of the back and distortion of the depth and (3) in renal studies, the lateral image of a poorly functioning kidney can be obscured by the radiation from the other, possibly hypertrophied kidney. Kidney depth estimations are by far the most commonly required and the parameters used in the formula method for estimating depth are age, weight and height. Raynaud *et al.,* (1968) based his estimations on weight, i.e. less than 10 kg–4.5 cm, 11 to 15kg–5 cm, 16 to 20 kg–5.5 cm, 21 to 30 kg–6 cm, 31 to 40 kg–6.5 cm, greater than 40 kg–7.5 to 8.5 cm for male and 7 to 8 cm for females depending on muscular development. Later, using data from lateral images Raynaud *et al.,* (1974) developed the following formulae:-

For 0–9 years: $D = 2.366 + 0.083W - 0.281H$
For 9–19 years: $D = 3.686 + 0.028W - 0.248H$
For over 19 years: $D = 1.017 + 0.049W + 2.198H$

Where D is depth (cm), W is weight (kg) and H is height (m).

Taux and Burke (1968) developed formulae obtained during renal biopsies:-

$$D = 8.82W - 0.36H - 0.06A + 61.08$$

Where D is depth (mm), W is weight (kg), H is height (cm) and A is age (years). Gordon *et al.,* (1987) measured the depth using lateral images and in 118 kidneys when the lateral images were considered to be reliable (i.e. no parallax, skin marker well placed and the kidneys were clearly seen), the directly measured depths were compared with the surface area, weight and height. They produced the formulae:

$$D = 2.82A + 1.42 \quad (r = 0.94)$$
$$D = 0.0742W + 2.03 \quad (r = 0.94)$$

Where D is depth (cm), A is surface area (m^2) and W is weight (kg).

Computer tomography images of the kidney were analysed by Kelly (1987) and depth estimations obtained from this method were compared with the weight of the patient. The formula described was:-

$$D = 0.0604W + 2.53$$

Where D is depth (cm) and W is weight (kg).

Various other techniques have been published for estimating kidney depths (Kawamura *et al.,* 1979; Morales *et al.,* 1984) and one which is currently being investigated at this hospital is the technique described by Wellman *et al.,* (1967) in which depth is related to the ratio of the counts in two energy windows. It is based on the principle that the primary energy spectrum of a radio-isotope changes as the radiation is attenuated. The degree of attenuation is inferred from the ratio of counts from the two windows. No additional imaging is required as the quantitation image is also used for the depth estimation. Calculations are performed by the computer and there is no need for lateral images or formulae.

The absolute uptake into an organ can be obtained without knowledge of the depth of the organ by taking posterior and anterior views and determining the attenuation coefficient for each patient directly by measuring the transmission fraction with a flood source (Thomas *et al.,* 1976; Myers, 1981). The activity in the organ (A) is then given by the equation:-

$$A = (I_a . I_p)^{1/2} . e^{(\mu_e(T/2))} . (F/C)$$

A is in MBq
I_a = Counts per min in anterior view
I_p = Counts per min in posterior view
T = Patients thickness in region of organ (cm)
μ_e = Effective linear attenuation coefficient (cm^{-1})
C = System calibration factor (c/min/MBq)
F = Correction for self attenuation

The system calibration factor (C) has to be calibrated using models of different sizes and different depths. Although this is undoubtedly a good method for obtaining absolute uptake in organs, it is not very practicable as 4 different views are required including one with a flood source resting on the patient. A simpler method would be to measure the dose on the face of the camera and then through the patient at the level of the organ of interest. The geometric mean of these two counts (the square root of the product) would be equivalent to 100% of the injected activity at mid plane depth. The geometric mean counts of the anterior and posterior gamma camera images can then be used to obtain the organ uptake without knowledge of the patient thickness or assuming a particular attenuation coefficient. If the organ is more than a few centimetres thick, a correction factor

$$\frac{\sin h\ (\mu_e T/2)}{(\mu_e T/2)}$$

can be applied but it differs negligibly from 1.00 for organs such as the kidney. For thicker organ such as liver it may be as much as 1.20.

27.8 ABSORBED RADIATION DOSE

As has been previously stated, the main criterion in deciding the amount of radioactivity to administer is that it should be the minimum consistent with adequate diagnostic information from the procedure, thus ensuring that the minimum radiation dose is delivered to the patient. In order to obtain an estimate of the risks for each paediatric investigation, it is necessary to estimate absorbed radiation dose to the whole body and to specific organs. Radiation dosimetry has been dealt with in detail in a previous chapter, but in estimating absorbed dose in children, other factors have to be considered such as size of organ and the different biodistribution and kinetics of the radiopharmaceutical in children.

If the MIRD system is used, then the equations of Loevinger and Berman (1968, 1976) are applicable:-

$$\bar{D}(r_k \leftarrow r_h) = \frac{A_k}{m_k} \sum \Delta_i \phi_i (r_k \leftarrow r_h)$$

Where Δ_i is the mean energy of radiation emitted per nuclear transformation
$\bar{D}$ is the mean absorbed dose due to i-type radiation
r_h is the source activity
r_k is the target organ

ϕ_i depends on the gamma-ray energy and source to target configuration (absorbed fraction)
A_k is the accumulated activity in the target organ and
m_k is the mass of the target organ

The unit S(rad $\mu Ci^{-1}h^{-1}$) has been defined as the mean dose per unit accumulated activity and incorporates all the physical characteristics of the radiation and configuration of the source and target organs including the mass of the target organ, i.e.

$$S = \frac{\Sigma_i \Delta_i \phi_i (r_k \leftarrow r_h)}{M_k}$$

Hence

$$\bar{D}(r_k \leftarrow r_h) = (\tilde{A}_h S(r_k \leftarrow r_h)$$

and the dose can be calculated with just the knowledge of the S value and all the accumulated activity. The accumulated activity depends on the amount of activity administered, the rate of uptake and removal from the organ and the half life of the radioisotope and is given by the formula:

$$\tilde{A} = 1.44 T_e A_o$$

where $\tilde{A}$ is in MBqh
A_o is in the initial activity in the organ (MBq)
and T_e is the effective half life of the radiopharmaceutical.

Snyder *et al.,* (1974) and Loevinger and Berman (1976) have tabulated the S values in adults for various source and target organs for all radionuclides in common use assuming a 70 kg whole body mass and average adult organ sizes. But these values cannot be used in children because of their differing whole body weights and organ sizes and they cannot be obtained simply by multiplying by a weight factor as this would not take the source to target configuration into account. However, Poston (1976) has calculated the S values for selected radionuclides in neonates, 1 year old and 5 year olds for a number of organs, using information on weights and organ sizes of a series of standard children provided by Spector (1956) and Kereiakes *et al.,* (1965). The S factor for specific source to target configurations for Cr-51, Ga-67, Tc-99m, In-111, I-123, I-131, and Tl-201 are listed in Appendix A of the report number 73, NCRP (1983).

For children of other ages and weights, formula 1 should be used. The values for the absorbed fraction, based on the appropriate source to target geometries, can be obtained from MIRD pamphlet 3 (1968) and the values for the mean energy per transformation can be obtained from MIRD pamphlet 10 (1975) or ICRU 32 (1979). If the accumulated activity in the target organ and the mass of the target are known then the absorbed dose can be calculated.

In adults, the largest dose usually comes from the source organ when the source organ and target are one and the same. In children, particularly in neonates, a greater proportion of the dose is delivered to the target organ from other source organs as the target organ, being much smaller, absorbs much less radiation from itself.

There is adequate information available on radionuclide properties, but biological data on children are very limited. However, there are published tables giving estimates of organ mass in children (Spector, 1956; Kereiakes *et al.,* 1965; Documenta Geigy Scientific tables, 1972; ICRP, 1975) and blood volumes at various ages (Handmaker and Lowenstein, 1975). There are also many tables in the literature giving estimates of absorbed dose to the whole body and organs from most commonly used radiopharmaceuticals in paediatrics (Kereiakes, 1976b; Roedler *et al.,* 1978). Absorbed dose estimates have also been made for most paediatric investigations by the radiopharmaceutical Internal dose Information Centre at the Oak Ridge Associated Universities and many of these are tabulated in Paediatric Nuclear Medicine (1985) – see list for further reading). NCRP (1983) lists absorbed dose information for certain organs in the neonate, 1, 5, 10 and 15 year olds using S values derived for children. The report also gives absorbed dose estimates to the embryo and fetus following the administration of commonly used radiopharmaceuticals to the mother.

Although a great deal of work has been done in estimating absorbed radiation doses in the paediatric patient using paediatric "S" values (NCRP 1983), much of the work has been done using adult biokinetic data because paediatric biokinetic data is not always available. Clearly, the acquisition of paediatric biokinetic data must be given a high priority and a number of centres are now obtaining the biodistribution of different radiopharmaceuticals in children of various age groups.

REFERENCES

Alderson P.O., Secker-Walker R.H., Strominger D.B., Markham J., and Hill R.L. (1974a). *Pulmonary deposition of aerosols in children with cystic fibrosis.* J. Pediatr., **84**, 479.

Alderson P.O., Secker-Walker R.H., Strominger D.B., McAlister W.H., Hill R.L. and Markham J. (1974b). *Quantitative assessment of regional ventilation and perfusion in children with cystic fibrosis.* Radiology, **111**, 151.

Alavi A., Bond J.P., Kuhl D.E., and Creech R.H. (1974). *Scan detection of bone marrow infarcts in sickle cell disorders.* J. Nucl. Med., **15**, 1003–1010.

Boedecker R.A., Sty J.R., and Jona F.J. (1979). *Testicular scanning as a diagnostic aid in evaluating scrotal pain.* J. Pediatr., **74**, 760–762.

Broker F.H.L., Fellows K. and Treves S. (1978). *Wandering spleen in three children.* Paediatr. Radiol., **6**, 211–214.

Butterman G., Wolf I., and Pabst H.W. (1975). *Quantitative analysis of hepatograms using a gamma camera and labelled contrast media. In* Dynamic Studies with Radioisotopes in Medicine. IAEA Vienna.

Clayton G.W. and Kirkland R.T. (1978). *Cancer of the thyroid in children. In* Thyroid Cancer, edited by L.D. Greenfield, pp 207–221. West Palm Beach, Florida. CRC Press.

Conway J.J., and Vollert J. (1972). *The accuracy of radionuclide imaging in detecting pediatric dural fluid collections.* Radiology, **105**, 77–83.

Conway J.J., Luck S., Filmer R.B. and Belman A.B. (1974). *Radionuclide differentiation of a unilateral flank mass in the newborn period.* J. Nucl. Med., **15**, 485.

Conway J.J., and Jruglik G.D. (1976). *Effectiveness of direct and indirect radionuclide cystography in detecting vesicoureteral reflux.* J. Nucl. Med., **17**, 81–83.

Denays R., Tondeur M., Toppet V. *et al.,* (1990). *Cerebral Palsy: Initial Experience with Tc-99m-HMPAO SPECT of the Brain.* Radiology, **175(1)**, 111–116.

DHSS (1979). *Notes for guidance on the administration of radioactive substances to persons for purposes of diagnosis, treatment or research.* Department of Health and Social Security. H.M.S.O. London.

Documents Geigy Scientific Tables (1972). *CIBA-Geigy Ltd., Basle.*

Dubois D., and Dubois E.F. (1916). Clinical calorimetry: A formula to estimate the approximate surface area if height and weight be known. Arch. Intern Med., **17**, 863.

Enrlich C.P., papanicolaou N., Treves S., Hurwitz R.A., and Richards P. (1982). *Splenic scintigraphy using technetium-99m labelled heat denatured red blood cells in paediatric patients.* J. Nucl. Med., **23**, 209–213.

Fischer K.C., Shapiro S., and Treves S. (1977). *Visualization of the spleen with a bone seeking radionuclide in a child with sickle cell anemia.* Radiology, **122**, 398.

Gates G.F., Fishman L.S., and Segall H.D. (1982). *Assessment of cerebral perfusion in childhood strokes.* Clin. Nucl. Med., **7**, 502–511.

Gerhuld J.P., Klingensmith W.C., Kuni C.C., Lilly J.R., Silverman A., Fritzberg A.R. *et al.,* (1983). *Diagnosis of biliary atresia with radionuclide hepatobiliary imaging.* Radiology, **146**, 499–504.

Gierup J., von Hedenberg C., and Osterman A. (1975). *Acute nonspecific epididymitis in boys.* Scand. J. Urol. Nephrol., **9**, 5–7.

Gilday D.L., Paul D.J., and Paterson J. (1975). *Diagnosis of osteomyelitis in children by combined blood pool and bone imaging.* Radiology, **117**, 331.

Gilday D., and Ash J.M. (1976). *Benign bone tumours.* Semin, Nucl. Med., **6**, 33.

Gilday D.L. (1983). *Special clinical problems in pediatrics. In:* Clinical Nuclear Medicine, edited by K.E. Britton, M.N. Maisey and C.L. Gilday. p. 331 London: Chapman Hall.

Golden G.S., and Erenberg G. (1972). *Radionuclide brain scans in convulsive disorders.* Pediatrics, **49**, 787.

Gordon I., Anderson P.J., Orton M., Evans K. (1991).. *Estimation of Tc99m-MAG3 Renal Clearance in Children: Two Gamma Camera Techniques Compared with Multiple Blood Samples.* J. Nucl. Med., **32**, 1704–1708.

Gordon I., Evans K., Peters A.M., Kelly J. Morales B.N., Oldraich N. *et al.,* (1987). *The quantitation ot technetium-99m DMSA in pediatrics.* Nucl. Med. Comm., **8**, 661–670.

Graham J.P., Jr., Goodrich J.K., Robinson A.E., and Harris C. (1970). *Scintiangiocardiography in children.* Am. J. Cardiol., **25**, 387.

Handmaker H., and Lowenstein J.M. (1975). *Nuclear Medicine in Clinical Pediatrics, New York:* The Society of Nuclear Medicine Inc.

Herbst J.J. (1981). *Gastroesophageal reflux.* J. Pediatr., **98**, 859–870.

Heyman S., Kirkpatric J.A., Winter H.S. and Treves J. (1079). *An improved method for the diagnosis of gastroesophageal reflux and aspiration in children (milk scan).* Radiology, **131**, 479–482.

Heyman S., Crigler J.F., and Treves S. (1982). *Congenital hypthyroidism: Iodine-123 thyroid uptake and scintigraphy.* J. Pediatr., **101**, 571–574.

Holloway A.M., Jordan D.G., and Brock-Utne J.G. (1982). *Midazolam for the intravenous induction of anaesthesia in children.* Anaesth. and Inten. Care, **10**, 340.

Hurley P.J. and Wagner H.N. (1972). *Diagnostic value of brain scanning the children.* JAMA, **221**, 877–881.

Hurwitz J.J., Maisey M.N., and Welham R.A.N. (1975). *Quantitative lacrimal scintillography 1. Method and physical application.* Br. J. Ophthalmal, **59**, 308.

Hurwitz J.J., Maisey M.N., and Welham R.A.N. (1975b). *Quantitative lacrimal scintillography, II Lacrimal pathology.* Br. J. Ophthalmol., **59**, 313.

ICRP (1971). *International commission on Radiological Protection. Protection of the patient in radionuclide investigations.* Publication 17, Pergamon Press, New York.

ICRP (1975). *International Commission on Radiological Protection. Reference Man: Anatomical Physiological and Metabolic Characteristics.* Publication 23, Pergamon Press, New York.

ICRP International Commission on Radiological Protection. *The handling, storage, use and disposal of unsealed radionuclides in hospitals and medical research establishments.* Publication No. 25. Pergamon Press, New York.

IRR (1988). *The Ionising Radiation (Protection of Persons Undergoing Medical Examination or Treatment) Regulations 1988 (SI 1988 No. 778. HMSO, London).*

Kaul A., Oeff K., Roedler H.D., and Vogelsang T. (1973). *Radiopharmaceuticals-Biokinetic Data and Results of Radiation Dose Calculations.* Berlin: Klinikum Steglitz der Freien Univcesitat.

Kawamura J., Hosokawa S., Yoshida O., Fujita T., Ishii Y., and Torizuka K. (1978). *Validity of technetium-99m dimercaptosuccinic acid renal uptake for an assessment of individual kidney function.* J. Urol., **119**, 303–309.

Kawamura J., Hosokawa S., and Yoshida O. (1979). *Renal function studies using technetium-99m dimercaptusuccinic acid.* Clinic Nucl. med., **4**, 39–47.

Kelly J.P. (1087). *An assessment of errors and their correction in the measurement of absolute renal uptake of technetium-99m DMSA.* M.Sc. Thesis North East London Polytechnic, London.

Keramidus D.C., Coran A.G. and Zaleska R.W. (1974). *An experimental model for assessing the radiopertechnetate diagnosis of gastric mucosa in Meckel's diverticulum.* J. Pediatr. Surg., **9**, 879–883.

Kereiakes J.G., Seltzer R., Blackburn B. and Saenger E. (1965). *Radionuclide doses to infants and children: a plea for a standard child.* health Phys., **11**, 999.

Kereiakes J.G., Wellman H.N., Simmonds G. and Saenger E.L. (1972). *Radiopharmaceutical dosimetry in pediatrics.* Semin. Nucl. Med., **2**, 316.

Kereiakes J.G., Simmonds G.H. and Feller P.A. (1972a). *Whole body and critical organ dosimetry for technetium-99m labelled pharmaceuticals. In* Biophysical Aspects of the Medical Uses of Technetium-99m, AAPM Monograph I. p 101, New York: American Association of Physicists in Medicine.

Kereiakes J.G., Feller P.A., Ascoli F.A., Thomas S.R., Gelfand M.L., and Saenger E. (1976b). *Pediatric radiopharmaceutical dosimetry in Radiopharmaceutical Dosimetry Symposium.* Edited by Cloutier R.J., Coffey J.L., Snyder W.S., Watson E.E. and Hamilton D.R., p. 73. New Publication (FDA) 76-8044. National Technical Information Service, Springfield, Virginia.

Koenigsberg M., Freeman L.M., and Blaufox M.D. (1978). *Radionuclide and Ultrasound Evaluation of renal Morphology and Function. In* Pediatric Kidney Disease, edited by Edelman, Little, Brown and Boston. Chapter 1, 236.

Kogan S.J., Lufker L.G. and Perex L.A. (1979). *The value of the negative radionuclide scrotal scan in the management of the acute inflamed scrotum in children.* J. Urol., **122**, 223–225.

Loevinger R. and Berman M. (1968). *A schema for absorbed dose calculations for biologically distributed radionuclides.* MIRD Supplement No. 1, pamphlet No. 1 J. Nucl. Med., **9**, 7.

Loevinger R. and Bermabn M. (1976). *A revised schema for calculating the absorbed dose from biologically distributed radionuclides. MIRD pamphlet No. 1.* Revised. Society of Nuclear Medicine, New York.

Majd M., Reba R.C. and Altman R.P. (1981). *Hepatobiliary scintigraphy with technetium-99m PIPIDA in the evaluation of neonated jaundice.* Pediatrics, **67**, 140–145.

Martin G.I., Kutner F.R. and Moses L. (1976). *Diagnosis of Meckel's diverticulum by radioisotope scanning.* Pediatrics, **571**, 11–12.

Mason D.T., Ashburn W.L. and Harbert J.C. (1968). *Rapid-sequence visualisation of the heart and great vessels in many using the wide-field Anger scintillation camera.* Circulation, **39**, 19.

Mayes J.S.E., Babich J.W., Carter R., *et al.,* (1989). *Quantitative Study of Radioiodinated Metaiodobenzylguanidine Uptake in Children with Neuroblastoma: Correlation with Tumour Histopathology.* J. Nucl. Med. **30(4)**, 474–480.

McDonald P., Tarar R., Gilday D.C. and Reilly B.J. (1974). *Some radiological observations in renal vein thrombosis.* Am. J. Roentgenol, **120**, 368.

MIRD Pamphlet No E. Brownell G.L., Ellett W.H. and Reddy A.R. (1968). *Absorbed fractions for photon dosimetry.* J. Nucl. Med. Supplement No 1. Society of Nuclear Medicine, New York.

MIRD Pamphlet No 10. (1975). *Radionuclide decay schemes and nuclear parameters for use in radiation dose estimations.* Ibid.

Mishkin F. (1972). *Brain scanning in children.* Sem. Nucl. Med. **2**, 328–342.

Morales B.R., Evans K and Gordon I. (1984). *Absolute quantitation of Technetium-99m DMSA in Paediatrics.* Nucl. Med. Comm. **5**, 212.

Myers M.J., Lavender J.P., de Oliviera J.B. and Masieri A. (1981). *A simplified method of quantitating organ uptake using a gamma camera.* Brit. J. Rad., **541**, 062–1067.

NCRP (1983). *Protection in Nuclear Medicine and Ultrasound Diagnostic Procedures in Children. Report No. 73 (NCRP, Bethesda, MD).*

NRCP. (1983). *National Council on Radiation Protection and Measurements. Bethesda Maryland USA.* Protection in nuclear medicine and ultrasound diagnostic procedure in children. Report No 73.

Odell G.B. N. and Boitnott J.K. (1974). *Evaluation of jaundice In:* Pediatric Nuclear Medicine. Editors James A.E., Wagner H.N. and Cook R.E., Saunders W.B., Philadelphia.

Pieretti R., Gilday D.L. and Jeffs R. (1974). *Differential kidney scan in pediatric urology.* Urology, **4**, 665.

Poston J. (1976). *The effects of body and organ size on absorbed dose: there is no standard patient. In:* Radiopharmaceuticals Dosimetry Symposium. Editors: Cloutier R.J., Coffey J.L., Snyder W.J., Watson E.E. and Hamilton D.R. HEW Publication (FDA) 76-8044. National Technical Information service. Springfield, Virginia.

Robinson A.E., Goodrich J.K. and Spock A. (1969). *Inhalation and perfusion radionuclide studies of pediatric chest disease.* Radiol., **93**, 1123.

Roedler H.O., Kaul A. and Hine G.J. (1978). *Internal radiation dose in diagnostic nuclear medicine.* Hoffman, Berlin.

Rosen P.R. and Treves S. (1984). *The relationship of gastro-esophageal reflux and gastric emptying infants and children.* J. Nucl. Med., **255**, 71–574.

Rosenfield N. and Treves S. (1974). *Liver spleen scanning in pediatrics.* Pediatrics, **53**, 692–701.

Rosenthal L. (1966). *Radionuclide venography using Technetium-99m Pertechnetate and the gamma ray scintillation camera.* Am. J. Roentgen, **97**, 874.

Rosenthall L. (1974). *Gastrointestinal imaging: Imaging the liver in pediatrics. In:* Pediatric Nuclear Medicine. Editors; James A.E., Wagner H.N. and Cooke R.E., Saunders W.B., Philadelphia.

Rossomondo R.M., Carlton W.H., Trueblood J.H. and Thoma P.R. (1972). *A new method of evaluating lachrimal drainage.* Arch. Ophthalmol., **88**, 523.

Sampson C.B. (1980). *A study of paediatric radiopharmaceuticals in America.* Br. J. Pharm. Pract. Jan. 17–25.

Sampson C. B. (1981). *Radiopharmacy at Gt Ormond Street.* Pharm. J. Nov. 654–656.

Siddiqui A.R. Oseas R.S., Wellman H.N., Doerr D.R. and Baehner R.L. (1979). *Evaluation of bone marrow scanning with Technetium-99m sulphur colloid in pediatric oncology.* J. Nucl. Med. **20**, 379–386.

Signer E. and Fridrich R. (1975). *Gastric emptying in newborns and young infants.* Acta. Paed. Scand., **64**, 525–530.

Spector W. (1956). *Handbook of Biological Data.* W.B. Saunders, Philadelphia. p. 162.

Spencer R.P. and Benever C. (1970). *Growth of the human liver; a preliminary scan study.* J. Nucl. Med., **11**, 660–662.

Tauscher J.W., Bryant D.R. and Gruenther R.C. (1978). *False positive scan for Meckels diverticulum.* J. Paed., **92**, 1022–1023.

Thomas S.R., Maxon H.R. and Kereiakes J.G. (1976). *In-vivo quantitation of lesion radioactivity using external counting methods.* Med. Phys., **3**, 253–255.

Treves S. and Spencer R.P. (1973). *Liver and spleen scintigraphy in children.* Semin. Nucl. Med., **3**, 137–150.

Valvo J.R., Caldamone A.A., O'Mara R. and Rabinowitz R. (1982). *Nuclear imaging in the pediatric acute scrotum.* Am. J. Dis. Child., **136**, 831–835.

Viers E.R., (1966). *Disorders of the nasolacrimal apparatus in infants and children.* J. Ped. Ophthalmol., **3**, 22.

Vivian G.C. (1983). *Dynamic renal scintigraphy in infants and children. MSc Thesis.* Institute of Nuclear Medicine, Middlesex Hospital London and Hospital for Sick Children, Gt Ormond St, London.

Walker W. (1976). *Splenectomy in childhood: a review in England and Wales.* Br. J. Surg. **63**, 36–43.

Webster W.E., Alpert N.M., and Brownett G.L. (1974). *Radiation doses in pediatric nuclear medicine and diagnostic X-ray procedures. In:* Pediatric Nuclear Medicine, edited by A.E. James, H.N. Wagner and R.E. Cook. p. 34, Philadelphia: W.B. Saunders Company.

Wellington H., August G.P., Randolph J.G., Schisgall R.M., and Chandra R. (1982). *Solitary thyroid nodules in children and adolescents.* J. Pediatric Surg., **17**, 225–229.

Wellman H.N., Kereiakes J.G., Yeager T.B., Karches G.J., and Saenger E.L., (1967). *A sensitive technique for measuring thyroidal uptake of iodine-131.* J. Nucl. Med., **8**, 86–96.

Wine C.R., Nahrwold D.L., and Waldhausen J.A., (1974). *Role of the technetium scan in the diagnosis of Meckel's diverticulum.* J. Pediatr. Surg. **9**, 855–888.

Worm A.M., Holten I., and Taaning E. (1980). *Nuclear imaging of pulmonary metastases in thyroid carcinoma.* Acta Radiol Oncol., **19**, 401–403.

FURTHER READING

Pediatric Nuclear Medicine (1974). Edited A.E. James, H.N. Wagner and R.E. Cooke, W.B. Saunders and Company, Philadelphia.

Nuclear Medicine in Clinical Pediatrics (1975). Editors: H. Handmaker and J.M. Lowenstein. The Society of Nuclear Medicine, New York.

Atlas of Pediatric Nuclear Medicine (1978). Editors: P.O. Alderson, O.L. Gilday and H.N. Wagner, C.V. Mosby, Company. St Louis.

Pediatric Nuclear Medicine (1985). Editor: S.T. Treves. Springer Verlag. New York. Berlin.

Diagnostic Imaging in Paediatrics (1988). Editor: Gordon I. Chapman and Hall, London.

Goldstone K.E., Jackson P.C., Myers M.J., and Simpson A.E. (1991). *In: Radiation Protection in Nuclear Medicine and Pathology. Report No. 63. Chapter 4.* Published by The Institute of Physical Sciences in Medicine.

ICRP Publication 56. *Age-Dependent Doses to Members of the Public from Intake of Radionuclides: Part 1. Vol. 20 No. 2. 1989.*

Appendix A

Summary of Decay Parameters of Some Commonly Used Radionuclides

CHROMIUM-51

Half-life: 27.8 days
Photon Energy(MeV): 0.323–9%
Type of Decay: Electron Capture 100%

DECAY TABLE

Time elapsed (days)	*Percentage activity remaining*	*Decay factor*
1	97.54	1.02
2	95.14	1.05
3	92.79	1.08
4	90.51	1.10
5	88.28	1.13
6	86.11	1.16
7	**83.98**	**1.19**
8	81.92	1.22
9	79.90	1.25
10	77.93	1.28
11	76.01	1.32
12	74.14	1.35
13	72.32	1.38
14	**70.53**	**1.42**
15	68.80	1.45
16	67.10	1.49
17	65.45	1.52
18	63.84	1.57
19	62.27	1.61
20	60.73	1.65
21	**59.24**	**1.69**
22	57.78	1.73
23	56.36	1.77
24	54.97	1.82
25	53.62	1.86
26	52.30	1.91
27	51.01	1.96
28	**49.75**	**2.01**
29	48.53	2.06
30	47.33	2.11
31	46.17	2.17
32	45.03	2.22
33	43.92	2.28
34	42.84	2.33
35	**41.78**	**2.39**
36	40.75	2.45
37	39.75	2.51
38	38.77	2.58
39	37.82	2.64
40	36.89	2.71
41	35.98	2.78
42	**35.09**	**2.85**
43	34.23	2.92
44	33.38	3.00
45	32.56	3.07
46	31.76	3.15
47	30.98	3.23
48	30.22	3.31
49	**29.47**	**3.39**
50	28.75	3.48
51	28.04	3.57
52	27.35	3.66
53	26.67	3.75
54	26.02	3.84
55	25.38	3.94
56	**24.75**	**4.04**
57	24.14	4.14
58	23.55	4.25
59	22.97	4.35
60	22.40	4.46
61	21.85	4.58
62	21.31	4.69
63	**20.79**	**4.81**
64	20.28	4.93
65	19.78	5.06
66	19.29	5.18

Time elapsed (days)	*Percentage activity remaining*	*Decay factor*
67	18.81	5.31
68	18.35	5.45
69	17.90	5.59
70	**17.46**	**5.72**
71	17.03	5.87
72	16.61	6.02
73	16.20	6.17
74	15.80	6.32
75	15.41	6.50
76	15.03	6.65
77	**14.66**	**6.82**
78	14.30	6.99
79	13.95	7.17
80	13.61	7.35
81	13.27	7.53
82	12.94	7.72
83	12.63	7.91
84	**12.31**	**8.12**

GALLIUM-67

Half-life: 78 hours
Photon Energy (MeV): 0.092–42%
0.182–24%
0.206–2.5%
0.30 –22%
0.39 –7%
Type of Decay: Electron Capture 100%
Internal Conversion: 29%

DECAY TABLE

Time elapsed (hours)	*Percentage activity remaining*	*Decay factor*
1	99.12	1.00
2	98.24	1.02
3	97.37	1.03
4	96.51	1.04
5	95.66	1.05
6	94.81	1.06
7	93.97	1.06
8	93.14	1.07
9	93.32	1.08
10	91.51	1.09
11	90.69	1.10
12	89.89	1.11
13	89.09	1.12
14	88.30	1.13
15	87.52	1.14

Time elapsed (hours)	*Percentage activity remaining*	*Decay factor*
16	86.75	1.15
17	85.98	1.16
18	85.22	1.17
19	84.77	1.18
20	83.72	1.19
21	82.98	1.20
22	82.25	1.22
23	81.52	1.23
24	**80.80**	**1.24**

Time elapsed (days)	*Percentage activity remaining*	*Decay factor*
1	80.80	1.238
2	65.28	1.532
3	52.75	1.896
4	42.62	2.346
5	34.43	2.904
6	27.82	3.594
7	**22.48**	**4.450**
8	18.16	5.506

INDIUM-111

Half-life: 67.2 hours
Photon Energy (MeV): 0.173–87%
0.247–94%
Type of Decay: Electron Capture 100%
Internal Conversion: 13%
6%

DECAY TABLE

Time elapsed (hours)	*Percentage activity remaining*	*Decay factor*
1	99.0	1.01
2	98.0	1.02
3	97.0	1.03
4	96.0	1.04
5	95.0	1.05
6	94.0	1.06
7	93.0	1.07
8	92.0	1.09
9	91.1	1.10
10	90.2	1.11
11	89.3	1.12
12	88.4	1.13
13	87.6	1.14
14	86.6	1.15
15	85.7	1.17
16	84.8	1.18
17	83.9	1.19
18	83.1	1.20
19	82.2	1.22
20	81.4	1.23
21	80.5	1.24
22	79.7	1.25
23	78.9	1.27
24	**78.1**	**1.28**

Time elapsed (days)	*Percentage activity remaining*	*Decay factor*
1	78.1	1.28
2	61.0	1.64
3	47.6	2.10
4	37.2	2.69
5	29.0	3.45
6	22.7	4.41
7	**17.7**	**5.65**

INDIUM-113m

Half-life: 1.7 hours
Photon Energy (MeV): 0.392–62%
Type of Decay: Isomeric Transition 100%
Internal Conversion: 38%

DECAY TABLE

Time elapsed (hours)	*Percentage activity remaining*	*Decay factor*
0.25	90.3	1.11
0.50	81.6	1.23
0.75	73.7	1.36
1.00	66.5	1.50
1.25	60.1	1.66
1.50	54.2	1.84
1.75	49.0	2.04
2.00	44.2	2.26
2.25	40.0	2.50
2.50	36.1	2.77
2.75	32.6	3.07
3.00	29.4	3.40
3.25	26.6	3.76
3.50	24.0	4.17
3.75	21.7	4.61
4.00	19.6	5.10
4.25	17.7	5.66
4.50	16.0	6.26
4.75	14.4	6.94
5.00	13.0	7.68
5.25	11.8	8.50
5.50	10.6	9.42
5.75	9.6	10.43
6.00	8.7	11.55
6.25	7.8	12.79
6.50	7.1	14.16
6.75	6.4	15.68
7.00	5.8	17.36
7.25	5.2	19.22
7.50	4.7	21.28
7.75	4.2	23.57
8.00	3.8	26.10

Appendix A

IODINE-123

Half-life: 13 hours
Photon Energy (MeV): 0.16–84%
Type of Decay: Electron Capture 100%
Internal Conversion: 16%

DECAY TABLE

Time elapsed (hours)	*Percentage activity remaining*	*Decay factor*
0.25	98.68	1.01
0.50	97.37	1.03
0.75	96.08	1.04
1.00	94.81	1.05
2.00	89.89	1.11
3.00	85.22	1.17
4.00	80.80	1.24
5.00	76.60	1.31
6.00	72.63	1.38
7.00	68.86	1.45
8.00	65.28	1.53
9.00	61.89	1.62
10.00	58.68	1.70
11.00	55.63	1.80
12.00	52.75	1.90
13.00	50.00	2.00
14.00	47.41	2.11
15.00	44.95	2.22
16.00	42.62	2.35
17.00	40.40	2.47
18.00	38.31	2.61
19.00	36.32	2.75
20.00	34.43	2.90
21.00	32.65	3.06
22.00	30.95	3.23
23.00	29.34	3.41
24.00	27.82	3.59
48.00	7.74	12.92
72.00	2.15	46.44

IODINE-125

Half-life: 60 days
Photon Energy (MeV): 0.035– 7%
0.027–138%
Type of Decay: Electron Capture 100%
Interval Conversion: 93%

DECAY TABLE

Time elapsed (weeks)	*Percentage activity remaining*	*Decay factor*
1	92.23	1.08
2	85.07	1.17
3	78.46	1.27
4	72.36	1.38
5	66.74	1.49
6	61.56	1.62
7	56.78	1.76
8	52.36	1.90
9	48.30	2.07
10	44.54	2.24
11	41.08	2.43
12	37.89	2.63
13	34.95	2.86
14	32.23	3.10
15	29.73	3.36
16	27.42	3.65
17	25.29	3.95
18	23.33	4.29
19	21.51	4.65
20	19.84	5.04
21	18.30	5.46
22	16.88	5.92
23	15.57	6.42
24	14.36	6.96
25	13.24	7.55
26	12.21	8.19
27	11.27	8.87
28	10.39	9.62
29	9.58	10.44
30	8.84	11.31

Time elapsed (days)	*Percentage activity remaining*	*Decay factor*
1	98.85	1.01
2	97.72	1.02
3	96.60	1.04
4	95.49	1.05
5	94.39	1.06
6	93.30	1.07
7	**92.23**	**1.08**

IODINE-131

Half-life:	8.04 days
Particle Energies (MeV):	0.25– 2.8%
	0.33– 9.3%
	0.61–87.2%
	0.81– 0.7%
Photon Energies (MeV):	0.08– 2.2%
	0.28– 6.3%
	0.36–79%
	0.64– 9.3%
	0.72– 2.8%
Type of Decay:	Beta
Internal Conversion:	4.5%
	0.4%
	1.5%

DECAY TABLE

Time elapsed (days)	*Percentage activity remaining*	*Decay factor*
1	91.74	1.09
2	84.16	1.19
3	77.21	1.29
4	70.83	1.41
5	64.98	1.54
6	59.61	1.68
7	**54.69**	**1.83**
8	50.17	1.99
9	46.03	2.17
10	42.23	2.37
11	38.74	2.58
12	35.54	2.81
13	32.60	3.07
14	**29.61**	**3.38**
15	27.44	3.64
16	25.17	3.97
17	23.09	4.33
18	21.19	4.71
19	19.44	5.14
20	17.83	5.61
21	**16.36**	**6.11**
22	15.01	6.66
23	13.77	7.26
24	12.63	7.91
25	11.59	8.63
26	10.63	9.40
27	9.75	10.26
28	**8.95**	**11.17**

PHOSPHORUS-32

Half-life:	14.3 days
Photon Energy (MeV):	1.71–100%
Type of Decay:	Beta

DECAY TABLE

Time elapsed (days)	*Percentage activity remaining*	*Decay factor*
1	95.27	1.05
2	90.76	1.10
3	86.47	1.16
4	82.38	1.21
5	78.48	1.27
6	74.76	1.34
7	**71.23**	**1.40**
8	67.86	1.47
9	64.65	1.55
10	61.59	1.62
11	58.67	1.70
12	55.90	1.79
13	53.25	1.88
14	**50.73**	**1.97**
15	48.33	2.07
16	46.05	2.17
17	48.37	2.07
18	41.79	2.39
19	39.81	2.51
20	37.93	2.64
21	**36.13**	**2.77**
22	34.43	2.90
23	32.80	3.05
24	31.24	3.20
25	29.77	3.36
26	28.36	3.52
27	27.02	3.70
28	**25.74**	**3.89**

SELENIUM-75

Half-life:	120 days
Photon Energy (MeV):	0.024– 0%
	0.066– 1%
	0.096– 3%
	0.12 –15%
	0.14 –54%
	0.20 – 1.5%
	0.27 –56%
	0.28 –23%
	0.31 – 1.4%
	0.40 –12.5%
Type of Decay:	Electron Capture 100%
Internal Conversion:	5%, 0.3%, 3%, 0.6%, 1.5%

DECAY TABLE

Time elapsed (days)	*Percentage activity remaining*	*Decay factor*
2	98.9	1.01
4	97.7	1.02
6	96.6	1.03
8	95.5	1.04
10	94.4	1.06
12	93.3	1.07
14	92.2	1.09
16	91.2	1.10
18	90.1	1.11
20	89.1	1.12
22	88.1	1.14
24	87.1	1.15
26	86.1	1.16
28	85.1	1.18

Time elapsed (weeks)	*Percentage activity remaining*	*Decay factor*
5	81.7	1.21
6	78.5	1.28
7	75.3	1.33
8	72.4	1.39
9	69.5	1.45
10	66.7	1.49
11	64.1	1.56
12	61.6	1.61
13	59.1	1.69
14	56.9	1.75
15	54.5	1.85
16	52.4	1.92
17	50.3	2.00
18	48.3	2.08
19	46.4	2.17
20	44.5	2.27

TECHNETIUM-99m

Half-life:	6 hours
Photon Energies (MeV):	0.14–90.1%
	0.002
Type of Decay:	Isomeric Transition 100%
Internal Conversion:	9.9%, 98.6%

DECAY TABLE

Time elapsed (hours)	*Percentage activity remaining*	*Decay factor*
0.25	97.09	1.03
0.50	94.34	1.06
0.75	91.74	1.09
1.00	89.29	1.12
1.25	86.96	1.15
1.50	84.03	1.19
1.75	81.30	1.23
2.00	79.36	1.26
2.25	76.92	1.30
2.50	74.63	1.34
2.75	72.46	1.38
3.00	70.52	1.42
3.25	68.49	1.46
3.50	66.67	1.50
3.75	64.94	1.54
4.00	62.89	1.59
4.25	60.98	1.64
4.50	59.52	1.68
4.75	57.80	1.73
5.00	56.18	1.78
5.25	54.64	1.83
5.50	52.91	1.89
5.75	51.28	1.95
6.00	50.00	2.00
7.00	44.54	2.24
8.00	39.69	2.52
9.00	35.36	2.82
10.00	31.50	3.17
11.00	28.06	3.56
12.00	25.00	4.00

THALLIUM-201

Half-life: 73.1 hours
Photon Energies (MeV): 0.135– 2.65%
0.167–10.16%
0.069–0.83 (X-rays)
Type of Decay: Electron Capture 100%
Internal Conversion: 9.15%, 19.2%, 95%

DECAY TABLE

Time elapsed (days)	*Percentage activity remaining*	*Decay factor*
1	79.36	1.26
2	63.29	1.58
3	50.50	1.98
4	40.16	2.49
5	32.05	3.12
6	25.51	3.92

YTTRIUM-90

Half-life: 64.1 hours
Particle Energy (MeV): 2.27–100%
Type of Decay: Beta

DECAY TABLE

Time elapsed (days)	*Percentage activity remaining*	*Decay factor*
4	96.15	1.04
8	91.74	1.09
12	87.71	1.14
16	84.03	1.19
20	80.64	1.24
24	76.92	1.30
28	74.07	1.35
32	70.92	1.41
36	67.57	1.48
48	59.52	1.68
60	52.33	1.91
72	45.97	2.17

Time elapsed (days)	*Percentage activity remaining*	*Decay factor*
4	35.48	2.81
5	27.38	3.65
6	21.13	4.73
7	16.31	6.13
8	12.59	7.94
9	9.71	10.30
10	7.50	13.33

XENON-133

Half-life: 5.3 days
Particle Energies (MeV): 0.27– 1%
0.35–99%
Photon Energies (MeV): 0.08 –35%
0.16 – 0.5%
0.031–47.4%
Type of Decay: Beta
Internal Conversion: 65%

DECAY TABLE

Time elapsed (days)	*Percentage activity remaining*	*Decay factor*
0.25	96.78	1.03
0.50	93.67	1.07
0.75	90.66	1.10
1.00	87.74	1.14
1.25	84.92	1.18
1.50	82.19	1.21
1.75	79.54	1.26
2.00	76.98	1.30
2.25	74.51	1.34
2.50	72.11	1.39
2.75	69.79	1.43
3.00	67.55	1.48
3.25	65.37	1.53
3.50	63.27	1.58
3.75	61.24	1.63
4.00	59.27	1.69
4.25	57.36	1.74
4.50	55.51	1.80
4.75	53.73	1.86
5.00	52.00	1.92
5.25	50.33	1.99
5.50	48.71	2.05
5.75	47.14	2.12
6.00	45.63	2.19
6.25	44.16	2.26
6.50	42.47	2.34
6.75	41.56	2.41
7.00	40.03	2.50

Appendix B

Mean Weight (kilogrammes) of Babies and Children

(Adapted with permission from Documenta Geigy Scientific Tables, 1975)

For calculating the weight of a child when only the age is known

Age	*Males Weight (kg)*	*Females Weight (kg)*
At birth	3.1	3.2
1 month	3.7	3.9
2 months	4.7	4.7
3 months	5.7	5.5
4 months	6.3	6.2
5 months	6.9	7.0
6 months	7.5	7.5
7 months	7.9	7.9
8 months	9.0	8.2
9 months	9.4	8.6
10 months	9.4	8.7
11 months	10.0	9.1
12 months	10.1	9.5
15 months	10.9	10.1
18 months	11.3	10.9
2 years	12.5	12.1
2.5 years	13.5	13.1
3 years	14.6	14.3
3.5 years	15.7	15.3
4 years	16.7	16.3
4.5 years	17.8	17.3
5 years	18.9	18.3
5.5 years	20.0	19.4

Age	*Males Weight (kg)*	*Females Weight (kg)*
6 years	21.0	20.6
6.5 years	22.1	21.8
7 years	23.2	23.5
7.5 years	24.3	25.2
8 years	25.3	26.7
8.5 years	26.4	27.8
9 years	27.5	28.8
9.5 years	28.6	30.0
10 years	30.5	31.5
10.5 years	32.7	33.0
11 years	35.0	34.8
11.5 years	37.3	36.8
12 years	39.5	39.0
12.5 years	41.8	41.4
13 years	44.1	44.3
13.5 Years	46.3	47.3
14 years	48.6	50.0
14.5 years	50.9	51.8
15 years	53.1	53.2
15.5 years	55.4	54.3
16 years	57.7	55.1
16.5 years	59.9	55.9
17 years	60.8	56.5

INDEX

Index

Index

Index

Index

Index

Index

Index